Molecular Research and Recent Advances in Diabetic Retinopathy

Molecular Research and Recent Advances in Diabetic Retinopathy

Guest Editors

Tomislav Bulum
Martina Tomić

MDPI

Basel • Beijing • Wuhan • Barcelona • Belgrade • Novi Sad • Cluj • Manchester

Guest Editors

Tomislav Bulum
Medical Faculty
University of Zagreb
Zagreb
Croatia

Martina Tomić
Vuk Vrhovac University Clinic
for Diabetes, Endocrinology
and Metabolic Diseases
Merkur University Hospital
Zagreb
Croatia

Editorial Office
MDPI AG
Grosspeteranlage 5
4052 Basel, Switzerland

This is a reprint of the Special Issue, published open access by the journal *Biomedicines* (ISSN 2227-9059), freely accessible at: https://www.mdpi.com/journal/biomedicines/special_issues/U8IAG94IGL.

For citation purposes, cite each article independently as indicated on the article page online and as indicated below:

Lastname, A.A.; Lastname, B.B. Article Title. *Journal Name* **Year**, *Volume Number*, Page Range.

ISBN 978-3-7258-7430-9 (Hbk)
ISBN 978-3-7258-7431-6 (PDF)
https://doi.org/10.3390/books978-3-7258-7431-6

Contents

About the Editors

Tomislav Bulum

Tomislav Bulum is employed at the Vuk Vrhovac University Clinic for Diabetes, Endocrinology, and Metabolic Diseases, University Hospital Merkur, Croatia's Referral Center for Diabetes, where he currently serves as a Specialist in Internal Medicine and a Subspecialist in Endocrinology and Diabetology. He received his PhD in 2010 from the Faculty of Science, University of Zagreb. Since 2016, he has been employed at the Medical School, University of Zagreb, where he currently holds the position of Associate Professor and Scientific Adviser. He lectures undergraduate courses as well as postgraduate specialist and PhD studies in biomedicine and health sciences at the Medical School, University of Zagreb. He has participated in multiple scientific and clinical projects in the field of type 1 and type 2 diabetes, with a particular focus on chronic diabetic complications. He has authored over 100 scientific papers published in Web of Science, Scopus, and Index Medicus-indexed journals, as well as over 100 scientific and professional abstracts, with his work cited over 1,000 times. He has served as a Guest Editor for over 10 Special Issues in first-quartile (Q1) journals, including *Biomedicines*, *Journal of Clinical Medicine*, *International Journal of Molecular Sciences*, *Diagnostics*, *Frontiers in Endocrinology*, and *Biology*. In 2023, he received the annual award from the Croatian Medical Chamber for scientific advancement in medicine and professional excellence. He is a member of the Croatian Academy of Medical Sciences.

Martina Tomić

Since 1998, Martina Tomić has been employed at the Vuk Vrhovac University Clinic, Merkur University Hospital, Zagreb, as an ophthalmologist and retina specialist, currently heading the Department for Diabetic Eye Complications. She graduated from the University of Zagreb School of Medicine in 1996, specializing in ophthalmology in 2005. Her master's thesis (2005) focused on physical activity's influence on metabolic regulation and hemorheology in type 1 diabetes, while her doctoral dissertation (2011) explored adiponectin's role in diabetic retinopathy. She holds the scientific titles of associate (2013) and senior scientific associate (2019) in biomedicine and health and earned the title of primarius in 2016. In 2019, she subspecialized in the posterior segment of the eye. She has contributed to several scientific projects, including a Croatian Ministry of Science project on chronic complications of diabetes (2007–2013) and a Croatian Science Foundation project on adipocytokine-modulated endothelial dysfunction (2015–2019). Her research focuses on diabetes-related diseases of the posterior segment of the eye, particularly diabetic retinopathy and macular edema, with numerous published articles and conference abstracts. She received the 2023 International Medis Award for her study on HDL cholesterol as a protective factor in diabetic retinopathy. She also serves as Guest Editor for journals such as *Biomedicines*, *Frontiers in Endocrinology*, and *Diagnostics*. As a lecturer at the Universities of Zagreb and Rijeka, she teaches courses on diabetes complications and retinal diseases, contributing chapters to academic textbooks. She is a member of several professional associations, including the European Association for Diabetic Eye Complications (EAsDEC).

biomedicines

MDPI

Article

DNA Methylation Profiles of *PSMA6*, *PSMB5*, *KEAP1*, and *HIF1A* Genes in Patients with Type 1 Diabetes and Diabetic Retinopathy

Zane Svikle [1], Natalia Paramonova [2], Emīls Siliņš [3], Leonora Pahirko [3], Līga Zariņa [1,4], Kristīne Baumane [1,4], Goran Petrovski [5] and Jelizaveta Sokolovska [1,*]

[1] Faculty of Medicine, University of Latvia, Jelgavas Street 3, LV 1004 Riga, Latvia; zane.svikle@gmail.com (Z.S.); bigzars@gmail.com (L.Z.); kbaumane75@gmail.com (K.B.)
[2] Institute of Biology, University of Latvia, Jelgavas Street 1, LV 1004 Riga, Latvia; natalia.paramonova@lu.lv
[3] Faculty of Physics, Mathematics and Optometry, University of Latvia, Jelgavas Street 3, LV 1004 Riga, Latvia; emils.silins@lu.lv (E.S.); leonora.pahirko@lu.lv (L.P.)
[4] Ophthalmology Department, Riga East University Hospital, Hipokrata Street 2, LV 1038 Riga, Latvia
[5] Center of Eye Research and Innovative Diagnostics, Department of Ophthalmology, Oslo University Hospital, Institute of Clinical Medicine, Faculty of Medicine, University of Oslo, 0372 Oslo, Norway; goran.petrovski@medisin.uio.no
* Correspondence: jelizaveta.sokolovska@lu.lv

Abstract: We explored differences in the DNA methylation statuses of *PSMA6*, *PSMB5*, *HIF1A*, and *KEAP1* gene promoter regions in patients with type 1 diabetes and different diabetic retinopathy (DR) stages. Study subjects included individuals with no DR (NDR, $n = 41$), those with non-proliferative DR (NPDR, $n = 27$), and individuals with proliferative DR or those who underwent laser photocoagulation (PDR/LPC, $n = 46$). DNA methylation was determined by Zymo OneStep qMethyl technique. The methylation of *PSMA6* (NDR 5.9 (3.9–8.7) %, NPDR 4.5 (3.8–5.7) %, PDR/LPC 6.6 (4.7–10.7) %, $p = 0.003$) and *PSMB5* (NDR 2.2 (1.9–3.7) %, NPDR 2.2 (1.9–3.0) %, PDR/LPC 3.2 (2.5–7.1) %, $p < 0.01$) differed across the groups. Consistent correlations were observed between the methylation levels of *HIF1A* and *PSMA6* in all study groups. DNA methylation levels of *PSMA6*, *PSMB5*, and *HIF1A* genes were positively correlated with the duration of diabetes, HbA1c, and albuminuria in certain study groups. Univariate regression models revealed a significant association between the methylation level z-scores of *PSMA6*, *PSMB5*, and *HIF1A* and severe DR (*PSMA6*: OR = 1.96 (1.15; 3.33), $p = 0.013$; *PSMB5*: OR = 1.90 (1.14; 3.16), $p = 0.013$; *HIF1A*: OR = 3.19 (1.26; 8.06), $p = 0.014$). *PSMB5* remained significantly associated with DR in multivariate analysis. Our findings suggest significant associations between the severity of DR and the DNA methylation levels of the genes *PSMA6*, *PSMB5*, and *HIF1A*, but not *KEAP1* gene.

Keywords: diabetic eye disease; epigenetics; proteasome

1. Introduction

Diabetic retinopathy (DR) is one of the most common complications of diabetes, and it has a significant impact on national and global health. In a US study conducted in 2021, an estimated 9.6 million people were found to have DR, with a prevalence rate of 26.43% among individuals with diabetes [1]. The pathogenetic mechanisms responsible for DR are not yet fully understood. At present, there is a deficiency in identifying susceptibility and probability of early indicators for DR and other microvascular complications of diabetes, and there is also a need for effective treatments to manage the progression of the disease during its initial stages.

Epigenetic alterations influence how genes are expressed without making changes to the underlying DNA sequence, adapting dynamically in response to environmental, developmental, and nutritional signals [2,3]. Recently, research has shown that epigenetic mechanisms play a role in diabetic complications [4], although there is not sufficient data about their implication in DR pathogenesis. The development of DR is multifactorial, and it is known to progress even after euglycemia is achieved [5], suggesting that epigenetics may play a role in the development and progression of DR. Indeed, global DNA methylation status was linked to retinopathy in a case–control study of 168 individuals with type 2 diabetes, demonstrating the strong relationship between DNA methylation and the regulation of gene transcription [6]. Moreover, patients with type 1 diabetes and proliferative DR (PDR) have displayed variations in the patterns of epigenetic factors, and this implies that certain changes in epigenetic markers could potentially serve as predictive indicators for the development of PDR and might be valuable as prospective biomarkers for DR screening [7]. Since disease outcomes are thought to be determined by a combination of genotypes, environmental exposures, and their interactions [8], DNA methylation may represent a potential biomarker of DR [9]. Some of the epigenetic modifications, being reversible, present important prospects for therapeutic intervention [10]. There is intense research interest in the development of non-invasive blood-based biomarkers for DR. However, the limited available data on this topic delay the development of diagnostic and disease-monitoring markers, which are related to the methylation statuses of genes in DR.

The ubiquitin–proteasome system plays a crucial role in regulating cell homeostasis through protein degradation [11]. Dysregulation of this system is implicated in various chronic diseases, including diabetes. Proteasomal gene *PSMA6* has been already identified as a gene with type 1 diabetes susceptibility [12], and *PSMB5* genetic variations were found in association with multiple sclerosis in Latvians [13].

Altered proteasome activity in response to hypoxia and oxidative stress under hyperglycemic conditions is observed in diabetes [14], potentially affecting the degradation of proteins involved in anti-oxidative and anti-hypoxic defense mechanisms, such as the Nrf2/Keap1 and hypoxia-inducible factor-1 (HIF-1) systems [15]. Under normal conditions, Keap1 facilitates the proteasomal degradation of Nrf2, but oxidative stress leads to Keap1 inactivation, stabilizing Nrf2 and promoting its anti-oxidative response [16]. In DR, epigenetic changes in the *KEAP1* gene can result in decreased Nrf2 expression, compromising the anti-oxidative response [17]. HIF-1, a key transcription factor in hypoxia responses, plays a critical role in maintaining oxygen homeostasis [18,19]. While HIF-1 alpha is established as a central stimulator of angiogenesis in the proliferative phase of DR, it plays a protective role during the early stages of DR, exhibiting anti-inflammatory, antiapoptotic, and anti-oxidative effects [20]. Notably, the *HIF-1A* Pro582Ser polymorphism, involved in resistance to hyperglycemia, is associated with protection against severe DR [21]. As the disease progresses, factors such as chronic hyperglycemia leading to the formation of advanced glycation end products (AGEs) and the chronic inflammatory state associated with diabetes can compromise HIF-1 function [22,23]. HIF-1 alpha undergoes hydroxylation and proteasomal degradation under normoxic conditions. However, under hypoxia or prolyl hydroxylase domain inhibition, HIF-1 alpha stabilizes, translocates into the nucleus, and activates downstream genes through hypoxia-responsive elements [24]. In experimental studies, inhibitors of proteasome activity have shown a beneficial impact on the progression of diabetic complications [25–28]. Noteworthily, there is evidence of distinct promoter methylation patterns in UPS genes in cancer [29,30], and in diabetology, the offspring of mothers with diabetes exhibit the altered methylation of UPS genes [31]. Numerous associations between proteasome system genes and autoimmune diseases, including type 1 diabetes, have previously been published in the Latvian population. Polymorphisms in *PSMA3*, *PSMA6*, and *PSMC6* were found to be associated with type 1 diabetes in Latvian patients [12]. Furthermore, correlations have been established between these proteasome gene polymorphisms and type 1 diabetes-susceptible genes involved in various pathways, including innate and adaptive immunity, antiviral response, insulin signaling, and glucose/energy metabolism, highlighting the complex interplay of these genes in type 1 diabetes pathogenesis [12]. This complex chain of associations highlights the importance of the proteasome system in the development of diabetes and its complications.

These findings underscore the significance of investigating UPS regulation and epigenetic modifications in understanding the DR pathogenesis. However, there is currently no published data on the association between the methylation status of genes associated with the ubiquitin–proteasome system and the hypoxia signaling axis and the severity of DR. Our study aimed to study the differences in the methylation statuses of the promoter parts of *PSMA6*, *PSMB5*, *HIF1A*, and *KEAP1* genes between patients with different DR stages and type 1 diabetes in Latvia.

2. Materials and Methods

2.1. Patients and Ethics

For the implementation of this study, patients in Latvia with type 1 diabetes were recruited in frames of the LatDiane study (a part of the international InterDiane consortium). Inclusion criteria for the study were as follows: patients with age $\geq$ 18 years and history and established treatment of type 1 diabetes (defined as an age of diagnosis younger than 40 years, with insulin treatment initiated within one year of diagnosis, and C-peptide levels below 0.3 nmol/L) [32]. Exclusion criteria were treatment with oral hypoglycemic medications for more than one year after diagnosis. The study protocol was approved by the Latvian Central Ethics Committee (clearance Nr. 1/19-10-01, issued on 1 October 2019). The recruitment of the study participants, biobanking, and sample storage were performed in agreement with the procedures of the Genome Database of the Latvian population [33] and are described in more detail in [34]. The study corresponds to the ethical standards defined in the 1964 Declaration of Helsinki and its later amendments. Written informed consent was obtained from all study participants before inclusion in the study.

2.2. Clinical Definitions

DR grading was based on the fundus oculi examination carried out by an ophthalmologist. Patients were stratified according to the DR status as follows: no retinopathy (NDR), non-proliferative retinopathy (NPDR), proliferative retinopathy (PDR), and patients after panretinal-laser photocoagulation (LPC). Furthermore, to increase the power of the study, subjects were stratified into three groups: patients with NDR; patients with NPDR; patients with PDR, and those after LPC (PDR/LPC).

The "smokers" group applied to patients currently smoking at least one cigarette per day, and smoking was self-reported in the questionnaire.

Body mass index (BMI) was calculated as weight (kg)/height (m)^2.

The definition of arterial hypertension was based on blood pressure values (systolic blood pressure $\geq$ 140 mmHg (18.7 kPa) or diastolic blood pressure $\geq$ 90 mmHg (12.0 kPa)) and the history of antihypertensive drug usage.

We defined cardiovascular disease as a history of stroke, amputation, peripheral vascular disease, acute myocardial infarction, or coronary bypass/percutaneous transluminal coronary angioplasty.

Diabetic nephropathy was defined as follows: macroalbuminuria or eGFR below 60 mL/min/1.73 m^2 or treatment with dialysis or kidney transplant. Albuminuria was determined using two out of three urine albumin-to-creatinine ratio measurements in the morning spot urine. The estimated glomerular filtration rate (eGFR) was calculated according to Chronic Kidney Disease Epidemiology Collaboration (CKD-EPI).

2.3. Biochemical Parameters

Total cholesterol, high- and low-density lipoprotein cholesterol, triglycerides, glycated hemoglobin (HbA1c), and the albumin/creatinine ratio in urine were measured in certified clinical laboratories.

2.4. Sampling of Blood for DNA Extraction and Serum Preparation

For serum preparation, peripheral venous blood was collected. The blood samples were incubated undisturbed for 30 min at room temperature and then centrifuged. The serum was removed from the pellet and transferred into fresh 2 mL tubes, frozen, and stored at −80 °C until analysis. Blood for DNA extraction was collected in EDTA tubes. DNA isolation from whole blood samples using the phenol–chloroform extraction method was carried out in the biobank setting, as previously described [33].

2.5. Targeted DNA Methylation Assessment

Bisulfite-free, restriction enzyme-dependent determination of the DNA methylation status in the promoter regions of *PSMA6, PSMB5, HIF1A,* and *KEAP1* genes was performed using real-time PCR procedure, following the instructions given in the manual (OneStep qMethyl™ Kit (Zymo research, Irvine, CA, USA)). The procedure involves two reactions for each investigated DNA sample: a "Test Reaction" and a "Reference Reaction". In the Test Reaction, DNA is digested with Methylation Sensitive Restriction Enzymes (MSREs), while DNA in the Reference Reaction remains undigested. Real-time PCR with the SYTO® 9 fluorescent dye (Thermo Fisher Scientific, Waltham, MA, USA) is then used to quantify the difference in the methylation status in both reactions. DNA methylation extent was calculated using threshold cycle or CT values and the following equation: $100 \times 2^{-\Delta CT}$, indicating methylation status in percentage values. UCSC Genome Browser on Human ((GRCh38/hg38, https://genome.ucsc.edu/) accessed on 27 October 2023) was used to determine the localization of CpG island and promoter regions of genes of interest. Primer design was performed with the online software Primer3plus (https://www.bioinformatics.nl/cgi-bin/primer3plus/, accessed on 27 October 2023 (Netherlands Bioinformatics Centre, Wageningen, The Netherlands)). To perform quantitative real-time polymerase chain reaction (RT-PCR) with methylation-sensitive restriction enzymes (MSREs), we designed primers that included two or more MSRE targeting sites in the amplicon flanking targeted CpG sites regions related to the promoter parts of the investigated genes (Supplementary Table S1). For each sample, 5 µL DNA (4 ng/µL) is added to achieve a final reaction volume of 20 µL (1 ng/µL concentration). Duplicate human methylated and non-methylated DNA standards with control MGMT primers, as well as positive controls, were used in each experiment to verify the accuracy of the reaction performed according to the standard procedure.

2.6. Statistical Analysis

Categorical data are presented as frequencies and percentages. Most of the variables analyzed violated the normality assumption (determined by the Shapiro–Wilk test), and continuous data are represented as medians with the interquartile range (Q1–Q3). Biomarker levels between DR groups (NDR, NPDR, PDR/LPC) were compared using the Kruskal–Wallis test. Post hoc analysis was performed using Dunn's test.

Analysis of covariance (ANCOVA) on ranks was conducted to assess differences in biomarker levels among retinopathy groups adjusted for age, sex, and BMI.

Logistic regression models were employed to evaluate the odds of severe DR (PDR/LPC) compared to patients in NDR and NPDR groups for predictors *PSMA6, PSMB5, KEAP1,* and *HIF1A* while adjusting for age, sex, smoking, and arterial hypertension.

Correlation analysis between biomarkers among DR groups was conducted using the Spearman correlation coefficient.

A p-value of less than 0.05 was considered statistically significant.

All statistical data analysis was performed using Statistical Software R version 4.3.0. ((http://www.r-project.org), accessed on 23 April 2024).

3. Results

3.1. Characteristics of Cohort

A total of 114 patients were analyzed in the study, 46.50% of them were male. The median age was 39 (30–49) years, duration of diabetes 22 (16–30) years, body mass index (BMI) 24.55 (22.22–27.98) kg/m^2, and waist/hip ratio 0.86 (0.78–0.93). Among all patients, 72 (63.20%) had arterial hypertension, 22 (19.30%) had diabetic nephropathy, 78 (68.40%)

had polyneuropathy, and 11 (9.60%) had cardiovascular diseases. In the entire cohort, the median HbA1c level was 8.75 (8.00–10.10) %, high-density lipoprotein cholesterol measured 1.58 (1.24–1.83) mmol/L, low-density lipoprotein cholesterol measured 2.91 (2.07–3.37) mmol/L, triglycerides measured 1.20 (0.80–1.65) mmol/L, the median estimated glomerular filtration rate (eGFR) was reported at 110.57 (91.15–120.53) mL/min/1.73 m^2, and the median albuminuria level was 1.10 (0.28–8.33) mg/mmol. The use of angiotensin-converting enzyme inhibitors/angiotensin II receptor blockers (ACEI/ARB) was reported by 43 (37.70%) of the patients, while 21 (18.40%) underwent statin therapy.

3.2. Characteristics of Patients with Different Severity of DR

Characteristics of the patients within the groups of retinopathies are demonstrated in Table 1. Patients within PDR/LPC group compared to NDR and NPDR groups had significantly longer diabetes duration, a higher prevalence of arterial hypertension and cardiovascular diseases, elevated serum triglyceride levels, lower eGFR, and a higher frequency of ACEI/ARB usage and statin therapy.

Table 1. Characteristics of patients stratified according to diabetic retinopathy status.

	NDR (n = 41)	NPDR (n = 27)	PDR/LPC (n = 46)	p-Value
Sex (female), n (%)	21 (51.22%)	12 (44.44%)	28 (61.87%)	0.372
Age, years	40 (30–47) [a,b]	31 (26–43) [b]	45 (35–51) [a]	**0.002**
Smokers, n (%)	9 (21.95%) [a]	14 (51.85%)	8 (17.39%) [a]	**0.004**
Duration of diabetes, years	19 (13–25) [a]	17 (13–21) [a]	28 (22–35)	**<0.001**
Body mass index, kg/m^2	26.60 (23.90–29.70)	22.80 (20.70–24.80) [a]	24.40 (22.02–27.40) [a]	**<0.001**
Waist/hip ratio	0.87 (0.77–0.94)	0.83 (0.80–0.88)	0.86 (0.78–0.95)	0.468
Arterial hypertension, n (%)	21 (51.22%) [a]	12 (44.44%) [a]	39 (84.78%)	**<0.001**
Diabetic nephropathy, n (%)	0 (0.00%)	6 (23.08%) [a]	16 (35.56%) [a]	**<0.001**
Polyneuropathy, n (%)	25 (60.98%)	18 (66.67%)	35 (76.09%)	0.310
Cardiovascular diseases, n (%)	1 (2.44%) [a]	0 (0.00%) [a]	10 (21.74%)	**<0.001**
HbA1c, %	8.30 (7.95–9.60) [a]	10.15 (8.72–11.17)	8.60 (8.02–9.70) [a]	**0.009**
Total cholesterol, mmol/L	5.32 (4.29–5.91)	4.78 (3.95–5.54)	5.20 (4.16–5.79)	0.378
High-density lipoprotein cholesterol, mmol/L	1.62 (1.26–1.91)	1.58 (1.24–1.76)	1.53 (1.21–1.90)	0.850
Low-density lipoprotein cholesterol, mmol/L	2.98 (2.33–3.42)	2.63 (1.84–3.26)	3.01 (2.07–3.34)	0.426
Triglycerides, mmol/L	0.96 (0.74–1.47) [a]	1.09 (0.79–1.81) [a,b]	1.32 (0.93–1.78) [b]	**0.047**
eGFR, mL/min/1.73 m^2	114.57 (108.26–124.13) [a]	118.53 (108.44–128.74) [a]	85.11 (64.17–105.30)	**<0.001**
Albuminuria, mg/mmol	0.39 (0.21–1.19)	2.58 (0.38–23.90) [a]	3.47 (0.48–17.57) [a]	**<0.001**
ACEI/ARB usage, n (%)	10 (24.39%) [a]	6 (22.22%) [a]	27 (58,70%)	**<0.001**
Statin usage, n (%)	4 (9.76%) [a]	2 (7.41%) [a]	15 (32.61%)	**0.006**

Continuous data are presented as medians with (Q1–Q3) with the corresponding Kruskal–Wallis test p-values. Categorical data are presented as frequencies (percentages) with the corresponding Chi-squared test p-value for the equality of proportions. [a,b]—indicates groups that, based on pairwise post hoc comparisons, did not exhibit significant differences (according to Dunn's or pairwise Chi-squared test). Entries with $p < 0.05$ are highlighted in bold. NDR—no diabetic retinopathy; NPDR—non-proliferative retinopathy; PDR/LPC—proliferative retinopathy/status after panretinal-laser photocoagulation; eGFR—estimated glomerular filtration rate (CKD-EPI); and ACEI/ARB—angiotensin-converting enzyme inhibitors/angiotensin II receptor blockers.

Among patients in NPDR, significantly younger age, higher prevalence of smokers, and higher levels of HbA1c were observed compared to both other groups. Patients in the

NDR group had significantly higher BMI and lower levels of albuminuria compared to NPDR and PDR/LPC groups. The prevalence of diabetic nephropathy was statistically significantly higher in the PDR/LPC group compared to the NDR group.

3.3. Association of DNA Methylation with DR Severity Stages

The level of methylation (%) in the promoter regions of the genes *HIF1A*, *PSMA6*, *PSMB5*, and *KEAP1* was compared in three study groups NDR, NPDR, and PDR/LPC. As demonstrated in Table 2 and Figure 1, only the levels of the methylation of *PSMA6* ($p = 0.003$) and *PSMB5* ($p < 0.01$) genes differed across the study groups.

Table 2. DNA methylation levels of promoter parts of genes across the groups of different retinopathy severity stages.

	NDR	NPDR	PDR/LPC	*p*-Value
HIF1A, %	4.7 (2.4–6.7)	3.8 (3.1–4.9)	4.9 (2.6–9.6)	0.216
KEAP1, %	4.7 (3.7–5.9)	4.7 (3.6–7.1)	4.6 (3.6–5.8)	0.973
PSMA6, %	5.9 (3.9–8.7) ^{a,b}	4.5 (3.8–5.7) ^{a}	6.6 (4.7–10.7) ^{b}	**0.003**
PSMB5, %	2.2 (1.9–3.7) ^{a}	2.2 (1.9–3.0) ^{a}	3.2 (2.5–7.1)	**<0.001**

The Kruskal–Wallis test was used to compare the differences in biomarkers between diabetic retinopathy groups. ^{a,b}—indicates groups that, based on pairwise post hoc comparisons using Dunn's test, did not exhibit significant differences. After adjusting for age, sex, and BMI (ANCOVA on ranks), the results remained consistent with the Kruskal–Wallis test. Entries with $p < 0.05$ are highlighted in bold. NDR—no diabetic retinopathy; NPDR—non-proliferative retinopathy; and PDR/LPC—proliferative retinopathy/status after panretinal-laser photocoagulation.

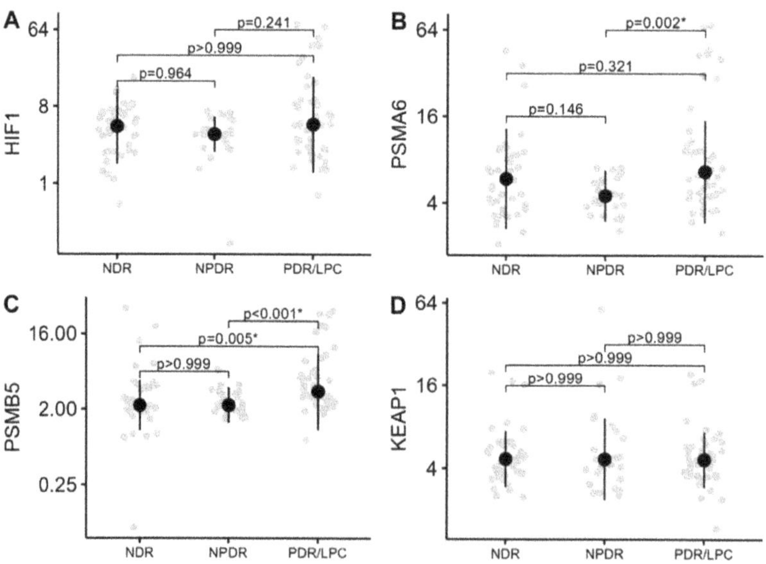

Figure 1. Methylation levels (%) of *HIF1A*, *PSMA6*, *PSMB5*, and *KEAP1* genes across the groups of DR severity stages. The median methylation levels (%) along with the interquartile range are highlighted. (**A**)—methylation of *HIF1A* gene; (**B**)—methylation of *PSMA6* gene; (**C**)—methylation of *PSMB5* gene; and (**D**)—methylation of *KEAP1* gene. The *y*-axis of the graphs is presented on a log scale. NDR—no diabetic retinopathy; NPDR—non-proliferative retinopathy; and PDR/LPC—proliferative retinopathy/status after panretinal-laser photocoagulation. *—statistically significant difference.

3.4. Correlations between DNA Methylation Levels and Clinical Parameters

Spearman correlation coefficients were calculated to assess the relationships between the methylation levels of genes *PSMA6, PSMB5, HIF1A,* and *KEAP1* among themselves and with other clinical parameters within the study groups stratified by DR severity stages. The results for parameters exhibiting significant correlations are summarized in Table 3.

Table 3. Correlations between DNA methylation levels (%) and clinical parameters.

	NDR			NPDR			PDR/LPC		
Variable	*HIF1A*	*PSMA6*	*PSMB5*	*HIF1A*	*PSMA6*	*PSMB5*	*HIF1A*	*PSMA6*	*PSMB5*
Duration of diabetes, years	**0.52 (<0.001)**	**0.43 (0.005)**	−0.04 (0.804)	−0.14 (0.493)	−0.04 (0.859)	0.05 (0.797)	0.14 (0.343)	−0.08 (0.588)	−0.08 (0.616)
HbA1c, %	−0.12 (0.465)	−0.09 (0.596)	**0.44 (0.005)**	−0.02 (0.91)	−0.08 (0.705)	−0.14 (0.483)	−0.12 (0.435)	−0.03 (0.84)	0.00 (0.993)
Albuminuria, mg/mmol	0.06 (0.728)	−0.15 (0.378)	0.24 (0.145)	0.07 (0.752)	−0.09 (0.701)	0.13 (0.554)	0.19 (0.278)	**0.45 (0.008)**	**0.45 (0.008)**
KEAP1	0.26 (0.102)	0.23 (0.145)	**0.46 (0.003)**	0.01 (0.977)	0.26 (0.187)	−0.07 (0.741)	0.08 (0.620)	0.17 (0.272)	0.12 (0.412)
HIF1A		**0.55 (<0.001)**	0.12 (0.463)		**0.39 (0.045)**	0.15 (0.44)		**0.45 (0.002)**	0.17 (0.26)
PSMA6			**0.35 (0.024)**			−0.01 (0.977)			**0.40 (0.006)**

Data are presented as Spearman correlation coefficient R (p-value). Entries with $p < 0.05$ are highlighted in bold. NDR/NPDR—no diabetic retinopathy/non-proliferative retinopathy; PDR/LPC—proliferative retinopathy/status after panretinal-laser photocoagulation.

In patients within the NDR group, positive correlations were observed between methylation levels of *HIF1A* and *PSMA6* (R = 0.55, $p < 0.001$), *PSMB5* and *KEAP1* (R = 0.46, $p = 0.003$), and *PSMA6* and *PSMB5* (R = 0.35, $p = 0.024$). Additionally, the duration of diabetes was positively correlated with *HIF1A* gene (R = 0.52, $p < 0.001$) and *PSMA6* gene methylation level (R = 0.43, $p = 0.005$). HbA1c was found to be positively correlated with *PSMB5* gene methylation level (R = 0.44, $p = 0.005$).

In the NPDR group, a positive correlation was observed between methylation levels of genes *HIF1A* and *PSMA6* (R = 0.39, $p = 0.045$).

In the PDR/LPC group, positive correlations were observed between methylation levels of genes *HIF1A* and *PSMA6* (R = 0.45, $p = 0.002$) and *PSMA6* and *PSMB5* (R = 0.40, $p = 0.006$). Moreover, albuminuria was observed to be positively correlated with *PSMA6* (R = 0.45, $p = 0.008$) and *PSMB5* methylation levels (R = 0.45, $p = 0.008$).

Overall, consistent correlation trends were observed exclusively between the methylation levels of genes *HIF1A* and *PSMA6* across all study groups. However, other correlations varied among the study groups.

3.5. Association of DNA Methylation with the Presence of DR Using Logistic Regression

Logistic regression models were constructed to examine the association between DNA methylation levels and the presence of severe DR (NDR and NPDR vs. PDR/LPC). All continuous predictors were standardized before analysis. The results are summarized in Table 4. Univariate regression analysis demonstrated significant effects of *PSMA6* (OR = 1.96 (1.15; 3.33), $p = 0.013$), *PSMB5* (OR = 1.90 (1.14; 3.16), $p = 0.013$), and *HIF1A* (OR 3.19 (1.26; 8.06), $p = 0.014$).

Multivariate regression models were fitted separately for each gene methylation level adjusted for age and sex (third column in Table 4) and additionally for smoking and arterial hypertension (fourth column in Table 4). Only *PSMB5* showed a trend towards a statistically significant effect (OR 1.75 (0.98; 3.12), $p = 0.057$) when adjusted for age and sex, and a statistically significant effect (OR 1.57 (1.04; 2.36), $p = 0.030$) when additionally adjusted for smoking and arterial hypertension. *HIF1A* demonstrated a trend towards statistical significance (OR 2.13 (0.95; 4.77), $p = 0.065$) when adjusted for age, sex, smoking and arterial hypertension.

Table 4. Results of logistic regression assessing the association between DNA methylation levels and severity of diabetic retinopathy.

Variables	Univariate Regression Results		Multivariate Regression Results [1]		Multivariate Regression Results [2]	
	OR (95% CI)	*p*-Value	OR (95% CI)	*p*-Value	OR (95% CI)	*p*-Value
PSMA6	**1.96 (1.15; 3.33)**	**0.013**	1.01 (0.50; 2.03)	0.983	1.00 (0.57; 1,78)	0.990
PSMB5	**1.90 (1.14; 3.16)**	**0.013**	1.75 (0.98; 3.12)	0.057	**1.57 (1.04; 2.36)**	**0.030**
KEAP1	0.84 (0.53; 1.34)	0.472	0.77 (0.42; 1.41)	0.395	0.74 (0.45; 1.22)	0.238
HIF1A	**3.19 (1.26; 8.06)**	**0.014**	2.00 (0.81; 4.93)	0.134	2.13 (0.95; 4.77)	0.065

Results of logistic regression analysis with the presence of severe diabetic retinopathy (no diabetic retinopathy and non-proliferative retinopathy vs. proliferative retinopathy/status post laser photocoagulation) as the response variable. Data are presented as odds ratios with 95% CI and *p*-values. Separate multiple regression models were fitted for each gene methylation level with the following adjustment variables: [1]—models adjusted for age and sex; [2]—models adjusted for age, sex, smoking, and arterial hypertension. All continuous predictors were standardized before analysis. Entries with $p < 0.05$ are highlighted in bold.

4. Discussion

In the present study, DNA methylation profiles of *PSMA6*, *PSMB5*, *KEAP1*, and *HIF1A* genes were analyzed in a Latvian cohort of 114 patients to examine the effect of methylation on different stages of retinopathy and to identify correlations with clinical and biochemical parameters.

According to the comparative analysis of the three study groups (NDR, NPDR, and PDR/LPC), methylation levels of genes *PSMA6* and *PSMB5* were found to be significantly higher in patients with PDR/LPC. In addition, in all studied DR groups, positive correlations were observed between the methylation levels of the *HIF1A* and *PSMA6* genes. According to data reported by Maghbooli et al., an increasing trend in global DNA methylation levels has also been observed with progressing retinopathy stages. In addition, gene promoter methylation levels found by us align with the reported global DNA methylation levels, ranging from 1.79% to 7.35% [6]. Subsequent studies have also consistently identified differential DNA methylation in specific genes associated with DR [35–37].

The molecular mechanism underlying increased proteasome gene promoter methylation in patients with severe DR possibly involves the epigenetic regulation of *PSMA6* and *PSMB5*, key subunits of the proteasome complex responsible for protein degradation [11,38]. Several studies have shown that severe oxidative stress induced by hyperglycemia decreases intracellular proteolysis, probably by generating damaged proteins that cannot be easily degraded and by damaging proteasomes [39]. The changes in DNA methylation also can be induced by hyperglycemia [40] and other metabolic by-products of diabetes that contribute to the development of diabetic complications in peripheral organs [41,42]. In the context of PDR, this methylation-induced regulation might impair the normal degradation of cellular proteins, leading to the accumulation of damaged or misfolded proteins [43]. Therefore, we can assume that the observed trend of increasing methylation profiles with advancing retinopathy stages in our study implies a cumulative effect of prolonged hyperglycemia and oxidative stress on the epigenetic regulation of these proteasomal genes. Notably, our cohort study in Latvia revealed a positive correlation between *PSMB5* methylation and HbA1c levels in the NDR group, suggesting a complex interaction involving glycemic control, epigenetic changes, and proteasome function. Methylation alterations under hyperglycemia conditions [40] can impact *PSMB5* transcription and, consequently, impact proteasome function, influencing cellular protein homeostasis [44–46]. Interestingly, no correlation between HbA1c and *PSMB5* gene methylation was observed in NPDR and PDR/LPC groups, which could be explained by confounding factors: higher levels of HbA1c, higher prevalence of other complications of diabetes, and more frequent usage of antihypertensive and hypolipidemic treatment in these groups [41–46]. Importantly, *PSMB5* gene methylation was identified in the current study as a significant predictor of severe DR and has the potential to become a clinically significant biomarker.

The consistent positive trends in the correlation between *HIF1A* and *PSMA6* methylation levels identified across all study groups in the current study can indicate a common regulatory mechanism. The ubiquitin–proteasome system is crucial for regulating the cellular response to hypoxia by controlling the stability of HIF-1 alpha. In normal oxygen conditions, HIF-1 alpha undergoes hydroxylation, ubiquitination, and degradation [47]; under hypoxic conditions, and reduced hydroxylation and impaired ubiquitin–proteasome degradation result in the stabilization of HIF-1 alpha [48,49]. This stabilized form translocates into the nucleus, thereby transactivating the transcription of downstream genes [50]. Other post-translational modifications, including methylation, can also regulate HIF signaling (reviewed in [51]).

Our results are consistent with previously published data on the utility of various DNA methylation changes in the diagnosis of autoimmune diseases associated with disease activity, progression, and clinical outcome. The promoter hypermethylation and associated silencing of the *C9orf72* gene occur in about 30% of amyotrophic lateral sclerosis and frontotemporal degeneration patients with a favorable prognosis [52]. Methylation levels of the *BDNF* gene can serve as a useful diagnostic marker in peripheral blood samples of children with autism spectrum disorder (ASD) [53]. In addition, the hypermethylation of a CpG site (cg20793532) in the *PPP2R2C* promoter can potentially be used as a blood biomarker for identifying adult patients with high-functioning ASD [54].

The significant alterations observed in Latvian patients with DR in the PDR/LPC group, including prolonged diabetes duration and changes in factors such as hypertension, diabetic nephropathy, cardiovascular disease, and elevated triglyceride levels, may also suggest a potential association with DNA methylation patterns [55,56]. In diabetic conditions, disruptions to metabolic homeostasis led to alterations in gene expression, affecting genes associated with oxidative stress, apoptosis, and inflammation [35,57,58]. Studies show that the duration of diabetes may correlate with changes in DNA methylation patterns [59]. They also aimed to identify specific genes and genomic regions that are affected by methylation changes associated with long-term diabetes. The Finnish Diabetic Nephropathy Study, with around 3000 diabetic patients, indicates an association between polymorphisms in the *SUV39H2* gene (which encodes histone methyltransferase) and diabetic microvascular complications, including retinopathy [60]. The development of diabetic complications may be associated with metabolic memory of previous glycemic exposure caused by epigenetic changes in target cells [61]. The higher utilization of ACEI/ARB and statin therapy observed in the Latvian PDR/LPC group may also be linked to DNA methylation levels. Qin et al. observed changes in longitudinal lipid and DNA methylation levels in the blood, after the initiation of statin treatment, with changes in DNA methylation responding primarily to changes in lipid levels rather than vice versa. Moreover, statin therapy has also been associated with changes in DNA methylation levels at certain CpGs (e.g., cg27243685 in the *ABCG1* gene) [62].

The positive correlation identified between albuminuria and methylation levels of *PSMA6* and *PSMB5* in our current study indicates a potential pathogenetic relationship between leakage of albumin following vascular damage and methylation status of these proteasome genes. According to previously published data, increased levels of global DNA methylation were also observed in diabetic patients with albuminuria compared to patients with normal albumin levels [59].

Therefore, our study's discovery of a positive association between DNA methylation level of certain genes and DR development indicates that an elevated DNA methylation status might pose a potential risk for DR. This observation aligns with previously reported data in other populations [63,64].

Univariate regression analysis in a DR cohort of Latvian patients revealed potential associations between severe DR and *PSMA6, PSMB5,* and *HIF1A* gene methylation. However, adjusting for covariates in multivariate regression models (Table 4) resulted in the loss of some associations. This indicates that covariates such as age, sex, smoking, and arterial hypertension may have contributed to differences in methylation more than DR status. In addition, the diminished associations in the multivariate analysis could result from the relatively small cohort, a limitation of this study. To address this issue and enhance associations related to DR progression, future studies may consider increasing the cohort size. Several other limitations of the present investigation should be emphasized. Methylation of CpG islands often occurs in parallel with histone modifications [65]. In the present study, we focused only on methylation status and did not evaluate the histone modification profile in the regions of the genes studied; thus, histone modifications may still play a role in changes in the expression of these genes in the blood cells of diabetic patients. Moreover, the present results do not exclude epigenetic mechanisms in the upstream signaling pathways that regulate the expression of these genes or in their other regions.

The limiting condition when using the Zymo OneStep qMethyl technique to determine the methylation sites of specific genes is the number of CpG sites in the amplicon. For a region that has many CpG sites, the current method cannot provide the exact quantitation of methylation percentage without creating a greater number of primers specific to each possible methylation pattern [66]. This can become potentially costly for sequences with a large number of CpG sites. However, if one only wants to determine whether a region is highly or lowly methylated, and to compare relative levels of methylation between experimental cohorts, conventional primers can hybridize to the sequence, and this method provides a simple and relatively inexpensive way to examine this question with reasonable confidence.

We believe that this study has provided a comprehensive understanding of promoter methylation of genes related to epigenetic regulation in the process of DR. By updating our knowledge of the mechanism of methylation regulation, we can integrate these data with genetics, protein expression, and function data.

5. Conclusions

The exploration of epigenetics in type 1 diabetes and DR is crucial for uncovering biomarkers and therapeutic targets. Our study revealed a positive correlation between methylation patterns of the promoter regions of the proteasomal genes *PSMA6* and *PSMB5* and the hypoxia signaling axis-related gene *HIF1A* in different DR groups, linking these patterns to clinical variables. These findings suggest a potential influence of disease progression and associated factors on the methylation status of investigated genes. While our results provide insights into the interplay of epigenetic processes in these conditions, further research is warranted to enhance our understanding of the underlying mechanisms and implications for inflammatory conditions in DR.

Supplementary Materials: The following supporting information can be downloaded at: https://www.mdpi.com/article/10.3390/biomedicines12061354/s1, Table S1: Primers and methodological details of the *PSMA6, PSMB5, HIF1A,* and *KEAP1* region-specific DNA methylation study.

Author Contributions: Z.S., N.P., G.P. and J.S. wrote the manuscript. E.S. and L.P. did the statistical analysis. L.Z. and K.B. performed the ophthalmological examination of patients in Latvia. N.P. was responsible for targeted DNA methylation assessment. All authors have read and agreed to the published version of the manuscript.

Funding: Research was funded in frames of the Baltic Research Programme's project Nr.EEA-RESEARCH-60 "Integrated model for personalized diabetic retinopathy screening and monitoring using risk-stratification and automated AI-based fundus image analysis (PerDiRe)" financially supported by the European Economic Area (EEA) Grants.

Institutional Review Board Statement: The study protocol was approved by The Latvian Central Ethics Committee; Nr. 1/19-10-01 (issued on 1 October 2019). The study is in line with the ethical standards defined in the 1964 Declaration of Helsinki and its later amendments.

Informed Consent Statement: Written informed consent was obtained from all study participants prior to inclusion in the study.

Data Availability Statement: The data underlying this article are available in the article and its online Supplementary Materials.

Conflicts of Interest: N.P., E.S., L.P., L.Z., K.B. and G.P. report no conflicts of interest. Z.S. reports educational grants from Sanofi, MSD, Novo Nordisk, AstraZeneca, and Lilly, lecture fee from KRKA Latvia, and fees from LYL love your life outside of the submitted work. J.S. reports lecture fees and educational grants from Sandoz, Sanofi, MSD, Novo Nordisk, AstraZeneca, and Grindex outside of the submitted work.

References

1. Lundeen, E.A.; Burke-Conte, Z.; Rein, D.B.; Wittenborn, J.S.; Saaddine, J.; Lee, A.Y.; Flaxman, A.D. Prevalence of Diabetic Retinopathy in the US in 2021. *JAMA Ophthalmol.* **2023**, *141*, 747–754. [CrossRef]
2. Chen, Y.; Hong, T.; Wang, S.; Mo, J.; Tian, T.; Zhou, X. Epigenetic modification of nucleic acids: From basic studies to medical applications. *Chem. Soc. Rev.* **2017**, *46*, 2844–2872. [CrossRef] [PubMed]
3. Surguchov, A. α-Synuclein and Mechanisms of Epigenetic Regulation. *Brain Sci.* **2023**, *13*, 150. [CrossRef] [PubMed]
4. Khullar, M.; Cheema, B.S.; Raut, S.K. Emerging Evidence of Epigenetic Modifications in Vascular Complication of Diabetes. *Front. Endocrinol.* **2017**, *8*, 237. [CrossRef] [PubMed]
5. Testa, R.; Bonfigli, A.R.; Prattichizzo, F.; La Sala, L.; De Nigris, V.; Ceriello, A. The "Metabolic Memory" Theory and the Early Treatment of Hyperglycemia in Prevention of Diabetic Complications. *Nutrients* **2017**, *9*, 437. [CrossRef] [PubMed]
6. Maghbooli, Z.; Hossein-Nezhad, A.; Larijani, B.; Amini, M.; Keshtkar, A. Global DNA methylation as a possible biomarker for diabetic retinopathy. *Diabetes Metab. Res. Rev.* **2015**, *31*, 183–189. [CrossRef] [PubMed]
7. Agardh, E.; Lundstig, A.; Perfilyev, A.; Volkov, P.; Freiburghaus, T.; Lindholm, E.; Rönn, T.; Agardh, C.-D.; Ling, C. Genome-wide analysis of DNA methylation in subjects with type 1 diabetes identifies epigenetic modifications associated with proliferative diabetic retinopathy. *BMC Med.* **2015**, *13*, 182. [CrossRef] [PubMed]
8. Hunter, D.J. Gene–environment interactions in human diseases. *Nat. Rev. Genet.* **2005**, *6*, 287–298. [CrossRef] [PubMed]
9. Feinberg, A.P. The Key Role of Epigenetics in Human Disease Prevention and Mitigation. *N. Engl. J. Med.* **2018**, *378*, 1323–1334. [CrossRef]
10. Kato, M.; Natarajan, R. Epigenetics and epigenomics in diabetic kidney disease and metabolic memory. *Nat. Rev. Nephrol.* **2019**, *15*, 327–345. [CrossRef]
11. Thibaudeau, T.A.; Smith, D.M. A practical review of proteasome pharmacology. *Pharmacol. Rev.* **2019**, *71*, 170–197. [CrossRef] [PubMed]
12. Sjakste, T.; Paramonova, N.; Osina, K.; Dokane, K.; Sokolovska, J.; Sjakste, N. Genetic variations in the PSMA3, PSMA6 and PSMC6 genes are associated with type 1 diabetes in latvians and with expression level of number of UPS-related and T1DM-susceptible genes in HapMap individuals. *Mol. Genet. Genom.* **2016**, *291*, 891–903. [CrossRef] [PubMed]
13. Kalnina, J.; Paramonova, N.; Sjakste, N.; Sjakste, T. Study of association between polymorphisms in the PSMB5 (rs11543947) and PSMA3 (rs2348071) genes and multiple sclerosis in Latvians. *Biopolym. Cell* **2014**, *30*, 305–309. [CrossRef]
14. Aghdam, S.Y.; Sheibani, N. The Ubiquitin-Proteasome System and Microvascular Complications of Diabetes. *Ophthalmic Vis. Res.* **2013**, *8*, 244–256. [PubMed]
15. Chapple, S.J.; Siow, R.C.M.; Mann, G.E. Crosstalk between Nrf2 and the proteasome: Therapeutic potential of Nrf2 inducers in vascular disease and aging. *Int. J. Biochem. Cell Biol.* **2012**, *44*, 1315–1320. [CrossRef]
16. Miyata, T.; Suzuki, N.; van Ypersele de Strihou, C. Diabetic nephropathy: Are there new and potentially promising therapies targeting oxygen biology? *Kidney Int.* **2013**, *84*, 693–702. [CrossRef] [PubMed]
17. Mishra, M.; Zhong, Q.; Kowluru, R.A. Epigenetic modifications of Keap1 regulate its interaction with the protective factor Nrf2 in the development of diabetic retinopathy. *Investig. Opthalmol. Vis. Sci.* **2014**, *55*, 7256–7265. [CrossRef] [PubMed]
18. Catrina, S.; Zheng, X. Disturbed hypoxic responses as a pathogenic mechanism of diabetic foot ulcers. *Diabetes Metab. Res. Rev.* **2016**, *32* (Suppl. 1), 179–185. [CrossRef] [PubMed]
19. Choudhry, H.; Harris, A.L. Advances in Hypoxia-Inducible Factor Biology. *Cell Metab.* **2018**, *27*, 281–298. [CrossRef]
20. Cheng, L.; Yu, H.; Yan, N.; Lai, K.; Xiang, M. Hypoxia-Inducible Factor-1α Target Genes Contribute to Retinal Neuroprotection. *Front. Cell. Neurosci.* **2017**, *11*, 20. [CrossRef]
21. Ekberg, N.R.; Eliasson, S.; Li, Y.W.; Zheng, X.; Chatzidionysiou, K.; Falhammar, H.; Gu, H.F.; Catrina, S.-B. Protective effect of the *HIF-1A* Pro582Ser polymorphism on severe diabetic retinopathy. *J. Diabetes Res.* **2019**, *2019*, 2936962. [CrossRef]

22. Han, X.; Ma, W.; Zhu, Y.; Sun, X.; Liu, N. Advanced glycation end products enhance macrophage polarization to the M1 phenotype via the HIF-1α/PDK4 pathway. *Mol. Cell. Endocrinol.* **2020**, *514*, 110878. [CrossRef]
23. Zhou, X.; Yu, D.; Sun, X.; Huang, W.; Xu, Y.; Li, C.; Zhang, Y. Hypoxia-inducible Factor-1α in Diabetic Foot Ulcers: Plain but Not Simple. *Gene Expr.* **2023**, *22*, 306–320. [CrossRef]
24. Hirakawa, Y.; Tanaka, T.; Nangaku, M. Mechanisms of metabolic memory and renal hypoxia as a therapeutic target in diabetic kidney disease. *J. Diabetes Investig.* **2017**, *8*, 261–271. [CrossRef]
25. Gao, C.; Huang, W.; Kanasaki, K.; Xu, Y. The role of ubiquitination and sumoylation in diabetic nephropathy. *BioMed Res. Int.* **2014**, *2014*, 160692. [CrossRef] [PubMed]
26. Huang, W.; Yang, C.; Nan, Q.; Gao, C.; Feng, H.; Gou, F.; Chen, G.; Zhang, Z.; Yan, P.; Peng, J.; et al. The Proteasome Inhibitor, MG132, Attenuates Diabetic Nephropathy by Inhibiting SnoN Degradation In Vivo and In Vitro. *BioMed Res. Int.* **2014**, *2014*, 684765. [CrossRef] [PubMed]
27. Luo, X.; Pan, J.; Wang, L.; Wang, P.; Zhang, M.; Liu, M.; Dong, Z.; Meng, Q.; Tao, X.; Zhao, X.; et al. Epigenetic regulation of lncRNA connects ubiquitin-proteasome system with infection-inflammation in preterm births and preterm premature rupture of membranes. *BMC Pregnancy Childbirth* **2015**, *15*, 35. [CrossRef]
28. Luo, Z.-F.; Qi, W.; Feng, B.; Mu, J.; Zeng, W.; Guo, Y.-H.; Pang, Q.; Ye, Z.-L.; Liu, L.; Yuan, F.-H. Prevention of diabetic nephropathy in rats through enhanced renal antioxidative capacity by inhibition of the proteasome. *Life Sci.* **2011**, *88*, 512–520. [CrossRef] [PubMed]
29. Mokarram, P.; Kavousipour, S.; Sarabi, M.M.; Mehrabani, G.; Fahmidehkar, M.A.; Shamsdin, S.A.; Alipour, A.; Naini, M.A. MGMT-B gene promoter hypermethylation in patients with inflammatory bowel disease—A novel finding. *Asian Pac. J. Cancer Prev.* **2015**, *16*, 1945–1952. [CrossRef]
30. Mokarram, P.; Shakiba-Jam, F.; Kavousipour, S.; Sarabi, M.M.; Seghatoleslam, A. Promoter Methylation Status of Two Novel Human Genes, UBE2Q1 and UBE2Q2, in Colorectal Cancer: A New Finding in Iranian Patients. *Asian Pac. J. Cancer Prev.* **2015**, *16*, 8247–8252. [CrossRef]
31. West, N.A.; Kechris, K.; Dabelea, D. Exposure to Maternal Diabetes in Utero and DNA Methylation Patterns in the Offspring. *Immunometabolism* **2013**, *1*, 1–9. [CrossRef] [PubMed]
32. Ahola, A.J.; Radzeviciene, L.; Zaharenko, L.; Bulum, T.; Skrebinska, S.; Prakapiene, E.; Blaslov, K.; Roso, V.; Rovite, V.; Pirags, V.; et al. Association between symptoms of depression, diabetes complications and vascular risk factors in four European cohorts of individuals with type 1 diabetes—InterDiane Consortium. *Diabetes Res. Clin. Pract.* **2020**, *170*, 108495. [CrossRef] [PubMed]
33. Rovite, V.; Wolff-Sagi, Y.; Zaharenko, L.; Nikitina-Zake, L.; Grens, E.; Klovins, J. Genome Database of the Latvian Population (LGDB): Design, Goals, and Primary Results. *J. Epidemiol.* **2018**, *28*, 353–360. [CrossRef] [PubMed]
34. Sokolovska, J.; Dekante, A.; Baumane, L.; Pahirko, L.; Valeinis, J.; Dislere, K.; Rovite, V.; Pirags, V.; Sjakste, N. Nitric oxide metabolism is impaired by type 1 diabetes and diabetic nephropathy. *Biomed. Rep.* **2020**, *12*, 251–258. [CrossRef] [PubMed]
35. Kowluru, R.A.; Santos, J.M.; Mishra, M. Epigenetic modifications and diabetic retinopathy. *BioMed Res. Int.* **2013**, *2013*, 635284. [CrossRef] [PubMed]
36. Wu, J.; Liu, L.-L.; Cao, M.; Hu, A.; Hu, D.; Luo, Y.; Wang, H.; Zhong, J.-N. DNA methylation plays important roles in retinal development and diseases. *Exp. Eye Res.* **2021**, *211*, 108733. [CrossRef]
37. Kumari, N.; Karmakar, A.; Ganesan, S.K. Targeting epigenetic modifications as a potential therapeutic option for diabetic retinopathy. *J. Cell. Physiol.* **2020**, *235*, 1933–1947. [CrossRef] [PubMed]
38. Bard, J.A.; Goodall, E.A.; Greene, E.R.; Jonsson, E.; Dong, K.C.; Martin, A. Structure and Function of the 26S Proteasome. *Annu. Rev. Biochem.* **2018**, *87*, 697–724. [CrossRef]
39. Shang, F.; Taylor, A. Ubiquitin–proteasome pathway and cellular responses to oxidative stress. *Free Radic. Biol. Med.* **2011**, *51*, 5–16. [CrossRef]
40. Olsen, A.S.; Sarras, M.P.; Leontovich, A.; Intine, R.V. Heritable transmission of diabetic metabolic memory in zebrafish correlates with DNA hypomethylation and aberrant gene expression. *Diabetes* **2012**, *61*, 485–491. [CrossRef]
41. Intine, R.V.; Sarras, M.P.J. Metabolic memory and chronic diabetes complications: Potential role for epigenetic mechanisms. *Curr. Diabetes Rep.* **2012**, *12*, 551–559. [CrossRef] [PubMed]
42. Bansal, A.; Pinney, S.E. DNA methylation and its role in the pathogenesis of diabetes. *Pediatr. Diabetes* **2017**, *18*, 167–177. [CrossRef] [PubMed]
43. Fernandes, R.; Bento, C.F.; Matafome, P.; Sena, C.M.; Seiça, R.M.; Pereira, P. Atorvastatin-mediated protection of the retina in a model of diabetes with hyperlipidemia. *Can. J. Physiol. Pharmacol.* **2014**, *92*, 1037–1043. [CrossRef] [PubMed]
44. Svikle, Z.; Peterfelde, B.; Sjakste, N.; Baumane, K.; Verkauskiene, R.; Jeng, C.-J.; Sokolovska, J. Ubiquitin-proteasome system in diabetic retinopathy. *PeerJ* **2022**, *10*, e13715. [CrossRef] [PubMed]
45. Shruthi, K.; Reddy, S.S.; Chitra, P.S.; Reddy, G.B. Ubiquitin-proteasome system and ER stress in the brain of diabetic rats. *J. Cell. Biochem.* **2019**, *120*, 5962–5973. [CrossRef] [PubMed]
46. Homma, T.; Fujii, J. Emerging connections between oxidative stress, defective proteolysis, and metabolic diseases. *Free Radic. Res.* **2020**, *54*, 931–946. [CrossRef] [PubMed]
47. Lee, F.S.; Percy, M.J. The HIF pathway and erythrocytosis. *Annu. Rev. Pathol. Mech. Dis.* **2011**, *6*, 165–192. [CrossRef] [PubMed]

48. Nakayama, K.; Frew, I.J.; Hagensen, M.; Skals, M.; Habelhah, H.; Bhoumik, A.; Kadoya, T.; Erdjument-Bromage, H.; Tempst, P.; Frappell, P.B.; et al. Siah2 regulates stability of prolyl-hydroxylases, controls HIF1α abundance, and modulates physiological responses to hypoxia. *Cell* **2004**, *117*, 941–952. [CrossRef] [PubMed]
49. Choi, H.J.; Song, B.-J.; Gong, Y.-D.; Gwak, W.J.; Soh, Y. Rapid degradation of hypoxia-inducible factor-1α by KRH102053, a new activator of prolyl hydroxylase 2. *Br. J. Pharmacol.* **2008**, *154*, 114–125. [CrossRef] [PubMed]
50. Catrina, S.-B.; Zheng, X. Hypoxia and hypoxia-inducible factors in diabetes and its complications. *Diabetologia* **2021**, *64*, 709–716. [CrossRef]
51. Koyasu, S.; Kobayashi, M.; Goto, Y.; Hiraoka, M.; Harada, H. Regulatory mechanisms of hypoxia-inducible factor 1 activity: Two decades of knowledge. *Cancer Sci.* **2018**, *109*, 560–571. [CrossRef] [PubMed]
52. Liu, E.Y.; Russ, J.; Wu, K.; Neal, D.; Suh, E.; McNally, A.G.; Irwin, D.J.; Van Deerlin, V.M.; Lee, E.B. C9orf72 hypermethylation protects against repeat expansion-associated pathology in ALS/FTD. *Acta Neuropathol.* **2014**, *128*, 525–541. [CrossRef] [PubMed]
53. Kundakovic, M.; Gudsnuk, K.; Herbstman, J.B.; Tang, D.; Perera, F.P.; Champagne, F.A. DNA methylation of BDNF as a biomarker of early-life adversity. *Proc. Natl. Acad. Sci. USA* **2015**, *112*, 6807–6813. [CrossRef] [PubMed]
54. Kimura, R.; Nakata, M.; Funabiki, Y.; Suzuki, S.; Awaya, T.; Murai, T.; Hagiwara, M. An epigenetic biomarker for adult high-functioning autism spectrum disorder. *Sci. Rep.* **2019**, *9*, 13662. [CrossRef] [PubMed]
55. Ahmed, S.A.H.; Ansari, S.A.; Mensah-Brown, E.P.K.; Emerald, B.S. The role of DNA methylation in the pathogenesis of type 2 diabetes mellitus. *Clin. Epigenet.* **2020**, *12*, 104. [CrossRef] [PubMed]
56. Li, K.Y.; Tam, C.H.T.; Liu, H.; Day, S.; Lim, C.K.P.; So, W.Y.; Huang, C.; Jiang, G.; Shi, M.; Lee, H.M.; et al. DNA methylation markers for kidney function and progression of diabetic kidney disease. *Nat. Commun.* **2023**, *14*, 2543. [CrossRef]
57. Giacco, F.; Brownlee, M. Oxidative stress and diabetic complications. *Circ. Res.* **2010**, *107*, 1058–1070. [CrossRef] [PubMed]
58. Volkmar, M.; Dedeurwaerder, S.; Cunha, D.A.; Ndlovu, M.N.; Defrance, M.; Deplus, R.; Calonne, E.; Volkmar, U.; Igoillo-Esteve, M.; Naamane, N.; et al. DNA methylation profiling identifies epigenetic dysregulation in pancreatic islets from type 2 diabetic patients. *EMBO J.* **2012**, *31*, 1405–1426. [CrossRef] [PubMed]
59. Maghbooli, Z.; Larijani, B.; Emamgholipour, S.; Amini, M.; Keshtkar, A.; Pasalar, P. Aberrant DNA methylation patterns in diabetic nephropathy. *J. Diabetes Metab. Disord.* **2014**, *13*, 69. [CrossRef]
60. Syreeni, A.; El-Osta, A.; Forsblom, C.; Sandholm, N.; Parkkonen, M.; Tarnow, L.; Parving, H.-H.; McKnight, A.J.; Maxwell, A.P.; Cooper, M.E.; et al. Genetic Examination of SETD7 and SUV39H1/H2 Methyltransferases and the Risk of Diabetes Complications in Patients with Type 1 Diabetes. *Diabetes* **2011**, *60*, 3073–3080. [CrossRef]
61. Villeneuve, L.M.; Natarajan, R. Epigenetics of diabetic complications. *Expert Rev. Endocrinol. Metab.* **2010**, *5*, 137–148. [CrossRef] [PubMed]
62. Qin, X.; Wang, Y.; Pedersen, N.L.; Tang, B.; Hägg, S. Dynamic patterns of blood lipids and DNA methylation in response to statin therapy. *Clin. Epigenet.* **2022**, *14*, 153. [CrossRef] [PubMed]
63. Zhang, X.; Zhao, L.; Hambly, B.; Bao, S.; Wang, K. Diabetic retinopathy: Reversibility of epigenetic modifications and new therapeutic targets. *Cell Biosci.* **2017**, *7*, 42. [CrossRef] [PubMed]
64. Cai, C.; Meng, C.; He, S.; Gu, C.; Lhamo, T.; Draga, D.; Luo, D.; Qiu, Q. DNA methylation in diabetic retinopathy: Pathogenetic role and potential therapeutic targets. *Cell Biosci.* **2022**, *12*, 186. [CrossRef] [PubMed]
65. Fan, S.; Zhang, M.Q.; Zhang, X. Histone methylation marks play important roles in predicting the methylation status of CpG islands. *Biochem. Biophys. Res. Commun.* **2008**, *374*, 559–564. [CrossRef]
66. Kurdyukov, S.; Bullock, M. DNA Methylation Analysis: Choosing the Right Method. *Biology* **2016**, *5*, 3. [CrossRef]

biomedicines

MDPI

Article

The Association between Diabetic Retinopathy and Macular Degeneration: A Nationwide Population-Based Study

Hsin-Ting Lin [1,2], Cai-Mei Zheng [3,4,5,6], Cheng-Hung Tsai [7], Ching-Long Chen [1,2], Yu-Ching Chou [7], Jing-Quan Zheng [6,8], Yuh-Feng Lin [2,3,5,6], Chia-Wei Lin [9,10,11], Yong-Chen Chen [12], Chien-An Sun [13,*] and Jiann-Torng Chen [1,2,*]

1 Department of Ophthalmology, Tri-Service General Hospital, National Defense Medical Center, Taipei 114, Taiwan; t72010@yahoo.com.tw (H.-T.L.); doc30881@mail.ndmctsgh.edu.tw (C.-L.C.)
2 Graduate Institute of Medical Sciences, National Defense Medical Center, Taipei 114, Taiwan; linyf@s.tmu.edu.tw
3 Division of Nephrology, Department of Internal Medicine, School of Medicine, College of Medicine, Taipei Medical University, Taipei 110, Taiwan; 11044@s.tmu.edu.tw
4 TMU Research Center of Urology and Kidney, Taipei Medical University, Taipei 110, Taiwan
5 Division of Nephrology, Department of Internal Medicine, Shuang Ho Hospital, Taipei Medical University, Taipei 235, Taiwan
6 Graduate Institute of Clinical Medicine, College of Medicine, Taipei Medical University, Taipei 110, Taiwan; 16044@s.tmu.edu.tw
7 School of Public Health, National Defense Medical Center, Taipei 114, Taiwan; martintsai0920@yahoo.com.tw (C.-H.T.); trishow@mail.ndmctsgh.edu.tw (Y.-C.C.)
8 Division of Pulmonary Medicine, Department of Internal Medicine, Shuang Ho Hospital, Taipei Medical University, Taipei 110, Taiwan
9 Department of Urology, Shuang Ho Hospital, Taipei Medical University, New Taipei City 110, Taiwan; sky02578@yahoo.com.tw
10 Department of Urology, School of Medicine, College of Medicine, Taipei Medical University, Taipei 110, Taiwan
11 Department of Urology, Tri-Service General Hospital, National Defense Medical Center, Taipei 114, Taiwan
12 Department of Medicine, College of Medicine, Fu Jen Catholic University, New Taipei City 242, Taiwan; 137159@mail.fju.edu.tw
13 Department of Public Health, College of Medicine, Fu Jen Catholic University, New Taipei City 242, Taiwan
* Correspondence: 040866@mail.fju.edu.tw (C.-A.S.); jt66chen@gmail.com (J.-T.C.); Tel.: +886-2-29053432 (C.-A.S.); +886-2-87923311 (J.-T.C.)

Abstract: Objective: Age-related macular degeneration (AMD), particularly its exudative form, is a primary cause of vision impairment in older adults. As diabetes becomes increasingly prevalent in aging, it is crucial to explore the potential relationship between diabetic retinopathy (DR) and AMD. This study aimed to assess the risk of developing overall, non-exudative, and exudative AMD in individuals with DR compared to those without retinopathy (non-DR) based on a nationwide population study in Taiwan. Methods: A retrospective cohort study was conducted using the Taiwan National Health Insurance Database (NHIRD) (2000–2013). A total of 3413 patients were placed in the study group (DR) and 13,652 in the control group (non-DR) for analysis. Kaplan–Meier analysis and the Cox proportional hazards model were used to calculate the hazard ratios (HRs) and adjusted hazard ratios (aHRs) for the development of AMD, adjusting for confounding factors, such as age, sex, and comorbid conditions. Results: Kaplan–Meier survival analysis indicated a significantly higher cumulative incidence of AMD in the DR group compared to the non-DR group (log-rank test, $p < 0.001$). Adjusted analyses revealed that individuals with DR faced a greater risk of overall AMD, with an aHR of 3.50 (95% CI = 3.10–3.95). For senile (unspecified) AMD, the aHR was 3.45 (95% CI = 3.04–3.92); for non-exudative senile AMD, it was 2.92 (95% CI = 2.08–4.09); and for exudative AMD, the aHR was 3.92 (95% CI = 2.51–6.14). Conclusion: DR is a significant risk factor for both overall, senile, exudative, and non-exudative AMD, even after adjusting for demographic and comorbid conditions. DR patients tend to have a higher prevalence of vascular comorbidities; however, our findings indicate that the ocular pathologies inherent to DR might have a more significant impact on the progression to AMD. Early detection and appropriate treatment of AMD is critically important among DR patients.

Keywords: diabetes mellitus (DM); diabetic retinopathy (DR); non-diabetic retinopathy (non-DR); age-related macular degeneration (AMD); Taiwan National Health Insurance Database (NHIRD)

1. Introduction

Diabetic retinopathy (DR) and age-related macular degeneration (AMD) are important retinal degenerative disorders that represent a growing concern among aging societies. These conditions exhibit overlapping pathological processes, such as retinal edema and progressive inflammation within the central macula. The hyperglycemic environment of diabetes mellitus activates inflammatory cells and increases the production of reactive oxygen species (ROS) and pro-inflammatory cytokines (e.g., IL-6, TNF-α, macrophage migration inhibitory factor (MIF), etc.) [1,2]. In addition, diabetes is characterized by the elevated release of substances, such as angiotensin II, prostaglandins (PGs), and vascular endothelial growth factor (VEGF), all of which are implicated in causing retinal vascular alterations [3]. These inflammatory and vascular changes are common underlying mechanisms that are pivotal in the progression of DR and AMD [4–6].

The balance between pro-inflammatory and anti-inflammatory pathways is crucial in managing the progression of both DR and AMD in diabetic patients. An imbalance between these pathways, marked by a deficiency in anti-inflammatory bioactive lipids and an accumulation of inflammatory cytokines, exacerbates the progression of these conditions [7–9]. Retinal pigment epithelial (RPE) cells, which protect against AMD and DR, counteract the production of ROS, inflammatory cytokines, and adhesion molecules through the secretion of pigment epithelium-derived factor (PEDF) [10,11]. However, in the context of diabetes, hyperglycemia disrupts the function of these RPE cells, impeding their PEDF production, which, in turn, can initiate retinal edema, DR, and AMD [12,13].

In Taiwan, an aging society, there is an increasing prevalence of both DR and AMD among elderly diabetic patients. While DR and AMD share common pathophysiological pathways, the epidemiological relationship between DR and AMD is still a subject of debate. Some studies have identified a link between DM and AMD [14,15], while others have not observed a significant correlation [16,17]. DM itself related positively with early AMD among elderly Korean patients [18], whereas a similar relation was noted between DR and neovascular AMD in a multicenter, population-based European study [19]. Herein, we used our population-based database to explore the incidence and risks for different types of AMD among patients with and without DR.

2. Methods

2.1. Data Source

Taiwan's National Health Insurance (NHI) was launched by the Taiwan Department of Health in 1995, providing comprehensive medical care coverage. A total of 23,832,551 Taiwanese residents, accounting for approximately 99% of the population in Taiwan, have joined the program. The Longitudinal Health Insurance Database (LHID), which is part of the NHI Research Database (NHIRD), contains data for one million randomly sampled patients from the Registry for Beneficiaries of the NHIRD. The database exhibits no statistically significant differences in terms of age, sex, or healthcare costs when compared to all NHI enrollees. Diagnoses in the database were assigned by qualified clinical physicians based on laboratory, imaging, and pathological data and following the International Classification of Diseases, Ninth Revision, Clinical Modification (ICD-9-CM). Personal identification numbers were encrypted to safeguard patient privacy before the electronic files were released for study.

2.2. Study Population

We conducted a population-based retrospective cohort study based on the LHID 2000. Following the ICD-9-CM format, AMD has several types, such as senile (unspecified), non-exudative, exudative, familial, juvenile, congenital, cystic AMD, etc. (Table 6), and we chose the most often cited codes by Ophthalmologists, which are senile (unspecified) (362.50) AMD, non-exudative (362.51) AMD, and exudative (362.52) AMD, to represent all types of AMD for reasonable convenience of further analysis. This study design will result in inconsistency of codes cited by Ophthalmologists and will be listed as a study limitation. We selected patients (aged ≥55 years old) who were newly diagnosed with diabetic retinopathy (DR) using ICD-9-CM codes 362.01 and 362.02 between 2000 and 2006 as the study cohort. To only include new cases, individuals who had previously received any DR and diabetes mellitus (DM) diagnoses, using ICD-9-CM code 250, in the medical claim data before 2000 were excluded. Additionally, DR patients with a history of age-related macular degeneration (AMD) using ICD-9-CM codes 362.50, 362.51, and 362.52 before the index date were excluded (*n* = 211). For each patient diagnosed with DR, we randomly selected four patients without diabetic retinopathy (non-DR) as the control group from the same database who were matched for age and sex. The non-DR group also excluded individuals with a history of AMD before the index date. Overall, our final sample for analysis included 3413 subjects with DR (the study group) and 13,652 subjects without DR (the control group). The study flowchart is shown in Figure 1. Both the study and control groups were followed to detect the occurrence of AMD. All subjects were observed until a diagnosis of AMD, death, or 31 December 2013, whichever occurred first. Our study was approved by the Institutional Review Board of Fu Jen Catholic University (FJU-IRB NO: C104014).

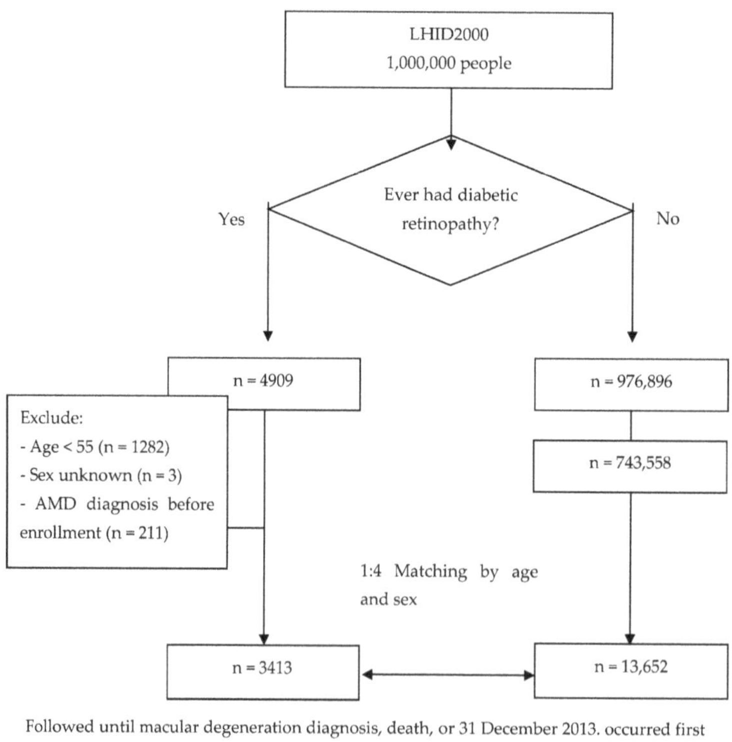

Figure 1. Study flowchart. AMD = age-related macular degeneration, LHID = Longitudinal Health Insurance Database.

Histories of comorbidities present in both the study group and control group, such as hypertension (ICD-9 codes 401, 402, 403, 404, and 405), hyperlipidemia (ICD-9-CM codes

272.0, 272.1, 272.2, and 272.4), coronary artery disease (CAD; ICD-9-CM codes 410, 411, 412, 413, and 414), stroke (ICD-9-CM codes 430, 431, 432, 433, 434, 435, 436, 437, and 438), chronic obstructive pulmonary disease (COPD; ICD-9-CM codes 490, 491, 492, 493, 494, 495, and 496), and liver cirrhosis/chronic hepatitis (ICD-9-CM code 571), were included in this study to control for their potential confounding effects.

2.3. Statistical Analysis

Chi-square tests were used to analyze categorical variables, including demographics and comorbidities, while continuous variables were assessed with two-sample *t*-tests. Kaplan–Meier curves were used to depict cumulative AMD incidence and Cox regression was used to estimate AMD risk, adjusted for age, sex, and comorbidities and stratified by age and sex to determine DR and AMD association. Data were analyzed via SAS 9.4 and SPSS 22.0, with $p < 0.05$ set as the significance level.

3. Results

The baseline demographic information and comorbidity conditions of patients in the diabetic retinopathy (DR) group ($N = 3413$) and the non-diabetic retinopathy (non-DR) group ($N = 13{,}652$) are presented in Table 1. The mean age in the DR group (67.1 years) was significantly higher than that in the non-DR group (66.5 years) ($p < 0.001$); however, there were no significant differences in age and gender between groups. DR patients had significantly higher rates of comorbidities, including hypertension, hyperlipidemia, coronary artery disease (CAD), stroke, chronic obstructive pulmonary disease (COPD), and liver cirrhosis/chronic hepatitis, compared to the non-DR group (all $p < 0.001$) (Table 1). Table 2 shows the occurrence and hazard ratios of all types of AMD for both the DR and non-DR groups. There was a higher incidence rate of AMD (16.77 per 10,000 person years (PYs)) in the DR group compared to the incidence rate of 5.36 per 10,000 PYs in the non-DR group. After adjusting for age, sex, and comorbid conditions, individuals with DR still had a significantly higher risk (aHR 3.50, 95% CI = 3.10–3.95) of overall AMD compared to those without DR (see Table 2). The incidence of AMD increased with age in both groups, but the association was stronger in the DR group across all age categories, with the highest risk observed in patients over 85 years old. The incidence rates of AMD were higher for both genders in the DR group, with males showing a slightly higher risk than females. Markedly, the DR group had a significantly higher HR and aHR than the non-DR group, regardless of its comorbid conditions.

Table 1. Baseline demographic status and comorbidity comparison between non-diabetic retinopathy and diabetic retinopathy groups.

Variable	Non-DR Group $N = 13{,}652$ (%)	DR Group $N = 3413$ (%)	*p*-Value
Age, years (SD) *	66.5 (7.9)	67.1 (7.2)	<0.001
55–65	5812 (42.6)	1453 (42.6)	1.000
65–75	5832 (42.7)	1458 (42.7)	
75–85	1868 (13.7)	467 (13.7)	
≥85	140 (1.0)	35 (1.0)	
Sex			1.000
Female	7732 (56.6)	1933 (56.6)	
Male	5920 (43.4)	1480 (43.4)	
Comorbidity			
Hypertension	6252 (45.8)	2354 (69.0)	<0.001
Hyperlipidemia	2593 (19.0)	950 (27.8)	<0.001
CAD	2412 (17.7)	1356 (39.7)	<0.001
Stroke	1405 (10.3)	1029 (30.2)	<0.001
COPD	3955 (29.0)	1265 (37.1)	<0.001
Liver cirrhosis and chronic hepatitis	1566 (11.5)	601 (17.6)	<0.001

* Independent *t*-test. Abbreviations: SD: standard deviation; non-DR: non-diabetic retinopathy; DR: diabetic retinopathy; CAD: coronary artery disease; COPD: chronic obstructive pulmonary disease.

Table 2. Incidence and estimated hazard ratios of all types of age-related macular degeneration (AMD) (ICD-9 codes 362.50, 362.51, 362.52).

Variable	Non-DR Group			DR Group			HR (95% CI)	p-Value	aHR (95% CI)	p-Value
	Event	PYs	Rate	Event	PYs	Rate				
DR	704	131,328	5.36	514	30,644	16.77	3.14 (2.80–3.52)	<0.001	3.50 (3.10–3.95)	<0.001
Demographic										
Age group										
55–65	252	57,141	4.41	218	13,412	16.25	3.70 (3.09–4.44)	<0.001	4.17 (3.44–5.06)	<0.001
65–75	380	56,031	6.78	210	13,117	16.01	2.37 (2.00–2.81)	<0.001	2.62 (2.19–3.12)	<0.001
75–85	70	16,959	4.13	81	3805	21.29	5.06 (3.67–6.96)	<0.001	5.69 (4.02–8.07)	<0.001
≥85	2	1196	1.67	5	311	16.08	10.18 (1.97–52.53)	0.006	16.64 (1.29–214.78)	0.031
Sex										
Female	451	74,920	6.02	297	17,648	16.83	2.81 (2.42–3.25)	<0.001	3.14 (2.69–3.66)	<0.001
Male	253	56,408	4.49	217	12,996	16.70	3.72 (3.10–4.46)	<0.001	4.15 (3.42–5.04)	<0.001
Comorbidity										
Hypertension										
No	311	71,194	4.37	210	9739	21.56	4.95 (4.15–5.89)	<0.001	5.44 (4.53–6.53)	<0.001
Yes	393	60,133	6.54	304	20,905	14.54	2.24 (1.93–2.60)	<0.001	2.57 (2.20–3.00)	<0.001
Hyperlipidemia										
No	569	106,311	5.35	408	22,157	18.41	3.44 (3.03–3.91)	<0.001	3.71 (3.25–4.25)	<0.001
Yes	135	25,016	5.40	106	8488	12.49	2.34 (1.82–3.02)	<0.001	2.68 (2.06–3.49)	<0.001
CAD										
No	534	108,276	4.93	356	18,627	19.11	3.88 (3.39–4.43)	<0.001	4.24 (3.69–4.88)	<0.001
Yes	170	23,052	7.37	158	12,017	13.15	1.80 (1.45–2.23)	<0.001	2.11 (1.69–2.63)	<0.001
Stroke										
No	657	118,136	5.56	457	21,689	21.07	3.80 (3.37–4.28)	<0.001	3.72 (3.29–4.22)	<0.001
Yes	47	13,191	3.56	57	8955	6.37	1.80 (1.22–2.65)	0.003	1.75 (1.17–2.60)	0.006
COPD										
No	460	93,850	4.90	356	19,227	18.52	3.77 (3.29–4.34)	<0.001	4.19 (3.62–4.87)	<0.001
Yes	244	37,478	6.51	158	11,417	13.84	2.14 (1.75–2.62)	<0.001	2.45 (1.99–3.01)	<0.001
Liver cirrhosis and chronic hepatitis										
No	616	116,796	5.27	429	25,350	16.92	3.21 (2.84–3.64)	<0.001	3.56 (3.12–4.05)	<0.001
Yes	88	14,531	6.06	85	5294	16.06	2.69 (2.00–3.62)	<0.001	3.11 (2.29–4.24)	<0.001

Model adjusted for age, sex, low income, hypertension, hyperlipidemia, CAD, stroke, COPD, and liver cirrhosis and chronic hepatitis. Abbreviations: DR: diabetic retinopathy; AMD: age-related macular degeneration; CAD: coronary artery disease; COPD: chronic obstructive pulmonary disease; PYs: person years; rate: incidence rate per 10,000 person years; HR: hazard ratio; aHR: adjusted hazard ratio.

Table 3 shows the comparative risks of senile (unspecified) AMD based on DR status. The non-DR group ($n = 13{,}652$) had an incidence rate of 4.78 per 10,000 PYs compared to the DR group ($n = 3413$) with an incidence rate of 14.65 per 10,000 PYs. The aHR for senile AMD in the DR group was 3.45 (95% CI: 3.04–3.92) compared to the non-DR group. Aging and the male gender were correlated with significantly higher risks than other demographic factors. A significant increase in AMD was noted in the DR group regardless of the presence or absence of comorbid conditions, such as hypertension, CAD hyperlipidemia, stroke, COPD, or cirrhosis/chronic hepatitis. These findings substantiate DR as a significant predictor of senile AMD, independent of demographic factors and comorbid conditions. Table 4 examines the incidence and hazard ratios of non-exudative senile AMD in DR compared to non-DR groups. A higher incidence rate of non-exudative AMD was observed in the DR group (1.89 per 10,000 person years) compared to the non-DR group (0.69 per 10,000 person years). The incidence rates increased with age in both the DR and non-DR groups. In the DR group, the incidence rate was markedly higher with aging, particularly in the 65–75 and ≥85 age groups. Like in overall AMD, male patients with DR had a higher incidence rate of non-exudative AMD compared to female patients with DR. Patients in DR had significantly higher incidence rates of AMD than their non-DR counterparts, regardless of their comorbid conditions (Table 4).

Table 3. Incidence and estimated hazard ratios of senile (unspecified) age-related macular degeneration (AMD) (ICD-9 code 362.50).

Variable	Non-DR Group			DR Group			HR (95% CI)	p-Value	aHR (95% CI)	p-Value
	Event	PYs	Rate	Event	PYs	Rate				
DR	629	131,665	4.78	455	31,053	14.65	3.08 (2.73–3.47)	<0.001	3.45 (3.04–3.92)	<0.001
Demographic										
Age group										
55–65	225	57,239	3.93	191	13,591	14.05	3.58 (2.96–4.35)	<0.001	4.04 (3.29–4.97)	<0.001
65–75	342	56,210	6.08	185	13,309	13.90	2.30 (1.92–2.75)	<0.001	2.55 (2.12–3.08)	<0.001
75–85	60	17,020	3.53	76	3830	19.84	5.51 (3.93–7.74)	<0.001	6.19 (4.28–8.94)	<0.001
≥85	2	1196	1.67	3	322	9.32	5.95 (0.99–35.64)	0.051	4.16 (0.28–61.35)	0.298
Sex										
Female	411	75,133	5.47	269	17,840	15.08	2.77 (2.37–3.23)	<0.001	3.09 (2.63–3.34)	<0.001
Male	218	56,532	3.86	186	13,213	14.08	3.65 (3.00–4.44)	<0.001	4.12 (3.35–5.07)	<0.001
Comorbidity										
Hypertension										
No	271	71,318	3.80	188	9833	19.12	5.05 (4.19–6.08)	<0.001	5.57 (4.67–6.89)	<0.001
Yes	358	60,348	5.93	267	21,220	12.58	2.13 (1.82–2.50)	<0.001	2.45 (2.08–2.89)	<0.001
Hyperlipidemia										
No	499	106,574	4.68	362	22,457	16.12	3.45 (3.02–3.95)	<0.001	3.76 (3.26–4.34)	<0.001
Yes	130	25,091	5.18	93	8596	10.82	2.11 (1.62–2.75)	<0.001	2.41 (1.83–3.18)	<0.001
CAD										
No	481	108,488	4.43	314	18,803	16.70	3.77 (3.27–4.35)	<0.001	4.14 (3.57–4.80)	<0.001
Yes	148	23,177	6.39	141	12,249	11.51	1.82 (1.44–2.29)	<0.001	2.13 (1.68–2.69)	<0.001
Stroke										
No	587	118,404	4.96	408	21,952	18.59	3.76 (3.31–4.27)	<0.001	3.69 (3.23–4.21)	<0.001
Yes	42	13,262	3.17	47	9101	5.16	1.64 (1.08–2.49)	0.020	1.56 (1.01–2.40)	0.043
COPD										
No	416	94,032	4.42	316	19,484	16.22	3.67 (3.17–4.25)	<0.001	4.06 (3.47–4.75)	<0.001
Yes	213	37,633	5.66	139	11,569	12.01	2.14 (1.73–2.65)	<0.001	2.47 (1.98–3.07)	<0.001
Liver cirrhosis and chronic hepatitis										
No	555	117,040	4.74	376	25,674	14.65	3.10 (2.72–3.53)	<0.001	3.47 (3.02–3.98)	<0.001
Yes	74	14,625	5.06	79	5379	14.69	2.94 (2.14–4.04)	<0.001	3.30 (2.38–4.59)	<0.001

Model adjusted for age, sex, low income, hypertension, hyperlipidemia, CAD, stroke, COPD, and liver cirrhosis and chronic hepatitis. Abbreviations: DR: diabetic retinopathy; AMD: age-related macular degeneration; CAD: coronary artery disease; COPD: chronic obstructive pulmonary disease; PYs: person years; rate: incidence rate per 10,000 person years; HR: hazard ratio; aHR: adjusted hazard ratio.

Table 4. Incidence and estimated hazard ratios of non-exudative age-related macular degeneration (AMD) (ICD-9 code 362.51).

Variable	Non-DR Group			DR Group			HR (95% CI)	p-Value	aHR (95% CI)	p-Value
	Event	PYs	Rate	Event	PYs	Rate				
DR	93	134,162	0.69	63	33,404	1.89	2.73 (1.98–3.76)	<0.001	2.92 (2.08–4.09)	<0.001
Demographic										
Age group										
55–65	29	58,124	0.50	26	14,503	1.79	3.59 (2.12–6.10)	<0.001	4.17 (2.37–7.34)	<0.001
65–75	51	57,578	0.89	26	14,321	1.82	2.06 (1.28–3.30)	0.003	2.06 (1.27–3.37)	0.004
75–85	13	17,247	0.75	9	4254	2.12	2.79 (1.19–6.53)	0.018	3.65 (1.45–9.18)	0.006
≥85	0	1213	0.00	2	326	6.13	NA	NA	NA	NA
Sex										
Female	52	76,773	0.68	30	19,251	1.56	2.31 (1.47–3.62)	0.001	2.51 (1.56–4.02)	0.001
Male	41	57,389	0.71	33	14,154	2.33	3.27 (2.07–5.18)	<0.001	3.45 (2.11–5.62)	<0.001
Comorbidity										
Hypertension										
No	43	71,997	0.60	25	10,349	2.42	4.07 (2.49–6.67)	<0.001	3.97 (2.36–6.67)	<0.001
Yes	50	62,164	0.80	38	23,055	1.65	2.05 (1.35–3.14)	0.001	2.40 (1.55–3.70)	<0.001
Hyperlipidemia										
No	79	108,192	0.73	47	24,076	1.95	2.67 (1.86–3.84)	<0.001	2.84 (1.94–4.16)	<0.001
Yes	14	25,970	0.54	16	9328	1.72	3.22 (1.57–6.59)	0.001	3.18 (1.51–6.69)	0.002
CAD										
No	65	110,205	0.59	41	20,028	2.05	3.48 (2.35–5.14)	<0.001	3.84 (2.59–5.77)	<0.001
Yes	28	23,957	1.17	22	13,376	1.64	1.42 (0.81–2.48)	0.217	1.71 (0.96–3.02)	0.067

Table 4. *Cont.*

Variable	Non-DR Group			DR Group			HR (95% CI)	*p*-Value	aHR (95% CI)	*p*-Value
	Event	PYs	Rate	Event	PYs	Rate				
Stroke										
No	88	120,519	0.73	57	23,436	2.43	3.35 (2.40–4.67)	<0.001	3.07 (2.17–4.36)	<0.001
Yes	5	13,642	0.37	6	9969	0.60	1.65 (0.50–5.41)	0.409	1.44 (0.43–4.87)	0.557
COPD										
No	55	95,300	0.58	38	20,842	1.82	3.17 (2.10–4.79)	<0.001	3.63 (2.33–5.67)	<0.001
Yes	38	38,861	0.98	25	12,562	1.99	2.04 (1.23–3.39)	0.006	2.23 (1.32–3.75)	0.003
Liver cirrhosis and chronic hepatitis										
No	75	119,043	0.63	53	27,608	1.92	3.06 (2.15–4.35)	<0.001	3.18 (2.19–4.62)	<0.001
Yes	18	15,118	1.19	10	5796	1.73	1.46 (0.67–3.15)	0.341	1.86 (0.84–4.15)	0.127

Model adjusted for age, sex, low income, hypertension, hyperlipidemia, CAD, stroke, COPD, and liver cirrhosis and chronic hepatitis. Abbreviations: DR: diabetic retinopathy; AMD: age-related macular degeneration; CAD: coronary artery disease; COPD: chronic obstructive pulmonary disease; PYs: person years; rate: incidence rate per 10,000 person years; HR: hazard ratio; aHR: adjusted hazard ratio; NA: not applicable.

A notably higher incidence rate of exudative AMD was observed in the DR group (1.37 per 10,000 person years) compared to the non-DR group (0.31 per 10,000 person years). The incidence rates of exudative AMD increased with age in both groups. However, the DR group exhibited significantly higher rates than non-DR over all age groups, especially in the 55–65 and 65–75 age groups. Males in the DR group had a higher incidence rate of exudative AMD compared to females in the same group. After adjusting for confounding factors, the aHRs of exudative AMD remained significantly higher in the DR group, and the risks were influenced by the presence of cardiovascular comorbid conditions, such as hypertension, hyperlipidemia, and CAD (Table 5). Table 6 presents types of age-related macular degeneration derived from ICD-9-CM Volume 2 Index entries containing backreferences to 362.50. Figures 2–5 illustrate the higher cumulative risk of all types of macular degeneration, senile (unspecified) AMD, non-exudative AMD, and exudative AMD in the DR group compared to that of the non-DR group.

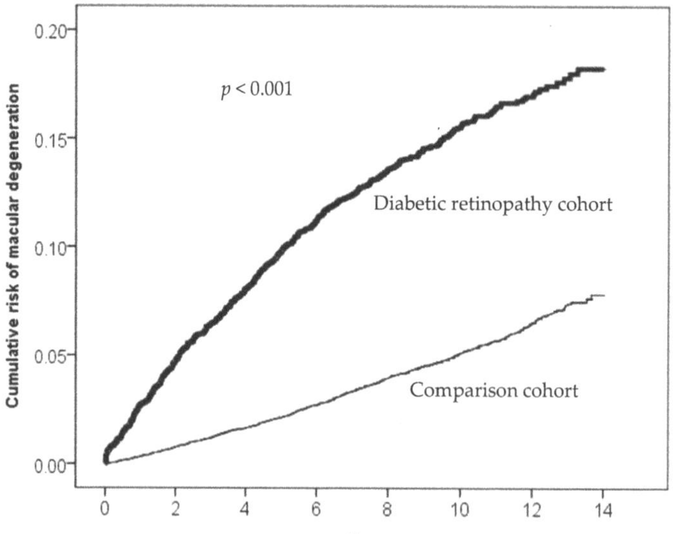

Figure 2. Cumulative risk of all types of AMD (age-related macular degeneration) (ICD-9 code 362.50, 362.51, and 362.52) in the DR group and the non-DR group.

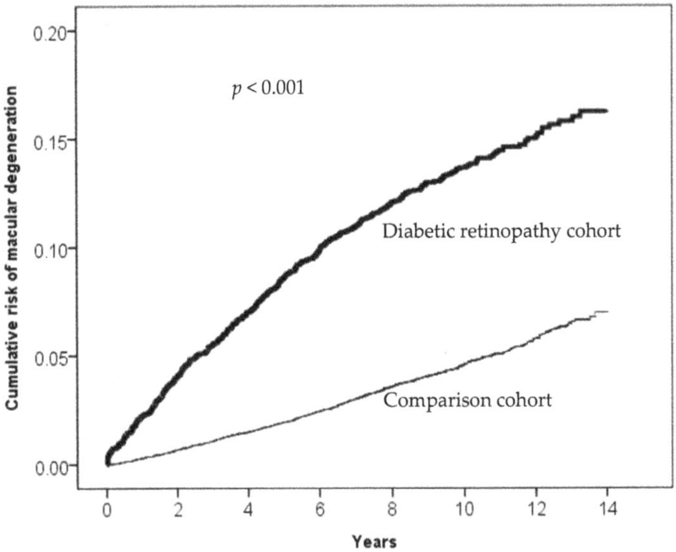

Figure 3. Cumulative risk of senile (unspecified) age-related macular degeneration (ICD-9 code 362.50) in the diabetic retinopathy cohort and the comparison cohort.

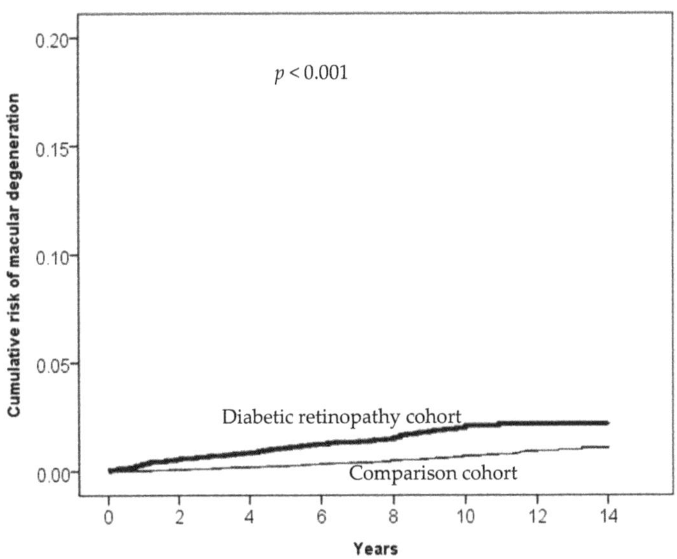

Figure 4. Cumulative risk of non-exudative age-related macular degeneration (ICD-9 code 362.51) in the diabetic retinopathy cohort and the comparison cohort.

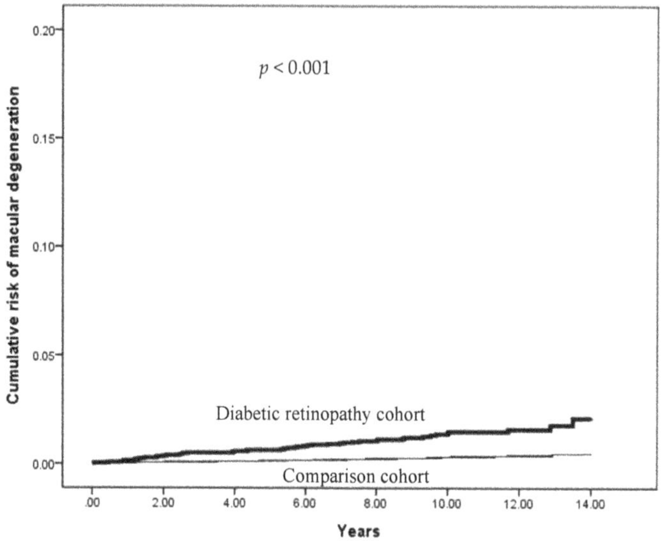

Figure 5. Cumulative risk of exudative age-related macular degeneration (ICD-9 code 362.52) in the diabetic retinopathy cohort and the comparison cohort.

Table 5. Incidence and estimated hazard ratios of exudative age-related macular degeneration (AMD) (ICD-9 code 362.52).

Variable	Non-DR Group			DR Group			HR (95% CI)	*p*-Value	aHR (95% CI)	*p*-Value
	Event	PYs	Rate	Event	PYs	Rate				
DR	42	134,395	0.31	46	33,545	1.37	4.38 (2.88–6.66)	<0.001	3.92 (2.51–6.14)	<0.001
Demographic										
Age group										
55–65	13	58,166	0.22	15	14,571	1.03	4.65 (2.21–9.78)	<0.001	4.20 (1.88–9.38)	0.001
65–75	22	57,716	0.38	24	14,371	1.67	4.33 (2.43–7.73)	<0.001	3.63 (1.97–6.71)	<0.001
75–85	7	17,300	0.40	7	4265	1.64	4.01 (1.41–11.45)	0.009	3.98 (1.32–12.02)	0.014
≥85	0	1213	0.00	0	338	0.00	NA	NA	NA	NA
Sex										
Female	21	76,917	0.27	20	19,315	1.04	3.83 (2.08–7.07)	<0.001	3.16 (1.65–6.07)	0.001
Male	21	57,478	0.37	26	14,230	1.83	4.98 (2.80–8.86)	<0.001	4.72 (2.55–8.74)	<0.001
Comorbidity										
Hypertension										
No	17	72,052	0.24	12	10,407	1.15	4.87 (2.33–10.21)	<0.001	4.67 (2.14–10.16)	0.001
Yes	25	62,343	0.40	34	23,138	1.47	3.66 (2.18–6.14)	<0.001	3.57 (2.09–6.10)	<0.001
Hyperlipidemia										
No	36	108,329	0.33	34	24,200	1.40	4.19 (2.62–6.70)	<0.001	3.77 (2.29–6.23)	<0.001
Yes	6	26,066	0.23	12	9345	1.28	5.68 (2.13–15.15)	0.001	4.66 (1.68–12.95)	0.003
CAD										
No	28	110,368	0.25	21	20,137	1.04	4.14 (2.35–7.28)	<0.001	4.11 (2.28–7.42)	<0.001
Yes	14	24,027	0.58	25	13,408	1.86	3.17 (1.65–6.11)	0.001	3.46 (1.78–6.75)	0.001
Stroke										
No	37	120,695	0.31	36	23,607	1.52	4.95 (3.13–7.84)	<0.001	4.19 (2.59–6.79)	<0.001
Yes	5	13,700	0.36	10	9938	1.01	2.78 (0.95–8.12)	0.062	2.71 (0.90–8.18)	0.077
COPD										
No	25	95,498	0.26	33	20,902	1.58	6.04 (3.59–10.15)	<0.001	4.64 (2.64–8.14)	<0.001
Yes	17	38,897	0.44	13	12,643	1.03	2.33 (1.13–4.80)	0.022	2.67 (1.27–5.64)	0.011
Liver cirrhosis and chronic hepatitis										
No	40	119,194	0.34	38	27,690	1.37	4.07 (2.61–6.34)	<0.001	3.41 (2.12–5.48)	<0.001
Yes	2	15,200	0.13	8	5856	1.37	10.53 (2.24–49.60)	0.003	12.02 (2.47–58.45)	0.002

Model adjusted for age, sex, low income, hypertension, hyperlipidemia, CAD, stroke, COPD, and liver cirrhosis and chronic hepatitis. Abbreviations: DR: diabetic retinopathy; AMD: age-related macular degeneration; CAD: coronary artery disease; COPD: chronic obstructive pulmonary disease; PYs: person years; rate: incidence rate per 10,000 person years; HR: hazard ratio; aHR: adjusted hazard ratio; NA: not applicable.

Table 6. ICD-9-CM Volume 2 Index entries containing backreference to 362.50; degeneration and degenerative.

Macula (Senile) (Unspecified) 362.50.
- non-exudative 362.51
- exudative 362.52
- atrophic 362.51
- best's 362.76
- congenital 362.75
- cystic 362.54
- cystoid 362.53
- disciform 362.52
- dry 362.51
- familial pseudoinflammatory 362.77
- hereditary 362.76
- hole 362.54
- juvenile 362.75
- pseudohole 362.54
- wet 362.52

4. Discussion

This population-based cohort study explored the risks of age-related macular degeneration (AMD) in senile (unspecified), exudative, and non-exudative forms in elderly patients with diabetic retinopathy (DR). The initial assessment of baseline characteristics, including age and gender, showed similar distributions between the DR and non-DR groups, as detailed in Table 1. This eliminates the potential impact of these variables on our findings. However, a notably higher prevalence of comorbidities, such as hypertension, hyperlipidemia, and coronary artery disease (CAD), was observed in patients with DR. These findings are in line with previous research underscoring the multifaceted nature of diabetes, with its extensive impact on various vascular diseases [20]. These vascular comorbidities are known to contribute to damage in retinal small vessel endothelial cells, thereby influencing the development and severity of DR, and might also have an impact on the development of AMD [21,22].

Our study revealed that DR patients have a significantly increased incidence of AMD, even after accounting for other variables. This higher incidence might be attributed to the chronic inflammation associated with DR, which leads to an increased expression of vascular endothelial growth factor (VEGF), a key factor in the development of AMD [23]. Consistent with previous studies, our research indicates that age is a significant risk factor for AMD, particularly in individuals older than 85, possibly due to hormonal variations, genetic predispositions, or other unknown factors [24–26]. Accordingly, we observed a higher occurrence of senile (unspecified) AMD in the DR group compared to the non-DR group, as shown in Table 3. The risk of AMD increases with age and is higher in men, regardless of DR status. Comorbid conditions, such as hypertension, hyperlipidemia, and CAD, further increase the risks of AMD. It appears that a complex interaction between DR and other systemic diseases influences the risk of AMD [27]. Overall, the data emphasize the need for regular eye examinations for AMD in individuals with DR.

Furthermore, individuals with DR were found to have a significantly higher likelihood of developing both non-exudative and exudative AMD compared to those without DR, as presented in Tables 4 and 5. Age and the male gender were identified as risk factors in both groups. The pathogenesis of exudative AMD often involves significant vascular components, which could be exacerbated by the presence of DR [28]. Although comorbidities like hypertension, hyperlipidemia, and CAD typically heighten the risks for AMD, their relative impact is less pronounced within the DR patient group. This suggests that DR-related pathophysiological changes might play a more dominant role in AMD development than individual systemic conditions. Chronic inflammation, oxidative stress, and impaired vascular function in DR are responsible for structural changes in the retinal pigment epithelium (RPE), which, in turn, increases the risk of AMD [29,30]. Pathways such as VEGF expression [31], impaired lipoprotein metabolism [32], and mitochondrial dysfunction [33] are common in the development of both DR and AMD. Our study highlights the importance of regular AMD monitoring and assessment among DR patients, irrespective of comorbid conditions.

The strength of our study lies in its comprehensive evaluation of demographic and comorbidity factors. This study included a large population sample size and examined various demographic variables, such as age and sex, as well as several comorbidities, including hypertension, hyperlipidemia, CAD, stroke, COPD, and liver cirrhosis and chronic hepatitis. Adjusting for these variables in the analysis not only enhances the robustness of the findings but also strengthens the evidence of the positive association between DR and AMD risk.

However, as our study is a retrospective data analysis, it is subject to inherent biases and limitations, including potential selection bias and the inability to establish causality. On the other hand, most Ophthalmologists cited senile (unspecified) AMD, which includes non-exudative AMD and exudative AMD, which results in large differences in patient numbers among different types of AMD. This inconsistency of citation by Ophthalmologists might result in a large difference in number among different types of AMD. Additionally, the study findings have been limited by the specified population and are not generalizable to other populations.

In conclusion, our study revealed a multifaceted relationship between DR and AMD. DR patients are more likely to have vascular conditions, which can contribute to the onset of all types of AMD. Here, we firstly provided the relation between DR and AMD, regardless of comorbid conditions, andsuggested that the inherent pathologies related to DR might have a greater impact on the progression to AMD than comorbid conditions. This is in contrast to the non-DR cohort, where a clearer correlation between comorbidities and the risk of AMD is observed. However, our study diverges in its emphasis on the heightened risk of non-exudative AMD in DR patients, a less explored aspect in previous studies. This discrepancy underscores the complexity of its association and the imperative for continued exploration in this field. Nevertheless, this study highlights the critical need for regular ocular monitoring in individuals with DR, with a particular focus on detecting AMD. Healthcare providers should maintain a heightened awareness of the increased risk of AMD in the DR population and emphasize the need for proactive and preventive eye care measures.

Author Contributions: Conceptualization, H.-T.L., C.-M.Z. and J.-T.C.; Methodology, H.-T.L. and C.-M.Z.; Formal analysis, C.-H.T.; Investigation, H.-T.L.; Resources, C.-L.C., Y.-C.C. (Yu-Ching Chou), J.-Q.Z., Y.-F.L., C.-W.L. and Y.-C.C. (Yo-Chang Chen); Data curation, H.-T.L. and C.-H.T.; Writing—original draft, H.-T.L., C.-M.Z. and C.-H.T.; Writing—review & editing, C.-L.C., C.-A.S. and J.-T.C.; Supervision, C.-A.S. and J.-T.C. All authors have read and agreed to the published version of the manuscript.

Funding: This research received no external funding.

Institutional Review Board Statement: The present study has been approved by the Institutional Review Board of Fu-Jen Catholic University (FJU-IRB No. C104014).

Informed Consent Statement: Patient consent was waived as this study was a retrospective cohort study conducted using the Taiwan National Health Insurance Database (NHIRD).

Data Availability Statement: Not applicable.

Conflicts of Interest: The authors declare no competing interests.

References

1. Donath, M.Y.; Shoelson, S.E. Type 2 diabetes as an inflammatory disease. *Nat. Rev. Immunol.* **2011**, *11*, 98–107. [CrossRef] [PubMed]
2. Pickup, J.C. Inflammation and activated innate immunity in the pathogenesis of type 2 diabetes. *Diabetes Care* **2004**, *27*, 813–823. [CrossRef]
3. Adamis, A.P.; Miller, J.W.; Bernal, M.T.; D'Amico, D.J.; Folkman, J.; Yeo, T.K.; Yeo, K.T. Increased vascular endothelial growth factor levels in the vitreous of eyes with proliferative diabetic retinopathy. *Am. J. Ophthalmol.* **1994**, *118*, 445–450. [CrossRef] [PubMed]
4. Kauppinen, A.; Paterno, J.J.; Blasiak, J.; Salminen, A.; Kaarniranta, K. Inflammation and its role in age-related macular degeneration. *Cell Mol. Life Sci.* **2016**, *73*, 1765–1786. [CrossRef] [PubMed]
5. Al-Kharashi, A.S. Role of oxidative stress, inflammation, hypoxia and angiogenesis in the development of diabetic retinopathy. *Saudi J. Ophthalmol.* **2018**, *32*, 318–323. [CrossRef] [PubMed]
6. Hollyfield, J.G.; Bonilha, V.L.; Rayborn, M.E.; Yang, X.; Shadrach, K.G.; Lu, L.; Ufret, R.L.; Salomon, R.G.; Perez, V.L. Oxidative damage-induced inflammation initiates age-related macular degeneration. *Nat. Med.* **2008**, *14*, 194–198. [CrossRef]
7. Kim, S.-Y.; Kim, Y.; Oh, Y. Inflammatory pathways in pathological neovascularization in retina and choroid: A narrative review on the inflammatory drug target molecules in retinal and choroidal neovascularization. *Ann. Eye Sci.* **2021**, *6*, 24. [CrossRef]
8. Ma, Q.; Shen, J.H.; Shen, S.R.; Das, U.N. Bioactive lipids in pathological retinopathy. *Crit. Rev. Food Sci. Nutr.* **2014**, *54*, 1–16. [CrossRef]
9. Elmasry, K.; Ibrahim, A.S.; Abdulmoneim, S.; Al-Shabrawey, M. Bioactive lipids and pathological retinal angiogenesis. *Br. J. Pharmacol.* **2019**, *176*, 93–109. [CrossRef]
10. Tombran-Tink, J.; Chader, G.G.; Johnson, L.V. PEDF: A pigment epithelium-derived factor with potent neuronal differentiative activity. *Exp. Eye Res.* **1991**, *53*, 411–414. [CrossRef]
11. Notari, L.; Miller, A.; Martinez, A.; Amaral, J.; Ju, M.; Robinson, G.; Smith, L.E.; Becerra, S.P. Pigment epithelium-derived factor is a substrate for matrix metalloproteinase type 2 and type 9: Implications for downregulation in hypoxia. *Investig. Ophthalmol. Vis. Sci.* **2005**, *46*, 2736–2747. [CrossRef] [PubMed]
12. Emerson, M.V.; Lauer, A.K. Emerging therapies for the treatment of neovascular age-related macular degeneration and diabetic macular edema. *BioDrugs* **2007**, *21*, 245–257. [CrossRef] [PubMed]
13. Rajappa, M.; Saxena, P.; Kaur, J. Ocular angiogenesis: Mechanisms and recent advances in therapy. *Adv. Clin. Chem.* **2010**, *50*, 103–121. [PubMed]
14. Mitchell, P.; Wang, J.J. Diabetes, fasting blood glucose and age-related maculopathy: The Blue Mountains Eye Study. *Aust. N. Z. J. Ophthalmol.* **1999**, *27*, 197–199. [CrossRef]
15. Clemons, T.E.; Milton, R.C.; Klein, R.; Seddon, J.M.; Ferris, F.L., 3rd; Age-Related Eye Disease Study Research, G. Risk factors for the incidence of Advanced Age-Related Macular Degeneration in the Age-Related Eye Disease Study (AREDS) AREDS report no. 19. *Ophthalmology* **2005**, *112*, 533–539. [CrossRef]
16. Hyman, L.; Schachat, A.P.; He, Q.; Leske, M.C. Hypertension, cardiovascular disease, and age-related macular degeneration. Age-Related Macular Degeneration Risk Factors Study Group. *Arch. Ophthalmol.* **2000**, *118*, 351–358. [CrossRef]
17. Risk factors for neovascular age-related macular degeneration. The Eye Disease Case-Control Study Group. *Arch. Ophthalmol.* **1992**, *110*, 1701–1708. [CrossRef]
18. Choi, J.K.; Lym, Y.L.; Moon, J.W.; Shin, H.J.; Cho, B. Diabetes mellitus and early age-related macular degeneration. *Arch. Ophthalmol.* **2011**, *129*, 196–199. [CrossRef] [PubMed]
19. Topouzis, F.; Anastasopoulos, E.; Augood, C.; Bentham, G.C.; Chakravarthy, U.; de Jong, P.T.; Rahu, M.; Seland, J.; Soubrane, G.; Tomazzoli, L.; et al. Association of diabetes with age-related macular degeneration in the EUREYE study. *Br. J. Ophthalmol.* **2009**, *93*, 1037–1041. [CrossRef] [PubMed]
20. Guo, V.Y.; Cao, B.; Wu, X.; Lee, J.J.W.; Zee, B.C. Prospective Association between Diabetic Retinopathy and Cardiovascular Disease—A Systematic Review and Meta-analysis of Cohort Studies. *J. Stroke Cerebrovasc. Dis.* **2016**, *25*, 1688–1695. [CrossRef] [PubMed]
21. Chase, H.P.; Garg, S.K.; Jackson, W.E.; Thomas, M.A.; Harris, S.; Marshall, G.; Crews, M.J. Blood pressure and retinopathy in type I diabetes. *Ophthalmology* **1990**, *97*, 155–159. [CrossRef]
22. Gillow, J.T.; Gibson, J.M.; Dodson, P.M. Hypertension and diabetic retinopathy—What's the story? *Br. J. Ophthalmol.* **1999**, *83*, 1083–1087. [CrossRef]
23. Penn, J.S.; Madan, A.; Caldwell, R.B.; Bartoli, M.; Caldwell, R.W.; Hartnett, M.E. Vascular endothelial growth factor in eye disease. *Prog. Retin. Eye Res.* **2008**, *27*, 331–371. [CrossRef] [PubMed]
24. Blasiak, J.; Pawlowska, E.; Sobczuk, A.; Szczepanska, J.; Kaarniranta, K. The Aging Stress Response and Its Implication for AMD Pathogenesis. *Int. J. Mol. Sci.* **2020**, *21*, 8840. [CrossRef] [PubMed]
25. Fritsche, L.G.; Loenhardt, T.; Janssen, A.; Fisher, S.A.; Rivera, A.; Keilhauer, C.N.; Weber, B.H. Age-related macular degeneration is associated with an unstable ARMS2 (LOC387715) mRNA. *Nat. Genet.* **2008**, *40*, 892–896. [CrossRef] [PubMed]
26. Shahid, H.; Khan, J.C.; Cipriani, V.; Sepp, T.; Matharu, B.K.; Bunce, C.; Harding, S.P.; Clayton, D.G.; Moore, A.T.; Yates, J.R.; et al. Age-related macular degeneration: The importance of family history as a risk factor. *Br. J. Ophthalmol.* **2012**, *96*, 427–431. [CrossRef] [PubMed]

27. Mehraban Far, P.; Tai, F.; Ogunbameru, A.; Pechlivanoglou, P.; Sander, B.; Wong, D.T.; Brent, M.H.; Felfeli, T. Diagnostic accuracy of teleretinal screening for detection of diabetic retinopathy and age-related macular degeneration: A systematic review and meta-analysis. *BMJ Open Ophthalmol.* **2022**, *7*, e000915. [CrossRef] [PubMed]
28. Wang, X.; Wang, T.; Lam, E.; Alvarez, D.; Sun, Y. Ocular Vascular Diseases: From Retinal Immune Privilege to Inflammation. *Int. J. Mol. Sci.* **2023**, *24*, 12090. [CrossRef] [PubMed]
29. Hein, T.W.; Potts, L.B.; Xu, W.; Yuen, J.Z.; Kuo, L. Temporal development of retinal arteriolar endothelial dysfunction in porcine type 1 diabetes. *Investig. Ophthalmol. Vis. Sci.* **2012**, *53*, 7943–7949. [CrossRef]
30. Haas, P.; Kubista, K.E.; Krugluger, W.; Huber, J.; Binder, S. Impact of visceral fat and pro-inflammatory factors on the pathogenesis of age-related macular degeneration. *Acta Ophthalmol.* **2015**, *93*, 533–538. [CrossRef]
31. Ho, A.C.; Scott, I.U.; Kim, S.J.; Brown, G.C.; Brown, M.M.; Ip, M.S.; Recchia, F.M. Anti-vascular endothelial growth factor pharmacotherapy for diabetic macular edema: A report by the American Academy of Ophthalmology. *Ophthalmology* **2012**, *119*, 2179–2188. [CrossRef] [PubMed]
32. Sasongko, M.B.; Wong, T.Y.; Nguyen, T.T.; Kawasaki, R.; Jenkins, A.J.; Shaw, J.; Robinson, C.; Wang, J.J. Serum apolipoproteins are associated with systemic and retinal microvascular function in people with diabetes. *Diabetes* **2012**, *61*, 1785–1792. [CrossRef] [PubMed]
33. Sorriento, D.; Pascale, A.V.; Finelli, R.; Carillo, A.L.; Annunziata, R.; Trimarco, B.; Iaccarino, G. Targeting mitochondria as therapeutic strategy for metabolic disorders. *Sci. World J.* **2014**, *2014*, 604685. [CrossRef] [PubMed]

biomedicines

MDPI

Article

Beneficial Effect of Sirolimus-Pretreated Mesenchymal Stem Cell Implantation on Diabetic Retinopathy in Rats

Nanyoung Kang [1], Ji Seung Jung [1], Jiyi Hwang [1], Sang-Eun Park [1], Myeongjee Kwon [1], Haerin Yoon [1], Jungyeon Yong [1], Heung-Myong Woo [2] and Kyung-Mee Park [1,*]

1 Laboratory of Veterinary Ophthalmology, College of Veterinary Medicine, Chungbuk National University, Cheongju 28644, Republic of Korea; rkdsksdud1@gmail.com (N.K.); wjdwltmd00@gmail.com (J.S.J.); wldml1013@gmail.com (J.H.); sangeunpark1992@gmail.com (S.-E.P.); k3clover@naver.com (M.K.); yun3038@naver.com (H.Y.); gold5181@naver.com (J.Y.)

2 Laboratory of Veterinary Surgery, College of Veterinary Medicine, Kangwon National University, Chuncheon 24341, Republic of Korea; woohm@kangwon.ac.kr

* Correspondence: parkkm@cbnu.ac.kr

Abstract: Background: Diabetic retinopathy (DR) is a vision-threatening complication that affects virtually all diabetic patients. Various treatments have been attempted, but they have many side effects and limitations. Alternatively, stem cell therapy is being actively researched, but it faces challenges due to a low cell survival rate. In this study, stem cells were pretreated with sirolimus, which is known to promote cell differentiation and enhance the survival rate. Additionally, the subconjunctival route was employed to reduce complications following intravitreal injections. Methods: Diabetes mellitus was induced by intraperitoneal injection of 55 mg/kg of streptozotocin (STZ), and DR was confirmed at 10 weeks after DM induction through electroretinogram (ERG). The rats were divided into four groups: intact control group (INT), diabetic retinopathy group (DR), DR group with subconjunctival MSC injection (DR-MSC), and DR group with subconjunctival sirolimus-pretreated MSC injection (DR-MSC-S). The effects of transplantation were evaluated using ERG and histological examinations. Results: The ERG results showed that the DR-MSC-S group did not significantly differ from the INT in b-wave amplitude and exhibited significantly higher values than the DR-MSC and DR groups ($p < 0.01$). The flicker amplitude results showed that the DR-MSC and DR-MSC-S groups had significantly higher values than the DR group ($p < 0.01$). Histological examination revealed that the retinal layers were thinner in the DR-induced groups compared to the INT group, with the DR-MSC-S group showing the thickest retinal layers among them. Conclusions: Subconjunctival injection of sirolimus-pretreated MSCs can enhance retinal function and mitigate histological changes in the STZ-induced DR rat model.

Keywords: diabetic retinopathy; sirolimus; mesenchymal stem cells; subconjunctival injection

1. Introduction

Diabetes mellitus (DM) is the most common endocrine disease in humans. As reported by the International Diabetes Federation in 2021, approximately 537 million adults (ages 20–79) have diabetes, constituting about 10.5% of the total global adult population. The prevalence of DM is continuously rising, with projections exceeding 780 million cases by 2045 [1]. DM leads to microvascular abnormalities, resulting in extensive damage to systemic tissues, including the eyes. Diabetic retinopathy (DR), a chronic microvascular complication of DM, impairs vision and affects nearly all patients with DM. Approximately 2% of all individuals with DM experience blindness due to DR, making it the leading cause of vision loss in adults over the age of 25 [2,3].

There are various methods to create a DM model, among which the administration of streptozotocin (STZ) is a commonly used approach. STZ induces the destruction of pancreatic β cells and is widely used experimentally to create a type 1 diabetes model [4,5].

STZ-induced DR typically develops after prolonged exposure to hyperglycemia levels above 150 mg/dL [6].

Exposure to DM conditions leads to various biochemical and metabolic abnormalities, including changes in the redox state of pyridine nucleotides, the accumulation of sorbitol, over-activation of protein kinase C, oxidative stress due to excessive free radical production, and alterations in hemodynamics. These pathogenic mechanisms play a crucial role in the progression of DR. Additionally, within weeks of the onset of diabetes, leukostasis occurs in the retinal capillaries, leading to capillary occlusion and local ischemia [7]. Retinal hypoxia results in the increased expression of vascular endothelial growth factor (VEGF) [8]. Elevated levels of VEGF induce angiogenesis and enhance retinal vessel permeability, causing disruption of the barrier between the retina and blood [8,9].

Current treatments for DR include retinal photocoagulation using lasers and intravitreal injections of anti-VEGF agents. However, due to its destructive nature, laser photocoagulation can result in permanent damage to retinal cells [10,11]. Anti-VEGF therapy has shown superior results in reducing vision loss and improving the rate of vision recovery compared to laser monotherapy. However, its effects are short-lived, necessitating continuous follow-up observation and injection therapy [10,12–14]. Additionally, cases of non-responsiveness to this therapy also occasionally occur. These methods target only vascular pathology, hence highlighting the need for the development of new treatments with different mechanisms [15,16].

Mesenchymal stem cells (MSCs) have the ability to differentiate into various cell lineages, thereby promoting tissue regeneration and enhancing function [17]. Furthermore, through paracrine effects, they can secrete immunomodulatory, anti-angiogenic, and neurotrophic factors [18]. They also support mitochondrial function, which is crucial in restoring retinal cell functionality [19]. Additionally, MSCs inhibit the secretion of pro-inflammatory cytokines and reduce oxidative damage [20]. Numerous studies have shown MSCs to be effective in treating retinal diseases, demonstrating their ability to prevent retinal capillary dropout, loss of ganglion cells, oxidative damage, and neovascularization [16,21,22].

However, the application of stem cells alone faces a significant challenge due to their low survival and adhesion rates [19]. This issue is particularly pronounced in hyperglycemic conditions, where an excessive accumulation of reactive oxygen species (ROS) can alter the regenerative abilities of MSCs, leading to decreased survival rates and reduced efficacy [23].

Therefore, there are attempts to enhance the success rate of stem cell therapies through pre-conditioning/treatment of the cells [24]. One such approach involves subjecting the stem cells to be transplanted to conditions similar to the harsh microenvironment of damaged tissues, such as hypoxia, thereby improving the cells' resistance to the stress of the host environment [25,26]. Another method involves pretreatment with drugs; there are already studies that have enhanced the efficacy of stem cells by pretreating them with tacrolimus, dexamethasone, and sirolimus [19,27–29].

Sirolimus, also known as rapamycin, was initially isolated from the bacterium *Streptomyces hygroscopicus* [30]. This drug functions by inhibiting the mammalian target of rapamycin, a key regulator of cell growth, proliferation, survival, protein synthesis, and autophagy [31,32]. Studies have shown that sirolimus enhances autophagy, regulates energy metabolism, reduces oxygen consumption, and ROS production and thereby promotes stem cell differentiation, increasing cell migration and survival rates [27,28].

Thus, the aim of this study is to investigate the therapeutic effects of sirolimus-pretreated MSC transplantation in the treatment of the STZ-induced DR rat model.

2. Materials and Methods

2.1. Animals

The research conducted was approved by the Institutional Animal Care and Use Committee (IACUC) at Chungbuk National University (Approval No. CBNUA-2032-

22-01), in accordance with the Association for Research in Vision and Ophthalmology statement for the Use of Animals in Ophthalmic and Vision Research.

Twenty-five male Sprague-Dawley rats, aged 8 weeks, were obtained from Nara Biotech (Pyeongtaek, Republic of Korea). They were housed in a conventional environment with a standard 12 h light/12 h dark cycle. The rats had free access to normal pellet chow (Experimental Rat & Mouse Diet, Purina, St. Louis, MO, USA) and water.

2.2. Measurements of Body Weight (BW) and Blood Glucose (BG)

All BW and BG measurements were conducted after a 6-h fasting period. The initial dataset was collected just before the diabetes induction. The second and third datasets were measured at 3 weeks and 10 weeks post-diabetes induction, respectively. The final measurements were taken at week 17 post-diabetes induction.

2.3. Diabetes Induction

DM was induced in the rats after an 8-h fasting period. This was achieved through an intraperitoneal injection of STZ (Sigma-Aldrich, St. Louis, MO, USA) in citrate buffer (pH 4.5) (Sigma-Aldrich) at a dose of 55 mg/kg. The intact control group (INT, eight rats, sixteen eyes) received an equivalent volume of citrate buffer via intraperitoneal injection [33].

DM was confirmed twenty-three days post-STZ injection when the BG exceeded 250 mg/dL, as measured by a commercial blood glucose meter (FORA G11, ForaCare, Moorpark, CA, USA). The seventeen diabetic rats were randomly divided into three groups: the diabetic retinopathy group (DR, seven rats, fourteen eyes); the DR group with subconjunctival MSC injection (DR-MSC, four rats, eight eyes); and the DR group with subconjunctival sirolimus-pretreated MSC injection (DR-MSC-S, six rats, twelve eyes).

2.4. Preparations and Injections of MSCs

Human umbilical cord blood-derived mesenchymal stem cells (hUCB-MSCs) were obtained from Kang Stem Biotech (Seoul, Republic of Korea). These cells were cultured using a KSB-3 Complete Medium® Kit (Kang Stem Biotech) with 10% fetal bovine serum (Thermo Fisher Scientific Inc., Waltham, MA, USA) in a humidified atmosphere containing 5% CO_2 at 37 °C. For the DR-MSC-S group, 100 nM of sirolimus dissolved in dimethyl sulfoxide (DMSO) (Sigma-Aldrich) was pretreated in the culture media for 24 h [19,34]. The same amount of DMSO, without sirolimus, was added to the culture media for the same duration for the DR-MSC group.

After 10 weeks of DM induction, subconjunctival MSC injections (1×10^5 MSCs in 10 μL phosphate-buffered saline; PBS) and sirolimus-pretreated MSC injections were performed using a 31G insulin syringe (Ultra-Fine II short needle, BD Biosciences, Franklin Lakes, NJ, USA). General anesthesia was induced by isoflurane (Terrell, Piramal Critical Care, Bethlehem, PA, USA) and topical anesthesia was induced by proparacaine (Alcaine, Alcon, Geneva, Switzerland). Then, disinfection of the surface of the globe was performed using 0.5% povidone iodine. In the INT and DR groups, 10 μL of PBS was injected using the same protocol. These injections were repeated twice, with an eight-day interval between administrations.

2.5. Electroretinography (ERG)

Ten weeks post-STZ injection, all the rats underwent 6 h of dark adaptation. ERG evaluations were then conducted after pupil dilation using topical 0.01% tropicamide and phenylephrine (Mydrin-P, Santen, Osaka, Japan). Flash and flicker stimuli (8.0 cd·s/m^2 at 2 Hz and 28.3 Hz, respectively) were utilized with the RETevet ERG system (LKC, Gaithersburg, MD, USA). The examination aimed to identify the presence of DR. Subsequent ERG assessments were performed fourteen weeks post-STZ injection to evaluate retinal function using the same protocol.

2.6. Histological Evaluation

Eighteen weeks post-STZ injection, three rats from each group were sacrificed, and their eyes were immediately removed and immersed in BioFix HD (BioGnost, Zagreb, Croatia). The eyes were bisected along the optic nerve, creating two equal halves, and the lenses and vitreous were removed. Following routine tissue processing, the eyes were then embedded in paraffin. The paraffin-embedded sections were stained using routine hematoxylin and eosin (H&E) staining. The thickness of the retinal tissue was measured at a magnification ×200.

2.7. Statistical Analysis

The data were analyzed using Prism 10 software (GraphPad Software, Boston, MA, USA). The results are presented as the mean ± standard deviation. Statistical significance between the groups was determined using an ordinary one-way analysis of variance. p values less than 0.01 were considered statistically significant.

3. Results

3.1. Assessment of BW and BG

The final measurements were taken at week 17 post-diabetes induction. A comparison of the BW and BG data was conducted across the INT, DR, DR-MSC, and DR-MSC-S groups. The averages of the BW for the INT, DR, DR-MSC, and DR-MSC-S groups were 589.50 ± 36.75 g, 234.20 ± 36.68 g, 262.50 ± 22.05 g, and 231.00 ± 26.76 g, respectively (Figure 1A). The averages of the BG were 98.75 ± 11.62 mg/dL, 540.70 ± 134.70 mg/dL, 429.50 ± 48.00 mg/dL, and 534.50 ± 102.70 mg/dL, respectively (Figure 1B). Prior to STZ administration, there were no significant differences in the BW and BG among the groups. However, post-diabetes induction by STZ, the INT group showed a significantly higher BW and a lower BG compared to the diabetic groups. No significant differences in the BW and BG were observed among the DR, DR-MSC, and DR-MSC-S groups at week 17. This suggests that subconjunctival administration of MSCs and sirolimus-pretreated MSCs did not demonstrate systemic therapeutic effects in DM.

3.2. Confirmation of DR with ERG

To confirm the induction of DR prior to the subconjunctival injections of the substance, ERG assessments were conducted at 10 weeks post-diabetes induction. The average flash b-wave amplitude in the INT group and the diabetes-induced groups was 153.2 ± 56.59 μV and 73.84 ± 21.25 μV, respectively (Figure 2A). The average flicker amplitude in the INT group and the diabetes-induced groups was 118.59 ± 32.29 μV and 66.41 ± 24.28 μV, respectively (Figure 2B). Both results were significantly lower in the diabetes-induced groups compared to the INT group ($p < 0.01$), confirming the induction of DR.

3.3. Retinal Function Evaluation with ERG

ERG measurements were repeated at 14 weeks post-diabetes induction, two weeks after the final substance administration, to evaluate changes in retinal function. The average flicker amplitudes in the INT, DR, DR-MSC, and DR-MSC-S groups were 147.00 ± 28.62 μV, 48.28 ± 17.03 μV, 88.27 ± 23.91 μV, and 107.30 ± 23.01 μV, respectively (Figure 3A). The DR-MSC group showed significantly higher values compared to the DR group ($p < 0.01$). The DR-MSC-S group demonstrated significantly higher values than both the DR and DR-MSC groups ($p < 0.01$), with no statistical difference from the INT group.

The average flash b-wave amplitudes in the INT, DR, DR-MSC, and DR-MSC-S groups were 173.30 ± 46.19 μV, 60.21 ± 22.31 μV, 89.53 ± 18.46 μV, and 148.50 ± 17.32 μV, respectively (Figure 3B). The DR-MSC-S group exhibited significantly higher values than both the DR and DR-MSC groups ($p < 0.01$).

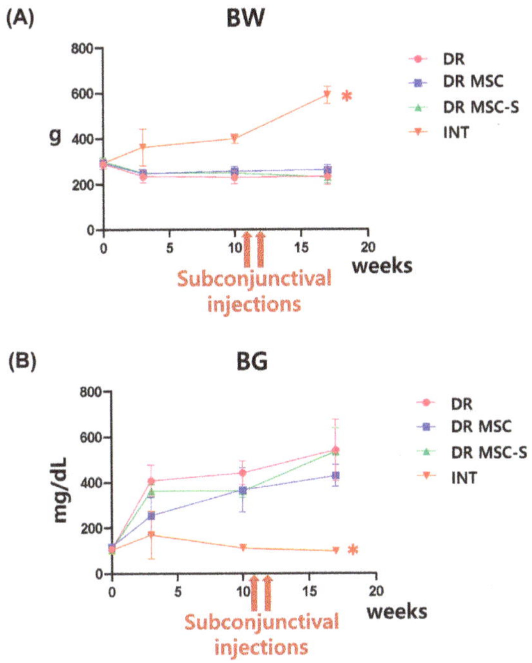

Figure 1. Changes in BW and BG over time. (**A**) A graph for BW changes over time (**B**) A graph for BG changes over time; subconjunctival administration was conducted at 11 and 12 weeks post-diabetes induction. There were no significant differences in BW and BG among the DR, DR-MSC, and DR-MSC-S groups at week 17. The INT group exhibited significantly higher BW and lower BG at all time points. * $p < 0.01$, INT, n = 8 rats; DR, n = 7 rats; DR-MSC, n = 4 rats; DR-MSC-S, n = 6 rats. Abbreviations: BW, body weight; BG, blood glucose; INT, intact control group; DR, diabetic retinopathy group; DR-MSC, DR group with subconjunctival MSC injection; DR-MSC-S, DR group with subconjunctival sirolimus-pretreated MSC injection.

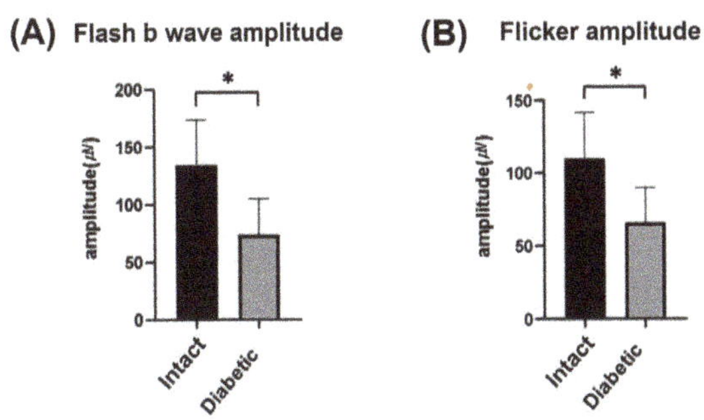

Figure 2. Comparison of electroretinogram results between intact and diabetic groups at week 10 post-diabetes induction. (**A**) Results of flash b-wave amplitude and (**B**) Results of flicker amplitude at 10 weeks post-diabetes induction; the diabetic group showed significantly lower values compared to the intact group, indicating the induction of diabetic retinopathy. * $p < 0.01$, Intact, n = 8 rats, 16 eyes; Diabetic, n = 17 rats, 34 eyes.

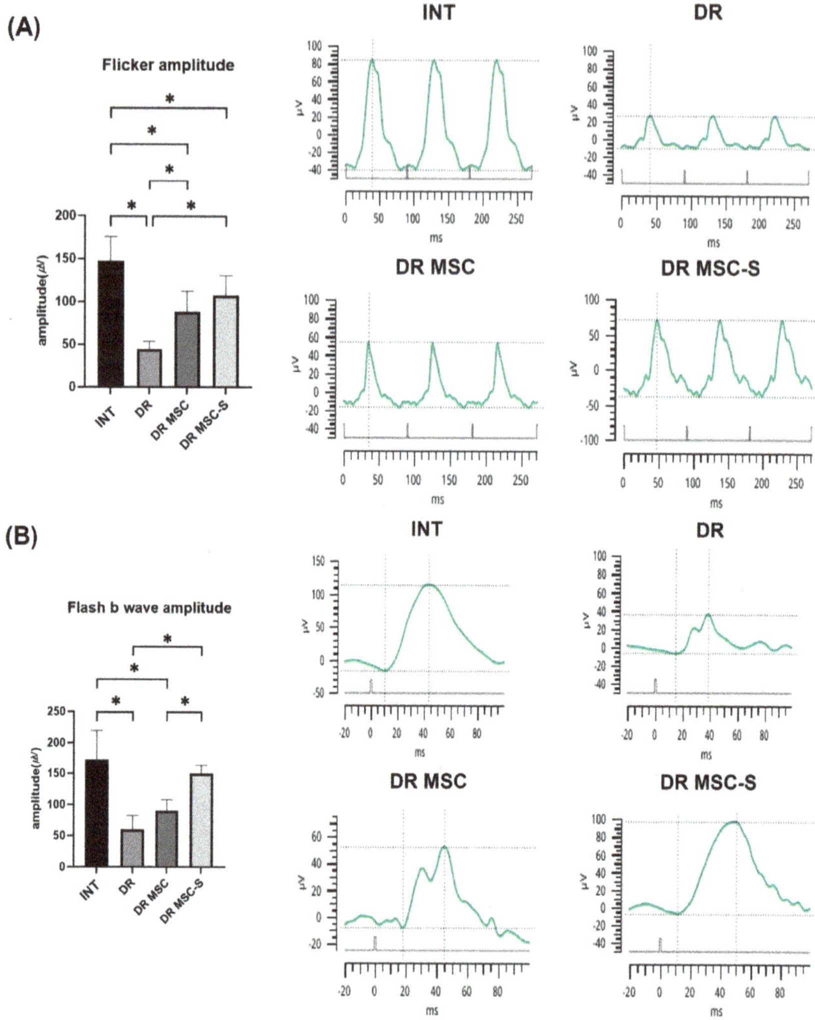

Figure 3. Comparative analysis of flicker and flash b-wave amplitudes in ERG across groups. (**A**) Flicker stimulus ERG results at 14 weeks post-diabetes induction; the DR-MSC and DR-MSC-S groups exhibited significantly greater amplitude than the DR group. (**B**) Flash stimulus ERG results at 14 weeks post-diabetes induction; the DR-MSC-S group showed significantly greater amplitude than both the DR and DR-MSC groups and did not differ statistically from the INT group. * $p < 0.01$. INT, n = 8 rats, 16 eyes; DR, n = 7 rats, 14 eyes; DR-MSC, n = 4 rats, 8 eyes; DR-MSC-S, n = 6 rats, 12 eyes. Abbreviations: ERG, electroretinogram; INT, intact control group; DR, diabetic retinopathy group; DR-MSC, DR group with subconjunctival MSC injection; DR-MSC-S, DR group with subconjunctival sirolimus-pretreated MSC injection.

3.4. Histological Evaluation of the Retina

Histological evaluation was conducted 7 weeks after the initial subconjunctival injections, which was 18 weeks post-diabetes induction. All the retinas were examined using H&E staining (Figure 4A). The total retinal thicknesses for the INT, DR, DR-MSC, and DR-MSC-S groups were 237.20 ± 13.71 μm, 179.60 ± 16.18 μm, 191.80 ± 18.78 μm, and 215.90 ± 12.04 μm, respectively. A decrease in the total retinal thickness was observed in the diabetic groups compared to the INT group. The DR-MSC-S group exhibited a significantly greater retinal thickness compared to the DR and DR-MSC groups ($p < 0.01$).

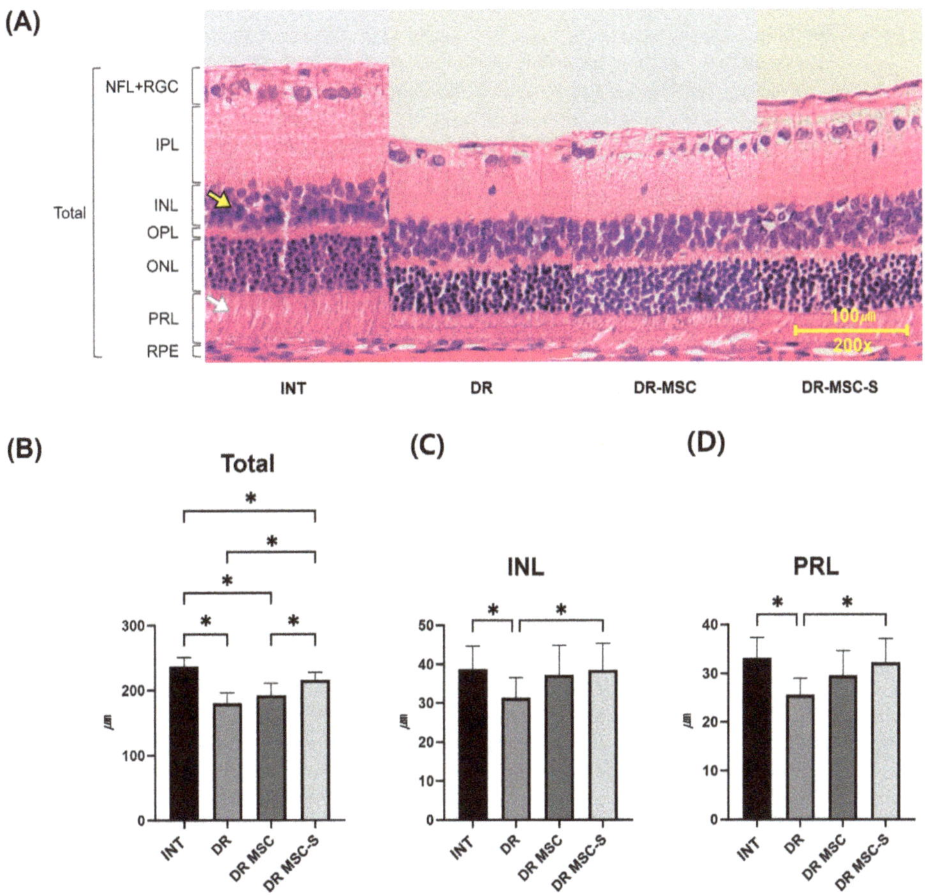

Figure 4. Comparison of histological evaluations of retina using H&E staining. (**A**) Total retinal layer of each group 7 weeks after the initial subconjunctival injections, which was 18 weeks post-diabetes induction (**B**) Results of total retinal thickness measuring; the DR-MSC-S had a significantly thicker retina compared to DR and DR-MSC groups. (**C**) Results of INL (yellow arrow) thickness measuring. The DR had the thinnest inner nuclear layer that showed significant difference with INT and DR-MSC-S. There were no statistical differences between INT, DR-MSC, and DR-MSC-S. (**D**) Results of PRL (white arrow) thickness measuring. The DR had the thinnest PRL that showed significant difference with INT and DR-MSC-S. There were no statistical differences between INT, DR-MSC, and DR-MSC-S. H&E staining, magnification ×200. * $p < 0.01$. INT, n = 8 rats, 16 eyes; DR, n = 7 rats, 14 eyes; DR-MSC, n = 4 rats, 8 eyes; DR-MSC-S, n = 6 rats, 12 eyes. Abbreviations: H&E, hematoxylin and eosin; NFL, nerve fiber layer; RGC, retinal ganglion cell layer; IPL, inner plexiform layer; INL, inner nuclear layer; OPL, outer plexiform layer; ONL, outer nuclear layer; PRL, photoreceptor layer; INT, intact control group; DR, diabetic retinopathy group; DR-MSC, DR group with subconjunctival MSC injection; DR-MSC-S, DR group with subconjunctival sirolimus-pretreated MSC injection.

The thickness of the inner nuclear layer (INL) for the INT, DR, DR-MSC, and DR-MSC-S groups was 38.70 ± 5.93 μm, 31.21 ± 5.30 μm, 37.17 ± 7.64 μm, and 38.45 ± 6.84 μm, respectively (Figure 4C). The thickness of the photoreceptor layer (PRL) for the INT, DR,

DR-MSC, and DR-MSC-S groups was 33.13 ± 4.19 μm, 25.43 ± 3.56 μm, 29.5 ± 5.13 μm, and 32.17 ± 4.93 μm, respectively (Figure 4D). Both layer thicknesses were significantly greater in the INT and DR-MSC-S groups compared to the DR group ($p < 0.01$).

4. Discussion

This study has demonstrated that subconjunctival injection of sirolimus-pretreated MSCs can increase the b-wave amplitude and flicker amplitude in ERG recordings from rats with DR while histologically mitigating the thinning of the retinal layers. These findings suggest that subconjunctival injections of sirolimus-pretreated MSCs may be therapeutically effective for DR.

Previous research indicates that DR develops three months after the intraperitoneal injection of STZ in rats, accompanied by thinning of the retinal layers and an increase in neovascularization [35,36]. In this study, a significant reduction in the ERG amplitude compared to the INT group was observed 10 weeks post-STZ injection, indicating the occurrence of DR, which was further supported by histological assessments showing reduced thickness of the total retinal layer.

Patients with DR are known to experience significant decreases in retinal function compared to their pre-disease state [37]. According to various studies measuring ERG in diabetic rats, the DR-induced groups exhibited a significantly reduced b-wave compared to the normal control [38–41]. Furthermore, flicker ERG recorded at a frequency of 30 Hz is reduced in amplitude in patients with moderate to severe DR [42]. Consistent with these findings, this study demonstrated a substantial decrease in both b-wave and flicker ERG amplitude in the DR-induced groups compared to the INT group. Nevertheless, an improvement in both amplitudes was observed in the DR-MSC-S group compared to the DR group, suggesting that sirolimus-pretreated MSCs may improve the retinal function of DR rats.

Histological changes in DR include thinning of the retinal layers, loss of retinal cells, formation of neovascularization, and increased inflammation [43,44]. Additionally, reductions in the thickness of the ganglion cell layer, INL, and PRL have been observed [45–48]. These changes suggest neurodegeneration and an increase in inflammatory and neurodegenerative markers has been reported in rats with DM induced by STZ [43]. Consistent with previous research, this study also observed a decrease in the total retinal thickness in the diabetic groups. However, the overall retinal thickness was greater in the DR-MSC-S group than in the DR and DR-MSC groups, and the thicknesses of the INL and PRL were also greater in the DR-MSC-S group compared to the DR group. These results indicate that subconjunctival injection of sirolimus-pretreated MSCs can mitigate histopathological changes in the retina.

A challenge in treating diabetic patients with MSCs is the reduced survival rate of MSCs in a hyperglycemic environment. Research has shown that MSCs cultured in serum from type 2 diabetic patients exhibit significantly decreased cell survival [49]. Various studies indicate that hyperglycemic conditions can lead to an increase in mitochondrial glucose metabolism, which through mitochondrial hyperpolarization induces the production of ROS [50–52]. Additionally, a chronic hyperglycemic environment can lead to the upregulation and activation of cyclooxygenase, which may increase not only oxidative stress but also inflammatory responses [53,54]. Excessive accumulation of ROS leads to mitochondrial damage, cell apoptosis, inflammation, and lipid peroxidation [55]. Consequently, persistently high glucose concentrations alter the potential regenerative capacity of MSCs and ultimately reduce their survival rate, lowering the success rate of treatment [19]. In this study, the DR-MSC group did not show significant differences from the DR group in the flash b-wave amplitude or histological evaluations, which could be attributed to the low survival rate of MSCs in a hyperglycemic environment.

In this study, the pretreating of stem cells with sirolimus, a technique already proven effective in several studies, was used. In mice, sirolimus has been shown to enhance autologous regeneration and hematopoiesis in hematopoietic stem cells [32]. Treatment with sirolimus-pretreated MSCs in a systemic lupus erythematosus mouse model alleviated clinical symptoms and extended survival, also enhancing the immunomodulatory function of MSCs [26]. Furthermore, pretreatment with sirolimus significantly increased autophagy activity and lysosome production in cells and reduced cell apoptosis under harsh conditions compared to untreated cells. The post-transplantation of sirolimus-pretreated cells markedly improved the repair and functional recovery in infarcted myocardium [56]. Additionally, numerous studies have used sirolimus via direct intraocular injection for retinal treatment, confirming its intraocular stability [57–60]. However, the concentration of sirolimus used in this study was significantly lower than that shown to be effective in previous research, suggesting a lower likelihood of direct effects from sirolimus.

Sirolimus can modulate inflammatory responses related to the generation of ROS and nitric oxide in cells [61]. Sirolimus-pretreated MSCs have shown increased survival or growth factor secretion in hypoxic and serum-deprivation conditions, increased production of survival or growth factors post-transplantation, and suppressed production of inflammatory cytokines [28]. These actions may account for the significantly higher results obtained by the DR-MSC-S group in the ERG and histological evaluations compared to the DR and DR-MSC groups.

Moreover, this study adopted the subconjunctival route instead of the commonly used intravitreal injection for DR treatment. Intravitreal injection has the advantage of delivering drugs directly to the vitreous and retina, but the technique is invasive with risks of increased intraocular pressure, infection, inflammation, potential damage to the lens, retinal toxicity, and detachment [62,63]. However, subconjunctival injection is less invasive and carries a lower risk of complications associated with intravitreal injections, making repeated administration feasible. Subconjunctival injections are generally thought to primarily deliver drugs to the anterior segment of the eye, but there are studies showing that effective drug delivery to the vitreous and retinal/vitreous layers is also possible [64,65]. Administering drugs or placing implants in the subconjunctival space can skip the barriers of the conjunctiva and cornea, resulting in enhanced permeability in the retina/choroidal region [63]. Nevertheless, subconjunctival injection results in a lower drug concentration reaching the posterior segment compared to intravitreal injection. There is a study showing that administering MSCs at weekly intervals is more effective in inhibiting disease progression than a single administration [66]. This study adopted a method of repeated administrations at 8-day intervals for a total of two times to enhance the therapeutic efficacy. Consequently, this study found subconjunctival injection to be effective in treating DR, with minimal systemic impact on the BW or BG.

In this study, the effectiveness of sirolimus-pretreated MSCs was evaluated, focusing on the functional improvement of the retina as measured by ERG and the histological assessment of retinal layer thickness. However, the evaluation was confined to a maximum duration of 7 weeks, indicating the necessity for further research into the long-term effects. Another limitation of this study is the absence of a comparative analysis between different concentrations of pretreated sirolimus as well as a lack of comparison between single and repeated administrations.

5. Conclusions

In conclusion, this study has demonstrated that DR rats treated with sirolimus-pretreated MSCs exhibit an increase in ERG amplitude. Additionally, there was a mitigation in the reduction of the retinal thickness at a histological level. These results suggest that sirolimus-pretreated MSCs can enhance retinal function and mitigate histological changes in rats with DR, indicating their potential for application in DR treatment. They also suggest that the subconjunctival route of administration can be effective for the treatment of retinopathy.

Author Contributions: Conceptualization and design, N.K. and K.-M.P.; investigation, N.K., J.S.J., J.H., S.-E.P., M.K., H.Y. and J.Y.; data curation, N.K.; writing—original draft preparation: N.K.; writing—review and editing, N.K., H.-M.W. and K.-M.P.; supervision, project administration, and funding acquisition, K.-M.P. All authors have read and agreed to the published version of the manuscript.

Funding: This study was supported by the "Regional Innovation Strategy (RIS)" through the National Research Foundation of Korea (NRF) funded by the Ministry of Education (MOE) (2021 RIS-001). This work was also supported by the Basic Research Lab Program (2022R1A4A1025557) funded by the Ministry of Science and ICT and the Korean Fund for Regenerative Medicine (KFRM) grant (the Ministry of Science and ICT, the Ministry of Health and Welfare) No. 22A0101L1-11. This work was also supported by the Korea Institute of Planning and Evaluation for Technology in Food, Agriculture, and Forestry (IPET) through the High Value-added Food Technology Development Program, funded by the Ministry of Agriculture, Food, and Rural Affairs (MAFRA) (321027-5).

Institutional Review Board Statement: The study conducted was approved by the Institutional Animal Care and Use Committee (IACUC) at Chungbuk National University (Approval No. CBNUA-2032-22-01) in accordance with the Association for Research in Vision and Ophthalmology statement for the Use of Animals in Ophthalmic and Vision Research.

Informed Consent Statement: Not applicable.

Data Availability Statement: The datasets analyzed during the current study are available from the corresponding author upon reasonable request.

Conflicts of Interest: The authors declare no conflicts of interest. The funders had no role in the design of the study; in the collection, analyses, or interpretation of the data; in the writing of the manuscript; or in the decision to publish the results.

List of Abbreviations

BG	Blood glucose
BW	Body weight
DM	Diabetes mellitus
DMSO	Dimethyl sulfoxide
DR	Diabetic retinopathy
DR-MSC	Diabetic retinopathy group with subconjunctival mesenchymal stem cell injection
DR-MSC-S	Diabetic retinopathy group with subconjunctival sirolimus-pretreated mesenchymal stem cell injection
ERG	Electroretinogram
H&E	Hematoxylin and eosin
hUCB-MSCs	Human umbilical cord blood-derived mesenchymal stem cells
INL	Inner nuclear layer
INT	Intact control group
IPL	Inner plexiform layer
MSCs	Mesenchymal stem cells
NFL	Nerve fiber layer
ONL	Outer nuclear layer
OPL	Outer plexiform layer
PBS	Phosphate-buffered saline
PRL	Photoreceptor layer
RGC	Retinal ganglion cell layer
ROS	Reactive oxygen species
STZ	Streptozotocin
VEGF	Vascular endothelial growth factor

References

1. Sun, H.; Saeedi, P.; Karuranga, S.; Pinkepank, M.; Ogurtsova, K.; Duncan, B.B.; Stein, C.; Basit, A.; Chan, J.C.N.; Mbanya, J.C.; et al. IDF Diabetes Atlas: Global, Regional and Country-Level Diabetes Prevalence Estimates for 2021 and Projections for 2045. *Diabetes Res. Clin. Pract.* **2022**, *183*, 109119. [CrossRef]
2. Barchetta, I.; Riccieri, V.; Vasile, M.; Stefanantoni, K.; Comberiati, P.; Taverniti, L.; Cavallo, M.G. High Prevalence of Capillary Abnormalities in Patients with Diabetes and Association with Retinopathy. *Diabet. Med.* **2011**, *28*, 1039–1044. [CrossRef]

3. Hammes, H.-P.; Feng, Y.; Pfister, F.; Brownlee, M. Diabetic Retinopathy: Targeting Vasoregression. *Diabetes* **2011**, *60*, 9–16. [CrossRef]
4. Rakieten, N.; Rakieten, M.L.; Nadkarni, M.V. Studies on the Diabetogenic Action of Streptozotocin (NSC-37917). *Cancer Chemother. Rep.* **1963**, *29*, 91–98. [PubMed]
5. Kolb-Bachofen, V.; Epstein, S.; Kiesel, U.; Kolb, H. Low-Dose Streptozocin-Induced Diabetes in Mice: Electron Microscopy Reveals Single-Cell Insulitis Before Diabetes Onset. *Diabetes* **1988**, *37*, 21–27. [CrossRef]
6. Quiroz, J.; Yazdanyar, A. Animal Models of Diabetic Retinopathy. *Ann. Transl. Med.* **2017**, *93*, 1272. [CrossRef]
7. Curtis, T.M.; Gardiner, T.A.; Stitt, A.W. Microvascular Lesions of Diabetic Retinopathy: Clues towards Understanding Pathogenesis? *Eye* **2009**, *23*, 1496–1508. [CrossRef] [PubMed]
8. Pande, G.S.; Tidake, P. Laser Treatment Modalities for Diabetic Retinopathy. *Cureus* **2022**, *14*, e30024. [CrossRef] [PubMed]
9. Kollias, A.N.; Ulbig, M.W. Diabetic Retinopathy. *Dtsch. Ärzteblatt Int.* **2010**, *107*, 75–83. [CrossRef]
10. Duh, E.J.; Sun, J.K.; Stitt, A.W. Diabetic Retinopathy: Current Understanding, Mechanisms, and Treatment Strategies. *JCI Insight* **2017**, *2*, e93751. [CrossRef]
11. Gupta, N.; Mansoor, S.; Sharma, A.; Sapkal, A.; Sheth, J.; Falatoonzadeh, P.; Kuppermann, B.D.; Kenney, M.C. Diabetic Retinopathy and VEGF. *Open Ophthalmol. J.* **2013**, *7*, 4–10. [CrossRef] [PubMed]
12. Elman, M.J.; Aiello, L.P.; Beck, R.W.; Bressler, N.M.; Bressler, S.B.; Edwards, A.R.; Ferris, F.L.; Friedman, S.M.; Glassman, A.R.; Miller, K.M.; et al. Randomized Trial Evaluating Ranibizumab Plus Prompt or Deferred Laser or Triamcinolone Plus Prompt Laser for Diabetic Macular Edema. *Ophthalmology* **2010**, *117*, 1064–1077. [CrossRef] [PubMed]
13. Brown, D.M.; Nguyen, Q.D.; Marcus, D.M.; Boyer, D.S.; Patel, S.; Feiner, L.; Schlottmann, P.G.; Rundle, A.C.; Zhang, J.; Rubio, R.G.; et al. Long-Term Outcomes of Ranibizumab Therapy for Diabetic Macular Edema: The 36-Month Results from Two Phase III Trials RISE and RIDE. *Ophthalmology* **2013**, *120*, 2013–2022. [CrossRef] [PubMed]
14. Gunasekaran, T., Jr.; Gunasekaran, Y.; Hui, P.T.; Gunasekaran, T. Review of Studies Comparing Panretinal Photocoagulation and Anti-Vascular Endothelial Growth Factor Therapy in the Treatment of Proliferative Diabetic Retinopathy. *Cureus* **2022**, *14*, e22471. [CrossRef] [PubMed]
15. Tremolada, G.; Turco, C.D.; Lattanzio, R.; Maestroni, S.; Maestroni, A.; Bandello, F.; Zerbini, G. The Role of Angiogenesis in the Development of Proliferative Diabetic Retinopathy: Impact of Intravitreal Anti-VEGF Treatment. *Exp. Diabetes Res.* **2012**, *2012*, 728325. [CrossRef] [PubMed]
16. Ezquer, M.; Urzua, C.A.; Montecino, S.; Leal, K.; Conget, P.; Ezquer, F. Intravitreal Administration of Multipotent Mesenchymal Stromal Cells Triggers a Cytoprotective Microenvironment in the Retina of Diabetic Mice. *Stem Cell Res. Ther.* **2016**, *7*, 42. [CrossRef]
17. Bharti, D.; Shivakumar, S.B.; Park, J.-K.; Ullah, I.; Subbarao, R.B.; Park, J.-S.; Lee, S.-L.; Park, B.-W.; Rho, G.-J. Comparative Analysis of Human Wharton's Jelly Mesenchymal Stem Cells Derived from Different Parts of the Same Umbilical Cord. *Cell Tissue Res.* **2018**, *372*, 51–65. [CrossRef]
18. Oh, J.Y.; Kim, M.K.; Shin, M.S.; Lee, H.J.; Ko, J.H.; Wee, W.R.; Lee, J.H. The Anti-Inflammatory and Anti-Angiogenic Role of Mesenchymal Stem Cells in Corneal Wound Healing Following Chemical Injury. *Stem Cells* **2008**, *26*, 1047–1055. [CrossRef]
19. Jo, H.H.; Goh, Y.S.; Kim, H.J.; Kim, D.H.; Kim, H.; Hwang, J.; Jung, J.S.; Kang, N.; Park, S.E.; Park, K.M.; et al. Tacrolimus Improves Therapeutic Efficacy of Umbilical Cord Blood-Derived Mesenchymal Stem Cells in Diabetic Retinopathy by Suppressing DRP1-Mediated Mitochondrial Fission. *Antioxidants* **2023**, *12*, 1727. [CrossRef] [PubMed]
20. Cui, Y.; Xu, N.; Xu, W.; Xu, G. Mesenchymal Stem Cells Attenuate Hydrogen Peroxide-Induced Oxidative Stress and Enhance Neuroprotective Effects in Retinal Ganglion Cells. *In Vitro Cell Dev. Biol. Anim.* **2017**, *53*, 328–335. [CrossRef] [PubMed]
21. Fiori, A.; Terlizzi, V.; Kremer, H.; Gebauer, J.; Hammes, H.-P.; Harmsen, M.C.; Bieback, K. Mesenchymal Stromal/Stem Cells as Potential Therapy in Diabetic Retinopathy. *Immunobiology* **2018**, *223*, 729–743. [CrossRef] [PubMed]
22. Rakoczy, E.P.; Rahman, I.S.A.; Binz, N.; Li, C.-R.; Vagaja, N.N.; de Pinho, M.; Lai, C.-M. Characterization of a Mouse Model of Hyperglycemia and Retinal Neovascularization. *Am. J. Pathol.* **2010**, *177*, 2659–2670. [CrossRef] [PubMed]
23. Kim, J.; Piao, Y.; Pak, Y.K.; Chung, D.; Han, Y.M.; Hong, J.S.; Jun, E.J.; Shim, J.-Y.; Choi, J.; Kim, C.J. Umbilical Cord Mesenchymal Stromal Cells Affected by Gestational Diabetes Mellitus Display Premature Aging and Mitochondrial Dysfunction. *Stem Cells Dev.* **2015**, *24*, 575–586. [CrossRef] [PubMed]
24. Moeinabadi-Bidgoli, K.; Babajani, A.; Yazdanpanah, G.; Farhadihosseinabadi, B.; Jamshidi, E.; Bahrami, S.; Niknejad, H. Translational Insights into Stem Cell Preconditioning: From Molecular Mechanisms to Preclinical Applications. *Biomed. Pharmacother.* **2021**, *142*, 112026. [CrossRef] [PubMed]
25. Lan, Y.-W.; Choo, K.-B.; Chen, C.-M.; Hung, T.-H.; Chen, Y.-B.; Hsieh, C.-H.; Kuo, H.-P.; Chong, K.-Y. Hypoxia-Preconditioned Mesenchymal Stem Cells Attenuate Bleomycin-Induced Pulmonary Fibrosis. *Stem Cell Res. Ther.* **2015**, *6*, 97. [CrossRef] [PubMed]
26. Oses, C.; Olivares, B.; Ezquer, M.; Acosta, C.; Bosch, P.; Donoso, M.; Léniz, P.; Ezquer, F. Preconditioning of Adipose Tissue-Derived Mesenchymal Stem Cells with Deferoxamine Increases the Production of pro-Angiogenic, Neuroprotective and Anti-Inflammatory Factors: Potential Application in the Treatment of Diabetic Neuropathy. *PLoS ONE* **2017**, *12*, e0178011. [CrossRef] [PubMed]
27. Li, C.; Ye, L.; Yang, L.; Yu, X.; He, Y.; Chen, Z.; Li, L.; Zhang, D. Rapamycin Promotes the Survival and Adipogenesis of Ischemia-Challenged Adipose Derived Stem Cells by Improving Autophagy. *Cell Physiol. Biochem.* **2018**, *44*, 1762–1774. [CrossRef]
28. Li, Z.; Wang, Y.; Wang, H.; Wu, J.; Tan, Y. Rapamycin-Preactivated Autophagy Enhances Survival and Differentiation of Mesenchymal Stem Cells After Transplantation into Infarcted Myocardium. *Stem Cell Rev. Rep.* **2020**, *16*, 344–356. [CrossRef]

29. Song, I.; Caplan, A.I.; Dennis, J.E. In Vitro Dexamethasone Pretreatment Enhances Bone Formation of Human Mesenchymal Stem Cells in Vivo. *J. Orthop. Res.* **2009**, *27*, 916–921. [CrossRef]
30. Vézina, C.; Kudelski, A.; Sehgal, S.N. RAPAMYCIN (AY-22, 989), A NEW ANTIFUNGAL ANTIBIOTIC. *J. Antibiot.* **1975**, *28*, 721–726. [CrossRef]
31. Lipton, J.O.; Sahin, M. The Neurology of MTOR. *Neuron* **2014**, *84*, 275–291. [CrossRef] [PubMed]
32. Chen, C.; Liu, Y.; Liu, Y.; Zheng, P. MTOR Regulation and Therapeutic Rejuvenation of Aging Hematopoietic Stem Cells. *Sci. Signal.* **2009**, *2*, ra75. [CrossRef]
33. Kim, H.; Goh, Y.-S.; Park, S.-E.; Hwang, J.; Kang, N.; Jung, J.S.; Kim, Y.-B.; Choi, E.-K.; Park, K.-M. Preventive Effects of Exosome-Rich Conditioned Medium from Amniotic Membrane-Derived Mesenchymal Stem Cells for Diabetic Retinopathy in Rats. *Transl. Vis. Sci. Technol.* **2023**, *12*, 18. [CrossRef]
34. Tanaka, Y.; Sonoda, S.; Yamaza, H.; Murata, S.; Nishida, K.; Hama, S.; Kyumoto-Nakamura, Y.; Uehara, N.; Nonaka, K.; Kukita, T.; et al. Suppression of AKT-MTOR Signal Pathway Enhances Osteogenic/Dentinogenic Capacity of Stem Cells from Apical Papilla. *Stem Cell Res. Ther.* **2018**, *9*, 334. [CrossRef] [PubMed]
35. Naderi, A.; Zahed, R.; Aghajanpour, L.; Amoli, F.A.; Lashay, A. Long Term Features of Diabetic Retinopathy in Streptozotocin-Induced Diabetic Wistar Rats. *Exp. Eye Res.* **2019**, *184*, 213–220. [CrossRef]
36. Gong, C.-Y.; Lu, B.; Hu, Q.-W.; Ji, L.-L. Streptozotocin Induced Diabetic Retinopathy in Rat and the Expression of Vascular Endothelial Growth Factor and Its Receptor. *Int. J. Ophthalmol.* **2013**, *6*, 573–577. [CrossRef]
37. Fenwick, E.K.; Pesudovs, K.; Rees, G.; Dirani, M.; Kawasaki, R.; Wong, T.Y.; Lamoureux, E.L. The Impact of Diabetic Retinopathy: Understanding the Patient's Perspective. *Br. J. Ophthalmol.* **2011**, *95*, 774. [CrossRef] [PubMed]
38. Deguchi, S.; Otake, H.; Nakazawa, Y.; Hiramatsu, N.; Yamamoto, N.; Nagai, N. Ophthalmic Formulation Containing Nilvadipine Nanoparticles Prevents Retinal Dysfunction in Rats Injected with Streptozotocin. *Int. J. Mol. Sci.* **2017**, *18*, 2720. [CrossRef]
39. He, M.; Long, P.; Guo, L.; Zhang, M.; Wang, S.; He, H. Fushiming Capsule Attenuates Diabetic Rat Retina Damage via Antioxidation and Anti-Inflammation. *Evid.-Based Complement. Altern. Med.* **2019**, *2019*, 5376439. [CrossRef]
40. Feng, Y.; Wang, R.; Xu, J.; Sun, J.; Xu, T.; Gu, Q.; Wu, X. Hydrogen-Rich Saline Prevents Early Neurovascular Dysfunction Resulting from Inhibition of Oxidative Stress in STZ-Diabetic Rats. *Curr. Eye Res.* **2013**, *38*, 396–404. [CrossRef]
41. Chang, J.Y.-A.; Yu, F.; Shi, L.; Ko, M.L.; Ko, G.Y.-P. Melatonin Affects Mitochondrial Fission/Fusion Dynamics in the Diabetic Retina. *J. Diabetes Res.* **2019**, *2019*, 8463125. [CrossRef]
42. McAnany, J.J.; Persidina, O.S.; Park, J.C. Clinical Electroretinography in Diabetic Retinopathy: A Review. *Surv. Ophthalmol.* **2022**, *67*, 712–722. [CrossRef]
43. Lelyte, I.; Ahmed, Z.; Kaja, S.; Kalesnykas, G. Structure–Function Relationships in the Rodent Streptozotocin-Induced Model for Diabetic Retinopathy: A Systematic Review. *J. Ocul. Pharmacol. Ther.* **2022**, *38*, 271–286. [CrossRef]
44. Yang, Y.; Mao, D.; Chen, X.; Zhao, L.; Tian, Q.; Liu, C.; Zhou, B.L.S. Decrease in Retinal Neuronal Cells in Streptozotocin-Induced Diabetic Mice. *Mol. Vis.* **2011**, *18*, 1411–1420.
45. Tao, Y.; Geng, L.; Xu, W.-W.; Qin, L.-M.; Peng, G.-H.; Huang, Y.-F. The Potential Utilizations of Hydrogen as a Promising Therapeutic Strategy against Ocular Diseases. *Ther. Clin. Risk Manag.* **2016**, *12*, 799–806. [CrossRef] [PubMed]
46. Zhang, Q.; Xiao, X.; Zheng, J.; Li, M.; Yu, M.; Ping, F.; Wang, T.; Wang, X. Compound Danshen Dripping Pill Inhibits Retina Cell Apoptosis in Diabetic Rats. *Front. Physiol.* **2018**, *9*, 1501. [CrossRef] [PubMed]
47. Liao, Y.-R.; Li, Z.-J.; Zeng, P.; Lan, Y.-Q. TLR7 Deficiency Contributes to Attenuated Diabetic Retinopathy via Inhibition of Inflammatory Response. *Biochem. Biophys. Res. Commun.* **2017**, *493*, 1136–1142. [CrossRef] [PubMed]
48. Ozkaya, A.; Alkin, Z.; Karakucuk, Y.; Karatas, G.; Fazil, K.; Erdogan, M.G.; Perente, I.; Taskapili, M. Thickness of the Retinal Photoreceptor Outer Segment Layer in Healthy Volunteers and in Patients with Diabetes Mellitus without Retinopathy, Diabetic Retinopathy, or Diabetic Macular Edema. *Saudi J. Ophthalmol.* **2017**, *31*, 69–75. [CrossRef] [PubMed]
49. Rezabakhsh, A.; Cheraghi, O.; Nourazarian, A.; Hassanpour, M.; Kazemi, M.; Ghaderi, S.; Faraji, E.; Rahbarghazi, R.; Avci, Ç.B.; Bagca, B.G.; et al. Type 2 Diabetes Inhibited Human Mesenchymal Stem Cells Angiogenic Response by Over-Activity of the Autophagic Pathway. *J. Cell. Biochem.* **2017**, *118*, 1518–1530. [CrossRef] [PubMed]
50. Yu, T.; Robotham, J.L.; Yoon, Y. Increased Production of Reactive Oxygen Species in Hyperglycemic Conditions Requires Dynamic Change of Mitochondrial Morphology. *Proc. Natl. Acad. Sci. USA* **2006**, *103*, 2653–2658. [CrossRef] [PubMed]
51. Brownlee, M. Biochemistry and Molecular Cell Biology of Diabetic Complications. *Nature* **2001**, *414*, 813–820. [CrossRef]
52. Nishikawa, T.; Edelstein, D.; Du, X.L.; Yamagishi, S.; Matsumura, T.; Kaneda, Y.; Yorek, M.A.; Beebe, D.; Oates, P.J.; Hammes, H.-P.; et al. Normalizing Mitochondrial Superoxide Production Blocks Three Pathways of Hyperglycaemic Damage. *Nature* **2000**, *404*, 787–790. [CrossRef] [PubMed]
53. Yaribeygi, H.; Atkin, S.L.; Sahebkar, A. A Review of the Molecular Mechanisms of Hyperglycemia-induced Free Radical Generation Leading to Oxidative Stress. *J. Cell. Physiol.* **2019**, *234*, 1300–1312. [CrossRef] [PubMed]
54. Helmersson, J.; Vessby, B.; Larsson, A.; Basu, S. Association of Type 2 Diabetes with Cyclooxygenase-Mediated Inflammation and Oxidative Stress in an Elderly Population. *Circulation* **2004**, *109*, 1729–1734. [CrossRef]
55. Kang, Q.; Yang, C. Oxidative Stress and Diabetic Retinopathy: Molecular Mechanisms, Pathogenetic Role and Therapeutic Implications. *Redox Biol.* **2020**, *37*, 101799. [CrossRef]

56. Gu, Z.; Tan, W.; Ji, J.; Feng, G.; Meng, Y.; Da, Z.; Guo, G.; Xia, Y.; Zhu, X.; Shi, G.; et al. Rapamycin Reverses the Senescent Phenotype and Improves Immuno-Regulation of Mesenchymal Stem Cells from MRL/Lpr Mice and Systemic Lupus Erythematosus Patients through Inhibition of the MTOR Signaling Pathway. *Aging (Albany NY)* **2016**, *8*, 1102–1114. [CrossRef]
57. Dugel, P.U.; Blumenkranz, M.S.; Haller, J.A.; Williams, G.A.; Solley, W.A.; Kleinman, D.M.; Naor, J. A Randomized, Dose-Escalation Study of Subconjunctival and Intravitreal Injections of Sirolimus in Patients with Diabetic Macular Edema. *Ophthalmology* **2012**, *119*, 124–131. [CrossRef]
58. Krishnadev, N.; Forooghian, F.; Cukras, C.; Wong, W.; Saligan, L.; Chew, E.Y.; Nussenblatt, R.; Ferris, F.; Meyerle, C. Subconjunctival Sirolimus in the Treatment of Diabetic Macular Edema. *Graefe's Arch. Clin. Exp. Ophthalmol.* **2011**, *249*, 1627. [CrossRef] [PubMed]
59. Li, H.; Zhang, Z.; Li, Y.; Su, L.; Duan, Y.; Zhang, H.; An, J.; Ni, T.; Li, X.; Zhang, X. Therapeutic Effect of Rapamycin-Loaded Small Extracellular Vesicles Derived from Mesenchymal Stem Cells on Experimental Autoimmune Uveitis. *Front. Immunol.* **2022**, *13*, 864956. [CrossRef]
60. Suri, R.; Neupane, Y.R.; Mehra, N.; Nematullah, M.; Khan, F.; Alam, O.; Iqubal, A.; Jain, G.K.; Kohli, K. Sirolimus Loaded Chitosan Functionalized Poly (Lactic-Co-Glycolic Acid) (PLGA) Nanoparticles for Potential Treatment of Age-Related Macular Degeneration. *Int. J. Biol. Macromol.* **2021**, *191*, 548–559. [CrossRef]
61. Tuñón, M.J.; Sánchez-Campos, S.; Gutiérrez, B.; Culebras, J.M.; González-Gallego, J. Effects of FK506 and Rapamycin on Generation of Reactive Oxygen Species, Nitric Oxide Production and Nuclear Factor Kappa B Activation in Rat Hepatocytes. *Biochem. Pharmacol.* **2003**, *66*, 439–445. [CrossRef] [PubMed]
62. Barar, J.; Javadzadeh, A.R.; Omidi, Y. Ocular Novel Drug Delivery: Impacts of Membranes and Barriers. *Expert Opin. Drug Deliv.* **2008**, *5*, 567–581. [CrossRef] [PubMed]
63. Kim, H.M.; Woo, S.J. Ocular Drug Delivery to the Retina: Current Innovations and Future Perspectives. *Pharmaceutics* **2021**, *13*, 108. [CrossRef] [PubMed]
64. Ghate, D.; Brooks, W.; McCarey, B.E.; Edelhauser, H.F. Pharmacokinetics of Intraocular Drug Delivery by Periocular Injections Using Ocular Fluorophotometry. *Investig. Opthalmol. Vis. Sci.* **2007**, *48*, 2230. [CrossRef]
65. Lee, T.W.-Y.; Robinson, J.R. Drug Delivery to the Posterior Segment of the Eye: Some Insights on the Penetration Pathways after Subconjunctival Injection. *J. Ocul. Pharmacol. Ther.* **2001**, *17*, 565–572. [CrossRef]
66. Ozeki, N.; Muneta, T.; Koga, H.; Nakagawa, Y.; Mizuno, M.; Tsuji, K.; Mabuchi, Y.; Akazawa, C.; Kobayashi, E.; Matsumoto, K.; et al. Not Single but Periodic Injections of Synovial Mesenchymal Stem Cells Maintain Viable Cells in Knees and Inhibit Osteoarthritis Progression in Rats. *Osteoarthr. Cartil.* **2016**, *24*, 1061–1070. [CrossRef]

biomedicines

MDPI

Article

Diagnostic Accuracy of Hand-Held Fundus Camera and Artificial Intelligence in Diabetic Retinopathy Screening

Martina Tomić [1], Romano Vrabec [1], Đurđica Hendelja [1], Vilma Kolarić [2], Tomislav Bulum [2,3,*] and Dario Rahelić [2,4,5]

1 Department of Ophthalmology, Vuk Vrhovac University Clinic for Diabetes, Endocrinology and Metabolic Diseases, Merkur University Hospital, Dugi dol 4a, 10000 Zagreb, Croatia
2 Department of Diabetes and Endocrinology, Vuk Vrhovac University Clinic for Diabetes, Endocrinology and Metabolic Diseases, Merkur University Hospital, Dugi dol 4a, 10000 Zagreb, Croatia
3 School of Medicine, University of Zagreb, Šalata 3, 10000 Zagreb, Croatia
4 School of Medicine, Catholic University of Croatia, Ilica 242, 10000 Zagreb, Croatia
5 School of Medicine, Josip Juraj Strossmayer University, Josipa Huttlera 4, 31000 Osijek, Croatia
* Correspondence: tomobulum@gmail.com

Abstract: Our study aimed to assess the role of a hand-held fundus camera and artificial intelligence (AI)-based grading system in diabetic retinopathy (DR) screening and determine its diagnostic accuracy in detecting DR compared with clinical examination and a standard fundus camera. This cross-sectional instrument validation study, as a part of the International Diabetes Federation (IDF) Diabetic Retinopathy Screening Project, included 160 patients (320 eyes) with type 2 diabetes (T2DM). After the standard indirect slit-lamp fundoscopy, each patient first underwent fundus photography with a standard 45° camera VISUCAM Zeiss and then with a hand-held camera TANG (Shanghai Zhi Tang Health Technology Co., Ltd.). Two retina specialists independently graded the images taken with the standard camera, while the images taken with the hand-held camera were graded using the DeepDR system and an independent IDF ophthalmologist. The three screening methods did not differ in detecting moderate/severe nonproliferative and proliferative DR. The area under the curve, sensitivity, specificity, positive predictive value, negative predictive value, positive likelihood ratio, negative likelihood ratio, kappa (κ) agreement, diagnostic odds ratio, and diagnostic effectiveness for a hand-held camera compared to clinical examination were 0.921, 89.1%, 100%, 100%, 91.4%, infinity, 0.11, 0.86, 936.48, and 94.9%, while compared to the standard fundus camera were 0.883, 83.2%, 100%, 100%, 87.3%, infinity, 0.17, 0.78, 574.6, and 92.2%. The results of our study suggest that fundus photography with a hand-held camera and AI-based grading system is a short, simple, and accurate method for the screening and early detection of DR, comparable to clinical examination and fundus photography with a standard camera.

Keywords: diabetic retinopathy; screening; slit-lamp fundoscopy; fundus camera; artificial intelligence

1. Introduction

Diabetes is one of the fastest-growing global health emergencies of the 21st century that has reached alarming levels and is projected to affect 783 million people by 2045 [1]. Diabetes is also a significant cause of disability and is still the leading cause of preventable blindness in the adult working population, nontraumatic amputations, and renal failure. Despite the growing awareness of diabetes, its complications continue to represent a significant public health problem with high health expenditure [1]. Diabetic retinopathy (DR) represents a crucial complication of diabetes leading to vision loss and, finally, blindness in the adult working population [2]. About 22% of patients with diabetes have DR, but over 10% have vision-threatening DR (VTDR), including proliferative DR (PDR) and diabetic macular edema (DME) [3]. By 2045, the number of people with DR and VTDR is projected to increase from 103.12 million and 47.37 million in 2020 to 160.50 million and 73.43 million, respectively.

In clinical settings, it is essential to diagnose DR in its early asymptomatic stages and to start on time with adequate therapy, preventing vision loss and blindness. Screening for DR is the best and most cost-effective method to avoid blindness [4,5]. However, screening every person with diabetes for DR with standard ophthalmological examinations is not optimal considering the limited number of ophthalmologists, and represents an inefficient use of resources. The minimum examinations for the screening of DR include a vision examination (before pupil dilation) and a retinal examination adequate for DR classification [6,7]. Several low-cost fundus cameras are widely available, and fundus photography telemedicine has become a good option for DR screening [8–10]. Fundus cameras can be handled by educated nurses or trained photographers taking high-quality retinal images that can further be reviewed for interpretation and DR grading by an ophthalmologist or an entirely artificial intelligence (AI)-based automated system [11]. In real-time, the trained system decides whether a person requires a referral to an ophthalmologist, and it is much cheaper than having ophthalmologists screen each person with diabetes. The first such AI-based automated system for DR identification was approved in April 2018 by the US Food and Drug Administration (FDA) [12], and since then, many other systems have been developed and introduced [13–15].

Recently, fuzzy-based image edge detection algorithms for blood vessel detection in retinal images have also become available [16]. The performance and accuracy of vessel segmentation approaches are based on a combination of image preprocessing techniques, global thresholding, and image postprocessing techniques [17,18]. A framework based on hybrid 2D–3D convolutional neural networks is developed to obtain a continuous 3D automated surface segmentation of the retinal layer, which is essential and challenging in analyzing optical coherence tomography (OCT) [19]. To overcome the lack of precision of these methods preventing medical professionals from completely trusting the results generated, explainable AI has been introduced to help increase the interpretability of the methods [20]. A systematic review investigating the test accuracy of AI-based grading of fundus images in DR screening suggests that AI-based systems are more sensitive than human graders and could be safe to use in clinical practice, but have variable specificity [21].

In July 2019, before the COVID-19 outbreak, the Republic of Croatia was, thanks to Professor Dario Rahelić, president of the Croatian Association for Diabetes and Metabolic Disorders and chair of the International Diabetes Federation (IDF) Young Leaders in Diabetes Programme, included in the IDF Diabetic Retinopathy Screening Project and for this purpose, received a hand-held fundus camera TANG, Shanghai Zhi Tang Health Technology Co., Ltd. (Shanghai China) (Fundoscope ID: EUR-04) (Figure 1) with DR screening software (DeepDR) that used the AI-based automated DR grading system for analyzing the retinal images captured by the camera. This IDF project and a partnership with the Fred Hollows Foundation highlighted the importance of integrating screening for DR ongoing care for people living with diabetes in developing countries worldwide and providing DR screening to all people with diabetes every one to two years [22]. The IDF also encouraged all people with diabetes who have not had their retinas screened in the past two years to speak to a health professional about receiving retinopathy screening as soon as possible.

As a part of the IDF Diabetic Retinopathy Screening Project, this study aimed to assess the role of a hand-held fundus camera and AI-based grading system in DR screening and determine its diagnostic accuracy in detecting DR compared with clinical examination and photography using the standard fundus camera.

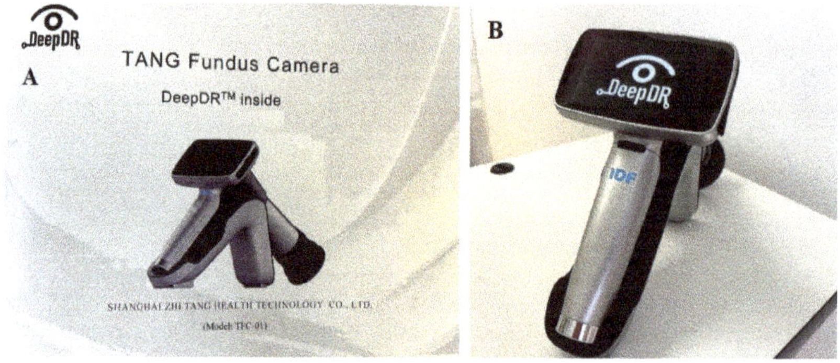

Figure 1. Instruction manual (**A**) and TANG hand-held fundus camera (**B**).

2. Materials and Methods

2.1. Study Design and Patients

This cross-sectional instrument validation study, as a part of the IDF Diabetic Retinopathy Screening Project, was conducted in Vuk Vrhovac University Clinic for Diabetes, Endocrinology and Metabolic Diseases, Merkur University Hospital in Zagreb, Croatia, following the Declaration of Helsinki and approved by the Hospital's Ethics Committee. All study participants received written and oral information about the study and signed the written informed consent.

A total of 160 patients (320 eyes) with type 2 diabetes (T2DM) consecutively referred to the ophthalmology department of the tertiary care specialist diabetes clinic over three months between September 2019 and December 2019 were randomly selected and included in the study by the first author, M.T., during her routine clinical work. At the inclusion visit, after signing the informed consent, the first author obtained a medical history regarding diabetes duration and other eye conditions and diseases. Patients with other posterior eye segment diseases (macular degeneration, the central retinal artery, vein, or branches occlusion) or anterior and posterior eye segment diseases that did not allow fundus visualization and photography (previous ocular trauma, acute infection, ocular surface diseases and irregularities, mature cataract, opacities, and vitreous hemorrhages) and patients with poor cooperation were not included in the study.

2.2. Ophthalmologic Retinal Examination and Fundus Photography

After signing the informed consent and pupil dilation with eye drops containing 0.5% tropicamide, each patient first underwent a standard clinical examination—indirect slit-lamp fundoscopy (Figure 2A)—then fundus photography with a standard 45° fundus camera VISUCAM Zeiss (Carl Zeiss Meditec AG, Goeschwitzer Str. 51-52, 07745 Jena, Germany (Figure 2B), and finally fundus photography with a hand-held fundus camera TANG (Shanghai Zhi Tang Health Technology Co., Ltd.) (Shanghai China) (Figure 2C,D).

A biomicroscopic indirect slit-lamp fundus examination and color fundus photography of two fields (macula-centered, optic disc-centered) of both eyes with a standard VISUCAM Zeiss camera was performed by the first author, M.T. Two-field 45° photographs consisted of the first field image (macula-centered) covering the temporal area and optic disc and the second field image (optic disc-centered) covering the nasal area [23,24]. Two-field photography has the advantage of detecting DR in the nasal retina that single-field photography could otherwise miss. After that, the first, M.T., and the second author, R.V., two medical retina specialists, independently graded the photographs and assigned a DR grade using the proposed international clinical diabetic retinopathy and diabetic macular edema disease severity ratings [25]. Since there was no case where the experts assigned different grades, there was no need for a third grader.

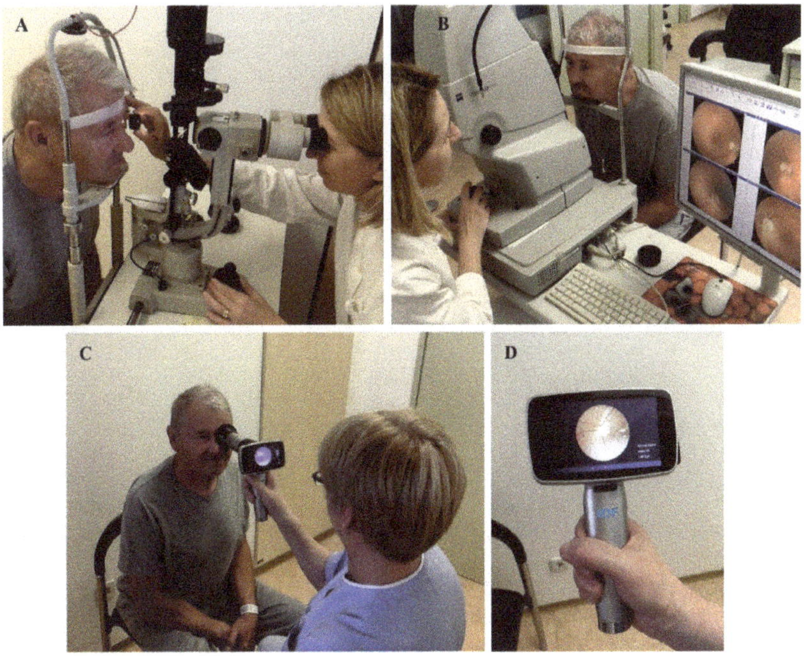

Figure 2. Standard clinical indirect slit-lamp fundus examination (**A**), photography with a standard (**B**) and a hand-held fundus camera (**C**,**D**).

Color fundus photography of two fields (macula-centered, optic disc-centered) of both eyes with a hand-held TANG camera was conducted, according to the IDF Diabetic Retinopathy Screening Project guidelines [26], by the ophthalmology nurse Đ.H. and graded using the AI-based automated software (DeepDR) and an independent IDF ophthalmologist from Brussels, Belgium. Fundus image reports from AI and the IDF ophthalmologist contained an image quality assessment, diagnosis, and advice. If the images were of sufficient quality, there were two possible results: (1) diagnose: no DR or mild nonproliferative DR (NPDR), and advice: regular follow-up; (2) diagnose: moderate/severe NPDR or PDR, and advice: refer to an ophthalmologist.

2.3. Statistical Analysis

Statistical analysis was performed, and the graphs were created using the software package Statistica™ 14.0.1 (TIBCO Software Inc., Palo Alto, CA, USA) and SPSS 23.0. (IBM, Armonk, NY, USA). The Kolmogorov–Smirnov test was used to evaluate the normality of data distribution, and the Leven test was used to evaluate the homogeneity of variance. The results were expressed as numbers or percentages for categorical variables and the mean $\pm$ SD or median (min-max) for continuous variables. For continuous data, the differences between groups were tested using the Kruskal–Wallis and one-way ANOVA tests. Scheffe's post-hoc test was used where needed. For categorical data testing, the Chi-square test was used. A receiver operating characteristic (ROC) curve, the area under the ROC curve (AUC), sensitivity and specificity, predictive values, likelihood ratios, kappa agreement, diagnostic odds ratio, and diagnostic effectiveness (accuracy) were used to assess the ability of the hand-held fundus camera TANG and AI-based grading system in DR screening and determine its diagnostic accuracy in detecting DR compared to clinical examination and photography using the standard fundus camera. To calculate all diagnostic accuracy measures, the examined eyes were divided into two groups: eyes with no retinopathy and those with any retinopathy (mild/moderate/severe NPDR/PDR). A p-value < 0.05 was considered statistically significant in all analyses.

3. Results

This study included 320 eyes of 160 T2DM (89 male/71 female) with a median age of 65 (45–83) years and a median diabetes duration of 14 (2–33) years. Their mean best-corrected visual acuity (BCVA) was 0.98 ± 0.10, and the mean intraocular pressure (IOP) was 15.21 ± 1.01 mmHg. Sixteen (5%) eyes had primary open-angle glaucoma and were regularly treated with local antiglaucoma medications. Thirty-six (11.25%) eyes had a clear crystalline lens, 230 (71.87%) had initial cataract, and 54 (16.88%) eyes were pseudophakic due to previous cataract surgery.

Based on the photography with a hand-held fundus camera, 202 (63.1%) eyes in this study had no DR, 58 (18.1%) had mild or moderate NPDR, and 60 (18.8%) eyes had severe NPDR or PDR. Their basic characteristics are presented in Table 1. The groups did not significantly differ in gender (Chi-square test, p = 0.058), age, and diabetes duration (Kruskal–Wallis test, p = 0.408, p = 0.161) nor in the mean IOP (one-way ANOVA test, p = 0.776), the prevalence of glaucoma, and the status of intraocular lens (Chi-square test, p = 0.612, p = 0.447). The only difference among the examined eyes was observed in BCVA (one-way ANOVA test, p = 0.027). The eyes with no retinopathy had significantly better BCVA than those with severe NPDR or PDR (Scheffe test, p = 0.029).

Table 1. The basic characteristics of 320 examined eyes of 160 T2DM divided into three groups according to the level of diabetic retinopathy.

	No DR	Mild/Moderate NPDR	Severe NPDR/PDR	p-Value
Gender (m/f)	50/50	73/27	80/20	0.058 [a]
Age (yrs.)	65 (48–83)	64(54–77)	62 (45–70)	0.408 [b]
Diabetes duration (yrs.)	12.5 (2–33)	14 (7–24)	15 (2–30)	0.161 [b]
BCVA (decimal)	0.98 ± 0.05	0.98 ± 0.08	0.89 ± 0.27	0.027 [c]
IOP (mmHg)	14.92 ± 2.29	15.27 ± 1.16	15.20 ± 0.68	0.776 [c]
Glaucoma (no/yes)	94/6	100/0	93/7	0.612 [a]
Lens (1/2/3)	16/68/16	7/80/13	0/87/13	0.447 [a]

Legend: Values are percentages, medians (min-max), or means ± SD. [a] indicates Chi-square test, [b] Kruskal–Wallis test, [c] one-way ANOVA test; BCVA best-corrected visual acuity; IOP intraocular pressure; Lens 1—eyes with clear crystalline lens, 2—eyes with initial cataract, 3—pseudophakic eyes.

After evaluation by AI and an IDF ophthalmologist, the images of 248 (77.5%) eyes taken by the hand-held camera were rated as good quality, while images of 72 (22.5%) eyes were of medium quality. Not a single image was considered low-quality or unreadable. Figures 3–5 present the images of the same patients taken by the standard (A) and hand-held fundus camera (B).

When comparing the reports of the hand-held camera with the standard clinical examination and the standard camera in DR degree assessment, there were no differences in detecting severe NPDR and PDR between the three methods (Table 2, Figure 6). However, the most significant discrepancy in DR degree assessment was in the eyes with no DR and those with signs of mild NPDR (single microaneurysms). Out of the 202 eyes with no DR screened by the hand-held camera, the signs of mild NPDR were detected in 22 (6.9%) eyes screened by the standard clinical examination and in 34 (10.6%) eyes by the standard camera.

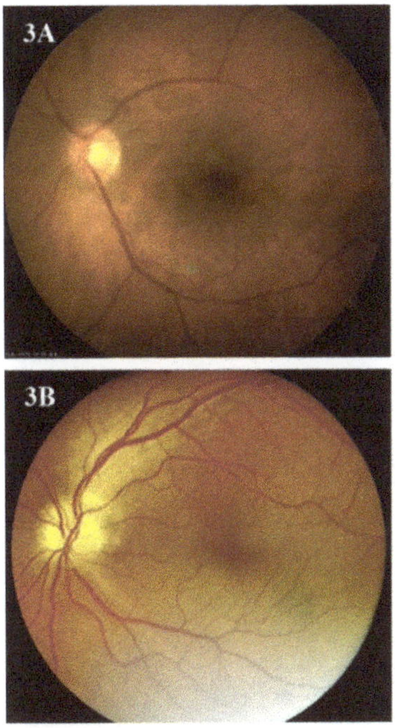

Figure 3. Images of the same patients taken by standard (**A**) and hand-held fundus camera (**B**).

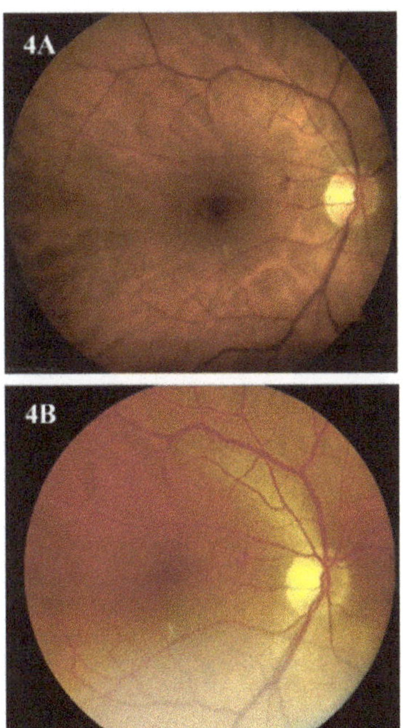

Figure 4. Images of the same patients taken by standard (**A**) and hand-held fundus camera (**B**).

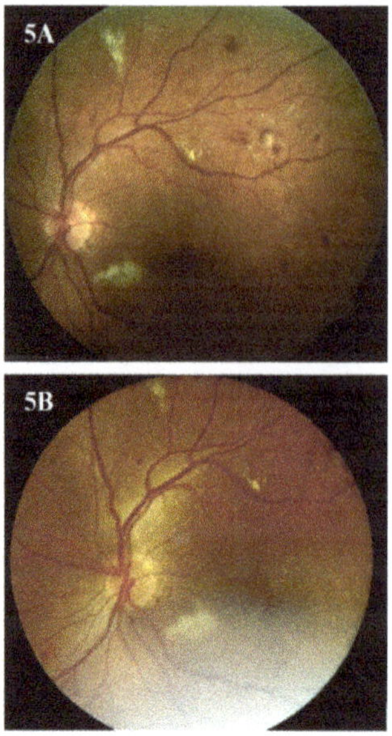

Figure 5. Images of the same patients taken by standard (**A**) and hand-held fundus camera (**B**).

Table 2. Diabetic retinopathy degree assessed by fundus photography with a hand-held fundus camera vs. standard clinical examination and photography with a standard fundus camera.

		Fundus Photography with a Hand-Held Fundus Camera		
		No Retinopathy	**Mild/Moderate NPDR**	**Severe NPDR/PDR**
Standard clinical examination	No retinopathy	180 (56.2)	0 (0)	0 (0)
	Mild/moderate NPDR	22 (6.9)	58 (18.1)	0 (0)
	Severe NPDR/PDR	0 (0)	0 (0)	60 (18.8)
Standard fundus camera	No retinopathy	168 (52.5)	0 (0)	0 (0)
	Mild/moderate NPDR	34 (10.6)	58 (18.1)	0 (0)
	Severe NPDR/PDR	0 (0)	0 (0)	60 (18.8)

N (%). Abbreviations: NPDR, nonproliferative diabetic retinopathy; PDR, proliferative diabetic retinopathy.

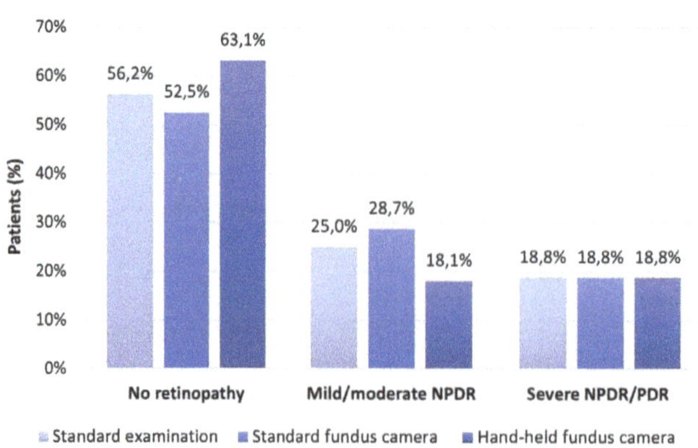

Figure 6. DR degree assessed by standard clinical examination, standard, and hand-held fundus camera.

In contrast to this useful clinical division of examined eyes into three groups, in the statistical calculation of all diagnostic accuracy measures, the examined eyes were divided into two grades: those with no retinopathy and those with any retinopathy (mild/moderate/severe NPDR/PDR). The shape of the ROC curves and the area under the curves (AUC) of 0.921 and 0.883 defined the excellent discriminative power of the hand-held fundus camera in DR detection compared to the standard clinical examination and very good discriminatory power compared to the standard fundus camera (Table 3, Figure 7).

Table 3. The area under the curve for diabetic retinopathy screening by fundus photography with a hand-held fundus camera vs. standard clinical examination and standard fundus camera.

	Fundus Photography with a Hand-Held Fundus Camera			
	Area	**Std. Error**	**95% CI**	***p***
Standard clinical examination	0.921	0.026	0.870–0.973	0.000
Standard fundus camera	0.883	0.030	0.824–0.942	0.000

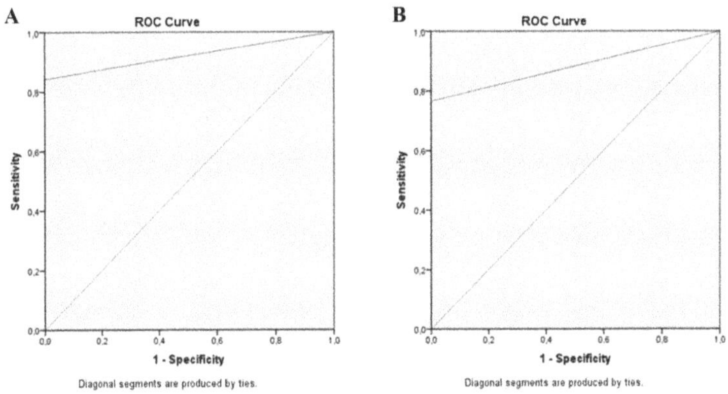

Figure 7. ROC curves of DR screening by photography with a hand-held fundus camera vs. standard clinical examination (**A**) and standard fundus camera (**B**). Blue line: ROC curve; green line: reference line.

Other diagnostic accuracy measures of DR detection by the hand-held camera compared to the standard clinical examination and standard fundus camera are shown in Table 4.

Photography with a hand-held camera had 89.1% and 83.2% sensitivity and 100% specificity in detecting DR compared to the clinical examination and standard camera. A positive predictive value (PPV) of 100% and a positive likelihood ratio (LR+) of infinity indicated absolute agreement between the hand-held camera and the other two methods in positively detecting patients with DR. In comparison, a negative predictive value (NPV) of 91.4% and 87.3% and negative likelihood ratio (LR−) of 0.11 and 0.17 implied almost perfect agreement between the hand-held camera and clinical examination and substantial agreement between the hand-held and standard camera in negatively noticing patients without DR. A kappa (κ) values of 0.86 and 0.78 and diagnostic odds ratio (DOR) values of 936.48 and 574.6 indicated almost perfect and significant agreement among the hand-held camera and clinical examination and the standard camera in detecting DR, presuming the excellent test performance of the hand-held camera. Finally, the diagnostic effectiveness (DE) of 94.9% compared to the clinical examination and 92.2% to the standard camera expressed the almost perfect accuracy of the hand-held camera in correctly classifying subjects (TP + TN) among all subjects.

Table 4. Diagnostic accuracy measures of diabetic retinopathy detection by the hand-held fundus camera vs. standard clinical examination and standard fundus camera.

Hand-Held Fundus Camera vs.	Standard Examination		Standard Fundus Camera	
	Estimate	95% CI	Estimate	95% CI
Sensitivity	89.1%	81.3–94.4%	83.2%	74.4–89.9%
Specificity	100%	93.9–100%	100%	93.9–100%
PPV	100%	95.9–100%	100%	95.7–100%
NPV	91.4%	85.9–94.9%	87.3%	81.7–91.4%
LR+	Infinity	NaN-Infinity	Infinity	NaN-Infinity
LR−	0.11	0.06–0.19	0.17	0.11–0.26
Kappa ± SE	0.86 ± 0.04	0.77–0.94	0.78 ± 0.05	0.69–0.88
DOR	936.48	54.2–16194.6	574.6	33.8–9743.5
DE	94.9%	90.3–97.8%	92.2%	86.9–95.8%

Abbreviations: PPV—positive predictive value; NPV—negative predictive value; LR+—positive likelihood ratio; LR−—negative likelihood ratio; Kappa—kappa agreement; DOR: diagnostic odds ratio; DE—diagnostic effectiveness (accuracy); NaN—the calculation cannot be performed because the values entered include one or more instances of zero.

4. Discussion

Generally, for each clinician, as well as for countries and their health systems, when choosing a method for diagnosing a disease, the diagnostic characteristics and costs of that method are fundamental. Diagnostic characteristics speak about the method's success in correctly discriminating between certain two conditions of interest (health and disease or two stages of a disease, etc.).

In this study, the main interest was to investigate and compare the diagnostic characteristics of the small hand-held camera and AI or teleophthalmology-based grading system with a standard clinical examination and standard fundus camera in detecting DR and discriminating those persons who need the referral. This applies especially to patients with severe NPDR and PDR requiring prompt further retinal diagnostics and treatments. However, in the present study, the number (percentage) of eyes with severe NPDR and PDR detected by the hand-held camera corresponded with absolute accuracy to those detected by the clinical examination and standard camera. There was also no discrepancy in detecting eyes with moderate NPDR, whereas the substantial distinction in DR degree assessment among methods was found in the eyes with no retinopathy and those with signs of mild NPDR (single microaneurysms). Out of the 320 eyes included in the study, the hand-held camera misdiagnosed the signs of mild NPDR in 22 (6.9%) eyes screened by the standard clinical examination and in 34 (10.6%) eyes by the standard camera. Still, in both conditions, with no DR and mild NPDR, the recommendation regarding the current diabetic retinopathy guidelines is the same: regular follow-up [6,7]. Furthermore, according to all diagnostic accuracy measures used in the present study, the hand-held camera demonstrated excellent to very good discriminative power in positively detecting patients with DR and negatively detecting those without it compared to the other two diagnostic methods. Compared to the standard clinical examination, the hand-held camera had an AUC of 0.921, a sensitivity of 89.1%, and a specificity of 100%, while compared to the standard fundus camera; these measures, except for a specificity of 100%, were slightly lower: the AUC was 0.883 and the sensitivity was 83.2%.

The diagnostic accuracy of DR screening using different mobile cameras or smartphones has been widely researched, and numerous authors from various institutions and countries have obtained similar results. One of the first of such studies, published in 2015 by Rajalakshmi R et al., compared DR detection by a smartphone with the seven standard field images taken by a digital fundus camera, and found a sensitivity of 92.7% and a specificity of 98.4% for detecting any DR degree by a smartphone, while for detecting the sight-threatening diabetic retinopathy (STDR) by smartphone, the sensitivity and specificity were 87.9% and 94.9% [27]. The same authors reported that 21.9% of the images taken by a smartphone were of good quality, and the remaining 66.8% were of medium-good quality, while 61.1% of the images taken by a standard fundus camera were of good quality, and 34.9% were of medium-good quality [27]. Zhang W et al. compared screening for DR using a portable, noncontact, nonmydriatic hand-held retinal camera and the images graded by five masked ophthalmologists to the dilated clinical exam, and observed that the overall sensitivity for identifying VTDR was 64–88% and the specificity was 71–90%, while the images were gradable in 86–94% of predilation and 94–97% of postdilation photos [28]. A scoping review and meta-analysis of nine diagnostic test accuracy studies published from January 2000 to November 2018 regarding the use of various smartphone ophthalmoscopy for detecting DR reported the pooled sensitivity and specificity for detecting any DR of 87% (95% CI 74–94%) and 94% (95% CI 81–98%) and referral-warranted DR of 91% (95% CI 86–94%) and 89% (95% CI 56–98%), while the AUC ranged from 0.879 to 0.979 and the DOR from 11.3 to 1225 [29]. In the present study, the DOR for detecting DR by a hand-held camera compared to the clinical examination was 936.48, and compared to the standard camera, it was 574.6. A comparative pilot study performed in rural and tribal India, another developing country, compared the images taken with a hand-held non-mydriatic fundus camera (Horus scope 200, Medical Imaging Innovation Solution Partner, Taiwan) by two different trained technicians and graded by a retinal specialist to the indirect ophthalmoscopy completed by expert ophthalmologists and found a sensitivity, specificity, PPV, and NPV of 54.8%, 92.1%, 59.6%, and 83.9%, while the kappa agreement for DR between both detection methods was 0.48 [30]. In the present study, PPV and LR+ were 100% and infinity when comparing the hand-held camera with both diagnostic methods, while NPV and LR- were 91.4% and 0.11 when comparing the hand-held camera with the clinical examination and 87.3% and 0.17 with the standard camera. The present study's kappa (κ) agreement for the comparison of the hand-held camera to clinical examination was 0.86 and 0.78 to the standard fundus camera.

In the Republic of Croatia, a country located in Central and Southeast Europe on the Adriatic Sea coast, with 327.785 adults having diabetes (8.5% of the population) [31], screening for DR is usually performed using dilated slit-lamp fundus examination only by ophthalmologists, mostly medical retina specialists, and fundus photography with a standard fundus camera is not used routinely for DR screening but only for fluorescein angiography and research purposes [32]. Also, no nurses/technicians, optometrists, new technologies such as small hand-held fundus cameras, electronic data transfer systems (including telemedicine), or AI and automated grading are introduced into DR screening in Croatia.

The hand-held fundus camera used in this study is the only one of its kind in Croatia, obtained thanks to Professor Rahelić and the IDF for the IDF Diabetic Retinopathy Screening Project which aimed to highlight the importance of integrating DR screening into routine care for people living with diabetes in developing countries. Furthermore, besides the first use of a hand-held fundus camera, this was the first time an ophthalmology nurse actively participated in DR screening in Croatia.

According to the current guidelines, screening for DR has become an important cost-effective part of diabetes care, which means that even if enough ophthalmologists are available, using ophthalmologists to screen every person with diabetes is usually not feasible and is likely to be an inefficient use of resources [6,7].

The present study determined that all three DR screening methods were simple, but the differences were in the duration of the procedure and the persons who performed them. The first author, M.T., an ophthalmologist—medical retina specialist—performed the standard clinical examination, which took the longest time, about 15–20 min for each patient. M.T. also conducted fundus photography with a standard 45° fundus camera, while Đ.H., an ophthalmology nurse, performed fundus photography with a hand-held fundus camera. Both photographing sessions lasted much shorter than the clinical examination, about 5 min each. All images (4 images of 160 subjects = 640 images in total) from the standard 45° fundus camera were subsequently and independently graded by M.T. and

R.V. in about 6 h (360 min), while the images (4 images of 160 subjects = 640 images in total) from the hand-held fundus camera were graded immediately by AI and after a few hours by an IDF independent ophthalmologist.

However, besides the DR degree report, AI and an IDF ophthalmologist also evaluated the image quality and rated 77.5% of them as good quality and 22.5% as medium quality. Not a single image taken by the hand-held camera was considered low-quality or unreadable. Yet, all images (100%) taken by the standard 45° fundus camera VISUCAM Zeiss were of good quality because that nonmydriatic fundus camera has been in the Vuk Vrhovac University Clinic for the last 15 years, and the images were taken by M.T., who is very experienced in working with it. In contrast, the hand-held fundus camera TANG was entirely new at the Vuk Vrhovac University Clinic, and the photographing was performed by the ophthalmology nurse Đ.H., who was completely inexperienced in photographing with fundus cameras because in Croatia, only ophthalmologists, medical retina specialists, perform fundus photography.

All these study results implied that DR's hand-held fundus camera assessment completed by a nurse and graded by AI or an external ophthalmologist was reliable and in agreement with those of the standard clinical examination and fundus photography with a standard camera performed by a medical retina specialist. With nurses' further education and active participation in the photography technique and improving the image quality, it could be expected that the images would be of better quality and that the method would be more accurate and reliable.

The crucial role of nurses/technicians in DR screening with the aim of reducing the prevalence of blindness due to diabetes and reducing diabetes-related costs has been confirmed and reported earlier in numerous scientific articles and reviews [33–36]. In many diabetes centers in Europe and worldwide, educated nurses/technicians especially, in addition to fundus photographing, grade the fundus images and refer each patient with suspicious and positive results to ophthalmologists for further diagnosis and treatment. During the DR screening, the nurses/technicians also continuously educate the patients about the importance of regular DR screening and maintain good control of risk factors, such as glycemia, hypertension, and dyslipidemia, to prevent vision loss and blindness due to diabetes.

Some limitations of the present study should be addressed. First, this study was cross-sectional, performed in a single health center, and included a small number of patients. Unfortunately, all of the above were consequences of the COVID-19 pandemic onset in December 2019, when authorities worldwide recommended implementing lockdown measures to preserve public health and control the transmission of the virus. With the COVID-19 outbreak, including more participants was impossible, and the IDF Diabetic Retinopathy Screening Project ended. Second, the difference in the fundus photography experience and skill between the first author, ophthalmologist M.T., and the nurse Đ.H. resulted in a higher percentage of medium-quality images taken by the hand-held camera. Third, comparing two standard diagnostic methods, clinical examination and photography using the standard fundus camera, with a new method using an entirely new camera during only three months resulted in a deviation from the expected agreement and lower accuracy of the tested method. Fourth, we did not incorporate different imaging modalities or sources to validate the method's versatility and explore the algorithm's resilience to potential adversarial attacks or noisy input data. Accordingly, a nuanced understanding of each element's contribution to the overall performance, aiding in identifying crucial components and possible areas, is missing.

5. Conclusions

Recently, several AI-based automated systems for DR identification have been developed and introduced. The results suggest that AI-based systems are more sensitive than human graders and could be safe to use in clinical practice. In the present study, the number (percentage) of eyes with severe NPDR and PDR detected by the hand-held fundus camera and AI-based grading system corresponded with absolute accuracy to those detected by the clinical examination and standard camera. There was also no discrepancy in detecting eyes with moderate NPDR, whereas the substantial distinction in DR degree assessment among methods was found in the eyes with no DR and those with signs of mild NPDR (single microaneurysms). In addition, the hand-held camera misdiagnosed the signs of mild NPDR in 22 (6.9%) eyes screened by the standard clinical examination and in 34 (10.6%) eyes by the standard camera. Compared to the standard clinical examination, the hand-held camera had an AUC of 0.921, a sensitivity of 89.1%, and a specificity of 100%. Implementing the DR screening using the small fundus cameras and active involvement of nurses/technicians in the DR screening process would enable all people with diabetes to be regularly screened for DR, and provide ophthalmologists—medical retina specialists—the proper time needed for further diagnostic procedures and treatments.

Author Contributions: Conception, design, clinical examination, fundus photography with a standard camera, grading the images and assigning a DR level; data acquisition, analysis, interpretation, writing the paper (M.T.); grading the images and assigning a DR level (R.V.); photographing with a hand-held fundus camera (Đ.H.); organization and support of the nurse's active participation in the project (V.K.); conception, design, data acquisition, writing a draft of the paper (T.B.); cooperation with the IDF Diabetic Retinopathy Screening Project manager (D.R.); conception, design, critical modification of the essential intellectual content of the paper, and final approval of the published manuscript (M.T., R.V., T.B. and D.R.). All authors have read and agreed to the published version of the manuscript.

Funding: This research received no specific grant from public, commercial, or not-for-profit funding agencies.

Institutional Review Board Statement: The study was conducted following the Declaration of Helsinki and approved by the Hospital's Ethics Committee (protocol number 04/38-299, approval date: 7 August 2019).

Informed Consent Statement: Informed consent was obtained from all subjects included in the study.

Data Availability Statement: The data presented in this study are available upon specific request from the corresponding author.

Conflicts of Interest: The authors declare no conflict of interest.

References

1. International Diabetes Federation. *IDF Diabetes Atlas*, 10th ed.; International Diabetes Federation: Brussels, Belgium, 2021; Available online: http://www.diabetesatlas.org/ (accessed on 1 October 2023).
2. Flaxman, S.R.; Bourne, R.R.A.; Resnikoff, S.; Ackland, P.; Braithwaite, T.; Cicinelli, M.V.; Das, A.; Jonas, J.B.; Keeffe, J.; Kempen, J.H.; et al. Global causes of blindness and distance vision impairment 1990–2020: A systematic review and meta-analysis. *Lancet Glob. Health* **2017**, *5*, e1221–e1234. [CrossRef] [PubMed]
3. Teo, Z.L.; Tham, Y.C.; Yu, M.; Chee, M.L.; Rim, T.H.; Cheung, N.; Bikbov, M.M.; Wang, Y.X.; Tang, Y.; Lu, Y.; et al. Global prevalence of diabetic retinopathy and projection of burden through 2045: Systematic review and meta-analysis. *Ophthalmology* **2021**, *128*, 1580–1591. [CrossRef] [PubMed]
4. Javitt, J.C.; Aiello, L.P. Cost-effectiveness of detecting and treating diabetic retinopathy. *Ann. Intern. Med.* **1996**, *124 Pt 2*, 164–169. [CrossRef] [PubMed]
5. Rohan, T.E.; Frost, C.D.; Wald, N.J. Prevention of blindness by screening for diabetic retinopathy: A quantitative assessment. *BMJ* **1989**, *299*, 1198–1201. [CrossRef] [PubMed]
6. Wong, T.Y.; Sun, J.; Kawasaki, R.; Ruamviboonsuk, P.; Gupta, N.; Lansingh, V.C.; Maia, M.; Mathenge, W.; Moreker, S.; Muqit, M.M.K.; et al. Guidelines on diabetic eye care: The international council of ophthalmology recommendations for screening, follow-up, referral, and treatment based on resource settings. *Ophthalmology* **2018**, *125*, 1608–16622. [CrossRef] [PubMed]
7. World Health Organization. *Regional Office for Europe (WHO/Europe). Diabetic Retinopathy Screening: A Short Guide: Increase Effectiveness, Maximize Benefits and Minimize Harm*; World Health Organization, Regional Office for Europe: Copenhagen, Denmark, 2020. Available online: https://apps.who.int/iris/handle/10665/336660 (accessed on 1 October 2023).
8. Garg, S.; Jani, P.D.; Kshirsagar, A.V.; King, B.; Chaum, E. Telemedicine and retinal imaging for improving diabetic retinopathy evaluation. *Arch. Intern. Med.* **2012**, *172*, 1677–1678. [CrossRef] [PubMed]

9. Shi, L.; Wu, H.; Dong, J.; Jiang, K.; Lu, X.; Shi, J. Telemedicine for detecting diabetic retinopathy: A systematic review and meta-analysis. *Br. J. Ophthalmol.* **2015**, *99*, 823–831. [CrossRef]
10. Jin, K.; Lu, H.; Su, Z.; Cheng, C.; Ye, J.; Qian, D. Telemedicine screening of retinal diseases with a handheld portable non-mydriatic fundus camera. *BMC. Ophthalmol.* **2017**, *17*, 89. [CrossRef]
11. Padhy, S.K.; Takkar, B.; Chawla, R.; Kumar, A. Artificial intelligence in diabetic retinopathy: A natural step to the future. *Indian J. Ophthalmol.* **2019**, *67*, 1004–1009. [CrossRef]
12. US Food and Drug Administration. *FDA Permits Marketing of Artificial Intelligence-Based Device to Detect Certain Diabetes-Related Eye Problems*; US Food and Drug Administration: Silver Spring, MD, USA, 2018. Available online: https://www.fda.gov/news-events/press-announcements/fda-permits-marketing-artificial-intelligence-based-device-detect-certain-diabetes-related-eye (accessed on 1 October 2023).
13. Bhaskaranand, M.; Ramachandra, C.; Bhat, S.; Cuadros, J.; Nittala, M.G.; Sadda, S.R.; Solanki, K. The value of automated diabetic retinopathy screening with the EyeArt system: A study of more than 100,000 consecutive encounters from people with diabetes. *Diabetes Technol. Ther.* **2019**, *21*, 635–643. [CrossRef]
14. Wang, X.N.; Dai, L.; Li, S.T.; Kong, H.Y.; Sheng, B.; Wu, Q. Automatic grading system for diabetic retinopathy diagnosis using deep learning artificial intelligence software. *Curr. Eye Res.* **2020**, *45*, 1550–1555. [CrossRef] [PubMed]
15. Wang, Y.; Shi, D.; Tan, Z.; Niu, Y.; Jiang, Y.; Xiong, R.; Peng, G.; He, M. Screening referable diabetic retinopathy using a semi-automated deep learning algorithm assisted approach. *Front. Med.* **2021**, *8*, 740987. [CrossRef] [PubMed]
16. Orujov, F.; Maskeliūnas, R.; Damaševičius, R.; Wei, W. Fuzzy based image edge detection algorithm for blood vessel detection in retinal images. *Appl. Soft Comput.* **2020**, *94*, 106452. [CrossRef]
17. Hu, K.; Zhang, Z.; Niu, X.; Zhang, Y.; Cao, C.; Xiao, F.; Gao, X. Retinal vessel segmentation of color fundus images using multiscale convolutional neural network with an improved cross-entropy loss function. *Neurocomputing* **2018**, *309*, 179–191. [CrossRef]
18. Jiang, Z.; Yepez, J.; An, S.; Ko, S. Fast, accurate and robust retinal vessel segmentation system. *Biocybern. Biomed. Eng.* **2017**, *37*, 412–421. [CrossRef]
19. Liu, H.; Wei, D.; Lu, D.; Li, Y.; Ma, K.; Wang, L.; Zheng, Y. Simultaneous Alignment and Surface Regression Using Hybrid 2D-3D Networks for 3D Coherent Layer Segmentation of Retina OCT Images. In *Medical Image Computing and Computer Assisted Intervention—MICCA 2021I*; Springer: Berlin/Heidelberg, Germany, 2021. [CrossRef]
20. Apon, T.S.; Hasan, M.M.; Islam, A.; Alam, G.R. Demystifying Deep Learning Models for Retinal OCT Disease Classification using Explainable AI. In Proceedings of the 2021 IEEE Asia-Pacific Conference on Computer Science and Data Engineering (CSDE), Brisbane, Australia, 8–10 December 2021. [CrossRef]
21. Zhelev, Z.; Peters, J.; Rogers, M.; Allen, M.; Kijauskaite, G.; Seedat, F.; Wilkinson, E.; Hyde, C. Test accuracy of artificial intelligence-based grading of fundus images in diabetic retinopathy screening: A systematic review. *J. Med. Screen.* **2023**, *30*, 97–112. [CrossRef] [PubMed]
22. The Fred Hollows Foundation, International Diabetes Federation. *Diabetes Eye Health: A Guide for Health Professionals*; International Diabetes Federation: Brussels, Belgium, 2015. Available online: www.idf.org/eyehealth (accessed on 1 October 2023).
23. Scanlon, P.H.; Malhotra, R.; Greenwood, R.H.; Aldington, S.J.; Foy, C.; Flatman, M.; Downes, S. Comparison of two reference standards in validating two field mydriatic digital photography as a method of screening for diabetic retinopathy. *Br. J. Ophthalmol.* **2003**, *87*, 1258–1263. [CrossRef]
24. Boucher, M.C.; Gresset, J.A.; Angioi, K.; Olivier, S. Effectiveness and safety of screening for diabetic retinopathy with two nonmydriatic digital images compared with the seven standard stereoscopic photographic fields. *Can. J. Ophthalmol.* **2003**, *38*, 557–568. [CrossRef]
25. Wilkinson, C.P.; Ferris, F.L., 3rd; Klein, R.E.; Lee, P.P.; Agardh, C.D.; Davis, M.; Dills, D.; Kampik, A.; Pararajasegaram, R.; Verdaguer, J.T.; et al. Proposed international clinical diabetic retinopathy and diabetic macular edema disease severity scales. *Ophthalmology* **2003**, *110*, 1677–1682. [CrossRef]
26. Shanghai Jiao Tong University. Project 27: Screening and Auxiliary Diagnosis System of Diabetic Retinopathy based on Artificial Intelligence. Available online: https://global.sjtu.edu.cn/en/studyatSJTU/session/436 (accessed on 1 October 2023).
27. Rajalakshmi, R.; Arulmalar, S.; Usha, M.; Prathiba, V.; Kareemuddin, K.S.; Anjana, R.M.; Mohan, V. Validation of smartphone-based retinal photography for diabetic retinopathy screening. *PLoS ONE* **2015**, *10*, e0138285. [CrossRef]
28. Zhang, W.; Nicholas, P.; Schuman, S.G.; Allingham, M.J.; Faridi, A.; Suthar, T.; Cousins, S.W.; Prakalapakornet, S.G. Screening for diabetic retinopathy using a portable, noncontact, nonmydriatic handheld retinal camera. *J. Diabetes Sci. Technol.* **2017**, *11*, 128–134. [CrossRef]
29. Tan, C.H.; Kyaw, B.M.; Smith, H.; Tan, C.S.; Tudor Car, L. Use of smartphones to detect diabetic retinopathy: Scoping review and meta-analysis of diagnostic test accuracy studies. *J. Med. Internet Res.* **2020**, *22*, e16658. [CrossRef] [PubMed]
30. Gajiwala, U.R.; Pachchigar, S.; Patel, D.; Mistry, I.; Oza, Y.; Kundaria, D.; Shamanna, B.R. Non-mydriatic fundus photography as an alternative to indirect ophthalmoscopy for screening of diabetic retinopathy in community settings: A comparative pilot study in rural and tribal India. *BMJ Open* **2022**, *12*, e058485. [CrossRef] [PubMed]
31. Poljičanin, T.; Buble, T. *National Diabetes Registry CroDiab—Report for 2021*; Croatian Institute of Public Health: Zagreb, Croatia, 2022.
32. Tomić, M.; Raštegorac, P.; Vrabec, R.; Poljičanin, T.; Rahelić, D. Telemedicine for diabetic retinopathy screening in Croatia: A dream that could become a reality. *Coll. Antropol.* **2020**, *44*, 175–179. [CrossRef]

33. Connolly, A.; Hosker, C. The nurse's role in screening for diabetic retinopathy. *Nurs. Times* **2001**, *97*, 40. Available online: https://www.nursingtimes.net/clinical-archive/diabetes-clinical-archive/the-nurses-role-in-screening-for-diabetic-retinopathy-29-03-2001 (accessed on 1 October 2023). [PubMed]
34. Kirkwood, B.J.; Coster, D.J.; Essex, R.W. Ophthalmic nurse practitioner led diabetic retinopathy screening. Results of a 3-month trial. *Eye* **2006**, *20*, 173–177. [CrossRef]
35. Spurr, S.; Bullin, C.; Bally, J.; Trinder, K.; Khan, S. Nurse-led diabetic retinopathy screening: A pilot study to evaluate a new approach to vision care for Canadian Aboriginal peoples. *Int. J. Circumpolar. Health* **2018**, *77*, 1422670. [CrossRef]
36. Boucher, M.C.; Nguyen, M.T.D.; Qian, J. Assessment of training outcomes of nurse readers for diabetic retinopathy telescreening: Validation study. *JMIR Diabetes* **2020**, *5*, e17309. [CrossRef]

biomedicines

MDPI

Article

SLC22A3 rs2048327 Polymorphism Is Associated with Diabetic Retinopathy in Caucasians with Type 2 Diabetes Mellitus

Emin Grbić [1], Mojca Globočnik Petrovič [2], Ines Cilenšek [3] and Danijel Petrovič [3,*]

1 Department of Physiology, Faculty of Medicine, University of Tuzla, 75000 Tuzla, Bosnia and Herzegovina; emin.grbic@untz.ba
2 Clinic of Ophthalmology, Ljubljana University Medical Centre, 1000 Ljubljana, Slovenia; mojca.globocnik@kclj.si
3 Institute of Histology and Embryology, Faculty of Medicine, University of Ljubljana, 1000 Ljubljana, Slovenia; ines.cilensek@mf.uni-lj.si
* Correspondence: daniel.petrovic@mf.uni-lj.si

Abstract: The Solute Carrier Family 22 Member 3 (SLC22A3) is a high-capacity, low-affinity transporter for the neurotransmitters norepinephrine, epinephrine, dopamine, serotonin, and histamine. SLC22A3 plays important roles in interorgan and interorganism small-molecule communication, and also regulates local and overall homeostasis in the body. Our aim was to investigate the association between the rs2048327 gene polymorphism and diabetic retinopathy (DR) in Slovenian patients with type 2 diabetes mellitus (T2DM). We also investigated SLC22A3 expression in the fibrovascular membranes (FVMs) of patients with proliferative DR (PDR). Our study involved 1555 unrelated Caucasians with T2DM with a defined ophthalmologic status: 577 of them with DR as the study group, and 978 without DR as the control group. The investigated polymorphisms were genotyped using the KASPar genotyping assay. The expression of SLC22A3 (organic cation transporter 3—OCT3) was examined via immunohistochemistry in human FVM from 16 patients with PDR. The C allele and CC genotype frequencies of the rs2048327 polymorphism were significantly higher in the study group compared to the controls. The logistic regression analysis showed that the carriers of the CC genotype in the recessive genetic models of this polymorphism have a 1.531-fold increase (95% CI 1.083–2.161) in the risk of developing DR. Patients with the C allele of rs2048327 compared to the homozygotes for the wild type T allele exhibited a higher density of SLC22A3 (OCT3)-positive cells ($10.5 \pm 4.5/\text{mm}^2$ vs. $6.1 \pm 2.7/\text{mm}^2$, respectively; $p < 0.001$). We showed the association of the rs2048327 *SLC22A3* gene polymorphism with DR in a Slovenian cohort with type 2 diabetes mellitus, indicating its possible role as a genetic risk factor for the development of this diabetic complication.

Keywords: SLC22A3; rs2048327; diabetic retinopathy; immunohistochemistry

1. Introduction

Diabetic retinopathy (DR) is one of the leading complications of diabetes that can cause visual impairment or blindness. A third of people with diabetes worldwide have DR, and a third of those people have retinopathy that could result in vision loss [1]. The development and progression of diabetic retinopathy are influenced by the type and duration of diabetes. Type 1 diabetes carries a higher relative risk of developing diabetic retinopathy than type 2, while type 2 diabetes carries a higher prevalence of diabetic macular edema [2]. Changes in the rheological properties of blood, as well as changes in the wall of retinal blood vessels, lead to capillary occlusion, hyperpermeability, and retinal ischemia. The combinations of these changes with inflammatory changes lead to the appearance and development of DR, with characteristic histological changes, the loss of pericytes, and the thickening of the basilar membrane. Microaneurysms, or locations where the capillary wall balloons outward, are pathognomonic [3], alongside retinal hemorrhages, macular edema, and retinal neovascularization.

In recent years, the role of diabetic retinal neurodegeneration is increasingly evident, not only as a biomarker for DR but also as a causal factor in the development of DR [4–6]. Retinal ganglion cell apoptosis, as the most important feature of neurodegeneration, occurs early in the disease course, presented as a thinner retinal inner layer by OCT imaging [7–11].

There are numerous biochemical signaling pathways at play among which the role of oxidative stress is crucial. Kang and Yang showed that hyperglycemia can cause oxidative stress through a series of pathways, including the polyol, protein kinase C, and hexosamine pathways, as well as an increased expression of advanced glycation end products (AGEs) and their receptors. This imbalance in cellular redox homeostasis is further exacerbated by the abnormal activity of nuclear factors like highly activated NF-κB, and the diminished activity of Nrf2, as well as hyperglycemia-induced mitochondrial dysfunction. These factors contribute to the overproduction of reactive oxygen species (ROS) in DR [12]. An overproduction of ROS leading to oxidative stress can upset the balance of the metabolic system and cause the dysfunction of the retinal neurovascular unit, resulting in apoptosis, inflammation, and the degeneration of both the vasculature and neurons. It may also promote the growth of new blood vessels (neovascularization). Additionally, oxidative stress can lead to epigenetic changes and alter the expression of genes involved in signal transduction [13–15].

Organic cation transporter 3 (OCT3, SLC22A3) is a high-capacity, low-affinity transporter for the neurotransmitters norepinephrine, epinephrine, dopamine, serotonin, and histamine. Corticosterone has a direct impact on inhibiting the OCT3-mediated transport of these neurotransmitters. Corticosteroid hormones can affect gene expression by acting on intracellular glucocorticoid receptors (GR) and mineralocorticoid receptors (MR), leading to a wide range of physiological and behavioral responses. In addition, corticosteroid hormones also have rapid effects on physiology and behavior through non-genomic mechanisms. Some of these mechanisms are dependent on GR or MR, while others are independent of these receptors. One such GR-independent mechanism involves the inhibition of monoamine transport mediated by "uptake2" transporters, including OCT3, as a result of corticosteroid action [16].

Dopamine and histamine are important neurotransmitters and neuromodulators in the retinal neurons [17,18].

Dopamine supplementation in diabetic rodent models prevents visual loss because dopamine levels in the retina are decreased [19,20]. According to a preclinical study in diabetic patients, neurodegeneration can be detected early on by electroretinography and treated with L-dopa to prevent it from progressing to clinically recognized retinopathy [21]. Dopamine was found to exert protective effects against microvascular leaking and pericyte and endothelial loss, as well as to inhibit hyperglycemia-induced oxidative stress and mitochondrial dysfunction in HRECs and mouse retinas; therefore, it affects the development of diabetic vasculopathy as well [22].

The Solute Carrier Family 22 Member 3 (SLC22A3 also known as organic cation transporter 3—OCT3, gene ID: 6581, OMIM: 604842, HGNC: 10967) is a protein-encoding gene located on chromosome 6 on the q arm at position 25.3 [23]. The protein encoded by this gene belongs to the SLC22 transporter family. The neuroendocrine, growth factor–cytokine, and other homeostatic systems, along with SLC22 transporters, play important roles in interorgan and interorganism small-molecule communication. These systems also regulate local and overall homeostasis in the body [24]. The SLC22 transporter family is divided into two major clades: OAT—organic anion transporters; OCT—organic cation transporters. Each of these clades can be further divided into three subclades, designated as OAT, OAT-like, OAT-related, OCT, OCTN (organic cation/carnitine transporter), and OCT/OCTN-related. The OCT subclade has three known members: OCT1, OCT2, and OCT3 (SLC22A1, SLC22A2, and SLC22A3). OCT3 is more widely expressed than OCT1 and OCT2. OCT3 expression is widespread and can be found in the skeletal muscle, heart, brain, placenta, cornea, retina, iris, liver, kidney, and vascular endothelial cells [24–27].

To date, the exact mechanism of action of OCT3 has not been fully elucidated. However, OCT3 is associated with liver fibrosis, hepatocellular carcinoma, colorectal carcinoma, and altered drug pharmacokinetics [28–31].

A few studies found an association between the rs2048327 polymorphism of the *SLC22A3 (OCT3)* gene and CHD (coronary heart disease) in the Iranian population, and CVD (cardiovascular disease) and low HDL concentration in the Canadian population [32]. In contrast to these studies, studies on the Chinese Han population found no association between the rs2048327 polymorphism and coronary heart disease. The same findings were supported by a second study that also included this population [33]. Possible reasons for the opposite results of the aforementioned studies may be due to the effects of epigenetic and environmental factors in the aforementioned populations. However, data on the polymorphism rs2048327 and its association with the DR, and prognostic and therapeutic significance are lacking.

The objective of this study was to investigate the association between the polymorphisms of the *SLC22A3* gene and the development of DR among patients with type 2 diabetes in the Slovenian population (Caucasians). Moreover, we investigated the association of the rs2048327 polymorphism of SLC22A3 gene expression in the FVMs of patients with T2DM and PDR.

2. Materials and Methods

2.1. Patients

In our case–control study, were enrolled 1555 unrelated Caucasians with T2DM, with a defined ophthalmologic status. The current American Diabetes Association criteria were used to identify patients with T2DM [34]. Between January 2010 and January 2023, participants were collected from the University Medical Center Ljubljana Diabetic Outpatient Clinic and Eye Clinic. After pupil dilation, as aforementioned, a senior eye specialist (M.G.P.) performed a fundus examination [35]. The study group consisted of 1555 subjects: 577 subjects with DR (cases) and the control group of 978 subjects with T2DM of more than a 10-year duration who had no clinical signs of DR.

Patients with overt nephropathy were not included in the study to avoid the confounding effect of impaired kidney function. Moreover, patients with other ocular diseases were excluded. The study was carried out in accordance with the Helsinki Declaration and received approval from the National Ethical Committee (number 118/12/2011). Following the acquisition of informed consent for study participation, a thorough interview was conducted.

2.2. Biochemical Analyses

Standard biochemical techniques were used to measure glucose, creatinine, total cholesterol, low-density lipoproteins (LDL), high-density lipoproteins (HDL), and triglycerides.

2.3. Genotyping

Using a Qiagen isolation kit, genomic DNA was extracted from 100 μL of whole blood. The rs2048327 polymorphism of the SLC22A3 gene was genotyped by LGC Biosearch Technologies using their own novel, fluorescence-based, competitive, allele-specific PCR (KASPar) assay. The details of the method used can be found at http://running-KASP-on-ABI-StepOne-and-StepOnePlus.pdf (accessed on 15 July 2023).

2.4. Immunohistochemistry

In this study, we investigated the expression of SLC22A3 in fibrovascular membranes (FVMs) obtained from 25 patients (mean age: 62.5 ± 14.3 years; 13 men and 12 women) with type 2 diabetes mellitus (T2DM) and proliferative diabetic retinopathy (PDR) during pars plana vitrectomy. A pars plana vitrectomy with fibrovascular membrane peeling was performed by an experienced surgeon (M.G.P.). Formalin-fixed paraffin-embedded (FFPE) tissue sections of the FVMs were prepared by cutting consecutive 5 μm sections from each paraffin block and mounting them on glass slides. Deparaffinization and dehydration were carried out using a series of alcohol solutions. To detect the SLC22A3 protein in our tissue samples, we performed immunohistochemistry using the i-View method with the Invitrogen SLC22A3 antibody (MA5-36158) on the Ventana Roche diagnostic system (Tucson, AZ, USA). To ensure the reliability of the staining procedure, positive and negative controls were included. Kidney tissue sections known to express SLC22A3 were used as positive controls, while brain tissue sections, which exhibited minimal or absent SLC22A3 expression, were used as negative controls.

Microscopic analysis was conducted to evaluate SLC22A3 expression in the fibrovascular membranes. The presence or absence of specific staining in the fibrovascular membranes was compared to the positive and negative control tissues. A quantitative assessment of SLC22A3 expression was performed by manually identifying and marking SLC22A3-positive cells. The area containing SLC22A3-positive cells was delineated, and the numerical areal density of SLC22A3-positive cells was calculated as the number of positive cells per square millimeter (mm^2) of the marked area. Data obtained from the stained tissue sections were analyzed qualitatively, and the expression and distribution of SLC22A3 in fibrovascular membranes were assessed. A statistical analysis was conducted using appropriate methods to determine the significance of any observed differences.

2.5. Statistical Analysis

The SPSS program for Windows version 24 (SPSS Inc., Chicago, IL, USA) was used for the statistical analyses. An unpaired Student's *t*-test was used to compare continuous clinical data, and the chi-square test was used to compare discrete variables. For continuous variables, data were presented as mean SD, while, for categorical variables, the number and percentage of patients were used. In the study, the normality of data distribution was ascertained using the Shapiro–Wilk test. Continuous variables were compared using an unpaired Student's *t*-test when normally distributed, and the Mann–Whitney U test when asymmetrically distributed. Continuous variables were reported as mean ± standard deviation when normally distributed, and as median values (interquartile range (IQR)) when asymmetrically distributed.

Additionally, a multiple logistic regression was used to incorporate all variables that by univariate analysis demonstrated significant differences. Statistical significance was set at $p < 0.05$.

3. Results

The clinical characteristics of the two groups are summarized in Table 1. The following parameters showed a statistically significant difference between the groups: waist circumference ($p < 0.006$), duration of T2D ($p < 0.001$), BMI ($p < 0.041$), insulin therapy ($p < 0.001$), CVD ($p < 0.001$), diabetic neuropathy ($p < 0.001$), diabetic foot ($p < 0.001$), and S-HbA1c ($p < 0.001$). However, there were no significant differences between the groups with respect to age, sex, systolic blood pressure, diastolic blood pressure, active smokers, fasting glucose, total cholesterol, HDL-cholesterol, LDL-cholesterol, and triglycerides. Patients in the case group had a larger waist circumference, a longer duration of T2D, a higher use of insulin, a higher percentage of diabetic complications such as diabetic neuropathy and diabetic foot, and higher HbA1c values compared to the control group.

Table 1. Clinical and laboratory characteristics of patients with DR (cases) and without DR (controls).

	Case (N = 577)	Control (N = 978)	*p* Value
Sex [M]	300 (52.0%)	541 (55.3%)	0.2
Age [years]	65.11 ± 8.91	64.77 ± 9.66	0.53
Waist circumference [cm]	108.39 ± 13.03	105.17 ± 12.32	0.006
Duration of T2D [years]	18.00 (13.00–25.00)	12.00 (8.00–16.00)	<0.001
Duration of DR [years]	11 (10.00–25.00)		
SBP [mmHg]	148.68 ± 21.26	148.24 ± 20.17	0.69
DBP [mmHg]	84.05 ± 10.22	83.49 ± 10.69	0.32
BMI	29.49 ± 4.88	29.99 ±4.47	0.041
Active smokers	54 (9.4%)	119 (12.2%)	0.089
Insulin therapy	432 (74.9%)	387 (39.6%)	<0.001
CVD	118 (20.5%)	352 (36.0%)	<0.001
Diabetic neuropathy	112 (19.4%)	96 (9.8%)	<0.001
Diabetic foot	41 (11.9%)	0 (0.0%)	<0.001
S-HbA1c [%]	7.90 (7.00–8.83)	7.50 (6.80–8.30)	<0.001
S-fasting glucose [mmol/L]	8.50 (6.70–10.50)	8.20 (6.80–9.80)	0.065
S-total cholesterol [mmol/L]	4.80 (4.00–5.60)	4.70 (4.00–5.70)	0.65
S-HDL [mmol/L]	1.10 (1.00–1.35)	1.10 (1.00–1.40)	0.27
S-LDL [mmol/L]	2.70 (2.10–3.50)	2.70 (2.10–3.40)	0.53
S-TG [mmol/L]	1.80 (1.20–2.50)	1.70 (1.20–2.60)	0.72

Abbreviations: SBP—systolic blood pressure; DBP—diastolic blood pressure; BMI—body mass index; CVD—cardiovascular diseases; HbA1c—glycated hemoglobin; S-HDL—serum-high-density lipoprotein; S-LDL—serum-low-density lipoprotein; S-TG—serum-triglycerides.

Data on the genotype distribution and allele frequency of the rs2048327 polymorphism of the *SLC22A3* gene are shown in Table 2. The univariate analysis showed a statistically significant difference in genotype distribution ($p < 0.008$), as well as in allele frequency ($p < 0.003$) between the case group and controls. The *SCL22A3* genotype distribution in cases and controls did not deviate significantly from Hardy–Weinberg equilibrium.

We used logistic regression analysis to assess whether the rs2048327 polymorphism was independently associated with DR after adjusting for waist circumference, duration of T2D, BMI, diabetic neuropathy, and HbA1c. The results in the two genetic models, co-dominant ($p < 0.013$) and recessive ($p < 0.016$), indicate the existence of a statistically significant association (Table 3). The statistical strength of the study was 0.80.

In the FVMs of diabetic patients with PDR, a significantly higher numerical areal density of OCT-3-positive cells (Figure 1) was found in patients with the C allele of rs2048327 (CC + TC genotypes) compared to the homozygotes for the wild type T allele ($10.5 \pm 4.5/\text{mm}^2$ vs. $6.1 \pm 2.7/\text{mm}^2$, respectively; $p < 0.001$).

Table 2. Genotype and allele frequencies of the rs2048327.

*SLC22A3*_rs2048327	Case (N = 577)	Control (N = 978)	*p* Value
Genotypes			
CC	85 (14.7%)	100 (10.2%)	
CT	284 (49.2%)	466 (47.6%)	0.008
TT	208 (36.0%)	412 (42.1%)	
Alleles			
C (MAF)	454 (39.3%)	666 (34.0%)	0.003
T	700 (60.7%)	1290 (66.0%)	
HWE (*p* value)	0.45	0.06	
dominant			
CC + CT	369 (64.0%)	566 (57.9%)	0.018
TT	208 (36.0%)	412 (42.1%)	
recessive			
CC	85 (14.7%)	100 (10.2%)	0.008
CT + TT	492 (85.3%)	878 (89.8%)	

Abbreviations: HWE—Hardy–Weinberg equilibrium; MAF—minor allele frequency.

Table 3. Association between rs2048327 and DR.

*SLC22A3*_rs2048327	CASES/CTRLs	Adjusted OR (95% CI)	*p*Value
co-dominant			
CC vs. TT	85/100 vs. 208/412	1.609 (1.104–2.345)	0.013
CT vs. TT	284/466 vs. 208/412	1.099 (0.860–1.403)	0.45
dominant			
[CC + CT] vs. TT	369/566 vs. 208/412	1.185 (0.938–1.499)	0.15
recessive			
CC vs. [CT + TT]	85/100 vs. 492/878	1.531 (1.083–2.161)	0.016

Adjusted for waist circumference, duration of T2D, BMI, diabetic neuropathy, S-HbA1c [%].

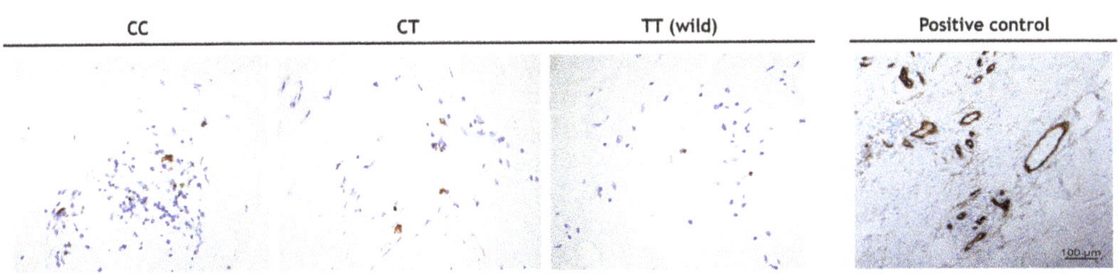

Figure 1. SLC22A3-positive cells in fibrovascular membranes from patients with PDR.

4. Discussion

The purpose of our study was to investigate the association between the rs2048327 of the *SLC22A3* gene and DR in the Slovene Caucasians with T2DM. Logistic regression analysis showed that there is an increased risk in carriers of the rs2048327 polymorphism for DR in two genetic models (co-dominant and recessive). The findings of our study should be compared to those of similar or related studies, and the potential for their use in clinical practice should be investigated.

This is the first report of any *SLC22A3* polymorphism on DR, a diabetic microvascular complication in T2DM. Many epidemiological studies have been conducted worldwide in the last few decades regarding the relationship between the rs2048327 *SLC22A3* gene polymorphism and other microvascular and vascular complications, such as diabetic nephropathy, cardiovascular disease (CVD), an coronary heart disease (CHD) [36].

In a study of unrelated Finnish patients with T1DM, an association was found between *SLC22A3* rs2048327 and diabetic nephropathy (DN) in men ($p < 0.03$) [36]. In their study, patients were divided into two samples: sample 1 (1086 patients) for the primary association analysis, and sample 2 (1252 patients) for replication. Patients were selected from all over Finland as part of the FinnDiane study. They also genotyped 165 non-diabetic Finns across the country. In the study, the age of onset of type 1 diabetes, the time of initiation of insulin therapy, and the fasting C peptide level were measured. According to the renal status, the patients were further divided into three groups, patients with normo-, micro-, and macroalbuminuria. In comparison with our study, the patients were younger and had a longer duration of diabetes, which is expected considering that type 1 diabetes mellitus appears earlier compared to in our subjects who have type 2 diabetes. It is also noticeable that out of the patients from the abovementioned study, 79.3% had hypertension in the microalbuminuria subgroup, and as many as 97.5% did in the macroalbuminuria subgroup. Similar to our study, in the aforementioned study, the group of cases includes mostly men. Regarding the rs2048327 *SLC22A3* gene polymorphism, by stratifying patients into those with HbA1c < 8.4% and HBA1c > 8.4%, an association with DN in men with HbA1c ≥ 8.4% was found, as well as allele frequency ($p < 0.03$), and genotype distribution ($p < 0.04$).

In a study on the Iranian population, which included 453 CHD patients and 453 non-CHD controls, the *SLC22A3* rs2048327 was significantly associated with an increased risk of CHD. A difference was found during the stratification analysis by gender, in male subjects from the case group compared to the control group, and in two genetic models: the additive (OR = 2.45; 95% CI: 1.17–5.11; $p = 0.017$) and recessive model (OR = 2.47; 95% CI: 1.21–5.06; $p = 0.013$). They also found that HDL concentration was 3.5 times lower in rs2048327 carriers [37]. In relation to our research, there is a difference in MAF frequency (minor allele frequency) between Iran and Slovenia (C allele frequency 29% and 35%). Also, in their research, no analysis of glycemic status was performed; but, despite this, the effect of rs2048327 on blood vessels was proven in the carriers of the C allele. Assuming that the effect of the rs2048327 polymorphism both in them and in us shows a possible association with changes in the blood vessels, it is possible that in our study there were changes in the blood vessels of the retina in the carriers of the C allele, with the influence of inadequately controlled glycemic status, which could ultimately favor the emergence and development of DR. Similar to the previous study, in a study on the Pakistani population, with 663 subjects of whom 78% were male, SLC22A3/rs2048327 showed an association with coronary stenosis ($p < 0.045$) in an additive genetic model [38]. In the aforementioned study, as in the previous two, there is a noticeably higher percentage of male respondents. The influence of gender is not negligible in the development of the mentioned events in conjunction with the rs2048327 polymorphism. Unfortunately, in the aforementioned studies, we do not have data on the diabetic status of the subjects. It is suggestive that in the mentioned studies, the rs2048327 polymorphism has an impact on changes in the blood vessels, and therefore we believe that it is possible that the mentioned polymorphism can also cause changes in retinal blood vessels, which could ultimately lead to DR in people with T2DM.

Contrary to previous studies, in the research on the Chinese Han population, no association of the rs2048327 polymorphism with the occurrence of CAD was found in any genetic model (recessive $p = 0.09$; dominant $p = 0.84$; additive $p = 0.44$) [39]. A similar finding was found in a study of Hispanics on the influence of the rs2048327 polymorphism on the occurrence of myocardial infarction ($p = 0.93$) [40]. Also, in another study on the Chinese Han population, a lower risk of developing CAD was found in carriers of the rs2048327 polymorphism ($p = 0.016$) [33]. The variance in sample size and population structure, failure to account for confounding factors, racial and ethnic differences, and the diversity of genetic and environmental backgrounds are some of the possible explanations for inconsistent results between populations. Additionally, the effects of population genotypes may vary among populations.

Additionally, our results suggest that the expression of SLC22A3 (OCT-3) is affected by the presence of the OCT-3 polymorphism (rs2048327), since the numerical areal density of rs2048327-positive cells was significantly higher in FVMs from DR patients carrying the C allele of rs2048327 compared to DR patients with the T allele, emphasizing the role of OCT-3 in the development of DR. To our knowledge, this is the first paper that investigated the expression of the OCT3 protein in the human retina. A similar paper was published analyzing the mouse retina [41]. A possible reason for the lack of works on this topic in humans is the difficulty in collecting samples for immunohistochemical analysis.

Our cross-sectional case–control study does, however, have some limitations. First of all, a relatively small but ethnically homogeneous cohort of cases and controls from Slovenia served as the research population. Secondly, in our study, there were differences in several parameters (for example, waist circumference, duration of T2D, BMI, diabetic neuropathy, HbA1c). By including each of these parameters in the logistic regression model, we attempted to reduce the impact of these differences. Thirdly, only one polymorphism of the SLC22A3 gene was studied. Therefore, more detailed research on larger samples with ethnically diverse subjects are needed to elucidate its role in the DR.

5. Conclusions

In our cross-sectional case–control study, we showed the association of the rs2048327 *SLC22A3* gene polymorphism with diabetic retinopathy in a Slovenian cohort with type 2 diabetes mellitus. In order to confirm the influence of the rs2048327 polymorphism on the occurrence and development of diabetic retinopathy, studies with a larger sample are necessary, as well as immunohistochemical analyses of the presence of the rs2048327 polymorphism on the retina in different populations.

Author Contributions: Conceptualization, D.P. and M.G.P.; methodology, I.C.; investigation, E.G.; resources, D.P.; writing—original draft preparation, E.G.; writing—review and editing, D.P. and I.C. All authors have read and agreed to the published version of the manuscript.

Funding: This work was supported by the program grants of the Slovenian Research Agency, ARRS P3-0326.

Institutional Review Board Statement: The study was carried out in accordance with the Helsinki Declaration and received approval from the National Ethical Committee (number 118/12/2011).

Informed Consent Statement: Informed consent was obtained from all subjects involved in the study.

Data Availability Statement: The data presented in this study are available on request from the corresponding author. The data are not publicly available due to privacy restrictions.

Conflicts of Interest: The authors declare no conflict of interest.

References

1. Gelcho, G.N.; Gari, F.S. Time to Diabetic Retinopathy and Its Risk Factors among Diabetes Mellitus Patients in Jimma University Medical Center, Jimma, Southwest Ethiopia. *Ethiop. J. Health Sci.* **2022**, *32*, 937. [CrossRef]
2. Nentwich, M.M.; Ulbig, M.W. Diabetic Retinopathy—Ocular Complications of Diabetes Mellitus. *World J. Diabetes* **2015**, *6*, 489. [CrossRef] [PubMed]
3. Ulbig, M.W.; Kollias, A.N. Diabetic Retinopathy: Early Diagnosis and Effective Treatment. *Dtsch. Arzteblatt Int.* **2010**, *107*, 75. [CrossRef]
4. Simó, R.; Stitt, A.W.; Gardner, T.W. Neurodegeneration in Diabetic Retinopathy: Does It Really Matter? *Diabetologia* **2018**, *61*, 1902. [CrossRef] [PubMed]
5. Garcia-Martin, E.; Cipres, M.; Melchor, I.; Gil-Arribas, L.; Vilades, E.; Polo, V.; Rodrigo, M.J.; Satue, M. Neurodegeneration in Patients with Type 2 Diabetes Mellitus without Diabetic Retinopathy. *J. Ophthalmol.* **2019**, *2019*, 1825819. [CrossRef]
6. Frydkjaer-Olsen, U.; Hansen, R.S.; Peto, T.; Grauslund, J. Structural Neurodegeneration Correlates with Early Diabetic Retinopathy. *Int. Ophthalmol.* **2018**, *38*, 1621–1626. [CrossRef] [PubMed]
7. Shi, R.; Guo, Z.; Wang, F.; Li, R.; Zhao, L.; Lin, R. Alterations in Retinal Nerve Fiber Layer Thickness in Early Stages of Diabetic Retinopathy and Potential Risk Factors. *Curr. Eye Res.* **2018**, *43*, 244–253. [CrossRef]

8. Kim, K.; Kim, E.S.; Yu, S.Y. Longitudinal Relationship Between Retinal Diabetic Neurodegeneration and Progression of Diabetic Retinopathy in Patients with Type 2 Diabetes. *Am. J. Ophthalmol.* **2018**, *196*, 165–172. [CrossRef]
9. Pinilla, I.; Idoipe, M.; Perdices, L.; Sanchez-Cano, A.; Acha, J.; Lopez-Galvez, M.I.; Cuenca, N.; Abecia, E.; Orduna-Hospital, E. Changes in total and inner retinal thicknesses in type 1 diabetes with no retinopathy after 8 years of follow-up. *Retina* **2020**, *40*, 1379–1386. [CrossRef]
10. Katsuyama, A.; Kusuhara, S.; Asahara, S.I.; Nakai, S.I.; Mori, S.; Matsumiya, W.; Miki, A.; Kurimoto, T.; Imai, H.; Kido, Y.; et al. En Face Slab Optical Coherence Tomography Imaging Successfully Monitors Progressive Degenerative Changes in the Innermost Layer of the Diabetic Retina. *BMJ Open Diabetes Res. Care* **2020**, *8*, e001120. [CrossRef]
11. Kim, K.; Kim, E.S.; Kim, D.G.; Yu, S.Y. Progressive Retinal Neurodegeneration and Microvascular Change in Diabetic Retinopathy: Longitudinal Study Using OCT Angiography. *Acta Diabetol.* **2019**, *56*, 1275–1282. [CrossRef]
12. Kang, Q.; Yang, C. Oxidative Stress and Diabetic Retinopathy: Molecular Mechanisms, Pathogenetic Role and Therapeutic Implications. *Redox Biol.* **2020**, *37*, 101799. [CrossRef] [PubMed]
13. Lin, W.J.; Kuang, H.Y. Oxidative Stress Induces Autophagy in Response to Multiple Noxious Stimuli in Retinal Ganglion Cells. *Autophagy* **2014**, *10*, 1692. [CrossRef]
14. Rodríguez, M.L.; Pérez, S.; Mena-Mollá, S.; Desco, M.C.; Ortega, Á.L. Oxidative Stress and Microvascular Alterations in Diabetic Retinopathy: Future Therapies. *Oxid. Med. Cell. Longev.* **2019**, *2019*, 4940825. [CrossRef] [PubMed]
15. Kowluru, R.A. Retinopathy in a Diet-Induced Type 2 Diabetic Rat Model and Role of Epigenetic Modifications. *Diabetes* **2020**, *69*, 689–698. [CrossRef]
16. Gasser, P.J.; Lowry, C.A. Organic Cation Transporter 3: A Cellular Mechanism Underlying Rapid, Non-Genomic Glucocorticoid Regulation of Monoaminergic Neurotransmission, Physiology, and Behavior. *Horm. Behav.* **2018**, *104*, 173–182. [CrossRef] [PubMed]
17. Nowak, J.Z.; Sek, B. Cyclic AMP Generating Systems in Vertebrate Retina: Effects of Histamine and an Established Retinal Modulator, Dopamine. *Agents Actions* **1991**, *33*, 138–142. [CrossRef]
18. Gastinger, M.J.; O'Brien, J.J.; Larsen, N.B.; Marshak, D.W. Histamine Immunoreactive Axons in the Macaque Retina. *Investig. Ophthalmol. Vis. Sci.* **1999**, *40*, 487–495.
19. Aung, M.H.; Park, H.N.; Han, M.K.; Obertone, T.S.; Abey, J.; Aseem, F.; Thule, P.M.; Iuvone, P.M.; Pardue, M.T. Dopamine Deficiency Contributes to Early Visual Dysfunction in a Rodent Model of Type 1 Diabetes. *J. Neurosci. Off. J. Soc. Neurosci.* **2014**, *34*, 726–736. [CrossRef]
20. Chesler, K.; Motz, C.; Vo, H.; Douglass, A.; Allen, R.S.; Feola, A.J.; Pardue, M.T. Initiation of L-DOPA Treatment After Detection of Diabetes-Induced Retinal Dysfunction Reverses Retinopathy and Provides Neuroprotection in Rats. *Transl. Vis. Sci. Technol.* **2021**, *10*, 8. [CrossRef]
21. Motz, C.T.; Chesler, K.C.; Allen, R.S.; Bales, K.L.; Mees, L.M.; Feola, A.J.; Maa, A.Y.; Olson, D.E.; Thule, P.M.; Iuvone, P.M.; et al. Novel Detection and Restorative Levodopa Treatment for Preclinical Diabetic Retinopathy. *Diabetes* **2020**, *69*, 1518–1527. [CrossRef]
22. Lee, Y.-J.; Jeon, H.-Y.; Lee, A.-J.; Kim, M.; Ha, K.-S. Dopamine Ameliorates Hyperglycemic Memory-Induced Microvascular Dysfunction in Diabetic Retinopathy. *FASEB J. Off. Publ. Fed. Am. Soc. Exp. Biol.* **2022**, *36*, e22643. [CrossRef]
23. SLC22A3 Gene—GeneCards | S22A3 Protein | S22A3 Antibody. Available online: https://www.genecards.org/cgi-bin/carddisp.pl?gene=SLC22A3&keywords=SLC22A3 (accessed on 17 January 2023).
24. Nigam, S.K. The SLC22 Transporter Family: A Paradigm for the Impact of Drug Transporters on Metabolic Pathways, Signaling, and Disease. *Annu. Rev. Pharmacol. Toxicol.* **2018**, *58*, 663. [CrossRef] [PubMed]
25. Solbach, T.F.; Grube, M.; Fromm, M.F.; Zolk, O. Organic Cation Transporter 3: Expression in Failing and Nonfailing Human Heart and Functional Characterization. *J. Cardiovasc. Pharmacol.* **2011**, *58*, 409–417. [CrossRef] [PubMed]
26. Zheng, P.-F.; Yin, R.-X.; Cao, X.-L.; Chen, W.-X.; Wu, J.-Z.; Huang, F. Effect of SYTL3-SLC22A3 Variants, Their Haplotypes, and G × E Interactions on Serum Lipid Levels and the Risk of Coronary Artery Disease and Ischaemic Stroke. *Front. Cardiovasc. Med.* **2021**, *8*, 713068. [CrossRef] [PubMed]
27. Koepsell, H. Organic Cation Transporters in Health and Disease. *Pharmacol. Rev.* **2020**, *72*, 253–319. [CrossRef] [PubMed]
28. Chen, E.C.; Liang, X.; Yee, S.W.; Geier, E.G.; Stocker, S.L.; Chen, L.; Giacomini, K.M. Targeted Disruption of Organic Cation Transporter 3 Attenuates the Pharmacologic Response to Metformin. *Mol. Pharmacol.* **2015**, *88*, 75–83. [CrossRef]
29. Nies, A.T.; Koepsell, H.; Winter, S.; Burk, O.; Klein, K.; Kerb, R.; Zanger, U.M.; Keppler, D.; Schwab, M.; Schaeffeler, E. Expression of Organic Cation Transporters OCT1 (SLC22A1) and OCT3 (SLC22A3) Is Affected by Genetic Factors and Cholestasis in Human Liver. *Hepatol. Baltim. Md* **2009**, *50*, 1227–1240. [CrossRef]
30. Vollmar, J.; Kim, Y.O.; Marquardt, J.U.; Becker, D.; Galle, P.R.; Schuppan, D.; Zimmermann, T. Deletion of Organic Cation Transporter Oct3 Promotes Hepatic Fibrosis via Upregulation of TGFβ. *Am. J. Physiol. Gastrointest. Liver Physiol.* **2019**, *317*, G195–G202. [CrossRef]
31. Yokoo, S.; Masuda, S.; Yonezawa, A.; Terada, T.; Katsura, T.; Inui, K.I. Significance of Organic Cation Transporter 3 (SLC22A3) Expression for the Cytotoxic Effect of Oxaliplatin in Colorectal Cancer. *Drug Metab. Dispos. Biol. Fate Chem.* **2008**, *36*, 2299–2306. [CrossRef]
32. Paquette, M.; Bernard, S.; Baass, A. SLC22A3 Is Associated with Lipoprotein (a) Concentration and Cardiovascular Disease in Familial Hypercholesterolemia. *Clin. Biochem.* **2019**, *66*, 44–48. [CrossRef] [PubMed]

33. Zhao, Q.; Wei, H.; Liu, D.; Shi, B.; Li, L.; Yan, M.; Zhang, X.; Wang, F.; Ouyang, Y.; Zhao, Q.; et al. PHACTR1 and SLC22A3 gene Polymorphisms Are Associated with Reduced Coronary Artery Disease Risk in the Male Chinese Han Population. *Oncotarget* **2016**, *8*, 658–663. [CrossRef]
34. Davies, M.J.; Aroda, V.R.; Collins, B.S.; Gabbay, R.A.; Green, J.; Maruthur, N.M.; Rosas, S.E.; Del Prato, S.; Mathieu, C.; Mingrone, G.; et al. Management of Hyperglycemia in Type 2 Diabetes, 2022. A Consensus Report by the American Diabetes Association (ADA) and the European Association for the Study of Diabetes (EASD). *Diabetes Care* **2022**, *45*, 2753–2786. [CrossRef] [PubMed]
35. Petrovic, M.G.; Kruzliak, P.; Petrovic, D. The Rs6060566 of the Reactive Oxygen Species Modulator 1 (Romo-1) Gene Affects Romo-1 Expression and the Development of Diabetic Retinopathy in Caucasians with Type 2 Diabetes. *Acta Ophthalmol.* **2015**, *93*, e654–e657. [CrossRef]
36. Sallinen, R.; Kaunisto, M.A.; Forsblom, C.; Thomas, M.; Fagerudd, J.; Pettersson-Fernholm, K.; Groop, P.H.; Wessman, M. Association of the SLC22A1, SLC22A2, and SLC22A3 Genes Encoding Organic Cation Transporters with Diabetic Nephropathy and Hypertension. *Ann. Med.* **2010**, *42*, 296–304. [CrossRef] [PubMed]
37. Najd Hassan Bonab, L.; Moazzam-Jazi, M.; Miri Moosavi, R.S.; Fallah, M.S.; Lanjanian, H.; Masjoudi, S.; Daneshpour, M.S. Low HDL Concentration in Rs2048327-G Carriers Can Predispose Men to Develop Coronary Heart Disease: Tehran Cardiometabolic Genetic Study (TCGS). *Gene* **2021**, *778*, 145485. [CrossRef]
38. Cheema, A.N.; Pirim, D.; Wang, X.; Ali, J.; Bhatti, A.; John, P.; Feingold, E.; Demirci, F.Y.; Kamboh, M.I. Association Study of Coronary Artery Disease-Associated Genome-Wide Significant SNPs with Coronary Stenosis in Pakistani Population. *Dis. Markers* **2020**, *2020*, 9738567. [CrossRef]
39. Lv, X.; Zhang, Y.; Rao, S.; Liu, F.; Zuo, X.; Su, D.; Wang, M.; Xia, M.; Guo, H.; Feng, D.; et al. Lack of Association between Four SNPs in the SLC22A3-LPAL2-LPA Gene Cluster and Coronary Artery Disease in a Chinese Han Population: A Case Control Study. *Lipids Health Dis.* **2012**, *11*, 128. [CrossRef]
40. Qi, L.; Ma, J.; Qi, Q.; Hartiala, J.; Allayee, H.; Campos, H. A Genetic Risk Score and Risk of Myocardial Infarction in Hispanics. *Circulation* **2011**, *123*, 374. [CrossRef]
41. Rajan, P.D.; Kekuda, R.; Chancy, C.D.; Huang, W.; Ganapathy, V.; Smith, S.B. Expression of the Extraneuronal Monoamine Transporter in RPE and Neural Retina. *Curr. Eye Res.* **2000**, *20*, 195–204. [CrossRef] [PubMed]

biomedicines

MDPI

Article

Spontaneous Neutrophil Extracellular Traps Release Are Inflammatory Markers Associated with Hyperglycemia and Renal Failure on Diabetic Retinopathy

Fátima Sofía Magaña-Guerrero [1], José Eduardo Aguayo-Flores [1], Beatriz Buentello-Volante [1], Karla Zarco-Ávila [1], Paola Sánchez-Cisneros [1], Ilse Castro-Salas [1], Enya De la Torre-Galván [1], José Luis Rodríguez-Loaiza [2], Aida Jiménez-Corona [3,4] and Yonathan Garfias [1,5,*]

1 Cell and Tissue Biology, Research Unit, Institute of Ophthalmology Conde de Valenciana, Mexico City 06800, Mexico; fatima.magana@institutodeoftalmologia.org (F.S.M.-G.); dreduardo_aguayo@hotmail.com (J.E.A.-F.); bbuentello@institutodeoftalmologia.org (B.B.-V.); karl120413@gmail.com (K.Z.-Á.); paoladejesussanchez@gmail.com (P.S.-C.); ilsecastrosalas@gmail.com (I.C.-S.); enyangelic@gmail.com (E.D.l.T.-G.)

2 Department of Retina, Institute of Ophthalmology Conde de Valenciana, Mexico City 06800, Mexico; jose.rodriguez@institutodeoftalmologia.org

3 Department of Ocular Epidemiology and Visual Health, Institute of Ophthalmology Conde de Valenciana, Mexico City 06800, Mexico; aidaajc@gmail.com

4 General Directorate of Epidemiology, Health Secretariat, Mexico City 01480, Mexico

5 Department of Biochemistry, Faculty of Medicine, Universidad Nacional Autónoma de México, Mexico City 04510, Mexico

* Correspondence: ygarfias@bq.unam.mx

Abstract: Diabetic retinopathy (DR) is the major microvascular complication of diabetes and causes vitreous traction and intraretinal hemorrhages leading to retinal detachment and total blindness. The evolution of diabetes is related to exacerbating inflammation caused by hyperglycemia and activation of inflammatory cells. Neutrophils are cells able to release structures of extracellular DNA and proteolytic enzymes called extracellular traps (NETs), which are associated with the persistence of inflammation in chronic pathologies. The purpose of the study was to determine the usefulness of neutrophil traps as indicators of DR progression in patients with type 2 diabetes (T2DM). We performed a case–control study of seventy-four cases classified into five groups (non-proliferative DR, mild, moderate, severe, and proliferative) and fifteen healthy controls. We found correlations between NETs and a diagnostic time of T2DM (r = 0.42; $p < 0.0001$), fasting glucose (r = 0.29; $p < 0.01$), glycated hemoglobin (HbA1c) (r = 0.31; $p < 0.01$), estimated glomerular filtration rate (eGFR) (r = −0.29; $p < 0.01$), and plasma osmolarity (r = 0.25; $p < 0.01$). These results suggest that due to NETs being associated with clinical indicators, such as HbA1c and eGFR, and that NETs are also associated with DR, clinical indicators might be explained in part through an NET-mediated inflammation process.

Keywords: hyperglycemia; diabetic retinopathy; immunopathology; inflammation markers; neutrophil; NETs

1. Introduction

Diabetic retinopathy (DR) is the main microvascular complication of diabetes and is one of the principal causes of blindness worldwide, affecting more than 93 million adults [1]. The changes that occur in the retinal tissue of patients with DR result from the development of five fundamental processes: (1) the formation of microaneurysms, (2) increased vascular permeability, (3) vascular occlusion, (4) the proliferation of neovessels and fibrous tissue in the retina and optic disc, and (5) the contraction of the vitreous and fibrovascular tissue [2].

The first ophthalmologically visible lesions appear during mild non-proliferative diabetic retinopathy (NPDR) involve the formation of capillary microaneurysms and continue with the presence or absence of diabetic macular edema (DME). DR progresses to being proliferative by the occlusion of terminal arterioles adjacent to areas with accumulations of aneurysms; at this stage, intraretinal hemorrhages and the formation of ischemic zones may occur. The secretion of proangiogenic factors and inflammatory cytokines in the retina promotes the growth of neovessels. Finally, due to the inflammatory process, contraction of the vitreous and adjacent fibrovascular tissue can lead to retinal detachment and blindness [3,4].

The development of DR is associated with permanent chronic inflammation caused by hyperglycemia and oxidative stress [5]. Neutrophils are inflammatory cells that are activated in the presence of microbial compounds, cytokines, and chemokines, among other inflammatory stimuli [6,7]. Activated neutrophils are defined as cells with a high expression of CD11b and CD66b and are able to perform inflammatory mechanisms such as degranulation, chemiotactic migration, and the release of neutrophil extracellular traps (NETs), among others [8,9]. NETs are structures formed by extracellular DNA decorated with proteolytic enzymes and modified proteins that are associated with the exacerbation of tissue damage in many pathologies such as sepsis [10], thrombosis [11], and autoimmune diseases such as systemic erythematosus lupus, rheumatoid arthritis, and psoriasis [12–14]. Thus, NETs are involved in inflammatory processes such as chronic obstructive pulmonary disease (COPD), cardiovascular risk, or risk of mortality in cancer [15–17].

In diabetic patients, hyperglycemia promotes NET release and high IL-6 serum levels, which are associated with nephropathy and cardiovascular complications [18]; similarly, diabetic patients have increased serum concentrations of NET compounds such as DNA histone complexes, elastase, and nucleosomes [19], suggesting that NETs and their molecular compounds could be biomarkers of diabetes [20]. The relationship between NETs and DR is not clearly understood, although some studies have reported an increased presence of circulating DNA histone and double DNA elastase complexes in DR patients compared to non-DR diabetic subjects [21,22].

The objective of this study was to evaluate the expression of neutrophil activation markers CD11b and CD66b, together with the spontaneous NET release on T2DM patients in different stages of DR to analyze the association of these inflammatory markers with hyperglycemia and renal failure and to elucidate whether these inflammatory markers are associated with DR development.

2. Materials and Methods

2.1. Reagents

Phosphate Buffer Solution (PBS, pH 7.2), Trypan blue, p-formaldehyde, poly-L-lysine, Triton 100X, Tween 20, Propidium iodide (PI), and Hank's Balanced Salt Solution (HBSS) were purchased from Sigma-Aldrich (Saint Louis, MI, USA). Bovine Serum Albumin (BSA) was obtained from Calbiochem (San Diego, CA, USA). Polymorphoprep was purchased from Alere Technologies AS (Jena, Germany). Purified antibody: human anti-neutrophil elastase antibody (NE) was purchased from Abcam (Cambridge, UK). FITC-conjugated anti-CD15, PE-conjugated anti-CD11b, BV450-conjugated anti-CD66b, and BD FACS Lysing 10X solutions were obtained from e-Bioscience, Beckton Dickinson (BD) (San Diego, CA, USA). An AlexaFluor-488-conjugated goat anti-rabbit antibody was obtained from LifeTechnologies (Eugene, OR, USA). Cell culture 24-well plastic plates were purchased from Corning Inc. (Corning, NY, USA).

2.2. Participants

This was a case–control study conducted at the Institute of Ophthalmology "Conde de Valenciana" Foundation; subjects were recruited from October 2020 to July 2022. Healthy individuals were defined as subjects without a diagnosis of T2DM or other pathologies such as autoimmune or renal diseases, hypertension, or active infections. The study was carried out by the tenets of the Helsinki Declaration and was approved by the Institutional

Review Boards of Research, Ethics, and Biosecurity of the "Conde de Valenciana" Institute of Ophthalmology (CEI-2020/01/01). All patients signed an informed consent form.

T2DM patients were defined according to the current ADA criteria. Patients from both sexes > 18 years were included. All patients that presented inflammatory-related diseases (except diabetes), such as active or chronic infections, were excluded, as well as immunocompromised subjects. Patients with media opacity or cataracts were also excluded. Patients in which biological samples were unsuitable to work with were eliminated from the study. The selection of the patients was performed sequentially. Healthy non-diabetic patients were included as the control subjects.

All patients underwent mydriatic fundus photography of both eyes; the images were acquired with the Optos P200DTx. Two retina specialists classified all patients according to the Diabetic Retinopathy Disease Severity Scale and the International Clinical Diabetic Retinopathy Disease Severity Scale in a blinded manner. T2DM participants were categorized into five groups: without DR; with mild non-proliferative diabetic retinopathy (NPMiDR); with moderate non-proliferative diabetic retinopathy (NPMDR); with severe non-proliferative diabetic retinopathy (NPSDR); and with proliferative diabetic retinopathy (DM-2 PDR).

Each participant donated 30 mL of peripheral blood. Urinalysis and hematic biometry were performed on each participant. Hemoglobin concentration, hematocrit, red blood cells, mean corpuscular volume, mean corpuscular hemoglobin, platelets and white blood cells (monocytes, lymphocytes, neutrophils, eosinophils and basophils), and a blood chemistry test that included glycated hemoglobin A1c (Hba1c), glucose, blood urea nitrogen (BUN), urea, uric acid, total protein, albumin, globulin, creatinine, cholesterol, triglycerides, alkaline phosphatase, electrolyte content, alanine aminotransferase (ALT), gamma-glutamyl transferase (GGT), high-density lipoproteins (HDLs), and low-density lipoproteins (LDLs) were tested.

The estimated Glomerular Filtration Rate (eGFR) was calculated using the Modification of Diet in Renal Disease (MDRD-6) formula. Plasma osmolarity refers to the serum concentration of osmotically active molecules, such as sodium (Na), potassium (K), glucose, and BUN. We use the following formula, $Osm = 2(Na + K) + (Glucose/18) + (BUN/2.8)$, to determine plasma osmolarity.

2.3. *Flow Cytometry Assays*

Complete peripheral blood was obtained from median cubital venipuncture and collected in sodium citrate anticoagulant tubes. Immediately, 0.1 mL of blood was transferred to polystyrene flow cytometer tubes, and 15 µL of the mix of antibodies FITC-CD15 (5 µL), PE-CD11b (5 µL) and BV450-CD66b (5 µL) were added; the tubes were incubated for 30 min at 4 °C in darkness. Afterward, 0.9 mL 1X of lysing and fixing solutions (BD FACS Lysing) were added to samples and incubated for 15 min at room temperature (RT) in darkness. Finally, 104 cells of the polymorphonuclear region were acquired on a BD FACS lyric flow cytometer (BD, San Diego, CA, USA); the acquired data were analyzed using FlowJo 10.0 v software (FlowJo LLC, Ashland, OR, USA).

2.4. *Peripheral Blood Polymorphonuclear (PMN) Cell Isolation*

Human PMNs were isolated using a density gradient method. Briefly, a sample of 20 mL of complete peripheral blood from individuals fasting for 6–8 h was collected in heparin tubes. The complete blood was placed on an equal volume of a polymorphoprep solution and centrifuged at 500× *g* for 35 min at RT. The PMN ring was collected and washed with 0.8 mL of ice-cold PBS (0.1 M). The remaining erythrocytes were lysed with a lysis solution (NH_4Cl 152.7 mM, Na_2EDTA 0.1 mM, $NaHCO_3$ 9.0 mM at pH 7.2–7.4) and washed with 0.1 M PBS as needed. The PMNs were suspended in Hank´s Balanced Salt Solution (HBSS) and kept on ice until further use. The trypan blue exclusion method was used to evaluate PMN viability. Cell purity was assessed by means of flow cytometry, obtaining ≥98% of CD11b and CD15+ double-positive cells.

2.5. Microscopy Staining of In Vitro NETs

The isolated PMNs from each subject were placed on poly-L-lysine pre-coated cover glasses in a 24-well plate with a density of 45 cells per well, incubated at 37 °C with an atmosphere of 5% of CO_2 for 20 min, and let to adhere. Subsequently, cells and the spontaneous release of NETs were fixed with a 4% p-formaldehyde solution for 10 min at RT and washed twice with 0.1 M PBS. The samples were incubated with constant shaking with a blocking solution (5%-BSA, 0.1% Triton 100X, and 0.1 M PBS) for 2 h at RT °C.

For the visualization of in vitro NET release, the samples were incubated overnight at 4 °C with constant shaking with a rabbit anti-human anti-neutrophil elastase antibody (NE) (1:100). Negative controls were performed, leaving out the primary antibody. After washing three times with 0.5 mL of PBS 0.05% tween 20 (PBS-T), the samples were incubated for 2 h with an Alexa 488 goat anti-rabbit IgG antibody (1:800) at RT °C. The samples were rinsed twice with PBS-T, and DNA visualization was performed with 25 µg/mL of propidium iodide (PI). Finally, the specimens were sealed, and the images were acquired with an ApoTome II microscope using ZEN 3.4 (blue edition) software from Carl Zeiss (Jena, Germany).

2.6. Image NET Analysis

To quantify NET area release, three random images from three independent assays were analyzed from each sample with an ApoTome II microscope using Carl Zeiss ZEN 3.4 (blue edition) software. A machine learning tool was designed for the detection and quantification of NETs, as previously described, with slight modifications [23]. Briefly, to perform a homogeneous analysis, we chose only fields with 80 nuclei-stained samples with IP. A deep learning module Intellesis Trainable Segmentation from Carl Zeiss ZEN 3.4 (blue edition) for the NET area quantification was used, excluding nuclei and background. The result was considered as the total area occupied by the NET release; data were expressed as mean ± SE.

2.7. Sample Size Calculation

The sample size was calculated using the mean difference of two independent groups, according to the results previously obtained by Lee, et al. [24]. A power analysis was conducted using G*power software (V 3.1.9.7, UCLA, Los Angeles, CA, USA) that was one-tailed, $(1 - \beta) = 0.80$, and $\alpha = 0.05$; determining that data from 15 patients in each group were required.

2.8. Statistical Analysis

Beforehand, the non-parametric distribution of the data was determined by Shapiro–Wilk and Kolmogorov–Smirnov tests. Data were analyzed with non-parametric Kruskal–Wallis tests, considering $p < 0.05$ as statistically significant. Linear regressions of variables were performed with a 95% confidence interval, and one-tail non-parametric Spearman's correlation tests were also performed. Graphics and statistical analysis were achieved using the Prism 8 GraphPad software (La Jolla, CA, USA). Finally, the association between the clinical scores with the area of NET release depending on each RD group was performed.

3. Results

3.1. Increased Activated Neutrophil Markers and Spontaneous NET Release Relationship with the Progression Time of Diabetes in Severe Stages of DR

Demographic data and clinical evaluation of the recruited subjects are shown in Table S1. Activated neutrophils CD15+ CD11b+ CD66b+ were found in DR groups. The population of CD15+ neutrophils of subjects with PDR had a significative higher expression of CD11b with respect to the groups with NPMiDR (** $p < 0.01$), NPSDR (* $p < 0.05$), and without T2DM (* $p < 0.05$) (Figure 1A, left panel). Similarly, in the analysis of CD66b expression on the CD15+ neutrophils population, we found that subjects with PDR had a significantly higher expression of CD66b markers with respect to subjects without

T2DM and patients without DR (* $p < 0.05$). The NPMDR group showed a significantly high expression (* $p < 0.05$) of CD66b with respect to the without DR group (Figure 1A, right panel). Our results indicate that CD15+ neutrophils of patients from the NPMDR and PDR groups present a state of activation and possible inflammation by the overexpression of CD11b and CD66b.

Additionally, we analyzed the capacity of spontaneous in vitro NET release of neutrophils in each recruited group. We found an increase in NET release in groups with any grade of DR compared with T2DM without DR and without T2DM groups (Figure 1B, left panel). The quantitative analysis showed higher NET release on NPMiDR (* $p < 0.05$), NPMDR (** $p < 0.01$), NPSDR (**** $p < 0.0001$), and PDR (** $p < 0.01$) with respect to the group without T2DM; we found significant differences on the increase in NET release in DR groups NPMDR (* $p < 0.05$), NPSDR (*** $p < 0.001$), and PDR (* $p < 0.05$) compared with the T2DM subjects without DR (Figure 1B, right panel). According to our results, the neutrophils of subjects with DR had an activated phenotype by the overexpression of CD11b and CD66b; similarly, the spontaneous in vitro NET release was higher in DR patients, suggesting a relationship between the activated/inflammatory profile of neutrophils and NETs in different stages of DR.

We were interested in analyzing the relationship between the diagnosis time of diabetes mellitus and the activation phenotype of neutrophils. As expected, NPDR in moderate and severe stages and PDR presented a higher time (*** $p < 0.001$) of the disease diagnosis in comparison with T2DM without DR (Figure 1C). In this way, we performed correlation analyses between the time of diabetes mellitus diagnosis and the expression values (MFI) of CD11b and CD66b, as well as NET release. Although we did not find a significant correlation between the CD11b value expression and T2DM diagnosis time, we found a positive correlation between the time of diagnosis of T2DM (** $p < 0.01$, $r = 0.1157$) and the expression of CD66b; similarly, the time of diagnosis of T2DM correlated with NET release (**** $p < 0.0001$, $r = 0.42$) (Figure 1D). The release of CD66b and NETs could be associated as biomarkers of the chronic inflammation of DR until its severe stages.

3.2. NETs Correlated with the Hyperglycemic and Renal Status on Severe Stages of DR

The hyperglycemia and renal status indicators correlated with the inflammatory environment caused by the spontaneous in vitro NET release. Glucose is an external stimulus able to induce NET release; in this context, we found significant ($p < 0.05$) high levels of fasting glucose in all diabetic groups in comparison with non-diabetic subjects (Figure 2A). Likewise, as expected, significantly increased values of HbA1c were found in all diabetic groups in comparison with non-diabetic subjects ($p < 0.05$) (Figure 2B).

We evaluated the correlation between two indicators of glycemic control, such as fasting glucose and HbA1c, with the in vitro NET release. We found a significant (** $p < 0.01$, $r = 0.2860$) positive correlation between fasting glucose (Figure 2A, right panel) and Hb1Ac (** $p < 0.01$, $r = 0.3139$) (Figure 2B, right panel) with NET release, suggesting that a scarce glycemic control is associated with the inflammatory environment promoting NET release, which might exacerbate the evolution of DR.

It is well-known diabetic subjects are more prone to present vascular complications than healthy individuals. In this sense, NETs have been associated with systemic vascular and thrombotic complications that could affect organs, including kidneys. To evaluate the renal function, we calculated the eGFR and plasma osmolarity. Interestingly, subjects with the most advanced stages of retinopathy such as NPMDR, NPSDR, and PDR had significantly ($p < 0.05$) lower eGFR values compared with non-diabetic subjects (Figure 2C). Contrariwise, osmolarity values were significantly ($p < 0.05$) upregulated among all diabetic patients, including those with and without different DR in different stages (Figure 2D).

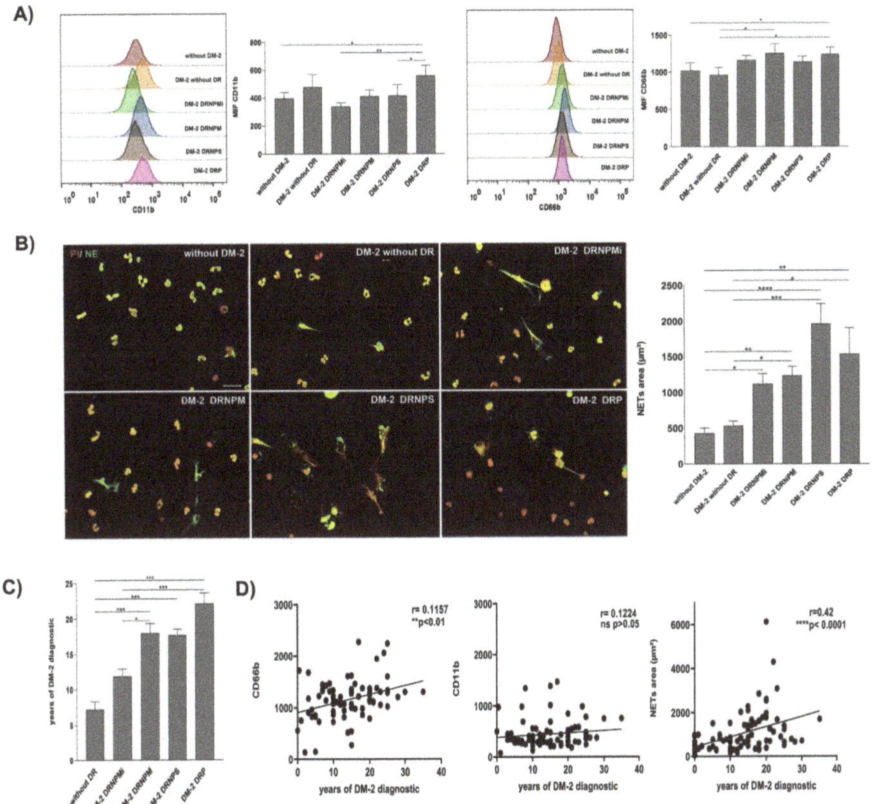

Figure 1. Increasingly activated neutrophil and spontaneous NET release relationship with the progression time of diabetes in severe stages of DR. Cytometry analysis of activation markers expression CD11b and CD66b on peripherical blood neutrophils (PBNs) of diabetic patients without retinopathy (DM-2), diabetic patients with a grade of non-proliferative retinopathy (mild (DM-2 NPMiDR); moderate (DM-2 NPMDR), or severe (DM-2 NPSDR), and diabetic patients with proliferative retinopathy (DM-2 PDR). A group of non-diabetic subjects (without DM-2) was recruited as a healthy healthy. Mean Fluorescence Intensity (MIF) was quantified for the expression of CD11b (left panel) and CD66b (right panel) in the PBN of diabetic patients with or without retinopathy (**A**). Micrographs of spontaneous NETs released (left panel) on diabetic patients with or without a grade of diabetic retinopathy. Neutrophil elastase (NE) staining in green was used to identify NET structures and iodide propidium in red (PI) was used to visualize extracellular DNA. The NETs are surrounded by a dashed white line. These images are representative of three random fields by the patient; scale bar = 20 μm (left panel) ((**B**), left panel). Graphical representation of the spontaneous NET area released in the groups of patients with or without retinopathy ((**B**), right panel). The spontaneous NET area was released in the groups of patients with a grade of retinopathy (DM-2 NPMiDR), (DM-2 NPMDR), (DM-2 NPSDR), and (DM-2 PDR). Data are representative from three random fields taken by the patient (n = 270). Graph of the progression of diabetic retinopathy dependent from the time of diagnosis of DM-2. The data are expressed as mean ± SE, * $p < 0.05$; ** $p < 0.001$; *** $p < 0.0001$; **** $p < 0.00001$, (n = 75) (**C**). Correlation graphs between the time of the diagnosis of DM-2 and expression of inflammatory markers CD11b and CD66b of the PBN and NETs-released area on the recruited groups. The time of the DM-2 diagnosis has a correlation with the expression of CD66b and the area of NETs released on recruited patients. The data are expressed as mean ± SE, * $p < 0.05$; ** $p < 0.001$; *** $p < 0.0001$; **** $p < 0.00001$, (n = 90) (**D**).

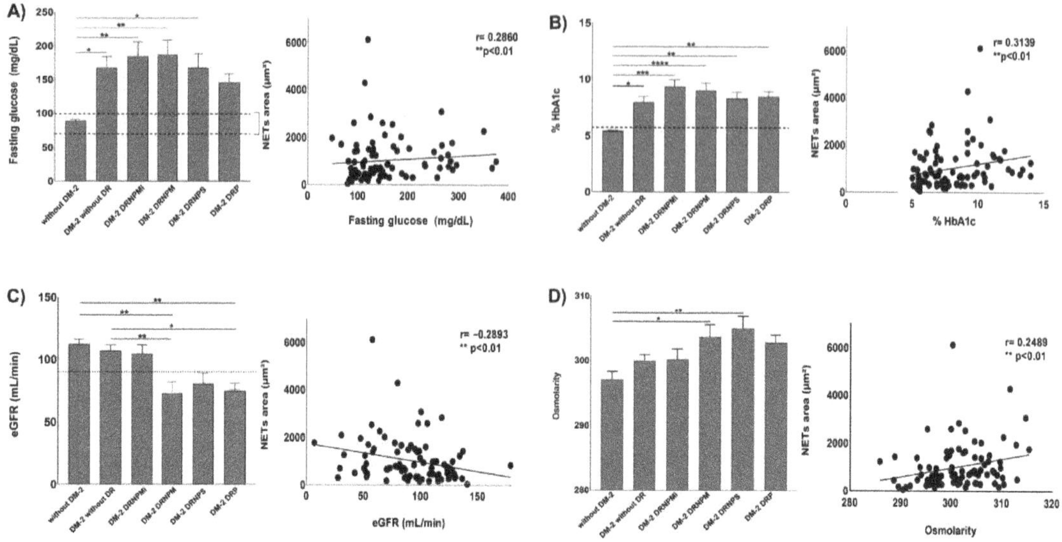

Figure 2. NETs are inflammatory markers correlated with hyperglycemia and renal failure in severe stages of DR. Graph of fast glucose on diabetic and retinopathy subjects; Spearman's correlation graph between the area of NETs released and fast glucose of diabetic and retinopathy subjects (**A**). Graph of glycated hemoglobin (HbA1c) of diabetic and retinopathy subjects; Spearman's correlation graph between the area of NETs released and HbA1c on diabetic and retinopathy subjects (**B**). Graph of estimated glomerular filtration rate (eGFR) of diabetic and retinopathy subjects; Spearman's correlation graph between the area of NETs released and eGFR on diabetic and retinopathy subjects (**C**). Graph of plasmatic osmolarity of diabetic and retinopathy subjects; Spearman's correlation graph between the area of NETs released and plasmatic osmolarity of diabetic and retinopathy subjects (**D**) The data are expressed as mean ± SE, * $p < 0.05$; ** $p < 0.001$; *** $p < 0.0001$; **** $p < 0.00001$ ($n = 90$). Dashed lines represent healthy normal values.

To analyze whether the clinical indicators, such as renal functions, such as eGFR and plasma osmolarity, had a relationship with the inflammatory environment caused by NETs, we performed correlation analyses between these indicators. The results showed a significantly negative correlation (** $p < 0.01$, r = −0.2893) between NET area and eGFR, indicating that the higher level of NET, the lesser eGFR values (Figure 2C, right panel); in contrast, plasma osmolarity showed a significantly (** $p < 0.001$, r = 0.2489) positive correlation with NET release (Figure 2D, right panel). Although proteinuria values were analyzed as another clinical indicator of renal status, no significant changes were found between the analyzed groups, and no correlation was observed respect with to NET release. These results suggest that increased inflammatory conditions caused by NET release can be related to an increased renal dysfunction in subjects with DR.

3.3. Risk Prognosis of DR Development by Association of the Spontaneous NET Release

As we have shown, NETs are associated with eGFR, HbA1c, and the diagnostic time of T2DM, and are differentially released in DR subjects. The associated risk of development of DR was calculated considering these clinical variables and the grade of NETs. A risk matrix was designed to categorize the three clinical risk variables: the diagnostic time of T2DM, the percentage of HbA1c, and the calculated eGFR, and were assigned a score at these categories (Figure 3). According to the risk matrix, a total score was obtained from these three variables, and four levels of risk were established as follows: low (0–1), mild-moderate (2–3), moderate–increased (4), and high (5–6) (Figure 3). These data indicate that the higher risk of development of DR is related to poor glycemic control, levels of

HbA1c > 9%, and eGFR values < 30 mL/min, in addition to a long time of T2DM > 9 years of diagnosis. On the other hand, the lower risk of DR development was associated with acceptable glycemic control, levels of HbA1c < 7%, eGFR values > 60 mL/min, and a DM-2 evolution of less than five years (Figure 3).

	score 0	score 1	score 2
Diagnostic time DM-2	<5 years	6-9 years	> 9 years
HbA1c	< 7.0%	7.1-9.0%	>9.1%
eGFR	> 60 ml/min	59-30 ml/min	<30 ml/min

Total score
low risk (0-1)
mild-moderated risk (2-3)
moderated increased risk (4)
high risk (5-6)

NETs release	DIABETIC RETINOPATHY RISK		
Low NETs 400-600	low	mild-moderated	high
Moderated NETs 601-1500	mild-moderated	moderated increased	high
High NETs >1500	moderated increased	high	high

Figure 3. Prognostic risk of DR development by the association of the spontaneous NET release and clinical score. Matrix risk of variables associated with the development of DR. Analysis of the categorized risk factors: diagnostic time of DM-2 (<5 years, 6–9 years, and >9 years); percentage of glycated hemoglobin (HbA1c) (<7.0%, 7.1–9.0%, and >9.1%); and the calculated eGFR (>60 mL/min, 59–30 mL/min, and <30 mL/min). The total score of the diagnostic time of DM-2, the percentage of glycated hemoglobin (HbA1c), and eGFR were ranked by four risk scores (low (0–1), mild–moderate (2–3), moderate–increased (4), and high (5–6)), which were associated with the level of NET release in each group with DR.

Data in the four risk categories of clinical variables were associated with in vitro NET release to know the impact on DR development. Interestingly, the low risk of developing DR remains related to a low score together with an NET release in a range between 400 and 600. In this category, we found subjects from the groups without T2DM and T2DM without DR. On the other hand, the high risk of developing DR is present when an increased risk score is maintained along with any degree of NET release. The risk of DR development toward a moderate state of NPDR is influenced by a grade of NET release ranging between 601 and 1500; mainly, the groups associated with these risks were the subjects with DRNPMi, DRNPM, and DRNPS (Figure 3). The results altogether allow us to suggest that in vitro NET release could be considered an indicator of the risk to development DR together with other clinical variables, such as diagnostic time DM-2, HbA1c, and eGFR values.

4. Discussion

Neutrophils are granulocytic cells that are activated by a myriad of stimuli such as cytokines and chemokines and damage-associated molecular patrons (DAMPs), among others. The activation of neutrophils in diabetic subjects is associated with hyperglycemia and high serum lipid concentrations [25,26]. Although the precise mechanisms of neutrophils in DR development are not well understood, their activity and proteolytic granule compounds are associated with DR development and other clinical complications of diabetes mellitus [27], mainly by their role in vascular leakage and endothelium damage [28,29]. The expression of CD11b and CD66b activation markers on monocytes and neutrophils is increased in T2DM patients, promoting and increasing the adhesive capacity of neutrophils and monocytes to the endothelium and enhancing vascular and systemic damage [30]. In the present study, we found that diabetic patients with MNPDR-moderated and PDR display an increased expression of CD11b and CD66b in the CD15+ neutrophil population, suggesting that prolongated inflammation on severe grades of DR can be related to enhanced neutrophil activation. The overexpression of CD11b and CD66b has been associated with the diagnosis of inflammatory processes, such as sepsis [31], as well as the increase in migration of tumor-associated neutrophils in gastric and esophageal adenocarcinoma. They have been recognized in both conditions as prognostic factors in the diagnosis of gastric cancer [32,33] and testicular germ cell tumor [34]. Thus, the increase in the expression of both CD11b and CD66b activation markers in neutrophils could be associated as a prognostic factor of severe stages of DR.

Neutrophil extracellular traps (NETs) are structures mainly formed by extracellular DNA decorated with nuclear-modified proteins and many proteins from granules of neutrophils. One of the diverse functions of NETs is to generate a degradant and oxidative microenvironment by their antimicrobial compounds; nevertheless, NETs also contribute to tissue damage in inflammatory and autoimmune disorders [16]. Interestingly, the peripheral neutrophils isolated from recruited subjects with NPDR and PRD showed a spontaneous capacity of NET release in vitro compared with diabetic subjects without DR and non-diabetic subjects. It is worth noting that although NET release is elevated in certain DR stages, NETs are not specific markers for diabetic retinopathy. Previously, age has been reported as a factor that influences NET release; neutrophils from young subjects are more prone to release NETs compared to neutrophils obtained from older subjects [35]. However, these findings are reported in stimulated neutrophils, and changes seen are due to failure in neutrophil activation mechanisms related to cell aging [36,37]. In the present study, although there are age differences between subjects, these differences do not impact the found data because we did not use an NET stimulator. We found changes in spontaneous NET release among subjects with DM-2 compared with diabetics with DR; all of them with similar ages.

According to our results, fasting glucose and the HbA1c of DR subjects correlated with the in vitro NET release. It has been reported that hyperglycemia is one external stimulus that is able to induce NET release in diabetic DR subjects [22,38]. In this sense, higher levels of fast glucose and HbA1c were found in all diabetic subjects, suggesting that NET release in diabetic subjects could be used as an indicator of disease deterioration.

It has been reported that chronic inflammation and progression of degenerative age-related eye diseases such as dry eye, glaucoma, age-related macular degeneration, and DR have an association with the participation of neutrophils in the progression and persistence of inflammatory conditions. In this way, reports have shown the overexpression of proinflammatory cytokines such as IL-6, IL-8, and IL1β and an increase in infiltrated neutrophils in diabetic rat retinas, as well as high concentrations of NET-related molecules, such as DNA protein complexes with myeloperoxidase (MPO) or neutrophil elastase (NE), on vitreous and the plasma of DR patients [21,22,39]. In this context, we found that spontaneous NETs released in the recruited groups of patients, as well as the increase in the activation markers CD11b and CD66b of neutrophils, were associated with the time to diagnose T2DM. This suggests that NETs and neutrophils would have a direct involvement in DR progression, maintaining an inflammatory environment.

The clinical values of eGFR involved in plasmatic osmolarity and renal function are indicators of clinical conditions and the state of diabetic patients. Multiple studies suggest that NETs have a strong association with the development of vascular complications and renal diseases [40,41]. In the present study, we found that decreased eGFR levels were present in subjects with moderate and severe NPDR and PDR; likewise, eGFR values had a negative linear correlation with NET area release. Comparably, the plasma osmolarity of subjects with moderate and severe DR was increased and similarly presented a linear correlation with NET release, indicating that NET inflammation could also be associated with renal complications in DR subjects.

Interestingly, we found that the clinical variables, HbA1c, eGFR, and time of T2DM diagnosis, together with the degree of NET release, are factors associated with the development of DR. According to our results, other works have reported some markers from NETs as factors associated with adverse clinical outcomes in atherosclerosis [42]. Similarly, other reports have associated some NET markers, such as citrullinated histone (H3Citr) and DNA extracellular with glucose, IL-6, and HbA1c, in the prediction of a prothrombotic state and hypofibrinolysis during T2DM [20]. Data obtained in this study are from Mexicans; thus, extrapolations to other populations have to be made prudently.

5. Conclusions

Neutrophil extracellular traps have an inflammatory mechanism of neutrophils that have a correlation with clinical variables such as HbA1c, eGFR, and time of diabetes diagnosis and are factors associated with the development of retinopathy.

Supplementary Materials: The following supporting information can be downloaded at https://www.mdpi.com/article/10.3390/biomedicines11071791/s1, Table S1: Demographic data and clinical evaluation of recruited subjects.

Author Contributions: Conceptualization, F.S.M.-G. and Y.G.; methodology, B.B.-V., F.S.M.-G., J.E.A.-F., K.Z.-Á., P.S.-C., I.C.-S. and E.D.l.T.-G.; formal analysis, J.L.R.-L., J.E.A.-F., F.S.M.-G., A.J.-C. and Y.G.; investigation, F.S.M.-G., I.C.-S., K.Z.-Á., P.S.-C., J.L.R.-L. and Y.G.; resources, Y.G.; writing—original draft preparation, F.S.M.-G., B.B.-V. and Y.G.; writing—review and editing, B.B.-V. and Y.G.; project administration F.S.M.-G. and B.B.-V.; funding acquisition, F.S.M.-G. and Y.G. All authors have read and agreed to the published version of the manuscript.

Funding: This research was sponsored by the Institute of Ophthalmology Conde de Valenciana Foundation and was funded by the Support Program for Research and Technological Innovation Projects of the Universidad Nacional Autónoma de México (UNAM-DGAPA-PAPIIT: IN203821), and the Ministry of Education, Science, Technology, and Innovation of México City (grant No. SECTEI 250/2019). J.E.A.-F. is a master's student at the Programa de Maestría en Ciencias de la Salud and has received a CONACyT Fellowship, CVU number 885311. F.S.M.-G. is the guarantor of this work; this author had full access to all the data in the study and takes responsibility for the integrity of the data and the accuracy of the data analysis.

Institutional Review Board Statement: The study was carried out according to the tenets of the Helsinki Declaration and was approved by the Institutional Review Boards of Research, Ethics, and Biosecurity of the "Conde de Valenciana" Institute of Ophthalmology (CEI-2020/01/01). All patients signed an informed consent form.

Informed Consent Statement: Informed consent was obtained from all subjects involved in the study. Written informed consent has been obtained from the patients to publish this paper.

Data Availability Statement: All data will be shared upon request.

Acknowledgments: The authors wish to acknowledge Mohamed Ali Pereyra Morales and Oscar Vivanco Rojas for their invaluable technical support.

Conflicts of Interest: The authors declare no conflict of interest.

References

1. Barquera, S.; Pedroza-Tobias, A.; Medina, C. Cardiovascular diseases in mega-countries: The challenges of the nutrition, physical activity and epidemiologic transitions, and the double burden of disease. *Curr. Opin. Lipidol.* **2016**, *27*, 329–344. [CrossRef] [PubMed]
2. Wang, W.; Lo, A.C.Y. Diabetic Retinopathy: Pathophysiology and Treatments. *Int. J. Mol. Sci.* **2018**, *19*, 1816. [CrossRef] [PubMed]
3. Wu, L. Classification of diabetic retinopathy and diabetic macular edema. *World J. Diabetes* **2013**, *4*, 290–294. [CrossRef] [PubMed]
4. Lechner, J.; O'Leary, O.E.; Stitt, A.W. The pathology associated with diabetic retinopathy. *Vis. Res.* **2017**, *139*, 7–14. [CrossRef]
5. Milne, R.; Brownstein, S. Advanced glycation end products and diabetic retinopathy. *Amino Acids* **2011**, *44*, 1397–1407. [CrossRef]

6. Kolaczkowska, E.; Kubes, P. Neutrophil recruitment and function in health and inflammation. *Nat. Rev. Immunol.* **2013**, *13*, 159–175. [CrossRef]
7. Rada, B. Neutrophil Extracellular Traps. *Methods Mol. Biol.* **2019**, *1982*, 517–528.
8. Cappenberg, A.; Kardell, M.; Zarbock, A. Selectin-Mediated Signaling—Shedding Light on the Regulation of Integrin Activity in Neutrophils. *Cells* **2022**, *11*, 1310. [CrossRef]
9. Zhou, H.; Liao, J.; Aloor, J.; Nie, H.; Wilson, B.C.; Fessler, M.B.; Gao, H.-M.; Hong, J.-S. CD11b/CD18 (Mac-1) Is a Novel Surface Receptor for Extracellular Double-Stranded RNA To Mediate Cellular Inflammatory Responses. *J. Immunol.* **2013**, *190*, 115–125. [CrossRef]
10. Czaikoski, P.G.; Mota, J.M.S.C.; Nascimento, D.C.; Sônego, F.; Castanheira, F.V.E.S.; Melo, P.H.; Scortegagna, G.T.; Silva, R.L.; Barroso-Sousa, R.; Souto, F.O.; et al. Neutrophil Extracellular Traps Induce Organ Damage during Experimental and Clinical Sepsis. *PLoS ONE* **2016**, *11*, e0148142. [CrossRef]
11. Perdomo, J.; Leung, H.H.; Ahmadi, Z.; Yan, F.; Chong, J.J.; Passam, F.H.; Chong, B.H. Neutrophil activation and NETosis are the major drivers of thrombosis in heparin-induced thrombocyto-penia. *Nat. Commun.* **2019**, *10*, 1322. [CrossRef]
12. Brinkmann, V.; Zychlinsky, A. Neutrophil extracellular traps: Is immunity the second function of chromatin? *J. Cell Biol.* **2012**, *198*, 773–783. [CrossRef]
13. Khandpur, R.; Carmona-Rivera, C.; Vivekanandan-Giri, A.; Gizinski, A.; Yalavarthi, S.; Knight, J.S.; Friday, S.; Li, S.; Patel, R.M.; Subramanian, V.; et al. NETs Are a Source of Citrullinated Autoantigens and Stimulate Inflammatory Responses in Rheumatoid Arthritis. *Sci. Transl. Med.* **2013**, *5*, 178ra40. [CrossRef]
14. Leffler, J.; Martin, M.; Gullstrand, B.; Tydén, H.; Lood, C.; Truedsson, L.; Bengtsson, A.A.; Blom, A.M. Neutrophil Extracellular Traps That Are Not Degraded in Systemic Lupus Erythematosus Activate Complement Exacerbating the Disease. *J. Immunol.* **2012**, *188*, 3522–3531. [CrossRef]
15. Dicker, A.J.; Crichton, M.L.; Pumphrey, E.G.; Cassidy, A.J.; Suarez-Cuartin, G.; Sibila, O.; Furrie, E.; Fong, C.J.; Ibrahim, W.; Brady, G.; et al. Neutrophil extracellular traps are associated with disease severity and microbiota diversity in patients with chronic obstructive pulmonary disease. *J. Allergy Clin. Immunol.* **2018**, *141*, 117–127. [CrossRef]
16. Kumar, S.; Gupta, E.; Kaushik, S.; Jyoti, A. Neutrophil Extracellular Traps: Formation and Involvement in Disease Progression. *Iran. J. Allergy Asthma Immunol.* **2018**, *17*, 208–220.
17. Seo, J.D.; Gu, J.-Y.; Jung, H.S.; Kim, Y.J.; Kim, H.K. Contact System Activation and Neutrophil Extracellular Trap Markers: Risk Factors for Portal Vein Thrombosis in Patients With Hepatocellular Carcinoma. *Clin. Appl. Thromb.* **2019**, *25*, 1076029618825310. [CrossRef]
18. Menegazzo, L.; Ciciliot, S.; Poncina, N.; Mazzucato, M.; Persano, M.; Bonora, B.; Albiero, M.; de Kreutzenberg, S.V.; Avogaro, A.; Fadini, G.P. NETosis is induced by high glucose and associated with type 2 diabetes. *Acta Diabetol.* **2014**, *52*, 497–503. [CrossRef]
19. Carestia, A.; Frechtel, G.; Cerrone, G.; Linari, M.A.; Gonzalez, C.; Casais, P.; Schattner, M. NETosis before and after Hyperglycemic Control in Type 2 Diabetes Mellitus Patients. *PLoS ONE* **2016**, *11*, e0168647. [CrossRef]
20. Bryk, A.H.; Prior, S.M.; Plens, K.; Konieczynska, M.; Hohendorff, J.; Malecki, M.T.; Butenas, S.; Undas, A. Predictors of neutrophil extracellular traps markers in type 2 diabetes mellitus: Associations with a pro-thrombotic state and hypofibrinolysis. *Cardiovasc. Diabetol.* **2019**, *18*, 49. [CrossRef]
21. Park, J.-H.; Kim, J.-E.; Gu, J.-Y.; Yoo, H.J.; Kim, Y.I.; Nam-Goong, I.S.; Kim, E.S.; Kim, H.K. Evaluation of Circulating Markers of Neutrophil Extracellular Trap (NET) Formation as Risk Factors for Diabetic Retinopathy in a Case-Control Association Study. *Exp. Clin. Endocrinol. Diabetes* **2016**, *124*, 557–561. [CrossRef] [PubMed]
22. Wang, L.; Zhou, X.; Yin, Y.; Mai, Y.; Wang, D.; Zhang, X. Hyperglycemia Induces Neutrophil Extracellular Traps Formation Through an NADPH Oxidase-Dependent Pathway in Diabetic Retinopathy. *Front. Immunol.* **2019**, *9*, 3076. [CrossRef] [PubMed]
23. Estúa-Acosta, G.A.; Buentello-Volante, B.; Magaña-Guerrero, F.S.; Flores, J.E.A.; Vivanco-Rojas, O.; Castro-Salas, I.; Zarco-Ávila, K.; García-Mejía, M.A.; Garfias, Y. Human Amniotic Membrane Mesenchymal Stem Cell-Synthesized PGE(2) Exerts an Immunomod-ulatory Effect on Neutrophil Extracellular Trap in a PAD-4-Dependent Pathway through EP2 and EP4. *Cells* **2022**, *11*, 2831. [CrossRef] [PubMed]
24. Lee, K.H.; Cavanaugh, L.; Leung, H.; Yan, F.; Ahmadi, Z.; Chong, B.H.; Passam, F. Quantification of NETs-associated markers by flow cytometry and serum assays in patients with thrombosis and sepsis. *Int. J. Lab. Hematol.* **2018**, *40*, 392–399. [CrossRef] [PubMed]
25. Joshi, M.B.; Ahamed, R.; Hegde, M.; Nair, A.S.; Ramachandra, L.; Satyamoorthy, K. Glucose induces metabolic reprogramming in neutrophils during type 2 diabetes to form constitutive extra-cellular traps and decreased responsiveness to lipopolysaccharides. *Biochim. Biophys. Acta (BBA)-Mol. Basis Dis.* **2020**, *1866*, 165940. [CrossRef]
26. Freitas, D.F.; Colón, D.F.; Silva, R.L.; Santos, E.M.; Guimarães, V.H.D.; Ribeiro, G.H.M.; de Paula, A.M.B.; Guimarães, A.L.S.; dos Reis, S.T.; Cunha, F.Q.; et al. Neutrophil extracellular traps (NETs) modulate inflammatory profile in obese humans and mice: Adipose tissue role on NETs levels. *Mol. Biol. Rep.* **2022**, *49*, 3225–3236. [CrossRef]
27. Shafqat, A.; Rab, S.A.; Ammar, O.; Al Salameh, S.; Alkhudairi, A.; Kashir, J.; Alkattan, K.; Yaqinuddin, A. Emerging role of neutrophil extracellular traps in the complications of diabetes mellitus. *Front. Med.* **2022**, *9*, 995993. [CrossRef]
28. Lessieur, E.M.; Liu, H.; Saadane, A.; Du, Y.; Tang, J.; Kiser, J.; Kern, T.S. Neutrophil-Derived Proteases Contribute to the Pathogenesis of Early Diabetic Retinopathy. *Investig. Opthalmology Vis. Sci.* **2021**, *62*, 7. [CrossRef]

29. Liu, H.; Lessieur, E.M.; Saadane, A.; Lindstrom, S.I.; Taylor, P.R.; Kern, T.S. Neutrophil elastase contributes to the pathological vascular permeability characteristic of diabetic retinopathy. *Diabetologia* **2019**, *62*, 2365–2374. [CrossRef]
30. Van Oostrom, A.J.; Van Wijk, J.P.; Sijmonsma, T.P.; Rabelink, T.J.; Cabezas, M.C. Increased expression of activation markers on monocytes and neutrophils in type 2 diabetes. *Neth. J. Med.* **2004**, *62*, 320–325.
31. Qiu, X.; Li, J.; Yang, X.; Tang, J.; Shi, J.; Tong, Y.; Qu, Y.; Mu, D. Is neutrophil CD11b a special marker for the early diagnosis of sepsis in neonates? A systematic review and meta-analysis. *BMJ Open* **2019**, *9*, e025222. [CrossRef]
32. Quaas, A.; Pamuk, A.; Klein, S.; Quantius, J.; Rehkaemper, J.; Barutcu, A.G.; Rueschoff, J.; Zander, T.; Gebauer, F.; Hillmer, A.; et al. Sex-specific prognostic effect of CD66b-positive tumor-infiltrating neutrophils (TANs) in gastric and esoph-ageal adenocarcinoma. *Gastric Cancer* **2021**, *24*, 1213–1226. [CrossRef]
33. Cong, X.; Zhang, Y.; Zhu, Z.; Li, S.; Yin, X.; Zhai, Z.; Zhang, Y.; Xue, Y. CD66b(+) neutrophils and alpha-SMA(+) fibroblasts predict clinical outcomes and benefits from postoperative chemotherapy in gastric adenocarcinoma. *Cancer Med.* **2020**, *9*, 2761–2773. [CrossRef]
34. Yamada, Y.; Nakagawa, T.; Sugihara, T.; Horiuchi, T.; Yoshizaki, U.; Fujimura, T.; Fukuhara, H.; Urano, T.; Takayama, K.; Inoue, S.; et al. Prognostic value of CD66b positive tumor-infiltrating neutrophils in testicular germ cell tumor. *BMC Cancer* **2016**, *16*, 898. [CrossRef]
35. Sabbatini, M.; Bona, E.; Novello, G.; Migliario, M.; Renò, F. Aging hampers neutrophil extracellular traps (NETs) efficacy. *Aging Clin. Exp. Res.* **2022**, *34*, 2345–2353. [CrossRef]
36. Wong, S.L.; Wagner, D.D. Peptidylarginine deiminase 4: A nuclear button triggering neutrophil extracellular traps in inflammatory diseases and aging. *FASEB J.* **2018**, *32*, 6258–6370. [CrossRef]
37. Xu, F.; Zhang, C.; Zou, Z.; Fan, E.K.Y.; Chen, L.; Li, Y.; Billiar, T.R.; Wilson, M.A.; Shi, X.; Fan, J. Aging-related Atg5 defect impairs neutrophil extracellular traps formation. *Immunology* **2017**, *151*, 417–432. [CrossRef]
38. Mikhalchik, E.V.; Lipatova, V.A.; Basyreva, L.Y.; Panasenko, O.M.; Gusev, S.A.; Sergienko, V.I. Hyperglycemia and Some Aspects of Leukocyte Activation In Vitro. *Bull. Exp. Biol. Med.* **2021**, *170*, 748–751. [CrossRef]
39. Martinez-Alberquilla, I.; Gasull, X.; Perez-Luna, P.; Seco-Mera, R.; Ruiz-Alcocer, J.; Crooke, A. Neutrophils and neutrophil extracellular trap components: Emerging biomarkers and thera-peutic targets for age-related eye diseases. *Ageing Res. Rev.* **2022**, *74*, 101553. [CrossRef]
40. Arneth, B.; Arneth, R. Neutrophil Extracellular Traps (NETs) and Vasculitis. *Int. J. Med. Sci.* **2021**, *18*, 1532–1540. [CrossRef]
41. Salazar-Gonzalez, H.; Zepeda-Hernandez, A.; Melo, Z.; Saavedra-Mayorga, D.E.; Echavarria, R. Neutrophil Extracellular Traps in the Establishment and Progression of Renal Diseases. *Medicina* **2019**, *55*, 431. [CrossRef] [PubMed]
42. Langseth, M.S.; Opstad, T.B.; Bratseth, V.; Solheim, S.; Arnesen, H.; Pettersen, A.; Seljeflot, I.; Helseth, R. Markers of neutrophil extracellular traps are associated with adverse clinical outcome in stable coronary artery disease. *Eur. J. Prev. Cardiol.* **2018**, *25*, 762–769. [CrossRef] [PubMed]

biomedicines

MDPI

Article

Relationship between Diabetic Nephropathy and Development of Diabetic Macular Edema in Addition to Diabetic Retinopathy

Yukihisa Suzuki [1,2,*] and Motohiro Kiyosawa [3]

1 Department of Ophthalmology, Japan Community Health Care Organization, Mishima General Hospital, Shizuoka 411-0801, Japan
2 Research Team for Neuroimaging, Tokyo Metropolitan Institute of Gerontology, Tokyo 173-0015, Japan
3 Jiyugaoka Kiyosawa Eye Clinic, Tokyo 152-0035, Japan; nra12337@nifty.com
* Correspondence: suzuki@f8.dion.ne.jp; Tel.: +81-55-975-3031; Fax: +81-55-973-3647

Abstract: This study aimed to examine the relationship between diabetic retinopathy (DR) and systemic factors. We evaluated 261 patients (143 men, 118 women, aged 70.1 ± 10.1 years) with type 2 diabetes. All participants underwent a fundus examination, fundus photography using spectral domain optical coherence tomography (SD-OCT), and blood tests. For glycated hemoglobin (HbA1c) levels, the average and highest values in the past were used. We observed DR in 127 (70 men and 57 women) of 261 patients. Logistic regression analyses revealed a significant correlation between DR development and the duration of diabetes (OR = 2.40; 95% CI: 1.50), average HbA1c level (OR = 5.57; 95% CI: 1.27, 24.4), highest HbA1c level (OR = 2.46; 95% CI: 1.12, 5.38), and grade of diabetic nephropathy (DN) (OR = 6.23; 95% CI: 2.70, 14.4). Regression analyses revealed a significant correlation between the severity of DR and duration of diabetes (t = −6.66; 95% CI: 0.21, 0.39), average HbA1c level (t = 2.59; 95% CI: 0.14, 1.02), and severity of DN (t = 6.10; 95% CI: 0.49, 0.97). Logistic regression analyses revealed a significant correlation between diabetic macular edema (DME) development and DN grade (OR = 2.22; 95% CI: 1.33, 3.69). DN grade correlates with the development of DR and DME, and decreased renal function predicts the onset of DR.

Keywords: diabetic macular edema; diabetic nephropathy; diabetic retinopathy; risk factors

1. Introduction

Diabetes is a disease that causes chronic hyperglycemia due to insufficient insulin secretion or insulin action. The number of people with diabetes worldwide was estimated at 420 million in 2015. This number is currently on the rise and is expected to reach 640 million by 2040 [1]. There are two main types of diabetes: insulin-dependent type 1 diabetes and non-insulin-dependent type 2 diabetes. In type 1 diabetes, almost no endogenous insulin is secreted due to the dysfunction of the insulin-producing beta cells. Type 2 diabetes is a disease in which endogenous insulin is secreted to some extent, but hyperglycemia occurs due to impaired insulin secretion or insulin resistance [2]. Complications of diabetes include retinopathy, nephropathy, and neuropathy, which can occur in both type 1 and type 2 diabetes.

Diabetic retinopathy (DR) is a microvascular complication caused by persistent hyperglycemia that is common in diabetic patients and is a major cause of blindness along with glaucoma and age-related macular degeneration [3]. DR is classified into non-proliferative DR and proliferative DR, according to the degree of disease progression, and may be complicated by macular edema. Patients with nonproliferative DR are typically asymptomatic. If proliferative DR develops, the patient may present with a sudden loss of vision due to a vitreous hemorrhage. In type 2 diabetes, the incidence with 5 years of evolution is 20%, while with 15 years of evolution, it reaches 80% [4]. The risk of developing DR is thought to be associated with the duration of diabetes, hypertension, hyperlipidemia, and glycated hemoglobin (HbA1c) levels [5]. HbA1c levels have been reported to be significantly associated with the progression of DR [6], and glycemic variability has been found to be associated with DR in type 2 diabetes [7]. In many patients with diabetes, HbA1c levels fluctuate from month to month and are thought to affect the retina over the next several decades. We thought it necessary to investigate the effects of the average HbA1c level and highest HbA1c level over the past years on the development and severity of retinopathy, respectively.

Macular edema (ME) can develop in various diseases such as uveitis [8], retinal vein occlusion [9], and diabetic macular edema [10] and is a major cause of vision loss. In macular edema, fluid leaking from capillaries accumulates in the subretinal or intraretinal region of the macula [11]. Diabetic macular edema (DME) also occurs with some frequency in non-proliferative DR and is a major cause of vision loss in such patients [12]. DME is defined as "retinal thickening within one disk diameter of the center of the macula or definite hard exudates in this region" [13]. The risk factors for developing DME include long-term diabetes, hypertension, and high HbA1c levels [14].

Diabetic nephropathy (DN) is also a major and important microvascular complication in diabetes [15]. DN is the leading cause of chronic kidney disease and accounts for 40% of new cases of end-stage renal disease each year. DN is characterized by persistent albuminuria and decreased glomerular filtration rate (GFR) and also causes elevated blood pressure. In patients with DN, persistent albuminuria reflects glomerular injury but may also reflect generalized endothelial dysfunction and widespread vascular injury [16,17]. Several studies have reported that DN is associated with the development and progression of DR [6,18]. DN generally causes body edema along with hypertension and proteinuria [19]. In patients with DN, hyperpermeability of the retinal blood vessels is expected to occur due to microvascular abnormalities, which are presumed to cause an increased leakage of serum into the extracellular space [20].

We hypothesized that DR development and severity are related not only to past average HbA1c levels but also to the highest HbA1c level. We also hypothesized that DME development is associated with DN. We investigated risk factors for developing DR and DME in patients with type 2 diabetes using logistic regression analyses.

2. Materials and Methods

2.1. Standard Protocol Approvals, Registrations, and Patient Consents

The study protocol was approved by the institutional ethics committee of the Japan Community Health Care Organization, Mishima General Hospital (protocol code: H30-005 and date of approval: 5 October 2018). All the procedures conformed to the tenets of the Declaration of Helsinki. All measurements in this study were performed at the Japan Community Health Care Organization Mishima General Hospital. Informed consent was obtained from all participants prior to participation in the study.

2.2. Subjects and Examination

This study is retrospective consecutive case series. Our study included 261 patients (143 men, 118 women, aged 70.1 $\pm$ 10.1 years) with type 2 diabetes who visited the Department of Ophthalmology, Mishima General Hospital. Type 1 diabetes and type 2 diabetes are inherently different pathologies [1,2]. It has been also reported that the incidence of DR differs between type 1 diabetes and type 2 diabetes [21,22], and in this study, only type 2 diabetes was focused on. Individuals with diabetes were classified as those with fasting plasma glucose >126 mg/dL or casual blood glucose >200 mg/dL and a previous diagnosis of diabetes by an internist. Inclusion criteria included patients who had regular medical examinations and required blood tests (HbA1c, creatinine) and urinalysis (urinary protein, urinary albumin). Patients with HbA1c data at least once every 6 months and at least the past 7 years were included (Figure 1). Exclusion criteria were lack of HbA1c data for the past 7 years and being unable to perform urinalysis due to chronic renal failure. We performed fundus examination and fundus photography using spectral-domain optical coherence tomography (SD-OCT) after mydriasis in all cases. OCT scans were acquired using an RS-3000 device (NIDEK, Gamagori, Japan), capturing an area of 9 × 9 mm^2 centered on the fovea. We performed fluorescein angiography to determine the grade of DR in patients with DR. In addition, the presence or absence of DME was determined from SD-OCT images. Blood tests (HbA1c, creatinine, LDL, triglyceride) and urinalysis (urinary protein, urinary albumin) were taken from ophthalmological examinations within 2 months, if available, or newly performed. The estimated glomerular filtration rate (eGFR) in each case was calculated from the blood creatinine level and age. Based on these data, we examined the stages of DR and DN in each case. The new Fukuda classification was used to diabetic retinopathy [23]. DR is divided into benign (type A) and malignant (type B), each of which is divided into five stages. Benign retinopathies include background retinopathy (A1 and A2) before proliferative changes and interrupted proliferative retinopathy (A3, A4, and A5) after photocoagulation or vitrectomy. Benign retinopathy includes background retinopathy (A1 and A2) and interrupted proliferative retinopathy (A3, A4, and A5) after photocoagulation or vitrectomy. DME is defined as a retinal thickening within 500 µm of the fovea or hard exudates at or within 500 µm of the fovea associated with adjacent retinal thickening or an area of retinal thickening that is one disc area or larger in size located one disc diameter (1500 µm) or less from the fovea [24]. We defined DME severity as none, mild (identified by retinal thickening or hard exudates in the posterior pole but distant from the center of the macula), moderate (characterized by retinal thickening or hard exudates approaching the center of the macula but not affected by the center), and severe (characterized by retinal thickening or hard exudates affecting the center of the macular) [25]. The diabetic nephropathy staging [26] was used for DN staging. The diabetic nephropathy staging classifies nephropathy into five stages from the 1st stage (early stage of nephropathy) to the 5th stage (dialysis therapy stage) using urinary albumin level or urinary protein level and eGFR. Urinary albumin levels were classified into A1 (less than 30 mg/day), A2 (30–299 mg/day), and A3 (300 mg/day or more) according to the KINGO CKD guideline 2012. We examined each patient for a history of ischemic heart disease and use of rennin-angiotensin-aldosterone system (RAS) inhibitors and sodium/glucose cotransporter (SGLT)-2 inhibitors.

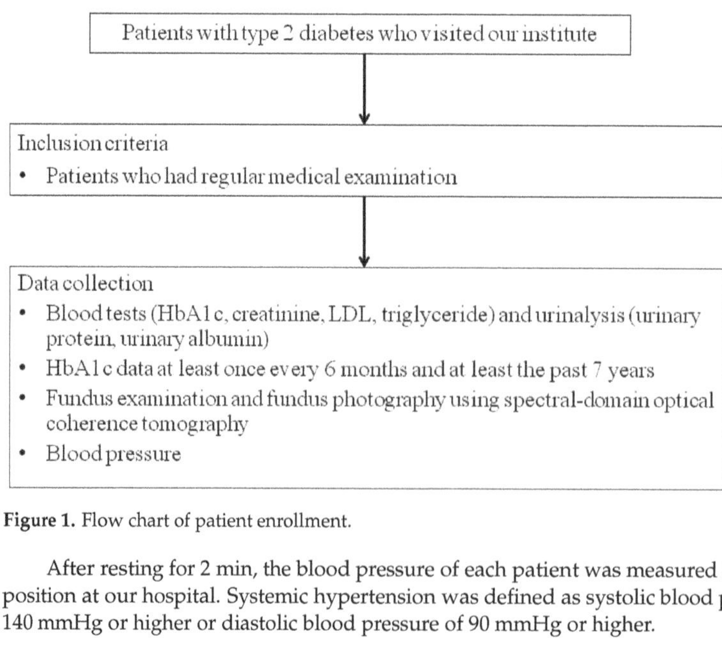

Figure 1. Flow chart of patient enrollment.

After resting for 2 min, the blood pressure of each patient was measured in a sitting position at our hospital. Systemic hypertension was defined as systolic blood pressure of 140 mmHg or higher or diastolic blood pressure of 90 mmHg or higher.

We collected data on blood tests (HbA1c, creatinine, LDL, triglyceride) and urinalysis (urinary protein, urinary albumin), fundus examination, and fundus photography using spectral-domain optical coherence tomography, and blood pressure. HbA1c data were collected at least once every 6 months and for at least the past 7 years.

2.3. Data Processing and Analysis of Risk Factors for Development and Severity of DR

The DR and DN stages in each case were converted into numerical values (retinopathy, 0–7, nephropathy, 1–5). We performed multivariable logistic regression analyses on all patients with type 2 diabetes to investigate the risk factors for developing DR. We selected the eye with more severe DR as the target eye for each patient. Cases with DR developing in only one eye were included in patients with DR. We used the Kolmogorov–Smirnov test to examine whether DR stage, average HbA1c level, high HbA1c level, and eGFR were normally distributed.

Multivariable logistic regression analyses were performed to determine the association between the parameters (gender, duration of diabetes, body mass index, systemic hypertension, average HbA1c level, highest HbA1c level, serum LDL, and serum triglyceride, DN stage, ischemic heart disease, and use of RAS inhibitors and SGLT-2 inhibitors) and a diagnosis of type 2 diabetes. Odds ratios (OR) and 95% confidence intervals (CI) were calculated for each factor. Statistical significance for all analyses was defined as $p < 0.05$.

We also performed a regression analysis between DR stage and the parameters (gender, duration of diabetes, body mass index, systemic hypertension, average HbA1c level, highest HbA1c level, serum LDL, and serum triglyceride, DN stage, ischemic heart disease, and use of RAS inhibitors and SGLT-2 inhibitors) in patients with DR. If the DR stages of the left and right eyes were different, the more severe stage was considered as the DR stage of the patient. The t-statistic and 95% CI were estimated for each factor. Statistical significance for all analyses was defined as $p < 0.05$.

These regression models were constructed by identifying potential confounding variables. All analyses were conducted using EZR [27] (Saitama Medical Center, Jichi Medical University, Saitama, Japan), a graphical user interface for R (The R Foundation for Statistical Computing, Vienna, Austria).

2.4. Analysis of Risk Factors for Developing DME

We performed multivariable logistic regression analyses on all patients with type 2 diabetes to investigate the risk factors for DME. Multivariable logistic regression analyses were performed to determine the association between the parameters (gender, duration of diabetes, body mass index, systemic hypertension, average HbA1c level, highest HbA1c level, serum LDL, serum triglyceride, DN stage, ischemic heart disease, and use of RAS inhibitors and SGLT-2 inhibitors) and the presence of DME. Cases with DME developing in only one eye were included in patients with DME. The t-statistic and 95% CI were estimated for each factor. Statistical significance for all analyses was defined as $p < 0.05$.

We also performed a regression analysis between DME stage and the parameters (gender, duration of diabetes, body mass index, systemic hypertension, average HbA1c level, highest HbA1c level, serum LDL, and serum triglyceride, DN stage, ischemic heart disease, and use of RAS inhibitors and SGLT-2 inhibitors) in patients. If the DME stages of the left and right eyes were different, the more severe stage was considered the DME stage of the patient. The t-statistic and 95% CI were estimated for each factor. Statistical significance for all analyses was defined as $p < 0.05$.

2.5. Data Availability

All data used for analysis are presented in the tables in this article. Data will be provided in anonymized form after ethics approval if requested by other investigators for purposes of replicating the results.

3. Results

3.1. Our Patients with Type 2 Diabetes

We observed 127 (70 men and 57 women) patients with DR and 134 (73 men and 61 women) without DR (Table 1). The diabetes duration was significantly longer in patients with DR than in patients without DR. The average and highest HbA1c levels were significantly higher in patients with DR than in patients without DR. In addition, eGFR was low in patients with DR, and the DN grade was also high in patients with DR. On the other hand, DME was observed in 64 (50.4%) patients with DR but not in patients without DR. There were no differences in body mass index, prevalence of systemic hypertension, serum LDL, and serum triglyceride.

Table 1. Demographic data of patients with type 2 diabetes.

	With DR	Without DR	*p* Value
Male:Female	70:57	73:61	0.9
Average year	68.9 ± 10.8	71.2 ± 9.4	0.8
Diabetes duration	12.0 ± 2.7	9.8 ± 2.0	<0.0000001
DME	64 (50.4%)	0 (0%)	<0.0000001
Body mass index	24.2 ± 4.8	24.0 ± 4.5	0.9
Hypertension	61 (48.0%)	51 (38.1%)	0.1
Average HbA1c	7.9 ± 1.3	6.9 ± 0.7	<0.0000001
Highest HbA1c	9.5 ± 2.0	7.7 ± 1.3	<0.0000001
Serum LDL	117.3 ± 34.8	115.9 ± 31.7	0.4
Serum triglyceride	151.6 ± 137.3	139.8 ± 69.3	0.4
eGFR	56.2 ± 26.4	67.1 ± 17.0	0.00008
DN stage	2.4 ± 1.2	1.4 ± 0.6	<0.0000001
Ischemic heart disease	9 (7.1%)	5 (3.7%)	0.2
RAS inhibitors	22 (17.3%)	38 (28.4%)	0.04
SGLT-2 inhibitors	20 (15.7%)	23 (17.2%)	0.8

DR: diabetic retinopathy, DME: diabetic macular edema, DN: diabetic nephropathy, HbA1c: glycated hemoglobin, LDL: low-density lipoprotein, eGFR: estimated glomerular filtration rate, RAS: rennin-angiotensin-aldosterone system, SGLT: sodium/glucose cotransporter.

3.2. Kolmogorov-Smirnov Test

The DR grade ($p < 0.001$), average HBA1c level ($p = 0.001$), and high HBA1c level ($p = 0.002$) were not normally distributed, while eGFR was normally distributed.

3.3. Risk Factors for the Development of DR

Multivariate logistic regression analyses revealed a significant correlation between DR development and the diabetes duration (OR = 2.77; 95% CI: 1.14, 2.39; $p = 0.009$), average HbA1c level (OR = 5.60; 95% CI: 1.36, 23.1; $p = 0.02$), highest HbA1c level (OR = 2.46; 95% CI: 1.12–5.38; $p = 0.02$), and DN stage (OR = 7.62; 95% CI: 2.63, 22.1; $p = 0.0002$) (Table 2). Univariate analysis revealed a significant correlation between DR development and the eGFR (OR = 0.98; 95% CI: 0.97, 0.99; $p = 0.0001$), albuminuria (OR = 5.23; 95% CI: 3.14, 8.71; $p < 0.00001$) (Table 3). No significant correlation was observed between DR development and the other parameters.

Table 2. Multivariate logistic regression analyses related to diabetic retinopathy development.

Factor	Odds Ratio	95% CI	*p* Value
Gender (male = 1, female = 0)	2.77	0.43, 17.9	0.3
Diabetes duration	1.65	1.14, 2.39	0.009
Body mass index	1.08	0.87, 1.32	0.5
Hypertension	0.42	0.09, 2.03	0.3
Average HbA1c	5.60	1.36, 23.1	0.02
Highest HbA1c	2.46	1.12, 5.38	0.02
Serum LDL	1.02	0.99, 1.04	0.2
Serum triglyceride	0.99	0.98, 1.00	0.07
DN stage	7.62	2.63, 22.1	0.0002
History of ischemic heart disease	0.55	0.03, 8.82	0.7
RAS inhibitors prescription	1.27	0.26, 6.18	0.8
SGLT-2 inhibitors prescription	1.57	0.30, 8.15	0.6

DN: diabetic nephropathy, HbA1c: glycated hemoglobin, LDL: low-density lipoprotein, RAS: rennin-angiotensin-aldosterone system, SGLT: sodium/glucose cotransporter.

Table 3. Univariate analysis with diabetic retinopathy development.

Factor	Odds Ratio	95% CI	*p* Value
eGFR	0.98	0.97, 0.99	0.0001
Albuminuria	5.23	3.14, 8.71	<0.00001
History of ischemic heart disease	0.55	0.03, 8.82	0.7
RAS inhibitors prescription	0.77	0.42, 1.40	0.4
SGLT-2 inhibitors prescription	1.55	0.79, 3.03	0.2

eGFR: estimated glomerular filtration rate RAS: rennin-angiotensin-aldosterone system, SGLT: sodium/glucose cotransporter.

3.4. Risk Factors for Severity of DR

Multivariate regression analyses revealed a significant correlation between DR severity and diabetes duration ($t = 4.97$; 95% CI: 0.15, 0.36; $p < 0.00001$), average HbA1c level ($t = 3.25$; 95% CI: 0.14, 1.02; $p = 0.002$), and DN stage ($t = 4.32$; 95% CI: 0.33, 0.89; $p = 0.00004$) (Table 4). Univariate analysis revealed a significant correlation between DR severity and the eGFR (OR = −4.96; 95% CI: −0.04, −0.020; $p < 0.00001$), albuminuria (OR = 0.19; 95% CI: 1.24, 1.99; $p < 0.00001$) (Table 5). No significant correlation was observed between the DR stage and the other parameters.

Table 4. Multivariate regression analyses related to severity of diabetic retinopathy.

Factor	*t*-Statistic	95% CI	*p* Value
Gender (male = 1, female = 0)	−1.35	−0.85, 0.16	0.4
Diabetes duration	4.97	0.15, 0.36	<0.00001
Body mass index	−0.32	−0.08, 0.05	0.8
Hypertension	−1.99	−1.01, 0.005	0.06
Average HbA1c	3.25	0.14, 1.02	0.002
Highest HbA1c	−0.87	−0.43, 0.17	0.4

Table 4. *Cont.*

Factor	*t*-Statistic	95% CI	*p* Value
Serum LDL	1.60	−0.002, 0.02	0.1
Serum triglyceride	−0.26	−0.002, 0.002	0.8
DN stage	4.32	0.33, 0.89	0.00004
History of ischemic heart disease	1.30	−0.35, 1.68	0.2
RAS inhibitors prescription	0.71	−0.39, 0.82	0.5
SGLT-2 inhibitors prescription	0.66	−0.45, 0.89	0.5

DN: diabetic nephropathy, HbA1c: glycated hemoglobin, LDL: low-density lipoprotein. RAS: rennin-angiotensin-aldosterone system, SGLT: sodium/glucose cotransporter.

Table 5. Univariate analysis with severity of diabetic retinopathy.

Factor	*t*-Statistic	95% CI	*p* Value
eGFR	−4.96	−0.04, −0.02	<0.00001
Albuminuria	0.19	1.24, 1.99	<0.00001
History of ischemic heart disease	1.67	−0.16, 1.91	0.1
RAS inhibitors prescription	0.27	−0.68, 0.39	0.6
SGLT-2 inhibitors prescription	1.55	0.79, 3.03	0.5

eGFR: estimated glomerular filtration rate, RAS: rennin-angiotensin-aldosterone system, SGLT: sodium/glucose cotransporter.

3.5. Risk Factors for the Development of DME

Multivariate logistic regression analyses revealed a significant correlation between DME development and the diabetes duration (OR = 1.33; 95% CI: 1.01, 1.75; $p = 0.04$), DN stage (OR = 2.80; 95% CI: 1.37, 5.72; $p = 0.005$) (Table 6). Univariate analysis revealed a significant correlation between DME development and the eGFR (OR = 0.98; 95% CI: 0.97, 0.99; $p = 0.009$), albuminuria (OR = 4.05; 95% CI: 2.30, 7.11; $p < 0.00001$) (Table 7). No significant correlation was observed between DME development and the other parameters.

Table 6. Multivariate logistic regression analyses related to diabetic macular edema development.

Factor	Odds Ratio	95% CI	*p* Value
Gender (male = 1, female = 0)	0.63	0.15, 2.61	0.5
Duration of diabetes	1.33	1.01, 1.75	0.04
Body mass index	0.95	0.79, 1.15	0.6
Hypertension	0.52	0.13, 2.04	0.3
Average HbA1c	5.52	1.27, 24.1	0.02
Highest HbA1c	0.75	0.35, 1.64	0.5
Serum LDL	1.01	0.93, 1.03	0.6
Serum triglyceride	1.00	0.99, 1.00	0.1
DN stage	2.80	1.37, 5.72	0.005
History of ischemic heart disease	2.63	0.27, 25.6	0.4
RAS inhibitors prescription	1.70	−0.27, 0.35	0.2
SGLT-2 inhibitors prescription	−0.12	−0.47, 0.22	0.2

DN: diabetic nephropathy, HbA1c: glycated hemoglobin, LDL: low-density lipoprotein. RAS: rennin-angiotensin-aldosterone system, SGLT: sodium/glucose cotransporter.

Table 7. Univariate analysis with diabetic macular edema development.

Factor	Odds Ratio	95% CI	*p* Value
eGFR	0.98	0.97, 0.99	0.009
Albuminuria	4.05	2.30, 7.11	<0.00001
RAS inhibitors prescription	0.76	0.36, 1.59	0.1
SGLT-2 inhibitors prescription	1.54	0.70, 3.37	0.3

eGFR: estimated glomerular filtration rate, RAS: rennin-angiotensin-aldosterone system, SGLT: sodium/glucose cotransporter.

3.6. *Risk Factors for Severity of DME*

Multivariate regression analyses revealed a significant correlation between DME severity and diabetes duration ($t = 2.57$; 95% CI: 0.02, 0.13; $p = 0.001$), average HbA1c level ($t = 2.54$; 95% CI: 0.08, 0.68; $p = 0.01$), and DN stage ($t = 2.48$; 95% CI: 0.04, 0.36; $p = 0.002$) (Table 8). Univariate analysis revealed a significant correlation between DR severity and the eGFR (OR = −2.44; 95% CI: −0.009, −0.001; $p = 0.02$), albuminuria (OR = 5.36; 95% CI: 0.26, 0.55; $p < 0.00001$) (Table 9). No significant correlation was observed between the DRE stage and the other parameters.

Table 8. Multivariate regression analyses related to severity of diabetic macular edema.

Factor	*t*-Statistic	95% CI	*p* Value
Gender (male = 1, female = 0)	−0.53	−0.37, 0.21	0.6
Diabetes duration	2.57	0.02, 0.13	0.001
Body mass index	−0.21	−0.04, 0.03	0.8
Hypertension	−1.07	−0.44, 0.13	0.3
Average HbA1c	2.54	0.08, 0.68	0.01
Highest HbA1c	−0.64	−0.22, 0.11	0.5
Serum LDL	0.95	−0.005, 0.005	0.07
Serum triglyceride	−1.92	−0.002, 0.0004	0.06
DN stage	2.48	0.04, 0.36	0.002
History of ischemic heart disease	−0.08	−0.56, 0.52	0.9
RAS inhibitors prescription	0.25	−0.27, 0.35	0.8
SGLT-2 inhibitors prescription	−0.70	−0.47, 0.22	0.5

DN: diabetic nephropathy, HbA1c: glycated hemoglobin, LDL: low-density lipoprotein. RAS: rennin-angiotensin-aldosterone system, SGLT: sodium/glucose cotransporter.

Table 9. Univariate analysis with severity of diabetic macular edema.

Factor	*t*-Statistic	95% CI	*p* Value
eGFR	−2.44	−0.009, −0.001	0.02
Albuminuria	5.36	0.26, 0.55	<0.00001
RAS inhibitors prescription	−0.86	−0.30, 0.12	0.4
SGLT-2 inhibitors prescription	0.30	−0.19, 0.26	0.8

eGFR: estimated glomerular filtration rate, RAS: rennin-angiotensin-aldosterone system, SGLT: sodium/glucose cotransporter.

3.7. *DME Prevalence by DR Grade*

Our patients included 134 patients with Fukuda classification A0, 3 patients with A1, 49 patients with A2, 34 patients with B1, 7 patients with B2, 23 patients with B4, and

3 patients with B5, respectively (Table 10). DME prevalence was 32.7% in A2, 58.8% in B1, 71.4% in B2, 87.0% in B4, and 100% in B5, respectively. Additionally, DME was not observed in A0 and A1.

Table 10. Patients with diabetic macular edema development by diabetic retinopathy grade.

Fukuda Classification	Patients (Male/Female)	DME (Male/Female)	Prevalence
A0	134 (73/61)	0 (0/0)	0%
A1	3 (3/0)	0 (0/0)	0%
A2	49 (26/23)	16 (8/8)	32.7%
B1	34 (21/13)	20 (10/10)	58.8%
B2	7 (4/3)	5 (2/3)	71.4%
B3	0 (0/0)	0 (0/0)	-
B4	23 (11/12)	20 (9/11)	87.0%
B5	3 (2/1)	3 (2/1)	100%

DME: diabetic macular edema.

4. Discussion

We observed 127 (70 men and 57 women) patients with DR and 134 (73 men and 61 women) without DR. The diabetes duration was longer in patients with DR than in patients without DR. The average and highest HbA1c levels were higher in patients with DR than in patients without DR. Multivariate logistic regression analyses revealed a significant correlation between DR development and the duration of diabetes (OR = 1.65), average HbA1c level (OR = 5.60), highest HbA1c level (OR = 1.17), and DN grade (OR = 7.62). Multivariate logistic regression analyses revealed a significant correlation between DR stage and diabetes duration, average HbA1c level, and DN stage. We observed a significant correlation between DME development and diabetes duration (OR = 1.33), average HbA1c level (OR = 5.52), and DN grade (OR = 2.80). Multivariate regression analyses revealed a significant correlation between DME stage and diabetes duration, average HbA1c level, and DN stage.

4.1. Pathophysiology of DR

The primary retinal vascular response to exposure to hyperglycemia is vasodilation and changes in blood flow. These responses are thought to be metabolic autoregulation to increase retinal metabolism in diabetic patients [28]. On the other hand, high glucose triggers apoptosis of capillary pericytes, resulting in the localized outpouching of the capillary walls. This process results in the formation of a microaneurysm, which is the earliest clinical manifestation of DR [29]. In parallel with this, endothelial cell apoptosis and basement membrane thickening in diabetic microvessels, which are associated with blood-retinal barrier (BRB) impairment, have been reported [30]. Furthermore, the loss of vascular pericytes and endothelial cells induces capillary occlusion and causes retinal ischemia. Retinal ischemia and hypoxia activate hypoxia-inducible factor 1 (HIF-1), leading to increased VEGF expression in the eye [31]. VEGF is a growth factor that induces angiogenesis and angiogenesis by stimulating the division, migration, and differentiation of vascular endothelial cells, and it is associated with the progression of PDR and DME. In addition, VEGF has a vascular hyperpermeability effect [32,33]. Adamis et al. [34] observed that VEGF was increased in the vitreous of patients with PDR. In the present study, the development of DR was associated with both the average and highest HbA1c levels, and the severity of DR was associated with the average HbA1c level. Song et al. [6] conducted a 3-year retrospective cohort study of 604 patients with type 2 diabetes. They observed that the mean HbA1c level was a significant predictor of DR progression, independent of the duration of diabetes and HbA1c-variability levels. In patients with type 2 diabetes mellitus, HbA1c variability such as microalbuminuria and decreased GFR is associated with DN initiation [35]. In recent studies, glycemic variability has been found to be strongly associated with DR in patients with type 2 diabetes [7]. It is unclear why HbA1c variations adversely affect the development of DR or DN, but one possible mechanism is associated with "metabolic memory" due to repeated exposure to glycemic instability [36], which can lead to increased oxidative stress [37]. If hyperglycemia continues for a certain period in the early stages of diabetes, it may be difficult to suppress the subsequent progression of complications even if hyperglycemia is corrected by subsequent treatment [38]. Concepts of "metabolic memory" include many factors such as mitochondrial DNA damage, activation of protein kinase C, polyol pathway, increased production of advanced glycation end products (AGEs), overexpression of AGE receptors, increased anion superoxide formation, glycation of mitochondrial proteins, and hexosamine influx alterations [39]. Kowluru et al. compared metabolites in the blood and urine of rats in which glycemic control was started immediately after the onset of diabetes and in a group in which control was delayed for 6 months. They observed that oxidative stressors such as lipid peroxides (LPO), 8-hydroxy-2-deoxyguanosine (8-OhdG), glutathione (GSH), and urinary nitric oxide (NO) increased in the control delay group, but these substances in the rapid control group were no different from those in healthy rats [40]. Ceriello et al. observed increased vascular endothelial dysfunction, inflammation, and oxidative stress in patients with high HbA1c levels, but these nearly normalized in patients with low HbA1c levels who normalized blood glucose [41]. These reports suggest that the early initiation of good glycemic control may reduce oxidative stress and associated damage in the body, but the damage may progress if treatment is delayed. Quagliaro et al. found that intermittent hyperglycemia increased nitrotyrosine and 8-hydroxydeoxyguanosine, a marker of oxidative stress, and observed increased apoptosis in human venous endothelial cells, compared to stable high glucose condition [42]. Horvath et al. [43] observed that excessive glycemic changes stimulated nitrotyrosine production and caused endothelial dysfunction in streptozotocin-induced diabetic rats. Alterations in the retinal nerve fiber layer (RNFL) have also been reported in DR. Wang et al. [44] examined peripapillary vessel density and RNFL thickness using swept-source optical coherence tomography angiography (SS-OCTA) imaging in patients with nonproliferative DR, and they observed that peripapillary capillary vessel density and RNFL thickness were significantly lower in the superior temporal quadrants compared with healthy. Moreover, Cao et al. [45] observed that peripapillary capillary vessel density and RNFL thickness were significantly lower also in diabetic patients without DR compared to normal controls using OCTA.

Higher HbA1c levels, longer duration of diabetes, and use of insulin therapy for treatment have been reported to be risk factors for DR, and these may reflect poor glycemic control. Wat et al. reported that hypertension was positively correlated with the prevalence and progression of DR [46]. However, obesity, hyperlipidemia, sex, and smoking have not been established with clear associations with DR, as different studies have reported different results [46].

4.2. Pathophysiology of DN

The pathophysiologic mechanisms that lead to DN are multifactorial [19]. In the early stages of DN, hyperglycemia causes the release of vasoactive mediators such as VEGF, NO, glucagon, insulin-like growth factor 1 (IGF-1), and prostaglandins [47–50]. This causes dilation of the arterioles, leading to a temporary increase in the glomerular filtration rate. On the other hand, hyperglycemia causes the increased production of reactive oxygen species (ROS), activation of protein kinase C (PKC), and increased advanced glycation end products (AGEs), leading to vascular endothelial cell damage [50]. Damage to glomerular blood vessels results in increased glomerular permeability to macromolecules, leading to proteinuria. The transformation of IGF-1 also causes the hypertrophy of renal cells and the accumulation of extracellular matrix [51]. Sustained hyperglycemia also activates the renin-angiotensin system to form angiotensin II, which is involved in the development of DN and concomitant hypertension [52].

In patients with type 1 diabetes and type 2 diabetes, high HbA1c levels, longer duration of diabetes, and systemic hypertension are associated with an increased risk of development and progression of DN [53,54], similar to DR. In addition, dyslipidemia, obesity, age, smoking, and genetic factors are also risk factors for the development and progression of DN [53–55]. In a previous study, lower low-density lipoprotein cholesterol (LDL-C) and triglyceride (TG) levels were associated with a reduced risk of progression from moderate to severe albuminuria or end-stage renal disease [56]. The onset and severity of DN take some time. Microalbuminuria occurs 5 to 10 years after the onset of diabetes, followed by macroalbuminuria in 20 years and end-stage renal disease in 30 years [57].

Many studies have reported a significant association between DR and DN [58–60], and Kotlarsky et al. [60] observed that DN precedes DR. High HbA1c levels, longer diabetes duration, and systemic hypertension are considered common risk factors for DR and DN. Therefore, it is predicted that DR and DN are likely to develop and progress in parallel in patients with these factors.

4.3. Pathophysiology of DME

In the present study, we observed DME in half of the patients with DR but not in patients without DR. On the other hand, patients who develop DR often already have DN, because DN tends to precede DR [60].

Several reports have investigated the relationship between DME and DN. Acan et al. [61] reported that DN is a risk factor for developing DME. Koo et al. [62] reported that the serous type of DME was associated with albuminuria. However, there have been several reports that DN did not significantly affect DME development or progression [18,63]. On the other hand, there have been reports that dialysis improves DME. Takamura et al. [64] observed that the central retinal thickness (CRT) values were decreased after hemodialysis initiation without ocular treatments for DME in most eyes. Theodossiadis et al. [65] reported that average macular thickness and total macular volume were also reduced after hemodialysis in patients with DME. The mechanism by which hemodialysis promotes subretinal fluid absorption is currently unknown, but it is believed that the mutual flow of the excess fluid between the retina and the choroidal tissue or the retinal pigment epithelium may have improved after hemodialysis [64]. On the other hand, it has been proposed that SGLT-2 inhibitors may be effective in treating DME. Tatsumi et al. [66] observed that the administration of SGLT-2 inhibitors significantly reduced CRT in patients with untreated DME. SGLT2 is thought to be present in retinal pericytes and mesangial cells, and it has been reported that SGLT2 inhibitors may protect the retina by acting directly on retinal pericytes [67]. Therefore, rather than a diuretic effect, this direct action on retinal pericytes may contribute to the reduction of macular edema.

Several theories have been proposed regarding the mechanisms through which DME develops. They include retinal pigment epithelial (RPE) pump impairment, oxygen tension, Starling's law, and BRB impairment. In areas with DME, microaneurysms and abnormal deep capillary networks are observed in the outer layer of the superficial nucleus, which is usually an avascular region [68]. The retinal pigment epithelium (RPE) has ion and fluid pumps for the reabsorption of subretinal fluid. This RPE pump is the sole extracellular fluid uptake mechanism in the fovea, and the dysfunction of this pump may be involved in the development of DME [69]. Decreased choroidal circulation may be the cause of RPE pump dysfunction [70]. An oxygen theory has also been proposed to explain the pathogenesis of DME [71]. Long-term hyperglycemia reduces retinal perfusion, resulting in a lower partial pressure of oxygen in the inner retina. Retinal arterioles dilate in an autoregulatory response, thus increasing the hydrostatic pressure within the capillaries and venules within the retina [72]. The resulting increase in intravascular pressure can damage capillaries [72]. In parallel, decreased retinal oxygen tension upregulates the synthesis of VEGF and other permeability factors and increases microvascular leakage.

VEGF is expressed not only by retinal cells but also by retinal pigment epithelium, glial cells, vascular endothelial cells, and pericytes under hypoxic conditions [73]. VEGF also causes endothelial hyperpermeability and endothelial cell proliferation [32]. VEGF is thought to play an important role in macular edema [74]. Funatsu et al. assessed fluorescence leakage in patients with DME and observed that VEGF levels in the vitreous humor were also elevated in patients with hyperfluorescence [75]. Therefore, the intravitreal injection of anti-VEGF agents (aflibercept and ranibizumab) has become the main treatment for DME, replacing conventional laser photocoagulation, vitrectomy, and steroid triamcinolone acetonide [76].

Starling's law, which relates hydrostatic and oncotic pressures opposing each other, has long been advocated. It is speculated that this law causes elevated intravascular pressure and increased vascular permeability, resulting in the flow of water, ions, and macromolecules from the intravascular space into the extravascular space [20]. BRB is composed of retinal vasculature and retinal pigment epithelium (RPE). Endothelial cells are responsible for maintaining the BRB, and damage to these cells increases vascular permeability [77].

We observed that the prevalence of DME increased as the DR grade progressed in this study (A2: 32.7%, B1: 58.8%, B2: 71.4%, B4: 87.0%, B5: 100%). DME is a frequent manifestation of DR and can occur during any stage of the disease [77]. However, de Faria et al. [24] reported that it occurs more frequently as the duration of diabetes and severity of DR increase (early DR: 0%, nonproliferative DR: 64%, preproliferative DR: 79%, proliferative DR: 84%). As DR progresses, damage to capillaries and BRB impairment increase in the macula, and it is thought that the prevalence of DME also increases.

We consulted previous systemic reviews to examine DR prevalence in patients with type 2 diabetes in a general cohort [78–83] (Table 11). The global DR prevalence was 22.2–34.6% [78–80], but those of China and India were lower [81,82]. The DR prevalence in this study was high, presumably because it included patients who were referred for the purpose of assessment and treatment of DR.

Table 11. Report on DR prevalence in patients with type 2 diabetes.

Report	DR Prevalence	Region	Year
Teo et al., 59 studies	22.3%	Global	2020
Yau et al., 35 studies	34.6%	Global	1980–2008
Cheloni et al., 10 studies	34.6%	Global	2008–2018
Song et al., 31 studies	18.5%	China	1990–2017
Brar et al., 10 studies	16.1%	India	1990–2021
Heiran et al., 109 studies	31%	Eastern Mediterranean	2019–2020
Present study	48.7%	Japan	2019–2022

DR: diabetic retinopathy.

4.4. Limitations

The blood pressure of each participant was measured at our institution but may not accurately reflect the usual blood pressure of each patient due to effects such as white-coat hypertension. Fundus findings in grades A1 and A2 and DME are reversible. Even if these findings had been temporarily present before, they may have disappeared at the time of examination. Diabetes onset time was estimated based on patient interviews and past medical records, but the duration of disease in each patient may have been longer because diabetes in its early stages is often asymptomatic.

Many patients with early-stage DR do not experience vision loss. Patients with diabetes require ophthalmology consultations to manage DR in parallel with medical treatment. However, many patients with diabetes only visit internal medicine, and the onset and progression of DR may be overlooked in such patients. The present study and previous studies [54] suggest a parallel progression of DR and DN. DN deterioration may be a predictor of DR onset and progression.

5. Conclusions

We observed that DR development involves the average HbA1c level, highest HbA1c level, and DN severity in addition to the duration of diabetes. DR severity correlated with the duration of diabetes, average HbA1c level, and DN severity. DN severity may be associated with DME development. Furthermore, DN progress may be a predictive indicator of DR development. Both DR and DN are microvascular complications of diabetes, and good long-term glycemic control may suppress the progression of both.

Author Contributions: Conceptualization, Y.S.; methodology, Y.S.; software, Y.S.; validation, Y.S., and M.K.; formal analysis, Y.S.; investigation, Y.S.; resources, Y.S.; data curation, Y.S.; writing—original draft preparation, Y.S.; writing—review and editing, M.K.; visualization, Y.S.; supervision, Y.S.; project administration, Y.S.; funding acquisition, Y.S. and M.K. All authors have read and agreed to the published version of the manuscript.

Funding: This research received no external funding.

Institutional Review Board Statement: This study protocol was approved by the Institutional Ethics Committee of the Japan Community Health Care Organization, Mishima General Hospital. All procedures conformed to the tenets of the Declaration of Helsinki. (Protocol code: H30-005 and date of approval: 5 October 2018).

Informed Consent Statement: All measurements in this study were performed in the Japan Community Health Care Organization, Mishima General Hospital. Informed consent was obtained from all subjects before participation in this study. Informed consent was obtained from all subjects involved in the study. Written informed consent has been obtained from the patients to publish this paper.

Data Availability Statement: All data used for analysis are presented in the tables in this article. Data will be shared after ethics approval if requested by other investigators for the purpose of replicating the results.

Acknowledgments: The authors would like to thank the nurses of Mishima General Hospital for their technical support.

Conflicts of Interest: The authors declare no conflict of interest.

References

1. International Diabetes Federation. *IDF Diabetes Atlas 2019*, 9th ed.; International Diabetes Federation: Brussels, Belgium, 2019; Available online: http://diabetesatlas.org (accessed on 12 April 2023).
2. Jameson, J.L.; Fauci, A.S.; Kasper, D.L.; Hauser, S.L.; Longo, D.L.; Loscalzo, J. *Harrison's Principles of Internal Medicine*, 20th ed.; McGraw Hill Education: New York, NY, USA, 2018.
3. Cheung, N.; Mitchell, P.; Wong, T.Y. Diabetic retinopathy. *Lancet* **2010**, *376*, 124–136. [CrossRef] [PubMed]
4. Moreno, A.; Lozano, M.; Salinas, P. Diabetic retinopathy. *Nutr. Hosp.* **2013**, *28* (Suppl. S2), 53–56. [CrossRef] [PubMed]
5. Lin, T.; Gubitosi-Klug, R.A.; Channa, R.; Wolf, R.M. Pediatric Diabetic Retinopathy: Updates in Prevalence, Risk Factors, Screening, and Management. *Curr. Diabetes Rep.* **2021**, *21*, 56. [CrossRef] [PubMed]
6. Song, K.H.; Jeong, J.S.; Kim, M.K.; Kwon, H.S.; Baek, K.H.; Ko, S.H.; Ahn, Y.B. Discordance in risk factors for the progression of diabetic retinopathy and diabetic nephropathy in patients with type 2 diabetes mellitus. *J. Diabetes Investig.* **2019**, *10*, 745–752. [CrossRef]
7. Lu, J.; Ma, X.; Zhang, L.; Mo, Y.; Ying, L.; Lu, W.; Zhu, W.; Bao, Y.; Zhou, J. Glycemic variability assessed by continuous glucose monitoring and the risk of diabetic retinopathy in latent autoimmune diabetes of the adult and type 2 diabetes. *J. Diabetes Investig.* **2019**, *10*, 753–759. [CrossRef]
8. Fardeau, C.; Champion, E.; Massamba, N.; LeHoang, P. Uveitic macular edema. *Eye* **2016**, *30*, 1277–1292. [CrossRef]
9. Iijima, H. Mechanisms of vision loss in eyes with macular edema associated with retinal vein occlusion. *Jpn. J. Ophthalmol.* **2018**, *62*, 265–273. [CrossRef]
10. Lee, R.; Wong, T.Y.; Sabanayagam, C. Epidemiology of diabetic retinopathy, diabetic macular edema and related vision loss. *Eye Vis.* **2015**, *2*, 17. [CrossRef]
11. Coscas, G.; Cunha-Vaz, J.; Soubrane, G. Macular edema: Definition and basic concepts. *Dev. Ophthalmol.* **2017**, *58*, 1–10. [CrossRef]
12. Ding, J.; Wong, T.Y. Current epidemiology of diabetic retinopathy and diabetic macular edema. *Curr. Diabetes Rep.* **2012**, *12*, 346–354. [CrossRef]
13. Early Treatment Diabetic Retinopathy Study Research Group. Treatment techniques and clinical guidelines for photocoagulation of diabetic macular edema. Early Treatment Diabetic Retinopathy Study Report Number 2. *Ophthalmology* **1987**, *94*, 761–774. [CrossRef] [PubMed]

14. Browning, D.J.; Stewart, M.W.; Lee, C. Diabetic macular edema: Evidence-based management. *Indian J. Ophthalmol.* **2018**, *66*, 1736–1750. [CrossRef] [PubMed]
15. Nagib, A.M.; Matter, Y.E.; Gheith, O.A.; Refaie, A.F.; Othman, N.F.; Al-Otaibi, T. Diabetic Nephropathy Following Posttransplant Diabetes Mellitus. *Exp. Clin. Transplant.* **2019**, *17*, 138–146. [CrossRef] [PubMed]
16. Deckert, T.; Feldt-Rasmussen, B.; Borch-Johnsen, K.; Jensen, T.; Kofoed-Enevoldsen, A. Albuminuria reflects widespread vascular damage. The Steno hypothesis. *Diabetologia* **1989**, *32*, 219–226. [CrossRef]
17. Ochodnicky, P.; Henning, R.; van Dokkum, R.P.E.; de Zeeuw, D. Microalbuminuria and endothelial dysfunction: Emerging targets for primary prevention of end-organ damage. *J. Cardiovasc. Pharmacol.* **2006**, *47* (Suppl. S2), S151–S162, discussion S72–S76. [CrossRef]
18. Jeng, C.J.; Hsieh, Y.T.; Yang, C.M.; Yang, C.H.; Lin, C.L.; Wang, I.J. Diabetic Retinopathy in Patients with Diabetic Nephropathy: Development and Progression. *PLoS ONE* **2016**, *11*, e0161897. [CrossRef]
19. Guo, M.F.; Dai, Y.J.; Gao, J.R.; Chen, P.J. Uncovering the Mechanism of Astragalus membranaceus in the Treatment of Diabetic Nephropathy Based on Network Pharmacology. *J. Diabetes Res.* **2020**, *2020*, 5947304. [CrossRef]
20. Miyamoto, K.; Khosrof, S.; Bursell, S.-E.; Moromizato, Y.; Aiello, L.P.; Ogura, Y.; Adamis, A.P. Vascular endothelial growth factor (VEGF)-induced retinal vascular permeability is mediated by intercellular adhesion molecule-1 (ICAM-1). *Am. J. Pathol.* **2000**, *156*, 1733–1739. [CrossRef]
21. Li, W.; Cheng, Z.; Song, Y.; Fang, Y.; Yang, M.; Zhang, M. Is diabetic retinopathy affected by diabetes type? A retrospective study using electronic medical record data from patients with latent autoimmune diabetes in adults, type 1 diabetes, and type 2 diabetes. *Acta Diabetol.* **2021**, *58*, 1503–1511. [CrossRef]
22. Matuszewski, W.; Baranowska-Jurkun, A.; Stefanowicz-Rutkowska, M.M.; Modzelewski, R.; Pieczyński, J.; Bandurska-Stankiewicz, E. Prevalence of Diabetic Retinopathy in Type 1 and Type 2 Diabetes Mellitus Patients in North-East Poland. *Medicina* **2020**, *56*, 164. [CrossRef]
23. Fukuda, M. Classification and treatment of diabetic retinopathy. *Diabetes Res. Clin. Pract.* **1994**, *24*, S171–S176. [CrossRef] [PubMed]
24. De Faria, J.M.L.; Jalkh, A.E.; Trempe, C.L.; Mcmeel, J.W. Diabetic macular oedema: Risk factors and concomitants. *Acta Ophthalmol. Scand.* **1999**, *77*, 170–175. [CrossRef] [PubMed]
25. Hwang, D.K.; Chou, Y.B.; Lin, T.C.; Yang, H.Y.; Kao, Z.K.; Kao, C.L.; Yang, Y.P.; Chen, S.J.; Hsu, C.C.; Jheng, Y.C. Optical coherence tomography–based diabetic macula edema screening with artificial intelligence. *J. Chin. Med. Assoc.* **2020**, *83*, 1034–1038. [CrossRef]
26. Wada, T.; Haneda, M.; Furuichi, K.; Babazono, T.; Yokoyama, H.; Iseki, K.; Araki, S.I.; Ninomiya, T.; Hara, S.; Suzuki, Y.; et al. The Research Group of Diabetic Nephropathy, Ministry of Health, Labour, and Welfare of Japan. Clinical impact of albuminuria and glomerular filtration rate on renal and cardiovascular events, and all-cause mortality in Japanese patients with type 2 diabetes. *Clin. Exp. Nephrol.* **2014**, *18*, 613–620. [CrossRef] [PubMed]
27. Kanda, Y. Investigation of the freely available easy-to-use software 'EZR' for medical statistics. *Bone Marrow Transplant.* **2013**, *48*, 452–458. [CrossRef]
28. Bek, T. Diameter changes of retinal vessels in diabetic retinopathy. *Curr. Diabetes Rep.* **2017**, *17*, 82. [CrossRef]
29. Ejaz, S.; Chekarova, I.; Ejaz, A.; Sohail, A.; Lim, C.W. Importance of pericytes and mechanisms of pericyte loss during diabetes retinopathy. *Diabetes Obes. Metab.* **2008**, *10*, 53–63. [CrossRef]
30. Beltramo, E.; Porta, M. Pericyte loss in diabetic retinopathy: Mechanisms and consequences. *Curr. Med. Chem.* **2013**, *20*, 3218–3225. [CrossRef]
31. Huang, H.; He, J.; Johnson, D.; Wei, Y.; Liu, Y.; Wang, S.; Lutty, G.A.; Duh, E.J.; Semba, R.D. Deletion of placental growth factor prevents diabetic retinopathy and is associated with Akt activation and HIF1alpha-VEGF pathway inhibition. *Diabetes* **2015**, *64*, 200–212. [CrossRef]
32. Antonetti, D.A.; Barber, A.J.; Hollinger, L.A.; Wolpert, E.B.; Gardner, T.W. Vascular endothelial growth factor induces rapid phosphorylation of tight junction proteins occludin and zonula occluden 1. A potential mechanism for vascular permeability in diabetic retinopathy and tumors. *J. Biol. Chem.* **1999**, *274*, 23463–23467. [CrossRef]
33. Rousseau, S.; Houle, F.; Landry, J.; Huot, J. p38 MAP kinase activation by vascular endothelial growth factor mediates actin reorganization and cell migration in human endothelial cells. *Oncogene* **1997**, *15*, 2169–2177. [CrossRef]
34. Adamis, A.P.; Miller, J.W.; Bernal, M.T.; D'Amico, D.J.; Folkman, J.; Yeo, T.K.; Yeo, K.T. Increased vascular endothelial growth factor levels in the vitreous of eyes with proliferative diabetic retinopathy. *Am. J. Ophthalmol.* **1994**, *118*, 445–450. [CrossRef] [PubMed]
35. Sugawara, A.; Kawai, K.; Motohashi, S.; Saito, K.; Kodama, S.; Yachi, Y.; Hirasawa, R.; Shimano, H.; Yamazaki, K.; Sone, H. HbA (1c) variability and the development of microalbuminuria in T2DM: Tsukuba Kawai Diabetes Registry 2. *Diabetologia* **2012**, *55*, 2128–2131. [CrossRef] [PubMed]
36. Ihnat, M.A.; Thorpe, J.E.; Ceriello, A. Hypothesis: The 'metabolic memory', the new challenge of diabetes. *Diabet. Med.* **2007**, *24*, 582–586. [CrossRef] [PubMed]
37. Monnier, L.; Mas, E.; Ginet, C.; Michel, F.; Villon, L.; Cristol, J.P.; Colette, C. Activation of oxidative stress by acute glucose fluctuations compared with sustained chronic hyperglycemia in patients with T2DM. *J. Am. Med. Assoc.* **2006**, *295*, 1681–1687. [CrossRef] [PubMed]

38. Russell, N.D.; Cooper, M.E. 50 years forward: Mechanisms of hyperglycaemia driven diabetic complications. *Diabetologia* **2015**, *58*, 1708–1714. [CrossRef]
39. Ceriello, A. The emerging challenge in diabetes: The "metabolic memory". *Vasc. Pharmacol.* **2012**, *57*, 133–138. [CrossRef]
40. Kowluru, R.A.; Abbas, S.N.; Odenbach, S. Reversal of hyperglycemia and diabetic nephropathy: Effect of reinstitution of good metabolic control on oxidative stress in the kidney of diabetic rats. *J. Diabetes Complicat.* **2004**, *18*, 282–288. [CrossRef]
41. Ceriello, A.; Esposito, K.; Ihnat, M.; Thorpe, J.; Giugliano, D. Long-term glycemic control influences the long-lasting effect of hyperglycemia on endothelial function in type 1 diabetes. *J. Clin. Endocrinol. Metab.* **2009**, *94*, 2751–2756. [CrossRef]
42. Quagliaro, L.; Piconi, L.; Assaloni, R.; Martinelli, L.; Motz, E.; Ceriero, A. Intermittent high glucose enhances apoptosis related to oxidative stress in human umbilical vein endothelial cells: The role of protein kinase C and NAD(P)H-oxidase activation. *Diabetes* **2003**, *52*, 2795–2804. [CrossRef]
43. Horvath, E.M.; Benko, R.; Kiss, L.; Murányi, M.; Pék, T.; Fekete, K.; Bárány, T.; Somlai, A.; Csordás, A.; Szabo, C. Rapid 'glycaemic swings' induce nitrosative stress, activate poly(ADP-ribose) polymerase and impair endothelial function in a rat model of diabetes mellitus. *Diabetologia* **2009**, *52*, 952–961. [CrossRef]
44. Wang, X.N.; Cai, X.; Li, T.T.; Long, D.; Wu, Q. Peripapillary vessel density and retinal nerve fiber layer thickness changes in early diabetes retinopathy. *Int. J. Ophthalmol.* **2022**, *15*, 1488–1495. [CrossRef] [PubMed]
45. Cao, D.; Yang, D.; Yu, H.; Xie, J.; Zeng, Y.; Wang, J.; Zhang, L. Optic nerve head perfusion changes preceding peripapillary retinal nerve fibre layer thinning in preclinical diabetic retinopathy. *Clin. Exp. Ophthalmol.* **2019**, *47*, 219–225. [CrossRef] [PubMed]
46. Wat, N.; Wong, R.L.; Wong, I.Y. Associations between diabetic retinopathy and systemic risk factors. *Hong Kong Med. J.* **2016**, *22*, 589–599. [CrossRef] [PubMed]
47. Ha, H.; Lee, H.B. Reactive oxygen species amplify glucose signaling in renal cells cultured under high glucose and in diabetic nephropathy. *Nephrology* **2005**, *10*, S7–S10. [CrossRef]
48. Lee, H.B.; Yu, M.I.-R.A.; Yang, Y.; Jiang, Z.; Ha, H. Reactive oxygen species-regulated signaling pathways in diabetic nephropathy. *J. Am. Soc. Nephrol.* **2003**, *14* (Suppl. S3), S241–S245. [CrossRef]
49. Forbes, J.M.; Cooper, M.E.; Oldfield, M.D.; Thomas, M.C. Role of advanced glycation end products in diabetic nephropathy. *J. Am. Soc. Nephrol.* **2003**, *14* (Suppl. S3), S254–S258. [CrossRef]
50. Thallas-Bonke, V.; Lindschau, C.; Rizkalla, B.; Bach, L.A.; Boner, G.; Meier, M.; Haller, H.; Cooper, M.E.; Forbes, J.M. Attenuation of extracellular matrix accumulation in diabetic nephropathy by advanced glycation end product cross-link breaker ALT-711 via a PKC-α-dependent pathway. *Diabetes* **2004**, *53*, 2921–2930. [CrossRef]
51. Cao, Z.; Cooper, M.E. Pathogenesis of diabetic nephropathy. *J. Diabetes Investig.* **2011**, *2*, 243–247. [CrossRef]
52. Funatsu, H.; Yamashita, H.; Nakanishi, Y.; Hori, S. Angiotensin II and vascular endothelial growth factor in the vitreous fluid of patients with proliferative diabetic retinopathy. *Br. J. Ophthalmol.* **2002**, *86*, 311–315. [CrossRef]
53. Tapp, R.J.; Shaw, J.E.; Zimmet, P.Z.; Balkau, B.; Chadban, S.J.; Tonkin, A.M.; Welborn, T.A.; Atkins, R.C. Albuminuria is evident in the early stages of diabetes onset: Results from the Australian Diabetes, Obesity, and Lifestyle Study (AusDiab). *Am. J. Kidney Dis.* **2004**, *44*, 792–798. [CrossRef] [PubMed]
54. Cederholm, J.; Eliasson, B.; Nilsson, P.M.; Weiss, L.; Gudbjörnsdottir, S. Steering Committee of the Swedish National Diabetes Register. Microalbuminuria and risk factors in type 1 and type 2 diabetic patients. *Diabetes Res. Clin. Pract.* **2005**, *67*, 258–266. [CrossRef] [PubMed]
55. Gambaro, G.; Bax, G.; Fusaro, M.; Normanno, M.; Manani, S.M.; Zanella, M.; Dangelo, A.; Fedele, D.; Favaro, S. Cigarette smoking is a risk factor for nephropathy and its progression in type 2 diabetes mellitus. *Diabetes Nutr. Metab.* **2001**, *14*, 337–342. [PubMed]
56. De Boer, I.H.; Rue, T.C.; Cleary, P.A.; Lachin, J.M.; Molitch, M.E.; Steffes, M.W.; Sun, W.; Zinman, B.; Brunzell, J.D.; White, N.H.; et al. Long-term renal outcomes of patients with type 1 diabetes mellitus and microalbuminuria: An analysis of the Diabetes Control and Complications Trial/Epidemiology of Diabetes Interventions and Complications cohort. *Arch. Intern. Med.* **2011**, *171*, 412–420. [CrossRef] [PubMed]
57. Lin, Y.C.; Chang, Y.H.; Yang, S.Y.; Wu, K.D.; Chu, T.S. Update of pathophysiology and management of diabetic kidney disease. *J. Formos. Med. Assoc.* **2018**, *117*, 662–675. [CrossRef] [PubMed]
58. Ahmed, M.H.; Elwali, E.S.; Awadalla, H.; Almobarak, A.O. The relationship between diabetic retinopathy and nephropathy in Sudanese adult with diabetes: Population based study. *Diabetes Metab. Syndr.* **2017**, *11* (Suppl. S1), S333–S336. [CrossRef]
59. Saini, D.C.; Kochar, A.; Poonia, R. Clinical correlation of diabetic retinopathy with nephropathy and neuropathy. *Indian J. Ophthalmol.* **2021**, *69*, 3364. [CrossRef]
60. Kotlarsky, P.; Bolotin, A.; Dorfman, K.; Knyazer, B.; Lifshitz, T.; Levy, J. Link between retinopathy and nephropathy caused by complications of diabetes mellitus type 2. *Int. Ophthalmol.* **2015**, *35*, 59–66. [CrossRef]
61. Acan, D.; Calan, M.; Er, D.; Arkan, T.; Kocak, N.; Bayraktar, F.; Kaynak, S. The prevalence and systemic risk factors of diabetic macular edema: A cross-sectional study from Turkey. *BMC Ophthalmol.* **2018**, *18*, 91. [CrossRef]
62. Koo, N.K.; Jin, H.C.; Kim, K.S.; Kim, Y.C. Relationship between the morphology of diabetic macular edema and renal dysfunction in diabetes. *Korean J. Ophthalmol.* **2013**, *27*, 98–102. [CrossRef]
63. Temkar, S.; Karuppaiah, N.; Takkar, B.; Bhowmik, D.; Tripathi, M.; Ramakrishnan, S.; Sharma, Y.R.; Vohra, R.; Chawla, R.; Venkatesh, P. Impact of estimated glomerular filtration rate on diabetic macular edema. *Int. Ophthalmol.* **2018**, *38*, 1043–1050. [CrossRef] [PubMed]

64. Takamura, Y.; Matsumura, T.; Ohkoshi, K.; Takei, T.; Ishikawa, K.; Shimura, M.; Ueda, T.; Sugimoto, M.; Hirano, T.; Takayama, K.; et al. Functional and anatomical changes in diabetic macular edema after hemodialysis initiation: One-year follow-up multicenter study. *Sci. Rep.* **2020**, *10*, 7788. [CrossRef] [PubMed]
65. Theodossiadis, P.G.; Theodoropoulou, S.; Neamonitou, G.; Grigoropoulos, V.; Liarakos, V.; Triantou, E.; Theodossiadis, G.P.; Vlahakos, D.V. Hemodialysis-induced alterations in macular thickness measured by optical coherence tomography in diabetic patients with end-stage renal disease. *Ophthalmologica* **2012**, *227*, 90–94. [CrossRef]
66. Tatsumi, T.; Oshitari, T.; Takatsuna, Y.; Ishibashi, R.; Koshizaka, M.; Shiko, Y.; Baba, T.; Yokote, K.; Yamamoto, S. Sodium-Glucose Co-Transporter 2 Inhibitors Reduce Macular Edema in Patients with *Diabetes mellitus*. *Life* **2022**, *12*, 692. [CrossRef] [PubMed]
67. Wakisaka, M.; Nagao, T. Sodium glucose cotransporter 2 in mesangial cells and retinal pericytes and its implications for diabetic nephropathy and retinopathy. *Glycobiology* **2017**, *27*, 691–695. [CrossRef]
68. Querques, G.; Bandello, F.; Souied, E.H. Abnormal deep retinal capillary networking and microaneurysms in the outer nuclear layer of diabetic eyes. *Ophthalmology* **2014**, *121*, 803–840. [CrossRef]
69. Browning, D.J. (Ed.) Diabetic macular edema. In *Diabetic Retinopathy, Evidence-Based Management*, 1st ed.; Springer Inc.: New York, NY, USA, 2010.
70. Nagaoka, T.; Kitaya, N.; Sugawara, R.; Yokota, H.; Mori, F.; Hikichi, T.; Fujio, N.; Yoshida, A. Alteration of choroidal circulation in the foveal region in patients with type 2 diabetes. *Br. J. Ophthalmol.* **2004**, *88*, 1060–1063. [CrossRef]
71. Stefánsson, E. Ocular oxygenation and the treatment of diabetic retinopathy. *Surv. Ophthalmol.* **2006**, *51*, 364–380. [CrossRef]
72. Lund-Andersen, H. Mechanisms for monitoring changes in retinal status following therapeutic intervention in diabetic retinopathy. *Surv. Ophthalmol.* **2002**, *47* (Suppl. S2), S270–S277. [CrossRef]
73. Dvorak, H.F.; Brown, L.F.; Detmar, M.; Dvorak, A.M. Vascular permeability factor/vascular endothelial growth factor, microvascular hyperpermeability, and angiogenesis. *Am. J. Pathol.* **1995**, *146*, 1029–1039.
74. Murata, T.; Nakagawa, K.; Khalil, A.; Ishibashi, T.; Inomata, H.; Sueishi, K. The relation between expression of vascular endothelial growth factor and breakdown of the blood-retinal barrier in diabetic rat retinas. *Lab. Investig.* **1996**, *74*, 819–825. [PubMed]
75. Funatsu, H.; Yamashita, H.; Ikeda, T.; Mimura, T.; Eguchi, S.; Hori, S. Vitreous levels of interleukin-6 and vascular endothelial growth factor are related to diabetic macular edema. *Ophthalmology* **2003**, *110*, 1690–1696. [CrossRef] [PubMed]
76. Funatsu, H.; Yamashita, H.; Noma, H.; Mimura, T.; Yamashita, T.; Hori, S. Increased levels of vascular endothelial growth factor and interleukin-6 in the aqueous humor of diabetics with macular edema. *Am. J. Ophthalmol.* **2002**, *133*, 70–77. [CrossRef] [PubMed]
77. Ciulla, T.A.; Amador, A.G.; Zinman, B. Diabetic retinopathy and diabetic macularoedema: Pathophysiology, screening, and novel therapies. *Diabetes Care* **2003**, *26*, 2653–2664. [CrossRef]
78. Teo, Z.L.; Tham, Y.C.; Yu, M.; Chee, M.L.; Rim, T.H.; Cheung, N.; Bikbov, M.M.; Wang, Y.X.; Tang, Y.; Lu, Y.; et al. Global Prevalence of Diabetic Retinopathy and Projection of Burden through 2045: Systematic Review and Meta-analysis. *Ophthalmology* **2021**, *128*, 1580–1591. [CrossRef]
79. Yau, J.W.Y.; Rogers, S.L.; Kawasaki, R.; Lamoureux, E.L.; Kowalski, J.W.; Bek, T.; Chen, S.J.; Dekker, J.M.; Fletcher, A.; Grauslund, J.; et al. Meta-Analysis for Eye Disease (META-EYE) Study Group. Global prevalence and major risk factors of diabetic retinopathy. *Diabetes Care* **2012**, *35*, 556–564. [CrossRef]
80. Cheloni, R.; Gandolfi, S.A.; Signorelli, C.; Odone, A. Global prevalence of diabetic retinopathy: Protocol for a systematic review and meta-analysis. *BMJ Open* **2019**, *9*, e022188. [CrossRef]
81. Song, P.; Yu, J.; Chan, K.Y.; Theodoratou, E.; Rudan, I. Prevalence, risk factors and burden of diabetic retinopathy in China: A systematic review and meta-analysis. *J. Glob. Health* **2018**, *8*, 010803. [CrossRef]
82. Brar, A.S.; Sahoo, J.; Behera, U.C.; Jonas, J.B.; Sivaprasad, S.; Das, T. Prevalence of diabetic retinopathy in urban and rural India: A systematic review and meta-analysis. *Indian J. Ophthalmol.* **2022**, *70*, 1945. [CrossRef]
83. Heiran, A.; Azarchehry, S.P.; Dehghankhalili, S.; Afarid, M.; Shaabani, S.; Mirahmadizadeh, A. Prevalence of diabetic retinopathy in the Eastern Mediterranean Region: A systematic review and meta-analysis. *J. Int. Med. Res.* **2022**, *50*, 3000605221117134. [CrossRef]

biomedicines

MDPI

Article

A Pilot Study of Implementing Diabetic Retinopathy Screening in the Oslo Region, Norway: Baseline Results

Ellen Steffenssen Sauesund [1,2,*], Øystein Kalsnes Jørstad [1], Cathrine Brunborg [3], Morten Carstens Moe [1,2], Maja Gran Erke [1], Dag Sigurd Fosmark [1,†] and Goran Petrovski [1,2,†]

1 Department of Ophthalmology, Oslo University Hospital, 0450 Oslo, Norway
2 Center for Eye Research and Innovative Diagnostics, Department of Ophthalmology, Institute of Clinical Medicine, Faculty of Medicine, University of Oslo, 0450 Oslo, Norway
3 Oslo Centre for Biostatistics and Epidemiology, Research Support Services, Oslo University Hospital, 0450 Oslo, Norway
* Correspondence: ellen.s.sauesund@gmail.com
† These authors contributed equally to this work.

Abstract: Purpose: to gain insight into the baseline parameters of a population with diabetes mellitus (DM) included in a pilot diabetic retinopathy (DR) screening program at Oslo University Hospital (OUH), Norway. Methods: This was a cross-sectional study of a cohort of adult patients (≥18 years) with type 1 or 2 DM (T1D and T2D). We measured the best-corrected visual acuity (BCVA), blood pressure (BP), heart rate (HR), intraocular pressure (IOP), height and weight. We also collected HbA1c, total serum cholesterol and urine-albumin, -creatinine and -albumin-to-creatinine ratio (ACR), as well as socio-demographic parameters, medications and previous screening history. We obtained color fundus photographs, which were graded by two experienced ophthalmologists according to the International Clinical Disease Severity Scale for DR. Results: The study included 180 eyes of 90 patients: 12 patients (13.3%) had T1D and 78 (86.7%) had T2D. In the T1D group, 5 patients (41.7%) had no DR, and 7 (58.3%) had some degree of DR. In the T2D group, 60 patients (76.9%) had no DR, and 18 (23.1%) had some degree of DR. None of the patients had proliferative DR. Of the 43 patients not newly diagnosed (time of diagnosis > 5 years for T1D and >1 years for T2D), 37.5% of the T1D patients and 5.7% of the T2D patients had previously undergone regular screening. Univariate analyses found for the whole cohort significant associations between DR and age, HbA1c, urine albumin-to-creatinine ratio, body mass index (BMI) and duration of DM. For the T2D group alone, there were significant associations between DR and HbA1c, BMI, urine creatinine, urine albumin-to-creatinine ratio and duration of DM. The analysis also showed three times higher odds for DR in the T1D group than the T2D group. Conclusions: This study underscores the need for implementing a systematic DR screening program in the Oslo region, Norway, to better reach out to patients with DM and improve their screening adherence. Timely and proper treatment can prevent or mitigate vision loss and improve the prognosis. A considerable number of patients were referred from general practitioners for not being followed by an ophthalmologist.Among patients not newly diagnosed with DM, 62.8% had never had an eye exam, and the duration of DM for these patients was up to 18 years (median: 8 years).

Keywords: diabetic retinopathy; diabetes mellitus; screening; Norway

1. Introduction

Diabetic retinopathy (DR) is a frequent complication of diabetes mellitus (DM) [1]. Still, it often remains asymptomatic until advanced disease has developed, which is one of the reasons for systematic DR screening programs. The retinal microvasculopathy of DM causes ischemia and hypoxia, the latter leading to the release of vascular endothelial growth factor (VEGF), which is able to induce both new vessel (NV) formation and edema.

These NVs may act as a source of low-grade bleeding and leakage of lipoproteins and fluid, infiltrating and changing the functional architecture of the retina. As the natural history of DR is well known, further sight-threatening lesions may ensue, such as hemorrhages, macular edema and more severely increased intraocular pressure (IOP) due to the fact of neovascular glaucoma and tractional retinal detachment.

DR is one of the leading causes of global blindness in those aged 50 years and older, and DR-related complications represent a main cause of impaired vision in patients aged 25–74 years [2,3]. DR is responsible for a severe economic burden and reduced quality of life [2,4]. In a pooled analysis comparing data from 35 populations [5], sight-threatening DR (STDR) (i.e., presence of preproliferative or proliferative DR, maculopathy or evidence of photocoagulation treatment) was estimated to affect 10.2% of DM patients. Data from England and Wales show a vision-saving effect of implementing a comprehensive program for regular retinal examinations. During a 10-year observation period, the proportion of newly blind people due to the fact of DM was reduced by approximately 20% [6]. Hence, there are reasons to assume that such an impact could be transferable to Norway and that a more personalized program for regular retinal examinations may further reduce the proportion of newly blind people. Still, the screening rate in Norway is only approximately 62% [7]. Regular retinal examinations to detect DR at an early stage is also known to be cost effective [8].

For people with a known DM for more than 20 years, 76% develop some degree of DR [5]. Other studies have shown that approximately 20% and 37% of patients with newly diagnosed T2D have already developed DR [9,10]. Accordingly, guidelines recommend the initiation of DR screening to begin at the time of T2D diagnosis.

The global prevalence of DM (age: 20–79 years) in 2021 was approximately 537 million (61 million in Europe alone), and the number is estimated to rise to 643 million (67 million in Europe) by 2030 and 783 million (69 million in Europe) by 2045 [11]. The National Diabetes registry for adults in Norway is incomplete (25% of GPs reporting), but it is estimated primarily by the Norwegian Prescription Database that approximately 316,000–345,000 persons (5.9–6.4% of the population) have DM, of whom 60,000 are undiagnosed [12]. Moreover, approximately 90% of DM patients in Norway are estimated to have T2D [13]. Data from The Norwegian Prescription Database show that 4.1% used blood-glucose-lowering drugs in 2020, representing a 70.3% increase from 2004 and a 32.1% increase from 2010 [14]. Because of the increasing prevalence of DM [11], it can be assumed that the prevalence of DR will further increase.

The living conditions in Norway have been ranked as high by a United Nations' Human Development Report [15], albeit a systematic national DR screening program as of yet has not been implemented. There is a lack of knowledge concerning the DM and DR prevalence, as well as risk factors in people with DM, in Oslo, Norway. This was incentive for a pilot study for baseline insight as a step towards establishing an optimal DR screening program.

2. Materials and Methods

This was a cross-sectional study of a cohort of adult patients (≥18 years of age) with T1D or T2D belonging to the region of OUH, Oslo, Norway. The patients were mainly referred from general practitioners after they received information concerning the project (12 patients were referred from another healthcare institution). The general practitioners were invited to refer patients without a known treatment-dependent DR and who were not already followed by an ophthalmologist. A total of 90 patients (180 eyes) were enrolled, and written informed consent was obtained from all participants. The patients were included in the period from December 2019 to January 2021. The Regional Committee for Medical and Health Research Ethics concluded that the project was outside the remit of the Norwegian Health Research Act (reference: 28857). The Institutional Data Protection Officer at OUH approved the study (reference: 20/00571).

The study took place at the Department of Ophthalmology, OUH. Best-corrected visual acuity (BCVA) was assessed using the Clear Chart 2 (Reichert Technologies, Depew, NY, USA) digital acuity test, which displays 5 letter optotypes per line and a logarithm of the minimal angle of resolution (logMAR) line size progression (i.e., each letter has a score of 0.02 logMAR). After one minute of rest, blood pressure (BP) and heart rate were measured in the left overarm using a calibrated automatic BP monitor (Riester, ri-champion N Automated Blood Pressure Monitor, Jungingen, Germany). Hypertension (HT) was defined as hypertension grade 2 according to the American Heart Association: systolic at least 140 or diastolic at least 90 mm Hg (≥140/90 mmHg). We measured the intraocular pressure (IOP) using an iCare ic 100 tonometer (Icare Finland Oy, Vantaa, Finland). Mean ocular perfusion pressure (MOPP) was calculated as two-thirds of the systemic mean arterial pressure (MAP) minus the IOP [16]. The MAP = diastolic blood pressure (DBP) + one-third (systolic blood pressure (SBP)−DBP). Prior to the imaging and fundus examination, the pupils were dilated with topical tropicamide 0.5%.

If not available from the referral, the following laboratory tests were performed at the department: HbA1c, total serum cholesterol and urine-albumin, -creatinine and -albumin-to-creatinine ratio (ACR).

Color fundus photography was performed using the CLARUS™ 700, Zeiss (Carl Zeiss Meditec AG, Jena, Germany). Fovea- and optic disc-centered images were obtained, both with a 133° field of view.

The fundus images were graded according to the International Clinical Disease Severity Scale for DR [17]: no DR, mild non-proliferative DR (NPDR), moderate NPDR, severe NPDR or proliferative DR. Both eyes were graded through consensus between two experienced ophthalmologists (E.S.S. and D.F.); the eye with the more severe retinopathy defined the individual grade.

Diabetic maculopathy based on fundus photography was classified as follows: no diabetic maculopathy (0), presence of microaneurysm(s) within 1 disc diameter from the foveola (1) and hard exudate(s) within 1 disc diameter from the foveola (2).

Socio-demographic parameters, such as gender, age, type of DM, duration of DM, use of tobacco and alcohol, body weight and body height (to determine BMI), were registered. We also documented medication history (type of DM medication, duration of insulin treatment and use of cholesterol lowering- and antihypertensive drugs) and previous history regarding DR screening.

We used the Mann–Whitney U test to investigate the differences between two groups for continuous variables and the Chi-square or Fisher's exact test (for small cell counts) to detect associations among categorical variables. All tests were two-sided, and a 5% significance level was defined. To investigate the factors associated with retinopathy, a generalized estimating equation (GEE) analysis was applied to adjust for intra-individual correlation (since both eyes of each individual were included). We used IBM SPSS Statistics 28.0 (IBM Corp., Armonk, NY, USA) for the data analyses.

3. Results

Altogether 180 eyes of 90 patients (61 males (67.8%) and 29 females (32.2%)) were included in the study.

The sizes of the T1D and T2D populations amounted to 12 (13.3%, 95% CI: 7.8, 21.9) and 78 (86.7%, 95% CI: 78.1, 92.2), respectively (Figure 1). There were 5 (41.7%, 95% CI: 19.3, 68.1) and 60 (76.9%, 95% CI: 83.2, 96.7) patients with no DR in the T1D versus the T2D group, while 7 (58.3%, 95% CI: 14.3, 47.6) and 18 (23.1%, 95% CI: 52.4, 85.7) patients had DR in the T1D and T2D groups, respectively. The distribution of the different grades of retinopathy were 5 (41.7%, 95% CI: 19.3, 68.1) and 12 (15.4%, 95% CI: 9.0, 25.0) with mild DR, 1 (8.3%,95% CI: 1.5, 35.4) and 4 (5.1%, 95% CI: 2.0, 12.5) with moderate DR, 1 (8.3%, 95% CI: 1.5, 35.4) and 2 (2.6%, 95% CI: 0.7, 8.9) with severe retinopathy in the T1D and T2D group, respectively; 0 had proliferative DR in either group.

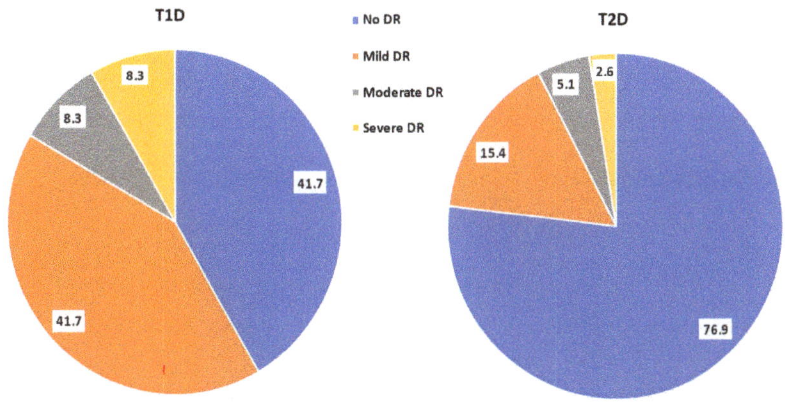

Figure 1. Pie chart (percentage frequency distribution) of the grades of diabetic retinopathy in the studied population having type 1 and type 2 diabetes mellitus (T1D and T2D).

Table 1 shows the demographic characteristics of the studied cohort where 12 (13.3%) had T1D and 78 (86.7%) had T2D. Among the T1D patients, 5 (41.7%) had no DR and 7 (58.3%) had DR, whereas 60 (76.9%) of the T2D patients had no DR and 18 (23.1%) had DR.

Table 1. Demographics of the studied population.

	T1D		T2D	
	No DR, *n* = 5	**DR, *n* = 7**	**No DR, *n* = 60**	**DR, *n* = 18**
Gender				
Male, *n* (%)	3 (60.0)	5 (71.4)	39 (65.0)	14 (77.8)
Female, *n* (%)	2 (40.0)	2 (28.6)	21 (35.0)	4 (22.2)
Age, (yrs, median (IQR))	38.0 (30.5, 54.0)	31.0 (22.0, 43.0)	54.0 (44.8, 62.0)	51.5 (37.3, 58.0)
Years since diagnosis, (median (IQR))	4.0 (0, 8.0)	17.0 (15.0, 23.0)	1.0 (0, 3.8)	11 (5.8, 14.3)
BMI ≥ 25, *n* (%)	2 (40.0)	2 (28.6)	49 (81.7)	13 (72.2)

For the T1D group, the median age was 38 (IQR 30.5, 54.0) for patients without DR and 31 (IQR 22.0, 43.0) for patients with DR. For the T2D group, the median age was 54 (IQR 44.8, 62.0) for patients without DR and 51.5 (IQR 37.3, 58.0) for patients with DR.

The median number of years since diagnosis of DM for the T1D patients having no DR was 4.0 (IQR: 0, 8.0) and having DR was 17.0 (IQR: 15.0, 23.0), while for the T2D patients it was 1.0 (IQR: 0, 3.8) and 11.0 (IQR: 5.8, 14.3), respectively.

Two T1D patients had obesity and DR (28.6%) (body mass index (BMI) ≥25), and two had obesity and no DR (40.0%); in the T2D group, obesity and DR was present in thirteen (72.2%) patients and obesity and no DR in forty-nine (81.7%) patients.

Table 2 shows the screening history of our study cohort. A total of 47 (52.2%) patients were newly diagnosed with DM (e.g., time since diagnosis was <5 years for patients with T1D and <1 year for patients with T2D): 4 (8.5%) T1D and 43 (91.5%) T2D. In the T1D group, 3 (75.0%) had non-DR and 1 (25.0%) had DR, while in the T2D group, 40 (93.0%) had non-DR and 3 (7.0%) had DR. Overall, 8.5% of the patients who were newly diagnosed with DM had DR.

Table 2. Screening history of the studied population.

	T1D		T2D		Total, n = 90
	No DR, n = 5	DR, n = 7	No DR, n = 60	DR, n = 18	
Patients newly diagnosed with DM **, n (%)	3 * (60.0)	1 (14.3)	40 (66.7)	3 (16.7)	47 (52.2)
Patients not newly diagnosed with DM *, n (%)**	2 (40.0)	6 (85.7)	20 (33.3)	15 (83.3)	43 (47.8)
Previous eye exam, n (%) of patients not newly diagnosed with DM	2 (100)	6 (100)	2 (10.0)	6 (40.0)	16 (37.2)
>2 years since last eye exam, n (%) of patients not newly diagnosed with DM	1 (50.0)	4 (66.7)	1 (50.0)	5 (83.3)	11 (68.8)
Patients followed-up as recommended, n (%) of patients not newly diagnosed with DM	1 (50.0)	2 (33.3)	1 (2.3)	1 (6.7)	5 (11.6)

* Two patients with T1D who were newly diagnosed had LADA. ** First visit within 1 year from diagnosis for patients with T2D and within 5 years for patients with T1D. *** First visit >5 years for patients with T1D and >1 year from diagnosis of patients with T2D.

A total of 43 (47.8%) patients were not newly diagnosed with DM (e.g., time since diagnosis > 5 years for patients with T1D and >1 year for patients with T2D); 8 (18.6%) of these patients had T1D and 35 (81.4%) had T2D. In the T1D group, 2 patients (25.0%) had no DR and 6 (75.0%) had DR, while in the T2D group, 20 patients (57%) had no DR and 15 (43%) had DR. Overall, 48.8% of the patients who were not newly diagnosed with DM had DR.

Of the 43 patients not newly diagnosed with DM, 16 (37.2%) had previously undertaken an eye exam. For 11 (68.8%) of the patients who had an eye exam, it was more than 2 years, with a maximum of 10 years since the last eye exam.

Twenty-seven (62.8%) patients not newly diagnosed with DM had not undertaken an eye exam (only T2D patients), and the duration of DM for these patients varied from 2 to 18 years (median 8 years); twelve (44.4%) of these patients had had DM for > 10 years.

With regard to antidiabetic drugs (Table 3), 9 out of 12 patients (75.0%) with TD1 used insulin, and the duration of insulin treatment ranged from 0 to 34 years; 8 out of 78 patients (10.3%) with T2D used insulin, and the duration of treatment ranged from 0 to 18 years; 3 out of 12 patients (25.0%) in the T1D group and 58 out of 78 patients (74.4%) in the T2D group used other antidiabetic medications (OAMs). Both insulin and OAMs were used by 4 out of 78 patients (5.1%) in the T2D group but none in the T1D group. None of the patients with T1D used glucagon-like peptide 1 analogues (GLP-1 analogues). In the T2D group, three patients (17.6%) with DR and four patients (7.8%) without DR used GLP agonists. None of the T1D patients used cholesterol-lowering medications, while 31 of the T2D patients (22 without DR (36.7%) and 9 with DR (50%)) used cholesterol medications. One patient in the T1D group having DR (14.1%) was on antihypertensive medication and in the T2D group forty patients (thirty-three without DR (55.0%) and seven with DR (38.9%)), respectively.

Table 4 shows the odds ratio for DR in the studied population (T1D and T2D) and in the T2D population alone.

The univariate analysis found for the whole cohort a significant association between DR and the following parameters: age increase of 1 year showed a 2% decrease ($p = 0.002$) in the odds ratio for DR; an increase of 11 mmol/mol HbA1c showed a 19% increase ($p = 0.003$) a 1-unit increase in the urine albumin-to-creatinine ratio showed a 1% increase ($p = 0.008$); a 1-unit increase in BMI showed a 6% decrease ($p < 0.001$); and a 1-year increase in DM duration showed a 13% increase ($p < 0.001$) in the odds ratio for DR.

Table 3. Diabetes, cholesterol-lowering and antihypertensive medications used in the studied population.

	T1D		T2D	
	No DR, $n = 5$	DR, $n = 7$	No DR, $n = 60$	DR, $n = 18$
Diabetes medication				
Insulin, n (%)	3 (60.0)	6 (85.7)	4 (6.7)	4 (22.2)
Years of insulin, median (range)	8.0 (0.0–8.0)	16.5 (1.0–34.0)	0 (0.0–11.0)	7.0 (3.0–18.0)
OAM * n (%)	2 ** (40.0)	1 ** (14.3)	43 (71.7)	15 (83.3)
OAM + insulin, n (%)	0 (0)	0 (0)	2 (3.3)	2 (11.1)
GLP analogues ***, n (%)	0 (0)	0 (0)	4 (7.8)	3 (17.6)
Cholesterol-lowering medications, n (%)	0 (0)	0 (0)	22 (36.7)	9 (50.0)
Antihypertensive medications, n (%)	0 (0)	1(14.3)	33 (55.0)	7 (38.9)

* OAM: other antidiabetic medication. ** Of the 3 patients in the T1D group not using insulin, 2 were newly diagnosed with LADA (2) and 1 not newly diagnosed had MODY3 (1). *** Glucagon-like peptide-1 analogues.

Table 4. Univariate analyses of the different parameters of the studied population.

	Total (T1D and T2D)		Only T2D	
	OR (95% CI)	p-Value	OR (95% CI)	p-Value
Age per 1 year	0.98 (0.96, 0.99)	**0.002**	0.99 (0.97, 1.01)	0.283
Male gender	1.40 (0.89, 2.19)	0.144	1.49 (0.88, 2.53)	0.137
HbA1c per 11 mmol/mol	1.19 (1.06, 1.34)	**0.003**	1.31 (1.15, 1.50)	**<0.001**
Total cholesterol	0.91 (0.74, 1.10)	0.322	0.99 (0.80, 1.22)	0.900
Urine creatinine	0.98 (0.95, 1.01)	0.268	0.95 (0.91, 0.997)	**0.036**
Urine albumin	1.001 (0.9999, 1.001)	0.101	1.001 (0.9999, 1.002)	0.524
Urine album-to-creatinine ratio	1.01 (1.003, 1.02)	**0.008**	1.01 (1.002, 1.02)	**0.016**
Microalbuminuria	0.95 (0.58, 1.56)	0.835	0.99 (0.58, 1.71)	0.989
BMI	0.94 (0.90, 0.97)	**<0.001**	0.92 (0.88, 0.97)	**0.001**
Duration of diabetes per 1 year	1.13 (1.09, 1.17)	**<0.001**	1.11 (1.07, 1.16)	**<0.001**
HT *	1.01 (0.66, 1.55)	0.948	0.86 (0.53, 1.39)	0.533
SBP	0.99 (0.98, 1.002)	0.104	0.99 (0.98, 1.001)	0.355
DBP	0.99 (0.97, 1.01)	0.351	1.00 (0.98, 1.02)	0.962
MAP	0.99 (0.97, 1.01)	0.162	0.995 (0.98, 1.02)	0.645
Type DM (1 vs. 2)	3.05 (1.75, 5.32)	**<0.001**		
Smoke (yes/no)	1.12 (0.64, 1.96)	0.695	0.45 (0.17, 1.22)	0.118
Smokeless tobacco (yes/no)	0.62 (0.34, 1.14)	0.124	0.80 (0.43, 1.51)	0.496
Alcohol	0.99 (0.92, 1.07)	0.853	0.92 (0.83, 1.02)	0.093
BCVA	1.29 (0.32, 5.26)	0.721	3.24 (0.71, 14.76)	0.129
IOP	0.97 (0.91, 1.04)	0.363	0.98 (0.91, 1.06)	0.657
MOPP	0.98 (0.96, 1.01)	0.210	0.99 (0.96, 1.03)	0.717

Note: Four patients had urine parameters missing, while 1 patient had HbA1c missing. * SBP $\geq$ 140 mmHg and/or DBP $\geq$ 90 mmHg.

The same analyses for the T2D population alone found a significant association between DR and the following parameters: an HbA1c increase of 11 mmol/mol showed a 31% increase ($p < 0.001$); an increase of 1 unit of BMI showed an 8% decrease ($p = 0.001$); and an increase of 1 year in DM duration showed an 11% increase ($p < 0.001$) in the odds ratio for DR.

There was a significant difference ($p < 0.001$) in the odds ratio for DR in the T1D versus the T2D group, with three times higher odds (OR 3.05) for DR in the T1D group.

Table 5 shows the presence of diabetic maculopathy based on fundus photos in the study cohort. None of the patients without DR had diabetic maculopathy; 43 eyes (23.9%) had DR, and in 27 (62.8%) of these eyes, diabetic maculopathy was also present.

In the T1D group, DR was found in 14 (58.3%) eyes, and 9 (64.3%) of these eyes had diabetic maculopathy based on fundus photos. All eyes with diabetic maculopathy had MA within 1 DD from the foveola, and one of these eyes (11.1%) also had hard exudates.

Table 5. Presence of diabetic maculopathy on fundus photo in the studied population.

	T1D Number of Eyes = 24		T2D Number of Eyes = 156		Total Number of Eyes = 180
	Number of Eyes with DR = 14		Number of Eyes with DR = 29		Total Number of Eyes with DR = 43
	OD	OS	OD	OS	
Diabetic maculopathy, ***n*** (%) of total eyes with DR in the same group	4 (28.6)	5 (35.7)	11 (37.9)	7 (24.1)	27 (62.8)
(1) Microaneurysm, *n* (%) of total eyes with DR and diabetic maculopathy in the same group	4 (100)	5 (100)	11(100)	7 (100)	27 (100)
(2) Hard exudates, *n* (%) of total eyes with DR and diabetic maculopathy in the same group	0	1 (0.2)	2 (18.2)	1 (14.3)	4(14.8)

In the T2D group, DR was found in 29 (18.6%) eyes, and 18 (62.1%) of these eyes had diabetic maculopathy based on fundus photos. All eyes with diabetic maculopathy had MA within 1 DD from the foveola, and three of these eyes (16.7%) also had hard exudates.

4. Discussion

The present pilot study provides us baseline screening information concerning the population with DM in the Oslo region, Norway. This is valuable for planning and establishing an optimal systematic screening system in this area of the country, and further, to establish a national screening system in Norway. The results from our pilot study demonstrate a lack of ophthalmological examinations and follow-ups for DM patients and the need for implementing a proper and systematic DR screening.

The majority of the 90 patients (180 eyes) recruited in our study came from general practitioners in the Oslo region, Norway. Approximately half of the patients were newly diagnosed with DM (time since diagnosis $\leq$5 years for patients with T1D and $\leq$1 year for patients with T2D). Two patients with T1D in this category had late autoimmune diabetes in the adults (LADA). Considering the group of patients without a newly diagnosed DM, nearly two-thirds of them had never had an eye exam performed. The duration time of DM for these patients varied from 2 to 18 years (median: 8 years), and 12 patients had DM > 10 years. Only 37% of the patients not newly diagnosed had a previous eye exam, and little over two-thirds of these patients had more than 2 years since their last eye exam. Implementing a proper and systematic DR screening in our region is needed for better reaching out to patients with DM, to improve timely follow-up and thereby reduce DR progression and vision loss.

The prevalence of any DR in patients with T1D and T2D were 58.3% (95% CI: 14.3, 47.6) and 23.1% (95% CI: 52.4, 85.7), respectively, which is similar to other population-based studies [10,18,19]. It is challenging, however, to compare the prevalence of DR among studies, since there are differences between grading protocols and populations. A Norwegian study, from 2012, by Kilstad et al. [7] found the prevalence of any DR in T1D to be 66%, which is higher than in our study, whereas the prevalence for any DR in T2D was 24%, which is in line with our study. Established treatment-dependent DR was an exclusion criterion in this study, and approximately half of the patients were newly diagnosed with DM, which could have affected the results obtained compared to other studies. In particular, the high proportion of newly diagnosed patients can be part of the explanation for why there were no cases of proliferative DR and few cases of severe DR. Still, another Norwegian study, from 2008, by Sundling et al. [20] reported an even lower prevalence of DR. However, this was a questionnaire-based survey study.

In other parts of Europe, Looker et al. [10] found the prevalence of DR in a population with newly diagnosed T2D in Scotland to be 19.3%. According to the Liverpool Diabetic Eye Study [18], the prevalence of DR was 45.7% and 25.3% for T1D and T2D, respectively, and the United Kingdom Prospective study (UKPDS) [21] found a prevalence of 37% for DR at diagnosis in a cohort of patients with T2D. In a cross-sectional study from Wales [19], the prevalence of any DR for T1D and T2D was 56.3% and 30.9%, respectively.

By comparison, a recent systematic review and meta-analysis showed that the prevalence of DR in patients with DM during 2020 was highest in the Middle East and North Africa (32.90%), North America and the Caribbean (33.30%), moderate in Southeast Asia (16.99%) and Western Pacific (19.20%) and lowest in South and Central America (13.37%) [22]. In China, the reported prevalence of DR in patients with DM in a relatively small cohort carried out between 2018 and 2019 was also high (40%) [23].

It is well known that the duration of DM is a major risk factor for DR [18,19,24–28], as also demonstrated by our study. Notably, each one-year increase in the duration of DM showed a 13% increase in the OR for DR (OR 1.13; 95% CI 1.09, 1.17; $p < 0.001$), and in the T2D group alone an increase of 1 year in duration of diabetes showed an 11% increase in the OR for DR (OR 1.11; 95% CI 1.07, 1.16; $p < 0.001$). In our cohort of patients, an age increase of 1 year showed a 2% decrease in the OR for DR (OR 0.98; 95% CI 0.96, 0.99; $p = 0.002$). This could be related to the younger age of the studied population in the T1D group and the higher number of patients with DR in this group itself. Other studies have also shown an association of DR with younger age [29,30]. No significant association was found between DR and age in the T2D population alone in our cohort.

For both groups T1D and T2D (OR 0.94; 95% CI 0.90, 0.97; $p < 0.001$) and for T2D alone (OR 0.92; 95% CI 0.88, 0.97; $p = 0.001$), there was an inverse association for DR with increased BMI, in accordance with other studies [31,32].

An increase of 11 mmol/mol HbA1c showed a 19% increase in the OR for DR for the whole cohort (OR 1.19; 95% CI 1.06, 1.34; $p = 0.003$) and a 31% increase for the T2D population alone (OR 1.31; 95% CI 1.15, 1.50; $p < 0.001$). This higher risk for DR with the increase in HbA1c is in line with multiple studies from several countries, both for T2D [21,27] and T1D [27,33–35].

For the urine creatinine level, a significant inverse association with DR was found in the T2D group (OR 0.95; 95% CI 0.91, 0.997; $p = 0.036$), which is in accordance with a population-based study of patients with T2D [36]. In both this study and others [37,38], the urine albumin-to-creatinine ratio showed a positive association with DR, similar to our cohort of both T1D and T2D grouped together (OR 1.01; 95% CI 1.003, 1.02; $p = 0.008$) but also in the T2D group alone (OR 1.01; 95% CI 1.002, 1.02; $p = 0.016$).

T1D is a known risk factor for DR [39,40], and we also found three times higher OR (OR 3.05; 95% CI 1.75, 5.32; $p < 0.001$) for DR in the T1D group compared to the T2D group. It needs to be taken into consideration the small number of T1D patients in our study cohort, which is a limitation of our study.

No significant association between DR and HT was found in our population; meanwhile, several other studies have found a positive association with HT [21,34,35,41]. Gender, total plasma cholesterol, urine albumin, microalbuminuria, HT, SBT, DBT, MAP, smoking, use of smokeless tobacco, alcohol, VA, IOP, BCVA and MOPP also did not show a significant association with DR.

Three-quarters of the patients with T1D and one-tenth of the patients with T2D were on insulin treatment. The three patients in the T1D group not on insulin treatment were two newly diagnosed patients with LADA and one not newly diagnosed patient with MODY3. In other population-based studies [7,42], 17–18% of the patients with T2D were on insulin treatment. The duration of the insulin treatment was the highest in the T1D group with DR, and the median duration of the insulin treatment in this group was more than double the time found in the T2D group with DR. In our pilot study, 67.8% used OAM, 4.4% were on insulin and OAM treatment and 7.8% were on GLP analogues. Regarding the percent of patients on GLP analogues, this is in accordance with a cohort study from the US, which included over a million patients with DM [43].

Diabetic maculopathy was found in more than one-third of the eyes examined in the T1D group and little over one-tenth of the eyes in the T2D group, with a total prevalence of 15%. The duration time of DM was 17 years in the T1D group with DR versus 11 years in the T2D group with DR. This and the limited number of patients in the T1D group can, to some extent, explain the impact on the divergent results obtained in the two groups. Compared to another cross-sectional study [44] of patients with T1D and T2D, the prevalence of diabetic maculopathy was lower in our study. The population included in the other study presented a longer duration of DM, patients and not eyes were observed, and the grading protocol was different from ours, which surely can affect the results.

5. Conclusions

This pilot study provides valuable baseline screening information concerning a DM population in the Oslo region, Norway. The results demonstrate a lack of ophthalmological examinations and follow-up for a considerable number of patients. Among the patients not newly diagnosed with DM, 62.8% had never had an eye exam; it was > 2 years since the last eye exam for 68.8% of the patients who had a previous eye exam. Implementing a systematic DR screening program is needed to better reach out to patients with DM and improve their screening adherence, thereby provide timely and proper treatment.

Author Contributions: Conceptualization, E.S.S., Ø.K.J., M.C.M., M.G.E., D.S.F. and G.P.; methodology, E.S.S., Ø.K.J., C.B., M.C.M., M.G.E., D.S.F. and G.P.; validation, E.S.S., D.S.F., C.B. and G.P.; investigation, E.S.S. and D.S.F.; writing—original draft preparation, E.S.S., Ø.K.J., C.B., M.C.M., M.G.E., D.S.F. and G.P.; writing—review and editing, E.S.S., Ø.K.J., C.B., M.C.M., M.G.E., D.S.F. and G.P.; visualization, E.S.S., C.B. and G.P.; supervision, Ø.K.J., M.G.E., D.S.F. and G.P. All authors have read and agreed to the published version of the manuscript.

Funding: Research was funded in the frames of the Baltic Research Programme's project Nr.EEA-RESEARCH-60 "Integrated model for personalized diabetic retinopathy screening and monitoring using risk-stratification and automated AI-based fundus image analysis (PerDiRe)" fi-nancially supported by the European Economic Area (EEA) Grants (Contract No. EEZ/BPP/VIAA/2021/8).

Institutional Review Board Statement: The Regional Committee for Medical and Health Research Ethics concluded that the project was outside the remit of the Norwegian Health Research Act (reference: 28857). The Institutional Data Protection Officer at OUH approved the study (reference: 20/00571).

Informed Consent Statement: Informed consent was obtained from all subjects involved in the study.

Data Availability Statement: Data from the project can be requested directly from the corresponding author.

Conflicts of Interest: The authors declare no conflict of interest.

References

1. Antonetti, D.A.; Klein, R.; Gardner, T.W. Diabetic retinopathy. *N. Engl. J. Med.* **2012**, *366*, 1227–1239. [CrossRef] [PubMed]
2. Leasher, J.L.; Bourne, R.R.; Flaxman, S.R.; Jonas, J.B.; Keeffe, J.; Naidoo, K.; Pesudovs, K.; Price, H.; White, R.A.; Wong, T.Y.; et al. Global Estimates on the Number of People Blind or Visually Impaired by Diabetic Retinopathy: A Meta-analysis from 1990 to 2010. *Diabetes Care* **2016**, *39*, 1643–1649. [CrossRef] [PubMed]
3. GBD Blindness and Vision Impairment Collaborators; Vision Loss Expert Group of the Global Burden of Disease Study. Causes of blindness and vision impairment in 2020 and trends over 30 years, and prevalence of avoidable blindness in relation to VISION 2020: The Right to Sight: An analysis for the Global Burden of Disease Study. *Lancet Glob. Health* **2021**, *9*, e144–e160. [CrossRef] [PubMed]
4. Mazhar, K.; Varma, R.; Choudhury, F.; McKean-Cowdin, R.; Shtir, C.J.; Azen, S.P. Severity of diabetic retinopathy and health-related quality of life: The Los Angeles Latino Eye Study. *Ophthalmology* **2011**, *118*, 649–655. [CrossRef] [PubMed]
5. Yau, J.W.Y.; Rogers, S.L.; Kawasaki, R.; Lamoureux, E.L.; Kowalski, J.W.; Bek, T.; Chen, S.-J.; Dekker, J.M.; Fletcher, A.; Grauslund, J.; et al. Global prevalence and major risk factors of diabetic retinopathy. *Diabetes Care* **2012**, *35*, 556–564. [CrossRef]
6. Rohan, T.E.; Frost, C.D.; Wald, N.J. Prevention of blindness by screening for diabetic retinopathy: A quantitative assessment. *BMJ* **1989**, *299*, 1198–1201. [CrossRef]
7. Kilstad, H.N.; Sjolie, A.K.; Goransson, L.; Hapnes, R.; Henschien, H.J.; Alsbirk, K.E.; Fossen, K.; Bertelsen, G.; Holstad, G.; Bergrem, H. Prevalence of diabetic retinopathy in Norway: Report from a screening study. *Acta Ophthalmol.* **2012**, *90*, 609–612.
8. Jones, S.; Edwards, R.T. Diabetic retinopathy screening: A systematic review of the economic evidence. *Diabet. Med.* **2010**, *27*, 249–256. [CrossRef]
9. Kohner, E.M.; Aldington, S.J.; Stratton, I.M.; Manley, S.E.; Holman, R.R.; Matthews, D.R.; Turner, R.C. United Kingdom Prospective Diabetes Study, 30: Diabetic retinopathy at diagnosis of non-insulin-dependent diabetes mellitus and associated risk factors. *Arch Ophthalmol.* **1998**, *116*, 297–303. [CrossRef]

10. Looker, H.C.; Nyangoma, S.O.; Cromie, D.; Olson, J.A.; Leese, G.P.; Philip, S.; Black, M.; Doig, J.; Lee, N.; on behalf of the Scottish Diabetic Retinopathy Screening Collaborative and the Scottish Diabetes Research Network Epidemiology Group; et al. Diabetic retinopathy at diagnosis of type 2 diabetes in Scotland. *Diabetologia* **2012**, *55*, 2335–2342. [CrossRef]
11. International Diabetes Federation. Diabetes Atlas, 10th ed. Brussels, Belgium. Available online: http://www.diabetesatlas.org (accessed on 24 August 2022).
12. Stene, L.C.; Ruiz, P.L.; Asvold, B.O.; Bjarko, V.V.; Sorgjerd, E.P.; Njolstad, I.; Hopstock, L.A.; Birkeland, K.I.; Gulseth, H.L. How many people have diabetes in Norway in 2020? *Tidsskr. Nor. Laegeforen.* **2020**, *140*. [CrossRef]
13. Bakke, A.; Cooper, J.G.; Thue, G.; Skeie, S.; Carlsen, S.; Dalen, I.; Løvaas, K.F.; Madsen, T.V.; Oord, E.R.; Berg, T.J.; et al. Type 2 diabetes in general practice in Norway 2005–2014: Moderate improvements in risk factor control but still major gaps in complication screening. *BMJ Open Diabetes Res. Care* **2017**, *5*, e000459. [CrossRef]
14. Available online: www.norpd.no/Prevalens.aspx (accessed on 24 August 2022).
15. Human Development Reports. Available online: https://worldpopulationreview.com/country-rankings/hdi-by-country (accessed on 24 August 2022).
16. Sehi, M.; Flanagan, J.G.; Zeng, L.; Cook, R.J.; Trope, G.E. Relative change in diurnal mean ocular perfusion pressure: A risk factor for the diagnosis of primary open-angle glaucoma. *Investig. Ophthalmol. Vis. Sci.* **2005**, *46*, 561–567. [CrossRef]
17. Wilkinson, C.P.; Ferris, F.L., III.; Klein, R.E.; Lee, P.P.; Agardh, C.D.; Davis, M.; Dills, D.; Kampik, A.; Pararajasegaram, A.; Verdaguer, J.T.; et al. Proposed international clinical diabetic retinopathy and diabetic macular edema disease severity scales. *Ophthalmology* **2003**, *110*, 1677–1682. [CrossRef]
18. Younis, N.; Broadbent, D.M.; Harding, S.P.; Vora, J.R. Prevalence of diabetic eye disease in patients entering a systematic primary care-based eye screening programme. *Diabet Med.* **2002**, *19*, 1014–1021
19. Thomas, R.L.; Dunstan, F.D.; Luzio, S.D.; Chowdhury, S.R.; North, R.V.; Hale, S.L.; Gibbins, R.L.; Owens, D.R. Prevalence of diabetic retinopathy within a national diabetic retinopathy screening service. *Br. J. Ophthalmol.* **2015**, *99*, 64–68.
20. Sundling, V.; Gulbrandsen, P.; Jervell, J.; Straand, J. Care of vision and ocular health in diabetic members of a national diabetes organization: A cross-sectional study. *BMC Health Serv. Res.* **2008**, *8*, 159.
21. Stratton, I.M.; Kohner, E.M.; Aldington, S.J.; Turner, R.C.; Holman, R.R.; Manley, S.E.; Matthews, D.R. UKPDS 50: Risk factors for incidence and progression of retinopathy in Type II diabetes over 6 years from diagnosis. *Diabetologia* **2001**, *44*, 156–163. [CrossRef]
22. Teo, Z.L.; Tham, Y.C.; Yu, M.; Chee, M.L.; Rim, T.H.; Cheung, N.; Bikbov, M.M.; Wang, Y.X.; Tang, Y.; Lu, Y.; et al. Global Prevalence of Diabetic Retinopathy and Projection of Burden through 2045: Systematic Review and Meta-analysis. *Ophthalmology* **2021**, *128*, 1580–1591. [CrossRef]
23. Yin, L.; Zhang, D.; Ren, Q.; Su, X.; Sun, Z. Prevalence and risk factors of diabetic retinopathy in diabetic patients: A community based cross-sectional study. *Medicine* **2020**, *99*, e19236. [CrossRef]
24. Al-Rubeaan, K.; Abu El-Asrar, A.M.; Youssef, A.M.; Subhani, S.N.; Ahmad, N.A.; Al-Sharqawi, A.H.; Alguwaihes, A.; Alotaibi, M.S.; Al-Ghamdi, A.; Ibrahim, H.M. Diabetic retinopathy and its risk factors in a society with a type 2 diabetes epidemic: A Saudi National Diabetes Registry-based study. *Acta Ophthalmol.* **2015**, *93*, e140–e147. [CrossRef] [PubMed]
25. Klein, R.; Klein, B.E.; Moss, S.E.; Davis, M.D.; DeMets, D.L. The Wisconsin epidemiologic study of diabetic retinopathy. II. Prevalence and risk of diabetic retinopathy when age at diagnosis is less than 30 years. *Arch. Ophthalmol.* **1984**, *102*, 520–526. [CrossRef] [PubMed]
26. Zhang, X.; Saaddine, J.B.; Chou, C.-F.; Cotch, M.F.; Cheng, Y.; Geiss, L.S.; Gregg, E.; Albright, A.L.; Klein, B.E.K.; Klein, R. Prevalence of diabetic retinopathy in the United States, 2005–2008. *JAMA* **2010**, *304*, 649–656. [CrossRef] [PubMed]
27. Matuszewski, W.; Stefanowicz-Rutkowska, M.M.; Szychlinska, M.; Bandurska-Stankiewicz, E. Differences in Risk Factors for Diabetic Retinopathy in Type 1 and Type 2 Diabetes Mellitus Patients in North-East Poland. *Medicina* **2020**, *56*, 177. [CrossRef]
28. Phillipov, G.; Alimat, A.; Phillips, P.J.; Drew, A.C. Screening for diabetic retinopathy. *Med. J. Aust.* **1995**, *162*, 518–520. [CrossRef]
29. Pan, C.W.; Wang, S.; Qian, D.J.; Xu, C.; Song, E. Prevalence, Awareness, and Risk Factors of Diabetic Retinopathy among Adults with Known Type 2 Diabetes Mellitus in an Urban Community in China. *Ophthalmic Epidemiol.* **2017**, *24*, 188–194. [CrossRef]
30. Kempen, J.H.; O'Colmain, B.J.; Leske, M.C.; Haffner, S.M.; Klein, R.; Moss, S.E.; Taylor, H.R.; Hamman, R.F. The prevalence of diabetic retinopathy among adults in the United States. *Arch. Ophthalmol.* **2004**, *122*, 552–563.
31. Lu, J.; Hou, X.; Zhang, L.; Jiang, F.; Hu, C.; Bao, Y.; Jia, W. Association between body mass index and diabetic retinopathy in Chinese patients with type 2 diabetes. *Acta Diabetol.* **2015**, *52*, 701–708. [CrossRef]
32. Sarrafan-Chaharsoughi, Z.; Manaviat, M.R.; Namiranian, N.; Yazdian-Anari, P.; Rahmanian, M. Is there a relationship between body mass index and diabetic retinopathy in type II diabetic patients? A cross sectional study. *J. Diabetes Metab. Disord.* **2018**, *17*, 63–69. [CrossRef]
33. Lind, M.; Pivodic, A.; Svensson, A.M.; Olafsdottir, A.F.; Wedel, H.; Ludvigsson, J. HbA(1c) level as a risk factor for retinopathy and nephropathy in children and adults with type 1 diabetes: Swedish population based cohort study. *BMJ* **2019**, *366*, l4894. [CrossRef]
34. Grauslund, J.; Green, A.; Sjolie, A.K. Prevalence and 25 year incidence of proliferative retinopathy among Danish type 1 diabetic patients. *Diabetologia* **2009**, *52*, 1829–1835. [CrossRef]
35. Klein, R.; Knudtson, M.D.; Lee, K.E.; Gangnon, R.; Klein, B.E. The Wisconsin Epidemiologic Study of Diabetic Retinopathy: XXII the twenty-five-year progression of retinopathy in persons with type 1 diabetes. *Ophthalmology* **2008**, *115*, 1859–1868. [CrossRef]

36. De Fine Olivarius, N.; Andreasen, A.H.; Vestbo, E.; Holstein-Rathlou, N.H.; Jorgensen, L.G.; Mogensen, C.E. Urinary creatinine concentration is inversely related to glycaemic control and the presence of some diabetic complications in patients with newly diagnosed Type 2 diabetes. *J. Diabetes Complicat.* **2006**, *20*, 45–50. [CrossRef]
37. Mujeeb, S.; Rodrigues, G.R.; Nayak, R.R.; Kamath, A.R.; Kamath, S.J.; Kamath, G. Urine protein: Urine creatinine ratio correlation with diabetic retinopathy. *Indian J. Ophthalmol.* **2021**, *69*, 3359–3363.
38. Lee, M.-K.; Han, K.-D.; Lee, J.-H.; Sohn, S.-Y.; Hong, O.-K.; Jeong, J.-S.; Kim, M.-K.; Baek, K.-H.; Song, K.-H.; Kwon, H.-S. Normal-to-mildly increased albuminuria predicts the risk for diabetic retinopathy in patients with type 2 diabetes. *Sci. Rep.* **2017**, *7*, 11757. [CrossRef]
39. Romero-Aroca, P.; Navarro-Gil, R.; Valls-Mateu, A.; Sagarra-Alamo, R.; Moreno-Ribas, A.; Soler, N. Differences in incidence of diabetic retinopathy between type 1 and 2 diabetes mellitus: A nine-year follow-up study. *Br. J. Ophthalmol.* **2017**, *101*, 1346–1351. [CrossRef]
40. Looker, H.C.; Nyangoma, S.O.; Cromie, D.T.; Olson, J.A.; Leese, G.P.; Black, M.W.; Doig, J.; Lee, N.; Lindsay, R.S.; A McKnight, J.; et al. Rates of referable eye disease in the Scottish National Diabetic Retinopathy Screening Programme. *Br. J. Ophthalmol.* **2014**, *98*, 790–795. [CrossRef]
41. Liu, L.; Quang, N.D.; Banu, R.; Kumar, H.; Tham, Y.-C.; Cheng, C.-Y.; Wong, T.Y.; Sabanayagam, C. Hypertension, blood pressure control and diabetic retinopathy in a large population-based study. *PLoS ONE* **2020**, *15*, e0229665. [CrossRef]
42. Taylor, R.H.; Jones, H.S.; Dodson, P.M.; Hamilton, A.P.; Kritzinger, E.E. Diabetic eye disease: A natural history study. *Eye* **1997**, *11*, 547–553. [CrossRef]
43. Eberly, L.A.; Yang, L.; Essien, U.R.; Eneanya, N.D.; Julien, H.M.; Luo, J.; Nathan, A.S.; Khatana, S.A.M.; Dayoub, E.J.; Fanaroff, A.C.; et al. Ethnic, and Socioeconomic Inequities in Glucagon-Like Peptide-1 Receptor Agonist Use Among Patients with Diabetes in the US. *JAMA Health Forum.* **2021**, *2*, e214182. [CrossRef]
44. Zander, E.; Herfurth, S.; Bohl, B.; Heinke, P.; Herrmann, U.; Kohnert, K.-D.; Kerner, W. Maculopathy in patients with diabetes mellitus type 1 and type 2: Associations with risk factors. *Br. J. Ophthalmol.* **2000**, *84*, 871–876. [CrossRef] [PubMed]

biomedicines

MDPI

Review

Advances in Structural and Functional Retinal Imaging and Biomarkers for Early Detection of Diabetic Retinopathy

Zhengwei Zhang [1,2,3], Callie Deng [3] and Yannis M. Paulus [3,4,*]

1 Department of Ophthalmology, Jiangnan University Medical Center, Wuxi 214002, China; zhengwz@med.umich.edu
2 Department of Ophthalmology, Wuxi No.2 People's Hospital, Wuxi Clinical College, Nantong University, Wuxi 214002, China
3 Department of Ophthalmology and Visual Sciences, University of Michigan, Ann Arbor, MI 48105, USA; calliede@med.umich.edu
4 Department of Biomedical Engineering, University of Michigan, 1000 Wall Street, Ann Arbor, MI 48105, USA
* Correspondence: ypaulus@med.umich.edu; Tel.: +1-734-232-8105; Fax: +1-734-936-3815

Abstract: Diabetic retinopathy (DR), a vision-threatening microvascular complication of diabetes mellitus (DM), is a leading cause of blindness worldwide that requires early detection and intervention. However, diagnosing DR early remains challenging due to the subtle nature of initial pathological changes. This review explores developments in multimodal imaging and functional tests for early DR detection. Where conventional color fundus photography is limited in the field of view and resolution, advanced quantitative analysis of retinal vessel traits such as retinal microvascular caliber, tortuosity, and fractal dimension (FD) can provide additional prognostic value. Optical coherence tomography (OCT) has also emerged as a reliable structural imaging tool for assessing retinal and choroidal neurodegenerative changes, which show potential as early DR biomarkers. Optical coherence tomography angiography (OCTA) enables the evaluation of vascular perfusion and the contours of the foveal avascular zone (FAZ), providing valuable insights into early retinal and choroidal vascular changes. Functional tests, including multifocal electroretinography (mfERG), visual evoked potential (VEP), multifocal pupillographic objective perimetry (mfPOP), microperimetry, and contrast sensitivity (CS), offer complementary data on early functional deficits in DR. More importantly, combining structural and functional imaging data may facilitate earlier detection of DR and targeted management strategies based on disease progression. Artificial intelligence (AI) techniques show promise for automated lesion detection, risk stratification, and biomarker discovery from various imaging data. Additionally, hematological parameters, such as neutrophil–lymphocyte ratio (NLR) and neutrophil extracellular traps (NETs), may be useful in predicting DR risk and progression. Although current methods can detect early DR, there is still a need for further research and development of reliable, cost-effective methods for large-scale screening and monitoring of individuals with DM.

Keywords: diabetes mellitus; early diabetic retinopathy; diagnostic tests; optical coherence tomography; optical coherence tomography angiography; combined measures; deep learning

1. Introduction

Diabetic retinopathy (DR) is a leading cause of preventable blindness globally, affecting approximately one-third of patients with diabetes [1,2], with vision-related quality of life (VRQoL) declining with the severity of DR [3]. A microvascular complication of both type 1 and type 2 diabetes, DR is characterized by progressive retinal vascular abnormalities and neurodegeneration [4] and disproportionately affects individuals in socioeconomically disadvantaged areas [5]. Multiple factors contribute to the onset of DR, including chronic hyperglycemia, oxidative stress, inflammation, the complement system, and gut microbiome. These processes lead to the development of various retinal lesions, such as microaneurysms, hemorrhages, hard exudates, cotton wool spots, and neovascularization. However, the precise mechanistic pathway remains an area of active investigation [6–9].

DR can progress through distinct stages, ranging from mild non-proliferative DR (NPDR) to more advanced proliferative DR (PDR), characterized by the abnormal growth of new blood vessels on the retinal surface or into the vitreous cavity. Diabetic macular edema (DME), a consequence of increased vascular permeability and fluid accumulation in the macula, can occur at any stage and is a leading cause of vision loss among individuals with DR [10]. The impact of DR extends beyond vision impairment, affecting individuals' quality of life, productivity, and overall well-being. Studies have shown that DR is associated with an increased risk of cardiovascular diseases, cognitive decline, and premature mortality [11,12].

Early detection and timely intervention are crucial in preventing the progression of DR and reducing the risk of vision loss and systemic cascading complications [13]. However, the initial stages of DR can be asymptomatic, making regular screening and comprehensive eye examinations essential for individuals not only diagnosed with diabetes mellitus (DM) but also those with euglycemic hyperinsulinemia or prediabetes/hyperglycemia [14–16]. A recent study, utilizing histological analysis and high-resolution in vivo imaging, demonstrated that subclinical DR is characterized by numerous alterations. These include changes in blood flow, vascular architecture, expression of contractile proteins, the function of pericytes and endothelial cells, glial activity and density (including astrocytes, Müller cells, and microglia), neuronal function, retinal cell counts, layer thickness, and choroidal thickness [17]. These collective subclinical changes likely contribute to the ultimate manifestation of clinically evident DR. The first sign of clinical DR—formation of microaneurysms—may represent a relatively late stage in the disease process. It is reasonable to deduce that the onset of clinically detectable DR lesions is preceded by a cascade of subclinical pathological events, underscoring the importance of identifying and monitoring these early alterations for timely intervention.

The significance of early detection of DR is twofold. From the ophthalmologist's perspective, advanced imaging modalities allow for the identification of subtle retinal and choroidal alterations at the earliest stages of the disease process. This knowledge guides the development of therapeutic interventions targeting these initial pathological events, enabling clinicians to promptly intervene and advise patients on stricter management of controllable risk factors. From the patient's perspective, convenient screening enables regular examination and early detection of DR, empowering patients to take a proactive role in managing their disease and preserving vision [18].

Advanced imaging and functional testing, combined with accurate risk stratification and personalized treatment planning, can improve visual outcomes for individuals with diabetes. This review synthesizes the latest advancements in multimodal imaging and functional testing for DR detection while highlighting the value of monitoring subclinical retinal alterations for early intervention.

The search strategy is as follows: Medline, Embase, and Google Scholar were searched until 1 April 2024. The keywords used in the search were "diabetic retinopathy", "prediabetes/hyperglycemia", and "early detection". The reference lists of relevant reviews and eligible articles identified from the electronic searches were manually examined to locate any pertinent studies that were not included in the electronic databases. Furthermore, the related articles cited in Google Scholar were also manually reviewed to identify any potentially relevant studies that had not been retrieved by the initial search.

2. Fundus Photography and Image Analysis

The retinal vasculature presents a uniquely accessible "window" for studying human microcirculation in vivo. Advancements in digital retinal photography and other imaging techniques have facilitated the precise characterization of retinal vascular changes in large populations. This non-invasive imaging approach has enabled researchers to investigate early retinal microvascular alterations as potential biomarkers for systemic microvascular diseases [19–21].

2.1. Conventional Color Fundus Photography

Conventional color fundus photography, capturing a field of view between 20° and 50°, has long been the standard method for screening and evaluating DR. This technique involves capturing images of the posterior retina using a tabletop fundus camera. In recent years, the emergence of portable and user-friendly imaging devices has made it easier to perform retinal screenings, particularly in remote or resource-limited settings [22,23]. The widespread availability of smartphones with advanced camera capabilities has led to the development of mobile phone-based fundus imaging systems (Figure 1) [24–28]. These systems typically involve attaching a lens or adaptor to a smartphone camera and transforming it into a portable fundus camera. This approach leverages the computational power and connectivity of smartphones, enabling telemedicine applications where retinal images can be captured and transmitted for remote evaluation by ophthalmologists or artificial intelligence (AI) systems [29,30].

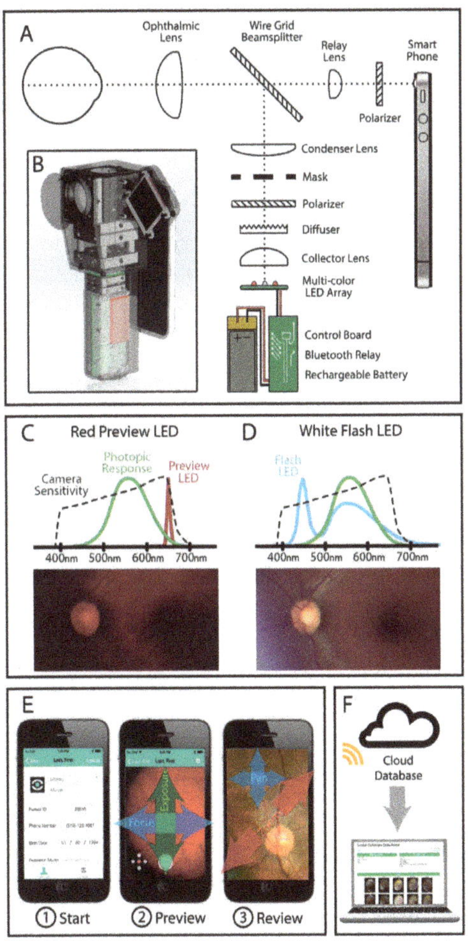

Figure 1. CellScope Retina schematic and workflow. (**A**) Schematic of the optical system. Light from LEDs is directed through a mask and forms an annulus that passes through the peripheral cornea,

focusing through the pupil. In propagating through the eye, the light becomes defocused, providing even illumination at the retina. Polarization filters minimize unwanted reflections from anterior ocular surfaces, enabling the smartphone to capture a clear image of the retina. (**B**) The compact optical system and custom-control electronics fit inside a handheld enclosure. (**C**) Red LED illumination of 655 nm peak emission is used for focusing on the retina, which is within the spectral range of the iPhone camera but outside the peak photopic response of the eye. (**D**) A white LED with a broad emission spectrum is flashed for recording images of the retina. LED spectra in (**C**,**D**) are from respective datasheets; photopic response is from the CIE 1931 standard [31]; phone response is approximate for a CMOS phone sensor. (**E**) Smartphone user interface enables (1) patient data capture, (2) preview during focus/alignment with swipe gestures adjusting camera settings, and (3) exam data review with pinch and swipe gestures for browsing stitched image montages. (**F**) Photos can be uploaded directly from the smartphone to a cloud database allowing remote diagnosis with a web interface. Reproduced with permission from Reference [24].

Up until now, color fundus photography remains a simple, accessible, and cost-effective technique for examining the retinal fundus. However, it is important to note that while the appearance of microaneurysms on color fundus photographs represents an early clinical manifestation, advanced multimodal imaging techniques and functional tests have revealed subclinical retinal alterations that occur long before the manifestation of these minimal fundus lesions [13,32,33]. A comparison of retinal imaging modalities, including their advantages, disadvantages, and key findings associated with early DR, are summarized (Table 1) and explored in further detail below. It is crucial for ophthalmologists to acknowledge that even in the absence of visible lesions in fundus photography, special attention is needed for high-risk diabetic patients with a disease duration exceeding 10 years. Alongside advising patients to undergo regular screening for potential complications, it is advisable to suggest auxiliary examinations for comprehensive evaluation and monitoring [34].

Table 1. A summary table comparing the advantages, disadvantages, and key findings in early DR for a variety of retinal imaging modalities.

Imaging Modality	Advantages	Disadvantages	Key Findings in Early DR
Conventional color fundus photography	The standard for evaluating and screening DR. Widely available, cost-effective, and easy to perform. Recent smartphone-based fundus imaging systems are low-cost and portable.	Unable to detect subclinical retinal alterations that occur prior to the appearance of microaneurysms. Limited field of view (between 20° and 50°), may miss peripheral lesions and requires pupil dilation.	Microaneurysms Retinal hemorrhages Macular edema Retinal venular widening Arteriolar tortuosity Venular tortuosity Decreased fractal dimension
Ultra-wide-field fundus photography	Extensive view of periphery (up to 200° in a single image), allowing for assessment of approximately 80% of retinal surface area. Enables detection of milder and earlier forms of DR affecting the periphery. Some systems offer true-color retinal images and artifact mitigation, enabling higher accuracy in detecting microaneurysms and retinal hemorrhages.	Higher cost and less readily available in clinical settings. May require specialized training to operate and interpret findings, particularly in peripheral regions which can appear distorted.	Peripheral retinal lesions and ischemia, in addition to the above findings seen in conventional fundus photography.

Table 1. *Cont.*

Imaging Modality	Advantages	Disadvantages	Key Findings in Early DR
Fundus fluorescein angiography (FFA)	Detailed visualization of blood vessel abnormalities and leakage.	Invasive, potential allergic reactions to dye, and requires skilled interpretation.	Microaneurysms Neovascularization (NV) Areas of non-perfusion (NP) Increased foveal avascular zone (FAZ) area
Optical coherence tomography (OCT)	High-resolution images of retinal layers, non-invasive, and quick. Provides quantitative measurements of retinal thickness and volume. Detects subtle retinal changes at early stages of the disease.	Higher cost and less ubiquitous than color fundus cameras. Limited field of view and may miss peripheral pathology. May require specialized training to interpret findings.	Faster rate of GC-IPL thinning Decreased pRNFL thickness Increased inner retinal reflectivity Decreased choroidal vascular index (CVI) Decreased choroidal thickness (ChT) Macular edema Intraretinal fluid or retinal thickening due to fluid accumulation
Optical coherence tomography angiography (OCTA)	Non-invasive, dye-free, and quick. High-resolution, depth-resolved angiographic images, including better visualization of capillary microvasculature compared to FFA. Provides a broader perspective of the fundus and quantitative features for assessing disease severity.	Higher cost and less ubiquitous. Artifacts may affect image quality. Barriers to widespread adoption include scan quality and lack of standardization of quantitative metrics between different commercial OCTA machines.	Decreased perfusion density of the deep capillary complex (DCC) Decreased mid-large choroidal vessel thickness and vessel density Foveal avascular zone (increased area, shape irregularity) Areas of non-perfusion (NP) Microaneurysms
Ultra-wide-field swept-source OCTA (SS-OCTA)	Extensive field of view, in addition to traditional OCTA advantages.	High cost, complex technology, and limited availability.	Early changes in vascular density of the superficial and deep vascular complexes in the peripheral retina, in addition to the above findings for OCTA.

2.2. Ultra-Wide-Field Fundus Photography

Recent advancements in fundus imaging enable physicians to capture a comprehensive view of the retina, covering up to 200° in a single image [35]. Clarus™ (CLARUS 500™, Carl Zeiss Meditec AG, Jena, Germany) and Optos® (Optos California®, Optos PLC, Dunfermline, UK) are currently the two most used ultra-wide-field (UWF) fundus imaging systems. Although the reliability in detecting signs of early DR is high for both devices [36], the Clarus™ system has demonstrated higher accuracy in detecting microaneurysms and retinal hemorrhages due to its capability of providing true-color retinal images and mitigating artifacts caused by eyelids and eyelashes [37]. Diabetic eyes exhibiting visible lesions exclusively in the periphery tend to present with a milder and earlier form of retinopathy in comparison to those with visible lesions present in either the central retina or spanning both the central and peripheral retina [38]. Therefore, comprehensive visualization and assessment of the peripheral retina are crucial for early detection, accurate severity staging, and prediction of DR progression [39–41]. In clinical practice, pupillary dilation and manual eyelid lifting have been reported to substantially increase the visible retinal area during UWF fundus imaging, enhancing the detection of retinal hemorrhages and microaneurysms [42]. To accurately detect early, subtle lesions, operators must pay close attention to the technique used when capturing UWF fundus images.

2.3. Advanced Fundus Image Analysis Techniques

2.3.1. Retinal Vascular Caliber

Pathophysiologic processes central to diabetes such as oxidative stress, endothelial dysfunction, inflammation, and hypertension can cause subclinical alterations in microvascular structure and perfusion. Abnormalities in retinal vessel caliber such as venular widening and microaneurysms can, therefore, serve as promising biomarkers for diabetic microvascular complications [43].

Wider retinal venular caliber has been correlated with an elevated risk of type 2 diabetes. In an extensive individual-level meta-analysis comprising 18,771 participants, retinal venular caliber was positively associated with an increased risk of developing diabetes over a median follow-up period of 10 years [21]. This correlation remained significant even after adjusting for potential confounders, including age, race/ethnicity, smoking status, body mass index (BMI), and hypertension, and was notably more pronounced in male participants. There was no significant correlation between retinal arteriolar caliber and incident type 2 diabetes [21]. In addition to predicting the risk of developing diabetes, studies suggest that venular caliber is significantly wider among type 2 diabetics with DR compared to non-DR [44]. However, the underlying mechanisms driving changes in retinal venular caliber in diabetes are not fully understood. Experimental data suggest that insulin resistance-induced microvascular dysfunction may prompt retinal venule dilation due to inflammation [44,45]. Monitoring changes in retinal vascular caliber could aid in the early detection of DR.

2.3.2. Tortuosity of Branch Retinal Artery

High glucose levels similarly precipitate changes in retinal vessel tortuosity. Increased vessel tortuosity, prevalent in various diseases and aging, serves as a critical indicator of retinal ischemia and DR progression [46]. Tortuosity reflects diabetes-induced hemodynamic alterations, including disrupted blood flow and endothelial dysfunction, alongside elevated vascular endothelial growth factor (VEGF) production.

Studies on the associations between retinal arteriolar tortuosity, venular tortuosity, and DR are mixed. In a study of 224 type 1 and 2 diabetic patients, Sasongko et al. reported that increased arteriolar tortuosity, not venular tortuosity, is associated with mild and moderate stages of DR [46]. Conversely, Forster et al. reported that greater venular tortuosity alone is associated with incident DR in adults with type 2 diabetes [47]. A recent study developed a prediction model for DR among type 2 diabetics and found that while arteriolar and venular tortuosity are both associated with DR, arteriolar tortuosity is significantly more predictive of DR [48].

Fundus photography-based studies investigating vessel tortuosity have primarily concentrated on the main retinal vessels, partly due to challenges in visualizing and analyzing branch retinal vessels in fundus images. A recent study involving high-resolution fundus images from diabetic patients across varying DR stages proposed that branch retinal vessels may be more closely related to the onset and progression of DR than main vessels [49]. Findings revealed a significant increase in branch artery tortuosity from no DR to evident DR and with increasing DR severity. Thus, branch retinal artery tortuosity appears to be a promising biomarker for early DR detection and precise evaluation, aiding in effective DR management strategies.

2.3.3. Fractal Dimension

Fractal dimension (FD) quantifies the complexity or density of vascular patterns in a two-dimensional space. It is more closely linked to microvascular than macrovascular diseases [48]. In DR, disease progression is marked by the formation of non-perfusion areas due to occluded microvasculature. This often leads to a simplified retinal vascular pattern and a decreased FD. However, some studies have reported an increase in FD in DR, highlighting the complexity of vascular changes throughout the disease's progression [50]. From moderate non-proliferative to proliferative stages characterized by neovascularization, FD may vary significantly. Observational studies in younger individuals with type 1 diabetes have shown an association between lower FD and proliferative DR [51,52]. In a prospective study of adults with type 2 diabetes, decreased FD at baseline was independently associated with the development of DR over a 10-year follow-up, even when accounting for other risk factors [47]. This was corroborated by a recent retrospective study, which identified decreased FD as one of five predictive variables for DR among type 2 diabetic patients, suggesting a potential role in early detection and assessment of DR [48].

3. Structural Imaging: OCT and OCTA

3.1. Structural Changes in Early DR

3.1.1. Retinal Neurodegeneration

The ganglion cell–inner plexiform layer (GC-IPL) is a vital neural layer in the retina. Changes detected in this layer can be indicative of neurodegeneration and can potentially occur in patients with DM even before the development of DR. This may be due to damage from chronically elevated blood sugar levels [53–55]. A 3-year longitudinal study confirmed significantly faster rates of GC-IPL thinning in eyes that developed incident DR compared to those that remained non-DR, although both groups showed decreased thickness [56].

Apart from the GC-IPL, the peripapillary retinal nerve fiber layer (pRNFL) and macular retinal nerve fiber layer (mRNFL) are other important retinal structural parameters that need to be considered for early detection of DR [57–60]. More recently, Hafner et al. reported a significant association between pRNFL but not mRNFL with parafoveal vessel density detected by OCTA [55]. This finding corroborated the result reported by the EUROCONDOR study, which demonstrated a strong correlation between narrower retinal arteriolar caliber and thinning of the pRNFL, reflecting the close relationship between microvascular abnormalities and neurodegeneration in the pathophysiology of diabetic retinopathy [61]. Therefore, monitoring GC-IPL and pRNFL thickness changes may offer a valuable window for early detection of DR.

3.1.2. Retinal Reflectivity

Structural OCT allows for quantitative assessment of retinal reflectivity, which holds potential in early diagnosis and prognostication of various retinal diseases, including DR [62,63]. Retinal reflectivity is a measure of the intensity of backscattered light from retinal tissues that can provide insights into structural and compositional changes associated with neurodegenerative processes and vascular impairment in early DR. Zhang et al. reported that outer retinal reflectivity was significantly reduced in non-DR diabetic patients when compared with normal controls, especially for the ellipsoid zone (EZ) [64]. Concurrently, other researchers investigated the role of inner retinal reflectivity. In a study conducted by Cetin et al. [65], diabetic patients without clinically evident DR exhibited a significant correlation between ganglion cell layer reflectivity and the extent of pericentral retinal thinning over time. Notably, this retinal thinning was more pronounced in the inner retinal layers, which comprise the ganglion cell and inner plexiform layers. However, a notable limitation of retinal reflectivity is the requirement for post-acquisition processing and analysis using third-party software (i.e., ImageJ, https://imagej.net/ij/). OCT images must be exported and imported into specialized software for quantitative analysis of reflectivity patterns, which can be time-consuming and impractical in clinical settings. If this functionality is integrated into commercial OCT devices in the future, it could streamline clinical applications.

3.1.3. Choroidal Vessel Index and Choroidal Thickness

Studies indicate that choroidal vascular index (CVI) and choroidal thickness (ChT) can be used to quantitatively assess changes in the structure and blood flow of the choroid, potentially serving as early biomarkers and severity indicators of DR [66–68]. Three studies with ultra-wide-field swept-source OCT (SS-OCT) revealed that diabetic patients exhibited significantly lower values of CVI and ChT compared to healthy individuals, with the difference being more pronounced in patients with early-stage DR than in those without clinical DR. Of note, the peripheral choroidal capillaries are more susceptible to the early microvascular insults induced by DM than the central choroidal region [69–71]. The observed reduction in choroidal vascularity and thinning of the choroid may precede clinically detectable retinal vascular changes.

Eyes that develop incident DR show significantly faster rates of ChT thinning compared to those that remain non-DR [56]. Remarkably, the peripheral choroidal alterations appear more pronounced than changes in the posterior pole during the early stages of DR. This discrepancy may represent a compensatory mechanism, wherein the choroid attempts to maintain adequate blood supply to the metabolically demanding posterior pole retina by redistributing flow from the periphery. These findings underscore the importance of closely monitoring peripheral choroidal changes, as they may serve as early indicators of the deleterious effects of diabetes on the choroidal–retinal complex.

3.2. *Vascular Changes in Early DR*

In contrast to fundus fluorescein angiography (FFA), which necessitates intravenous injection of a contrast agent, OCTA is a non-invasive, dye-free, three-dimensional imaging technique [72]. It not only allows visualization of capillaries across all retinal layers but also provides a broader perspective of the fundus, facilitating comprehensive examination and quantitative analysis [73]. Researchers have conducted numerous studies validating OCTA's ability to detect early signs of microvascular alterations. Additionally, it provides a quantitative assessment of disease severity, including conditions like DR and its associated complications [74–76]. Recently, a meta-analysis suggests retinal microvascular damage may precede clinical DR and can be detected early using OCTA [33].

3.2.1. Retinal and Choroidal Vascular Density and Perfusion

A study focused on retinal perfusion reported that the perfusion density of the deep capillary complex (DCC) was notably reduced in patients with diabetes, even in the absence of clinically detectable DR. Remarkably, the retinal capillary network outside the parafoveal region exhibited greater susceptibility to capillary perfusion deficits compared to the capillaries close to the fovea [77]. Investigating images of 12 mm $\times$ 12 mm scanning area obtained by swept-source OCTA (SS-OCTA), Qi and colleagues' study unveiled that structural and blood flow alterations in the choroid manifested before the onset of DR and preceded changes in the retinal microcirculation [78]. Of note, their findings highlighted that mid-large choroidal vessel thickness and density were more sensitive imaging biomarkers for the early clinical detection of DR compared to retinal vascular changes. Interestingly, the choriocapillaris remained unaffected in the pre-clinical and early stages of DR [78], possibly due to the necessity for compensatory blood supply. This finding was corroborated by results from another study [79]. These results suggest that parameters of choroidal blood vessels could serve as earlier indicators of diabetic fundus changes, potentially enabling more timely detection and intervention before retinal vascular complications arise.

While the aforementioned studies highlight that the choriocapillaris remains unaffected in the pre-clinical and early stages of DR, choriocapillaris perfusion metrics (quantitative flow deficit density, number, and size) in the macula from another study were reported to independently correspond to the severity of DR [80]. This suggests that although the choriocapillaris may not exhibit observable changes in the initial stages, its perfusion characteristics could serve as valuable biomarkers for evaluating the progression and severity of DR. Moreover, two studies reported a significant decrease in choriocapillaris perfusion of the central macular region (3 mm $\times$ 3 mm or 6 mm $\times$ 6 mm) in diabetic patients without DR when compared to age-matched non-diabetic controls. This reduction in choriocapillaris perfusion was observed despite an absence of detectable changes in macular retinal vessel parameters [81,82]. These findings suggest that decreased choriocapillaris perfusion in the macular region may serve as an early indicator of diabetic vasculopathy, potentially preceding clinically apparent retinal vascular alterations.

3.2.2. Ultra-Wide-Field SS-OCTA for Vascular Analysis

The TowardPi SS-OCT/OCTA commercial system (Medical Technology, Beijing, China) is a cutting-edge, high-resolution, and wide-field tomographic and angiography imaging platform [83]. Boasting an impressive A-scan rate of 400 KHz and an axial scan depth of 6 mm, this advanced system offers unprecedented capabilities. Remarkably, it can acquire wide-field tomography spanning 24 mm and comprehensive angiography information covering an extensive 24 × 20 mm area in a single rapid capture, taking only about 15 s (Figure 2). This innovative system combines high-speed imaging with an extensive field of view, enabling comprehensive and efficient examination of retinal and choroidal structures [84,85].

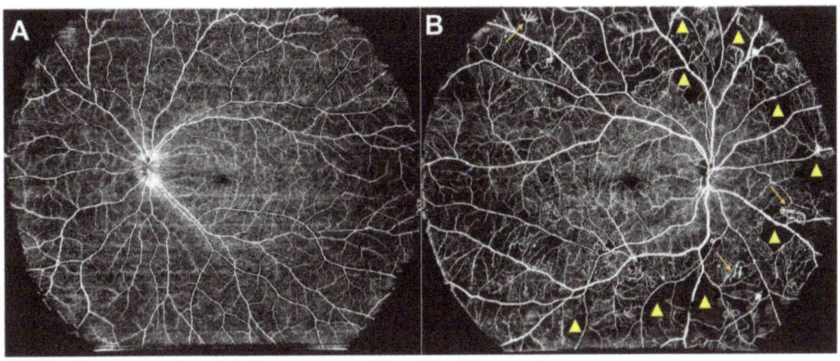

Figure 2. Ultra-wide-field swept-source optical coherence tomography angiography (SS-OCTA) imaging systems in a normal eye (**A**) and in a case of proliferative diabetic retinopathy (**B**). The triangles highlight areas of non-perfusion, while the arrows indicate the presence of retinal neovascularization. (Images courtesy of Dr. Jialiang Duan, The Second Hospital of Hebei Medical University, Shijiazhuang, Hebei, China).

An observational study demonstrated that the average vascular density (VD) of the superficial vascular complex (SVC) across all observed areas was significantly lower in DR eyes compared to normal controls [86]. However, only the most peripheral area (16–21 mm) exhibited a significant decrease in VD for the DM group relative to healthy individuals, with a good receiver operating characteristic (ROC) curve value (0.8353) to predict DR. The average VD of the deep vascular complex (DVC) in the outermost peripheral area (16–21 mm) was significantly reduced in the DM group compared to the normal controls. Surprisingly, no significant changes were observed in the thicknesses of the SVC or DVC nourishing segments in the peripheral retina. These findings suggest that alterations in peripheral choroidal blood flow, as reflected by vascular density changes, may serve as a more sensitive indicator for early detection of diabetic fundus changes than thickness measurements alone.

3.2.3. Foveal Avascular Zone

The foveal avascular zone (FAZ) is a specialized, capillary-free region at the center of the macula, which is essential for preserving high visual acuity. It appears as a circular or slightly oval-shaped area devoid of retinal vasculature. OCTA enables detailed, non-invasive visualization and quantitative analysis of the FAZ's size, perimeter, shape, and vascular density, facilitating early detection and monitoring of macular disorders affecting this critical area [74,87]. Although FAZ size can exhibit great inter-person variability among normal individuals (Figure 3) [88,89], longitudinal follow-up and monitoring of FAZ dimensions through OCTA may prove valuable in detecting and tracking the progression of DR [90,91]. By contrast, the FAZ circularity index serves as a relatively stable parameter that reflects the regularity of the FAZ shape [92,93], with a mean value of 1.12 to 1.32 in normal subjects [93,94]. With the progression of DR severity, the FAZ is recognized to exhibit increased tortuosity or irregularity in its shape [94]. This alteration in FAZ contour is attributed to localized capillary dropout at various points along its perimeter, resulting in an expanded and less circular outline. The change in the FAZ circularity index may serve as a valuable biomarker for monitoring the progression and severity of DR, especially in instances where longitudinal data are unavailable.

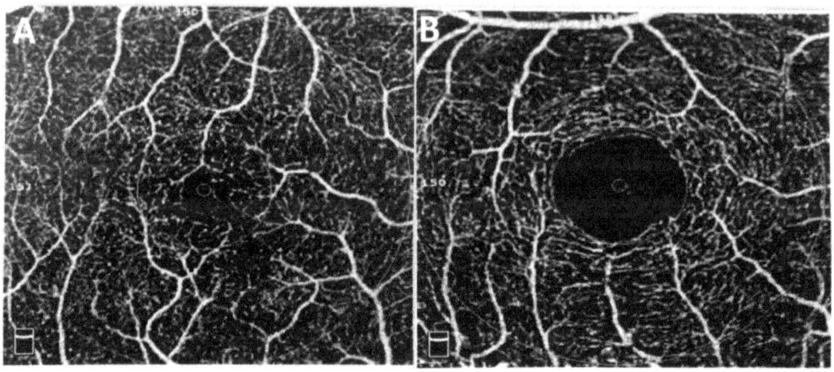

Figure 3. High inter-person variability among normal individuals in the foveal avascular zone (FAZ). (**A**) A woman with a spherical equivalent of +0.75 diopters and an axial length of 24.01 mm exhibited a FAZ area of 0.070 mm^2. (**B**) A man with a spherical equivalent of −3.50 diopters and an axial length of 23.97 mm showcased a notably larger FAZ area, measuring 0.671 mm^2.

4. Functional Tests

4.1. Multifocal Electroretinogram (mERG)

Multifocal electroretinography (mfERG) has been widely used to evaluate the retinal function of the macula. DR is largely caused by defects of the retinal deep capillary plexus in the inner nuclear layer, where the cell bodies of bipolar cells are located. It has been documented that the primary generators of mfERG are on and off bipolar cells [95]. Thus, mfERG is well suited for the study of DR. By precisely mapping localized retinal responses, mfERG can detect early neurodegenerative alterations associated with DR, even before clinically evident vascular lesions appear. By utilizing electroretinography (ERG), some studies have demonstrated that retinal dysfunction can be detected in children with DM without visual impairment or clinically evident DR [96,97]. Their findings suggest that hyperglycemia can induce neurodegenerative changes in the retina during the early stages of type 1 DM, even before the onset of overt vascular lesions or visual symptoms. These results highlight the potential of ERG or mfERG as sensitive functional tests for detecting subclinical retinal neurodegeneration, which may precede the microvascular complications of DR.

Recent mfERG studies have found that both reduced amplitudes and response delays are present in DM patients with or without clinical DR. Additionally, the degree of mfERG implicit time delays appears to be directly related to the severity of DR, and the locations of abnormal implicit times spatially align with anatomical abnormalities in the macula [98]. The areas of the retina that appeared visually normal in clinical examinations but exhibited functional abnormalities showed overall stability. However, after a one-year follow-up, these areas were found to be more susceptible to the development of microaneurysms compared to zones with a normal baseline implicit time [99]. In short, mfERG can be a valuable monitoring tool and effectively identify early abnormalities of the retina in DM patients without or with early stages of DR [100–102]. Notably, a mfERG study suggested that males may be more vulnerable to the neurodegenerative changes that preceded the development of background diabetic retinopathy in type 2 diabetes, compared to their female counterparts [103].

4.2. Microperimetry

Microperimetry (MP) is a visual function test that maps light sensitivity across the retina. Participants actively report their perception of light stimuli presented at various locations, generating a detailed decibel (dB) map of retinal function. Unlike other functional tests like electroretinography and standard perimetry, MP's ability to register the fundus allows for correlations between functional changes (light sensitivity) and the underlying retinal structure [104]. MP-3, the state-of-the-art model of fundus microperimetry, boasts a wider range of measurable parameters and eye tracking system. Early detection of DR can benefit from measuring retinal sensitivity, as documented in many studies [105]. It can reveal subtle declines in retinal sensitivity, even before structural changes are visible through ophthalmoscopy or OCT/OCTA. While the full implications of this finding are still being debated, microperimetry appears valuable for identifying early functional impairment in the diabetic retina. This technique excels at mapping the point-to-point relationship between retinal structure and function.

4.3. Multifocal Pupillographic Objective Perimetry

Multifocal pupillographic objective perimetry (mfPOP) is a rapid and objective visual field test that measures how pupils react to multiple light stimuli flashed simultaneously. This response can help track retinal dysfunction in diabetic patients, potentially reflecting the severity of underlying blood vessel damage in the retina [32,106,107]. Compared with subjective automated perimetry (SAP), Sabeti et al. found significant differences between the non-proliferative diabetic retinopathy for ObjectiveFIELD Analyzer (OFA; Konan Medical USA, Irvine, CA) mean defects (MDs) and pattern standard deviations (PSDs), but not for SAP MDs or PSDs [108].

4.4. Contrast Sensitivity

Contrast sensitivity (CS) goes beyond just detecting light intensity differences, providing a more comprehensive assessment of spatial vision. Research has shown it to be associated with overall health function [109]. Recently, Silva-Viguera et al. conducted a systematic review including a total of 21 studies published between 2010 and 2021 to evaluate whether CS assessment in patients with type 1 or type 2 diabetes could be a reliable test in early detection of DR [110]. The study concluded that individuals with DR exhibited a substantial reduction in CS across a wide range of spatial frequencies. The findings have been supported by recent research publications, which echo similar conclusions [111–113]. While some diabetic patients without clinically evident DR may also demonstrate decreased CS, this effect was less consistent, and the affected frequencies varied. These changes in visual function suggest that retinal neuronal damage may precede overt vascular lesions in DR, potentially enabling early detection through CS testing. However, longitudinal studies are warranted to establish CS as a reliable biomarker for predicting DR onset and progression, strengthening evidence for its application in early screening and monitoring [112].

4.5. Visual Evoked Potential Test

The visual evoked potential (VEP) test offers a functional assessment of the integrity of the optic nerve. Using the pattern-reversal VEP (PRVEP) test, the technique showing less variability in timing and waveform, El-Tawab et al. found a significant delay in P100 latencies of the patients with pre-clinical DR when compared with normal controls [114]. The findings indicated retinal ganglion cell dysfunction and demyelinating changes in the optic nerve pathway, which are consequences of microvascular insults caused by the hyperglycemic state in diabetes [115]. Although the VEP test is not routinely used for DR, it can be considered for early detection of DR in patients who are negative in other tests but need to rule out whether there is retinal dysfunction.

4.6. Retinal Vessel Reactivity

In current clinical practice, two stimuli prompt responses from retinal blood vessels, facilitating the assessment of vascular function: flicker light and gas perturbation. The Dynamic Vessel Analyzer (DVA, Imedos, Jena, Germany) is a commercially available system comprising a fundus camera and a video unit connected to a computer. This setup facilitates uninterrupted recording of the retina throughout the examination, with specialized software monitoring changes in retinal vessel diameter in real-time in response to diffuse luminance flicker [116]. It has been reported that prediabetic and diabetic individuals without DR exhibit significantly attenuated peak vasodilator responses and relative amplitude changes in retinal vein and artery diameters in response to the flickering light stimulus compared to healthy controls [117]. Further studies have demonstrated that the responses of retinal arterioles and venules to flickering light are diminished in subjects with DR, and this reduction progresses with more severe stages of DR [118]. Another prospective study unveiled that decreased dilatory responses of retinal arterioles and venules to flickering light are linked to a greater probability of DR progression within one year among adult patients with DM [119]. These findings may indicate endothelial dysfunction or disrupted neuro-regulation of retinal vascular tone in eyes affected by DM or DR, despite limited reports of negative results [120].

The other approach for evaluating retinal vascular responses is gas perturbation experiments that involve modifying the partial pressures of CO_2 and O_2 (PCO_2 and PO_2) within the bloodstream. The alterations in retinal microvascular blood flow signals can be captured by OCTA. Safi et al. assessed the retinal vascular response to hyperoxia in patients with diabetes at the pre-clinical stage of DR and compared it with normal controls. They found that impaired retinal vascular reactivity was apparent at this stage, with disturbances in the autoregulatory mechanism particularly pronounced in the parafoveal DCP [121]. This finding further underscored that the DCP experiences more severe microvascular damage than the SCP in patients with DM or DR at the early stage [122]. In another study on patients with mild to severe DR, findings revealed impaired retinal capillary reactivity across the full retinal layer to both hyperoxia and hypercapnia among individuals with DM in comparison to healthy controls [123]. However, the clinical practicality of this method is limited, and it may serve as a supplementary approach.

5. Combining Structural and Functional Data

Vascular and neurodegenerative changes occur early in the DR disease process, causing loss of function and cell death among retinal ganglion cells, with consequent GC-IPL and RNFL thinning. Numerous studies have looked at the integration of multimodal imaging data to elucidate the pathophysiologic relationship between retinal neurodegenerative and vascular changes prior to the appearance of DR. Emerging evidence points to early neuronal damage as a precursor to clinically visible retinopathy changes. Combining structural and functional imaging data may facilitate earlier detection of DR and targeted management strategies based on disease progression.

In a recent study, Boned-Murillo et al. examined patient eyes with type 2 diabetes using SS-OCT and microperimetry, correlating macular Early Treatment Diabetic Retinopathy Study (ETDRS) grid areas with corresponding microperimetry points [124]. Total retinal thinning was found at the parafoveal ring, with a reduction in both ganglion cell layer (GCL) and inner plexiform layer (IPL) thickness, suggesting ganglion cells have increased susceptibility to neurodegenerative and vascular effects in DM patients. Additionally, both mRNFL thickness and retinal sensitivity were decreased in patients with moderate DR with no DME. In particular, the RNFL thickness was significantly lower in the outer nasal area in ganglion cells and IPL among T2DM patients. While retinal sensitivity was correlated with RNFL thickness, there was no correlation between retinal sensitivity and thickness of the GCL combined with the IPL.

Topographic quantification of macular function using microperimetry has also shown utility in assessing mild DR, with studies successfully detecting functional impairment [125]. In mild DR eyes, studies suggest that mesopic macular dysfunction may be present with a preserved outer retinal thickness and a strong relationship between macular perfusion and photoreceptor function.

Several studies have also examined the relationship between OCTA-measured blood flow channels and functional parameters [126–128]. In a prospective observational study, Tsai et al. applied OCTA and microperimetry to examine the relationship between perifoveal vessel densities, FAZ areas, and retinal sensitivity in diabetic patients [126]. They found deep perifoveal vessel density was inversely correlated with the severity of DR and directly correlated with retinal sensitivity. Meanwhile, the superficial FAZ area was inversely correlated with retinal sensitivity. Further building on this, Levine et al. registered OCTA images with microperimetry of eyes stratified by severity of DR to quantitatively demonstrate a point-wise structure–function relationship between vessel density obtained from OCTA and retinal sensitivity in global and zonal spatial scales in the parafovea [128]. Notably, the study identified local regions of retinal flow impairments that were only evident in advanced DR and were most often accompanied by regions of functional loss, but not vice versa.

This suggests that local ischemia may not be the initial cause of retinal dysfunction in DR, but rather supports the neurodegenerative theory of DR. The neurodegenerative theory posits that DR primarily affects retinal neurons and the reaction of these retinal neurons to microenvironment stressors is responsible for vascular complications. This operates in contrast with the classic hypothesis of DR as primarily a retinal vascular disorder with pathogenesis rooted in glycosylation-induced microvascular damage that leads to ischemic neuronal injury. Significant research has been published suggesting both neurodegeneration and glial dysfunction precede microvascular changes in DR. Studies using mfERG to assess neuroglial dysfunction have shown an increase in implicit time is predictive for the development of visible vascular abnormalities over 1-year and 3-year periods [129,130].

Alterations in neuronal function measured by mfERG similarly precede clinical manifestation of structural changes in the ganglion cell complex and retinal vascular changes in prediabetics. Studies show a significant decrease in mfERG amplitude but no significant increase in implicit time among prediabetics [131,132]. This is partially corroborated by the EUROCONDOR study where mfERG P1 amplitude was seen to be more sensitive than the P1 implicit time [133]. Combining OCTA with mfERG data, Zagst et al. showed a significant positive correlation between FAZ area and mfERG amplitude [132].

Another study by Srinivasan et al. aimed to determine structural and functional differences between eyes with and without NPDR using OCTA and mfERG [100]. The group with mild or moderate NPDR had no statistically significant structural differences from those without DR. However, participants with mild to moderate NDPR had significantly lower mfERG implicit times and response densities in rings five and six, suggestive of abnormal neuronal function. In eyes without DR, lower macular vessel density and perfusion almost always corresponded to delayed implicit times and lower response densities. However, these correlations were not significant in the NDPR group, suggesting that other structural and functional correlates could exist in retinas with NPDR. These findings were expanded upon in a study by Santos et al. that more granularly stratified the NDR group and compared them to healthy controls [133]. DR was correlated with higher implicit times of mfERG rings 3–6 and lower response density. Structurally, diabetic patients with ETDRS <20 had significantly thinner GC-IPLs compared to non-diabetics. However, in retinas with ETDRS levels between 20 and 35, there was no significant relationship between GC-IPL thickness and ETDRS level.

6. Applications of Artificial Intelligence in DR Detection

Artificial intelligence (AI) such as deep learning (DL) algorithms can be trained on large datasets of retinal images labeled by ophthalmologists to provide automated DR diagnosis or risk assessment. Current applications of AI demonstrate remarkable sensitivity and specificity in detecting referable DR from retinal fundus photographs [134,135] and show the potential to help efficiently triage patients, optimize resource allocation, and reduce the burden on healthcare systems. A recent meta-analysis of 21 prospective studies investigating diagnostic performance of AI algorithms for DR showed a pooled sensitivity of 88% (87.5–88.4%), pooled specificity of 91.2% (99–91.3%), AUC of 0.98, and pooled diagnostic odds ratio of 206.80 (124.82–342.63) [136]. Higher quality studies in the analysis demonstrated less heterogeneity in performance. Studies with higher image quality, greater number of included eyes, patient sourcing from healthcare facilities, and high population representativeness yielded higher diagnostic efficacy. The integration of AI-based automated tools offers substantial benefits including reduced screening costs, improved accessibility to healthcare services, and facilitation of earlier interventions and treatments [137].

6.1. Milestones and Market Approvals for AI Algorithms

Historical milestones for applications of AI in DR include the 2016 Google deep learning DR validation study by Gulshan et al., which presented a deep convolutional neural network (CNN) trained on a vast dataset of 128,175 fundus photos to detect referable DR, defined as moderate or worse DR or referable DME [138]. In this retrospective study, photos were acquired in the US and three eye hospitals in India using a variety of cameras. Compared to the reference standard grading determined by a panel of US board-certified ophthalmologists, the DL model demonstrated sensitivities greater than 96% and specificities greater than 93% for detection of referable diabetic retinopathy. Concomitantly, Gargeya et al. developed a customized CNN for detecting DR and validated it against a larger dataset of color fundus photos from multiple independent sources, emphasizing the generalizability of their model. In addition to showing comparable sensitivity and specificity for the detection of referable DR, Gargeya et al. demonstrated the utility of a DL algorithm to detect mild DR, with sensitivities ranging from 74–90% and specificities ranging from 80–94% [139].

In 2018, the US Food and Drug Administration (FDA) approved IDx-DR (now rebranded as LumineticsCore), the first AI-powered medical device for analyzing retinal images in primary care settings for DR screening. In a multi-center pivotal trial for IDx-DR, Abramoff et al. prospectively enrolled 900 diabetic adult participants without a prior diagnosis of DR and acquired two-field retinal fundus photos centered on the disc and macula, using a Topcon TRC-NW400 camera (Topcon, Tokyo, Japan) [140]. Compared to the reference standard of experienced human graders using the ETDRS severity scale, the IDx-DR algorithm demonstrated a sensitivity of 87% and specificity of 91% for detecting more than mild DR (mtmDR), defined as ETDRS > 35.

To date, three AI algorithms for DR screening have been approved by the FDA: LumineticsCore (formerly known as IDx-DR), EyeArt, and AEYE-DS. Since its approval in 2018, the LumineticsCore algorithm has been improved to read previously ungradable images with higher processing speeds. EyeArt, a deep learning algorithm developed by Eyenuk and first FDA-cleared in 2020, was similarly designed to screen patients for referable DR based on the ETDRS standard (>35) using two-field color fundus photos. In a US multi-center pivotal trial, EyeArt applied the same protocol implemented by authors of IDx-DR to show 96% sensitivity and 88% specificity for detecting mtmDR [141]. Most recently, AEYE-DS, an algorithm created by AEYE Health, received FDA clearance in April 2024 as the first fully autonomous AI algorithm that diagnoses referable diabetic retinopathy from retinal images taken by a handheld camera. While the details of the pivotal studies have yet to be published as scientific manuscripts, in a recent press release

AEYE-DS was reported to have achieved sensitivities ranging from 92–93% and specificities between 89–94%, across two large-scale prospective phase 3 studies.

Several AI-based algorithms and devices have received class IIa approval in the European Union (EU), including LumineticsCore, EyeArt, RetmarkerDR by Retmarker, SELENA+ by eyRIS, Automated Retinal Disease Assessment (ARDA) by Verily Life Sciences LLC, Medios AI by Remidio, OphtAI by Evolucare, VUNO Med-Fundus AI by VUNO Inc., and RetCAD by Thirona (Table 2) [142,143].

Table 2. Ophthalmology AI devices approved for DR screening in the US and EU (class II, CE mark).

Model	Approval Year	Target Disease	Company	Markets Available
RetmarkerDR	2010	DR, AMD	Retmarker SA, Taveiro, Portugal	EU
Automated Retinal Disease Assessment (ARDA)	2016	Referable DR	Google LLC, Mountain View, CA, USA	EU
LumineticsCore (previously IDx-DR)	2018	Referable DR, DME	Digital Diagnostics Inc., Coralville, IA, USA	US, EU
OphtAI	2019	Referable DR, DME, AMD, glaucoma	Evolucare/ADCIS, Villers-Bretonneux, France	EU
SELENA+	2019, 2020	Referable DR, AMD, glaucoma	EyRIS Pte Ltd, Singapore	EU, Singapore
EyeArt	2015, 2020	Referable DR, AMD, glaucoma	Eyenuk, Inc., Woodland Hills, CA, USA	US, EU
VUNO Med-Fundus AI	2020	Referable DR, AMD, glaucoma	VUNO Inc., Seoul, Korea	EU, Korea, Singapore
RetCAD	2022	Referable DR, AMD	Thirona Retina BV, Nijmegen, Netherlands	EU
Medios AI	2023	Referable DR, glaucoma	Remidio Innovative Solutions Pvt Ltd., Karnataka, India	EU
AEYE-DS	2024	Referable DR	AEYE Health, Inc., New York, NY, USA	US

6.2. OCT/OCTA-Trained AI Algorithms

While the majority of DR screening algorithms have been developed for color fundus photos, recent studies have explored training AI algorithms on OCT and/or OCTA images [144,145], or UWF OCTA images [146]. Compared to fundus photography, OCTA has only recently been introduced into clinical eye care over the last 10 years and the availability of large, publicly available datasets remains relatively limited. However, given DR's nature as a retinal microvascular disease, OCTA's detailed microvascular insights significantly enhance diagnosis, particularly through metrics like the FAZ area and macular capillary density, which correlate with DR pathophysiology. OCTA's advantages over fluorescein angiography, such as its ability to image both deep and superficial vascular plexuses, non-invasiveness, ease of use, and compatibility with existing OCT platforms, make it an invaluable complement to standard OCT.

In a single-center, cross-sectional study based in South Korea, Ryu et al. developed a fully automated CNN-based classification algorithm that detects the onset of DR and referable status using raw OCTA images. Their model was able to detect early DR with an accuracy of 90–95%, sensitivity of 91–98%, and specificity of 85–93%, comparable to previously reported CNN models utilizing fundus photographs with fewer than 250 samples [147]. The study also explored the algorithm's performance across various image sizes and retinal slabs to pinpoint optimal configurations for DR classification, finding the end-to-end CNN classifier surpassed traditional machine learning approaches that relied on extracted local features from OCTA images. Another study achieved robust model performance by not only including the raw OCTA images but also extracting a binary map of the segmented retinal vascular network from OCTA images and calculating a distance map of blood vessels as additional processed inputs for the CNN model [148].

Sandhu et al. developed a novel machine learning algorithm for diagnosing and grading NPDR by integrating OCT and OCTA imaging data with basic clinical and demographic information from 111 patients [149]. Three pathophysiologic features were extracted from each layer on OCT: reflectivity, curvature, and thickness; four features were extracted from each OCTA plexus: blood vessel caliber, vessel density, size of FAZ, and the number of bifurcation and crossover points. Combined with clinical data, these seven image features were fed into a two-stage random forest classifier, which first determined the presence of DR and subsequently classified the severity of NPDR with 96% accuracy, 100% sensitivity, and 94% specificity. The model outperformed machine learning models trained on OCT or OCTA images alone, demonstrating the utility of combining OCT and OCTA imaging with patient data to improve the detection and classification of NPDR. As OCT technology becomes more ubiquitous, there may be significant potential for its application in DR screening.

6.3. *Potential Risks and Limitations*

A significant risk of AI models is the potential for bias. This can come in the form of data sampling and representation bias, where non-random sampling produces datasets that do not represent the diversity of the population. As a result, a model trained on a biased dataset may not generalize to data collected from a new population, performing poorly for certain subgroups [150]. For example, an algorithm trained predominantly on retinal images of a subgroup with lighter skin pigmentation and lower retinal pigment scores may not accurately diagnose retinal disease in individuals with darker skin pigmentation and higher retinal pigment scores [151]. Additionally, there is also potential for algorithmic bias, where bias is not present in the input data and is added purely by the algorithm. Bias can exacerbate existing healthcare disparities, particularly affecting under-represented and marginalized populations. To mitigate this risk, developers must ensure that training datasets are diverse and representative of the broader population.

The quality and variability of data used to train AI algorithms also pose significant challenges. Retinal images can vary widely based on the equipment used, the skill of the operator, and the conditions under which the images are taken. Variations in image quality can impact the performance of AI systems, potentially leading to false positives or negatives. Ensuring consistent, high-quality data for training and validation is essential but challenging in diverse clinical environments. Standardizing imaging protocols and using high-quality datasets can help improve the robustness of AI systems.

6.4. *Practical Implementation Challenges*

6.4.1. Integration into Clinical Workflows

Despite the proven accuracy and reliability of DL systems in detecting various ocular diseases, their integration into clinical practice faces hurdles, primarily due to concerns over the systems' interpretability and complexity. Efforts to improve neural network visualization techniques have progressed, offering insights into decision-making aspects of AI, although inconsistencies among visualization methods exist. Healthcare providers must ensure that these technologies complement rather than disrupt current practices. This requires a careful redesign of workflows to incorporate AI screening processes without overburdening healthcare professionals or causing delays in patient care. Medical professionals also need to be trained to use new AI systems, interpret the results, and understand the limitations of AI-based diagnostics. Addressing these concerns through comprehensive training programs and demonstrating the efficacy of AI systems through pilot projects and case studies can help mitigate resistance and build trust among healthcare providers.

6.4.2. Cost-Effectiveness

The initial cost of AI-based DR screening systems is another significant barrier. Although AI technologies can reduce long-term healthcare costs by enabling early detection and intervention, the upfront investment is substantial. This includes the cost of purchasing high-quality retinal imaging equipment, software licenses, and the necessary IT infrastructure to support AI applications.

An economic modeling study in Singapore suggested that the incorporation of an AI algorithm as an assistive tool in a large-scale DR screening program is associated with significant cost savings [152]. Using a decision tree model, the study compared traditional human assessment with two deep learning approaches: a semi-automated DL model as a triage filter before secondary human assessment, and a fully automated DL model without human assessment. From the health system perspective, the semi-automated screening model was the least expensive of the three models, costing USD 62 per patient per year, generating 19.5% in cost savings compared to the human assessment model.

Other economic modeling studies have reported that the implementation of automated systems for DR screening generates cost savings between 12% and 23.3% in the UK and US [153,154]. In a study analyzing the cost-effectiveness of AI for DR detection in rural China, where patients have limited access to skilled ophthalmologists, AI screening was determined to be cost-effective.

6.4.3. Infrastructure and Access

One of the foremost challenges in implementing AI for DR screening is the lack of necessary infrastructure, particularly in low-resource settings. High-quality retinal cameras, which are essential for capturing the detailed images required by AI algorithms, are often expensive and not readily available in these areas. These costs may be prohibitive, making it challenging to justify the investment despite the potential long-term benefits. Additionally, some low-resource settings lack reliable internet access, which is critical for cloud-based AI systems that require data transmission to central servers for analysis. In many low-resource settings, healthcare disparities already exist, and the introduction of advanced technologies risks widening these gaps if not implemented thoughtfully. Efforts must be made to ensure that AI-based screening programs are accessible to all patients, regardless of socioeconomic status or geographic location. This may involve subsidizing costs, providing mobile screening units, and developing user-friendly technologies that do not require extensive training or infrastructure.

Recent advancements include the integration of AI algorithms with smartphone-based imaging, facilitating reliable DR screening even in remote areas with high sensitivity and specificity (Tables 3 and 4) [28,155]. Multiple studies, including that by Tomic et al., have validated the effectiveness of hand-held cameras and AI grading systems in DR screening, demonstrating accuracy comparable to traditional clinical examinations [30,156]. However, significant sources of heterogeneity in diagnostic efficacy include variable experience levels of the camera operator, rates of ungradable images due to the inclusion of poor-quality images or media opacity-causing diseases, undilated patients, and overfitting due to small sample sizes. Smart-phone-based imaging presents transformative potential for DR screening, especially in resource-limited settings, by enabling efficient and accurate early detection and facilitating timely referral for treatment.

Table 3. Patient level sensitivity and specificity of all three graders as derived using a standard 2 × 2 matrix and Wilson confidence intervals. Reproduced with permission from Reference [28].

Grader Diagnosis	RWDR	No RWDR	Sensitivity (95% CI)	Specificity (95% CI)
		Grader 1		
RWDR	52	8	96.3% (86.2, 99.4)	42.9% (18.8, 70.4)
No RWDR	2	6		
		Grader 2		
RWDR	49	7	92.5% (80.9, 97.6)	50.0% (24.0, 76.0)
No RWDR	4	7		
		EyeArt® AI eye screening system		
RWDR	47	3	87.0% (74.5, 94.2)	78.6% (44.8, 94.3)
No RWDR	7	11		

RWDR, referral-warranted diabetic retinopathy; AI, artificial intelligence.

Table 4. Eye level sensitivity and specificity of all three graders as derived using a GEE logistic regression with an exchangeable working correlation matrix. Reproduced with permission from Reference [28].

Grader Diagnosis	RWDR	No RWDR	Sensitivity (95% CI)	Specificity (95% CI)
		Grader 1		
RWDR	83	14	94.0% (85.5, 97.7)	52.2% (33.4, 70.5)
No RWDR	5	17		
		Grader 2		
RWDR	77	10	89.5% (79.3, 95.0)	66.9% (48.8, 81.1)
No RWDR	9	21		
		EyeArt® AI eye screening system		
RWDR	69	8	77.8% (67.3, 85.7)	71.5% (48.7, 86.9)
No RWDR	19	23		

RWDR, referral-warranted diabetic retinopathy; AI, artificial intelligence.

7. Hematology

Research suggests that elevated levels of specific blood markers and cytokines may signal the early stages of DR. Hyperglycemia and the metabolic disruptions it causes trigger a cascade of harmful effects on the retina's neurovascular structure. These effects impact not only blood vessels but also the optic nerve, glial cells, and immune cells.

7.1. Neutrophil–Lymphocyte Ratio

The neutrophil–lymphocyte ratio (NLR), a new inflammatory marker, reflects both innate and adaptive immune responses. The NLR suggests abnormal immune system activity, potentially indicating subclinical inflammation. This type of low-grade inflammation is a common feature of chronic diseases, and individuals with diabetes often exhibit higher NLR levels [157]. Moreover, it has been reported that NLR could be used as a biomarker to predict the incidence of DR in the Scottish population [158]. More recently, El-Tawab et al. reported that NLR showed promise as a reliable marker for detecting DR even before symptoms appear. Studies have shown good sensitivity (89.29%) and specificity (84.37%) for NLR with a cut-off point ≥ 1.97 in identifying pre-clinical DR [114]. Therefore, routine NLR measurement in patients with type 2 diabetes could be beneficial. This simple test could help select individuals suspected of having pre-clinical DR, allowing for earlier intervention.

7.2. *Neutrophil Extracellular Traps (NETs)*

Beyond their role in fighting infection, neutrophil extracellular traps (NETs), webs of chromatin fibers and antimicrobial peptides released by neutrophils, have recently been implicated in the development of various non-infectious diseases, including diabetic retinopathy [159]. Neutrophil elastase (NE), a key component of NETs, has been linked to the early stages of DR. Research suggests it plays a role in capillary degeneration, retinal oxidative stress, and inflammation—all factors contributing to the development of diabetic retinopathy [160]. Like NLR, further research is warranted to identify the cutoff value of prompts for predicting DR occurrence in the early stage.

7.3. *Ethanolamine*

Ethanolamine, also known as monoethanolamine, aminoethanol, or glycinol, exists as free ethanolamine in normal human bodily fluids, such as blood, and its average concentration is about 1.6 μmol/L in the serum of individuals more than 18 years old as revealed in the Human Metabolome Database (https://hmdb.ca/metabolites/HMDB0000149, accessed on 25 March 2024). More recently, ethanolamine was found to significantly lower the serum of DR in individuals with glucose-well-controlled diabetes mellitus (GW-DR) compared to matched control patients and was identified and validated as a potential biomarker for new-onset DR in diabetic patients with well-controlled glycemia. The diagnostic accuracy of ethanolamine for GW-DR ranged from 83.6% to 100% in the discovery cohort and 83.2% to 96.0% in the validation cohort, demonstrating significant improvement over hemoglobin A1c (HbA1c) [161]. Similarly, in two large Asian cohorts, including 464 diabetic patients with various DR stages and 1405 diabetic patients without DR, lower ethanolamine levels in urinary metabolites were associated with DR outcome [162]. Future studies are warranted to investigate the combined analysis of serum and urinary ethanolamine levels to establish reference ranges for the early diagnosis of DR.

8. Conclusions and Future Directions

Currently, there is increasing acceptance of the concept that DR is a neurovascular disorder, characterized by dysfunction in the neurovascular unit (NVU) consisting of neurons, glial cells, and vascular cells [163–166]. The intricate interaction between neurons and glial cells in neurovascular coupling plays a critical role in preserving the normal homeostatic function of the NVU. Consequently, neurodegeneration and glial activation are recognized as primary events in the development of DR, frequently manifesting before the emergence of evident microangiopathy. This phenomenon has been consistently observed in both experimental models of DR and in the retinas of diabetic donors [167]. The pathogenesis of DR lies in the intricate interplay between components of the NVU, resulting in a complex interdependence of structural and functional changes.

An essential question arises: Which of these changes occur earlier and can be detected using current diagnostic methods with high diagnostic power for discriminating eyes of patients with DM who exhibit no to mild DR? This review has delved into this topic in detail, aiming to elucidate the early structural and functional alterations in DR. A preprint study proposed that by employing histological phenotyping and quantitative analysis of postmortem retina from diabetic donors without clinical DR, the observed disparity between localized capillary dropout and widespread neural loss within the inner nuclear layer (INL) suggests that microvascular loss might not directly lead to neurodegeneration during the early stages of DR. This indicated that diabetes could independently impact these two indicators [168]. Both our review and this article suggest that combining structural and functional examinations may represent the optimal strategy for enhancing early detection of DR. Healthcare institutions can implement both structural and functional examinations for patients at high risk of developing DR, tailoring the approach according to their respective capabilities and resources.

In the future, there is a pressing need for more effective, accessible, and reliable methods to facilitate early detection and longitudinal monitoring of DR progression. Of note, the ethical considerations and regulatory challenges associated with the clinical translation of novel approaches for early detection of DR should be kept in mind. Ethically, upholding patient safety through meticulous pre-clinical and clinical trials to rigorously evaluate the safety profile, potential risks, and adverse effects of novel approaches is of paramount importance. Moreover, equitable access to innovative treatments, transcending barriers of affordability and geographic constraints, must be addressed to prevent disparities in care. Consideration must also be given to the inclusion and protection of vulnerable populations, such as children and pregnant women. On the regulatory front, navigating the intricate approval processes, which demand comprehensive data demonstrating safety, efficacy, and quality, can be a protracted and complex endeavor.

Recently, a functional OCTA (fOCTA) system was developed and utilized in diabetic mice [169]. The results revealed that, in normal mice, retinal capillaries displayed a noticeable hyperemic response to flicker light stimulation, whereas diabetic mice exhibited a significant loss of functional hyperemia at an early stage of DR, despite showing few overt signs of retinopathy. If this non-invasive technology can be applied to patients in the future, retinal capillary functional hyperemia may hold strong potential to serve as more sensitive vascular biomarkers of early DR. New approaches have also been explored in animal models of DR for in vivo studies. Notably, Zhang et al. [170] developed an innovative adhesive fluorescent nanoprobe crafted from biodegradable materials. This nanoprobe was designed to detect alterations in VEGFR-2 expression within the retinal microcirculation, offering a non-invasive means of diagnosis. Through specific binding to retinal microvascular endothelial VEGFR-2, the nanoprobe effectively differentiated diabetic animals from their healthy counterparts, showcasing its potential for early detection in DR. Furthermore, novel imaging techniques should be developed and improved for early detection of DR, such as photoacoustic microscopy [171–178].

Additionally, efforts should be made to increase the accessibility and convenience of these technologies in real-world settings, particularly in resource-limited settings where the burden of DR is often highest [179]. This may involve the improvement in cost-effective, portable, and user-friendly imaging devices, as well as the integration of telemedicine and AI-assisted analysis for remote screening and monitoring. Longitudinal studies incorporating multimodal imaging and comprehensive clinical data should be undertaken to deepen our understanding of the complex pathophysiology of DR and enhance our ability to detect and monitor DR progression at an early stage. Such research endeavors may pave the way for personalized risk stratification and tailored therapeutic interventions, ultimately improving visual outcomes and vision-related quality of life for individuals with diabetes.

Author Contributions: Conceptualization, Z.Z. and Y.M.P.; methodology, Z.Z., C.D. and Y.M.P.; investigation, Y.M.P.; resources, Z.Z. and Y.M.P.; writing—original draft preparation, Z.Z. and C.D.; writing—review and editing, Y.M.P.; supervision, Y.M.P.; project administration, Z.Z. and Y.M.P.; funding acquisition, Z.Z. and Y.M.P. All authors have read and agreed to the published version of the manuscript.

Funding: This study was supported by the Top Talent Support Program for Young and Middle-aged People of Wuxi Health Committee (Grant No. BJ2023037), the Elderly Health Research Project of Jiangsu Province (Grant No. 2022043), the Research Project of Wuxi Commission of Health (Grant No. M202131), and the Social Development Project of Jiangsu Provincial Department of Science and Technology (Grant No. BE2022699). This work was also funded by grants from Fight for Sight, the International Retinal Research Foundation (YMP: FFSGIA16002), the Alcon Research Institute Young Investigator Grant (YMP), unrestricted departmental support from Research to Prevent Blindness, and the Helmut F. Stern Career Development Professorship in Ophthalmology and Visual Sciences (YMP).

Conflicts of Interest: The authors declare no conflicts of interest.

References

1. Teo, Z.L.; Tham, Y.C.; Yu, M.; Chee, M.L.; Rim, T.H.; Cheung, N.; Bikbov, M.M.; Wang, Y.X.; Tang, Y.; Lu, Y.; et al. Global Prevalence of Diabetic Retinopathy and Projection of Burden through 2045: Systematic Review and Meta-analysis. *Ophthalmology* **2021**, *128*, 1580–1591. [CrossRef] [PubMed]

2. Paulus, Y.M.; Gariano, R.F. Diabetic retinopathy: A growing concern in an aging population. *Geriatrics* **2009**, *64*, 16–20.
3. Zayed, M.G.; Karsan, W.; Peto, T.; Saravanan, P.; Virgili, G.; Preiss, D. Diabetic Retinopathy and Quality of Life: A Systematic Review and Meta-Analysis. *JAMA Ophthalmol.* **2024**, *142*, 199–207. [CrossRef] [PubMed]
4. Antonetti, D.A. The neuroscience of diabetic retinopathy. *Vis. Neurosci.* **2021**, *38*, E001. [CrossRef]
5. Tan, L.; Wang, J.; Han, J.; Sainsbury, C.; Denniston, A.K.; Crowe, F.L.; Toulis, K.A.; Karamat, M.A.; Yao, M.; Nirantharakumar, K. Socioeconomic Deprivation and the Risk of Sight-Threatening Diabetic Retinopathy (STDR): A Population-Based Cohort Study in the U.K. *Diabetes Care.* **2024**, *47*, 844–848. [CrossRef] [PubMed]
6. Li, H.; Liu, X.; Zhong, H.; Fang, J.; Li, X.; Shi, R.; Yu, Q. Research progress on the pathogenesis of diabetic retinopathy. *BMC Ophthalmol.* **2023**, *23*, 372. [CrossRef]
7. Jiang, F.; Lei, C.; Chen, Y.; Zhou, N.; Zhang, M. The complement system and diabetic retinopathy. *Surv. Ophthalmol.* **2024**, *69*, 575–584. [CrossRef]
8. Zhao, S.; Yan, Q.; Xu, W.; Zhang, J. Gut microbiome in diabetic retinopathy: A systematic review and meta-analysis. *Microb. Pathog.* **2024**, *189*, 106590. [CrossRef]
9. Young, B.K.; Bommakanti, N.; Yu, G.; Patel, T.P.; Azzouz, L.; Powell, C.; Paulus, Y.M. Retinal neovascularization as self-organized criticality on ultra-widefield fluorescein angiography imaging of diabetic retinopathy. *Eye* **2023**, *37*, 2795–2800. [CrossRef]
10. Wilkinson, C.P.; Ferris, F.L., 3rd; Klein, R.E.; Lee, P.P.; Agardh, C.D.; Davis, M.; Dills, D.; Kampik, A.; Pararajasegaram, R.; Verdaguer, J.T.; et al. Proposed international clinical diabetic retinopathy and diabetic macular edema disease severity scales. *Ophthalmology* **2003**, *110*, 1677–1682. [CrossRef]
11. Kropp, M.; Golubnitschaja, O.; Mazurakova, A.; Koklesova, L.; Sargheini, N.; Vo, T.K.S.; de Clerck, E.; Polivka, J., Jr.; Potuznik, P.; Polivka, J.; et al. Diabetic retinopathy as the leading cause of blindness and early predictor of cascading complications-risks and mitigation. *EPMA J.* **2023**, *14*, 21–42. [CrossRef] [PubMed]
12. Pedersen, H.E.; Sandvik, C.H.; Subhi, Y.; Grauslund, J.; Pedersen, F.N. Relationship between Diabetic Retinopathy and Systemic Neurodegenerative Diseases: A Systematic Review and Meta-analysis. *Ophthalmol. Retina.* **2022**, *6*, 139–152. [CrossRef] [PubMed]
13. Safi, H.; Safi, S.; Hafezi-Moghadam, A.; Ahmadieh, H. Early detection of diabetic retinopathy. *Surv. Ophthalmol.* **2018**, *63*, 601–608. [CrossRef] [PubMed]
14. Ebrahimi, M.; Sivaprasad, S.; Thompson, P.; Perry, G. Retinal Neurodegeneration in Euglycemic Hyperinsulinemia, Prediabetes, and Diabetes. *Ophthalmic Res.* **2023**, *66*, 385–397. [CrossRef] [PubMed]
15. Wang, T.; Kuang, L.; Yao, X.; Gan, R.; Chen, Q.; Yan, X. Association between prediabetes/hyperglycemia and retinal diseases: A meta-analysis. *Eur. J. Ophthalmol.* **2023**, *33*, 1687–1696. [CrossRef] [PubMed]
16. White, N.H.; Pan, Q.; Knowler, W.C.; Schroeder, E.B.; Dabelea, D.; Chew, E.Y.; Blodi, B.; Goldberg, R.B.; Pi-Sunyer, X.; Darwin, C.; et al. Risk Factors for the Development of Retinopathy in Prediabetes and Type 2 Diabetes: The Diabetes Prevention Program Experience. *Diabetes Care* **2022**, *45*, 2653–2661. [CrossRef]
17. Hein, M.; Qambari, H.; An, D.; Balaratnasingam, C. Current understanding of subclinical diabetic retinopathy informed by histology and high-resolution in vivo imaging. *Clin. Exp. Ophthalmol.* **2024**, *52*, 464–484. [CrossRef] [PubMed]
18. Aldahlawi, A.; Alamoudi, L.; Taher, N.; Alnabihi, A.N.; Almufarriji, N.; Alzahrani, R.; Talat, K. The Evaluation of Diabetic Patients' Awareness of Diabetic Retinopathy and Its Complications in the Western Region of Saudi Arabia. *Cureus* **2024**, *16*, e53090. [CrossRef] [PubMed]
19. Nguyen, T.T.; Wang, J.J.; Wong, T.Y. Retinal vascular changes in pre-diabetes and prehypertension: New findings and their research and clinical implications. *Diabetes Care* **2007**, *30*, 2708–2715. [CrossRef]
20. Diabetes Prevention Program Research Group. The prevalence of retinopathy in impaired glucose tolerance and recent-onset diabetes in the Diabetes Prevention Program. *Diabet Med.* **2007**, *24*, 137–144. [CrossRef]
21. Sabanayagam, C.; Lye, W.K.; Klein, R.; Klein, B.E.K.; Cotch, M.F.; Wang, J.J.; Mitchell, P.; Shaw, J.E.; Selvin, E.; Sharrett, A.R.; et al. Retinal microvascular calibre and risk of diabetes mellitus: A systematic review and participant-level meta-analysis. *Diabetologia* **2015**, *58*, 2476–2485. [CrossRef] [PubMed]
22. Piyasena, M.; Gudlavalleti, V.S.M.; Gilbert, C.; Yip, J.L.; Peto, T.; MacLeod, D.; Fonseka, C.; Kulatunga, A.; Bandutilake, B.; Dhanapala, M.; et al. Development and Validation of a Diabetic Retinopathy Screening Modality Using a Hand-Held Nonmydriatic Digital Retinal Camera by Physician Graders at a Tertiary-Level Medical Clinic: Protocol for a Validation Study. *JMIR Res. Protoc.* **2018**, *7*, e10900. [CrossRef] [PubMed]
23. Caceres, J.; Zhang, Y.; Boe, L.; Zhou, Y.; Besirli, C.; Paulus, Y.M.; Rosenthal, J.M. Diabetic Retinopathy Screening Using a Portable Retinal Camera in Vanuatu. *Clin. Ophthalmol.* **2023**, *17*, 2919–2927. [CrossRef] [PubMed]
24. Kim, T.N.; Myers, F.; Reber, C.; Loury, P.J.; Loumou, P.; Webster, D.; Echanique, C.; Li, P.; Davila, J.R.; Maamari, R.N.; et al. A Smartphone-Based Tool for Rapid, Portable, and Automated Wide-Field Retinal Imaging. *Transl. Vis. Sci. Technol.* **2018**, *7*, 21. [CrossRef] [PubMed]
25. Patel, T.P.; Kim, T.N.; Yu, G.; Dedania, V.S.; Lieu, P.; Qian, C.X.; Besirli, C.G.; Demirci, H.; Margolis, T.; Fletcher, D.A.; et al. Smartphone-Based, Rapid, Wide-Field Fundus Photography for Diagnosis of Pediatric Retinal Diseases. *Transl. Vis. Sci. Technol.* **2019**, *8*, 29. [CrossRef] [PubMed]
26. Tan, C.H.; Kyaw, B.M.; Smith, H.; Tan, C.S.; Tudor Car, L. Use of Smartphones to Detect Diabetic Retinopathy: Scoping Review and Meta-Analysis of Diagnostic Test Accuracy Studies. *J. Med. Internet Res.* **2020**, *22*, e16658. [CrossRef] [PubMed]

27. Li, P.; Paulus, Y.M.; Davila, J.R.; Gosbee, J.; Margolis, T.; Fletcher, D.A.; Kim, T.N. Usability testing of a smartphone-based retinal camera among first-time users in the primary care setting. *BMJ Innov.* **2019**, *5*, 120–126. [CrossRef] [PubMed]
28. Kim, T.N.; Aaberg, M.T.; Li, P.; Davila, J.R.; Bhaskaranand, M.; Bhat, S.; Ramachandra, C.; Solanki, K.; Myers, F.; Reber, C.; et al. Comparison of automated and expert human grading of diabetic retinopathy using smartphone-based retinal photography. *Eye* **2021**, *35*, 334–342. [CrossRef]
29. Natarajan, S.; Jain, A.; Krishnan, R.; Rogye, A.; Sivaprasad, S. Diagnostic Accuracy of Community-Based Diabetic Retinopathy Screening With an Offline Artificial Intelligence System on a Smartphone. *JAMA Ophthalmol.* **2019**, *137*, 1182–1188. [CrossRef]
30. Hasan, S.U.; Siddiqui, M.A.R. Diagnostic accuracy of smartphone-based artificial intelligence systems for detecting diabetic retinopathy: A systematic review and meta-analysis. *Diabetes Res. Clin. Pract.* **2023**, *205*, 110943. [CrossRef]
31. *ISO/CIE 11664-1:2019*; Colorimetry: CIE Standard Colorimetric Observers. British Standards Institute: London, UK, 2019.
32. Rai, B.B.; van Kleef, J.P.; Sabeti, F.; Vlieger, R.; Suominen, H.; Maddess, T. Early diabetic eye damage: Comparing detection methods using diagnostic power. *Surv. Ophthalmol.* **2024**, *69*, 24–33. [CrossRef] [PubMed]
33. Zhang, B.; Chou, Y.; Zhao, X.; Yang, J.; Chen, Y. Early Detection of Microvascular Impairments With Optical Coherence Tomography Angiography in Diabetic Patients Without Clinical Retinopathy: A Meta-analysis. *Am. J. Ophthalmol.* **2021**, *222*, 226–237. [CrossRef] [PubMed]
34. Vujosevic, S.; Toma, C.; Villani, E.; Nucci, P.; Brambilla, M.; Torti, E.; Leporati, F.; De Cilla, S. Longitudinal Microvascular and Neuronal Retinal Evaluation in Patients with Diabetes Mellitus Types 1 and 2 and Good Glycemic Control. *Retina* **2023**, *43*, 1723–1731. [CrossRef]
35. Patel, S.N.; Shi, A.; Wibbelsman, T.D.; Klufas, M.A. Ultra-widefield retinal imaging: An update on recent advances. *Ther. Adv. Ophthalmol.* **2020**, *12*, 2515841419899495. [CrossRef] [PubMed]
36. Stino, H.; Riessland, S.; Sedova, A.; Datlinger, F.; Sacu, S.; Schmidt-Erfurth, U.; Pollreisz, A. Comparison of two ultra-widefield color-fundus imaging devices for visualization of retinal periphery and microvascular lesions in patients with early diabetic retinopathy. *Sci. Rep.* **2022**, *12*, 17449. [CrossRef]
37. Hirano, T.; Imai, A.; Kasamatsu, H.; Kakihara, S.; Toriyama, Y.; Murata, T. Assessment of diabetic retinopathy using two ultra-wide-field fundus imaging systems, the Clarus(R) and Optos systems. *BMC Ophthalmol.* **2018**, *18*, 332. [CrossRef]
38. Santos, A.R.; Almeida, A.C.; Rocha, A.C.; Reste-Ferreira, D.; Marques, I.P.; Cunha-Vaz Martinho, A.; Mendes, L.; Santos, T.; Lewis, W.; Cunha-Vaz, J. Central and Peripheral Involvement of the Retina in the Initial Stages of Diabetic Retinopathy. *Retina* **2024**, *44*, 700–706. [CrossRef]
39. Oh, K.; Kang, H.M.; Leem, D.; Lee, H.; Seo, K.Y.; Yoon, S. Early detection of diabetic retinopathy based on deep learning and ultra-wide-field fundus images. *Sci. Rep.* **2021**, *11*, 1897. [CrossRef]
40. Ghasemi Falavarjani, K.; Tsui, I.; Sadda, S.R. Ultra-wide-field imaging in diabetic retinopathy. *Vis. Res.* **2017**, *139*, 187–190. [CrossRef]
41. Silva, P.S.; Cavallerano, J.D.; Haddad, N.M.; Kwak, H.; Dyer, K.H.; Omar, A.F.; Shikari, H.; Aiello, L.M.; Sun, J.K.; Aiello, L.P. Peripheral Lesions Identified on Ultrawide Field Imaging Predict Increased Risk of Diabetic Retinopathy Progression over 4 Years. *Ophthalmology* **2015**, *122*, 949–956. [CrossRef]
42. Jacoba, C.M.P.; Ashraf, M.; Cavallerano, J.D.; Tolson, A.M.; Tolls, D.; Pellegrini, E.; Fleming, A.; Sun, J.K.; Aiello, L.P.; Silva, P.S. Association of Maximizing Visible Retinal Area by Manual Eyelid Lifting With Grading of Diabetic Retinopathy Severity and Detection of Predominantly Peripheral Lesions When Using Ultra-Widefield Imaging. *JAMA Ophthalmol.* **2022**, *140*, 421–425. [CrossRef] [PubMed]
43. Ikram, M.K.; Cheung, C.Y.; Lorenzi, M.; Klein, R.; Jones, T.L.; Wong, T.Y. Retinal vascular caliber as a biomarker for diabetes microvascular complications. *Diabetes Care* **2013**, *36*, 750–759. [CrossRef] [PubMed]
44. Tsai, A.S.; Wong, T.Y.; Lavanya, R.; Zhang, R.; Hamzah, H.; Tai, E.S.; Cheung, C.Y. Differential association of retinal arteriolar and venular caliber with diabetes and retinopathy. *Diabetes Res. Clin. Pract.* **2011**, *94*, 291–298. [CrossRef]
45. Kolodjaschna, J.; Berisha, F.; Lung, S.; Schaller, G.; Polska, E.; Jilma, B.; Wolzt, M.; Schmetterer, L. LPS-induced microvascular leukocytosis can be assessed by blue-field entoptic phenomenon. *Am. J. Physiol. Heart Circ. Physiol.* **2004**, *287*, H691–H694. [CrossRef] [PubMed]
46. Sasongko, M.B.; Wong, T.Y.; Nguyen, T.T.; Cheung, C.Y.; Shaw, J.E.; Wang, J.J. Retinal vascular tortuosity in persons with diabetes and diabetic retinopathy. *Diabetologia* **2011**, *54*, 2409–2416. [CrossRef]
47. Forster, R.B.; Garcia, E.S.; Sluiman, A.J.; Grecian, S.M.; McLachlan, S.; MacGillivray, T.J.; Strachan, M.W.J.; Price, J.F.; Edinburgh Type 2 Diabetes Study Investigators. Retinal venular tortuosity and fractal dimension predict incident retinopathy in adults with type 2 diabetes: The Edinburgh Type 2 Diabetes Study. *Diabetologia* **2021**, *64*, 1103–1112. [CrossRef]
48. Wang, M.; Zhou, X.; Liu, D.N.; Chen, J.; Zheng, Z.; Ling, S. Development and validation of a predictive risk model based on retinal geometry for an early assessment of diabetic retinopathy. *Front. Endocrinol.* **2022**, *13*, 1033611. [CrossRef] [PubMed]
49. Song, Y.; Zhou, Z.; Liu, H.; Du, R.; Zhou, Y.; Zhu, S.; Chen, S. Tortuosity of branch retinal artery is more associated with the genesis and progress of diabetic retinopathy. *Front. Endocrinol.* **2022**, *13*, 972339. [CrossRef] [PubMed]
50. Cheung, C.Y.; Sabanayagam, C.; Law, A.K.; Kumari, N.; Ting, D.S.; Tan, G.; Mitchell, P.; Cheng, C.Y.; Wong, T.Y. Retinal vascular geometry and 6 year incidence and progression of diabetic retinopathy. *Diabetologia* **2017**, *60*, 1770–1781. [CrossRef]
51. Pedersen, K.B.; Broe, R.; Grauslund, J. Inter-Eye Agreement in Measurement of Retinal Vascular Fractal Dimension in Patients with Type 1 Diabetes Mellitus. *Ophthalmic Epidemiol.* **2016**, *23*, 131–135. [CrossRef]

52. Grauslund, J.; Green, A.; Kawasaki, R.; Hodgson, L.; Sjolie, A.K.; Wong, T.Y. Retinal vascular fractals and microvascular and macrovascular complications in type 1 diabetes. *Ophthalmology* **2010**, *117*, 1400–1405. [CrossRef] [PubMed]
53. Sohn, E.H.; van Dijk, H.W.; Jiao, C.; Kok, P.H.; Jeong, W.; Demirkaya, N.; Garmager, A.; Wit, F.; Kucukevcilioglu, M.; van Velthoven, M.E.; et al. Retinal neurodegeneration may precede microvascular changes characteristic of diabetic retinopathy in diabetes mellitus. *Proc. Natl. Acad. Sci. USA* **2016**, *113*, E2655–E2664. [CrossRef] [PubMed]
54. De Clerck, E.E.; Schouten, J.S.; Berendschot, T.T.; Kessels, A.G.; Nuijts, R.M.; Beckers, H.J.; Schram, M.T.; Stehouwer, C.D.; Webers, C.A. New ophthalmologic imaging techniques for detection and monitoring of neurodegenerative changes in diabetes: A systematic review. *Lancet Diabetes Endocrinol.* **2015**, *3*, 653–663. [CrossRef]
55. Hafner, J.; Karst, S.; Sacu, S.; Scholda, C.; Pablik, E.; Schmidt-Erfurth, U. Correlation between corneal and retinal neurodegenerative changes and their association with microvascular perfusion in type II diabetes. *Acta Ophthalmol.* **2019**, *97*, e545–e550. [CrossRef] [PubMed]
56. Huang, Y.; Zhang, N.; Bulloch, G.; Zhang, S.; Shang, X.; Chen, Y.; Liao, H.; Zhu, Z.; Wang, W. Rates of Choroidal and Neurodegenerative Changes Over Time in Diabetic Patients Without Retinopathy: A 3-Year Prospective Study. *Am. J. Ophthalmol.* **2023**, *246*, 10–19. [CrossRef] [PubMed]
57. Vujosevic, S.; Midena, E. Retinal layers changes in human preclinical and early clinical diabetic retinopathy support early retinal neuronal and Muller cells alterations. *J. Diabetes Res.* **2013**, *2013*, 905058. [CrossRef]
58. Peng, P.H.; Lin, H.S.; Lin, S. Nerve fibre layer thinning in patients with preclinical retinopathy. *Can. J. Ophthalmol.* **2009**, *44*, 417–422. [CrossRef] [PubMed]
59. van Dijk, H.W.; Verbraak, F.D.; Kok, P.H.; Stehouwer, M.; Garvin, M.K.; Sonka, M.; DeVries, J.H.; Schlingemann, R.O.; Abramoff, M.D. Early neurodegeneration in the retina of type 2 diabetic patients. *Investig. Ophthalmol. Vis. Sci.* **2012**, *53*, 2715–2719. [CrossRef] [PubMed]
60. Wanek, J.; Blair, N.P.; Chau, F.Y.; Lim, J.I.; Leiderman, Y.I.; Shahidi, M. Alterations in Retinal Layer Thickness and Reflectance at Different Stages of Diabetic Retinopathy by En Face Optical Coherence Tomography. *Investig. Ophthalmol. Vis. Sci.* **2016**, *57*, OCT341–OCT347. [CrossRef]
61. Frydkjaer-Olsen, U.; Soegaard Hansen, R.; Simo, R.; Cunha-Vaz, J.; Peto, T.; Grauslund, J.; Eurocondor. Correlation between Retinal Vessel Calibre and Neurodegeneration in Patients with Type 2 Diabetes Mellitus in the European Consortium for the Early Treatment of Diabetic Retinopathy (EUROCONDOR). *Ophthalmic Res.* **2016**, *56*, 10–16. [CrossRef]
62. Kessler, L.J.; Auffarth, G.U.; Bagautdinov, D.; Khoramnia, R. Ellipsoid Zone Integrity and Visual Acuity Changes during Diabetic Macular Edema Therapy: A Longitudinal Study. *J. Diabetes Res.* **2021**, *2021*, 8117650. [CrossRef]
63. Guyon, B.; Elphege, E.; Flores, M.; Gauthier, A.S.; Delbosc, B.; Saleh, M. Retinal Reflectivity Measurement for Cone Impairment Estimation and Visual Assessment After Diabetic Macular Edema Resolution (RECOVER-DME). *Investig. Ophthalmol. Vis. Sci.* **2017**, *58*, 6241–6247. [CrossRef]
64. Zhang, F.; Du, Z.; Zhang, X.; Wang, Y.; Chen, Y.; Wu, G.; Liang, Y.; Cao, D.; Zhao, J.; Fang, Y.; et al. Alterations of outer retinal reflectivity in diabetic patients without clinically detectable retinopathy. *Graefes Arch. Clin. Exp. Ophthalmol.* **2024**, *262*, 61–72. [CrossRef]
65. Cetin, E.N.; Parca, O.; Akkaya, H.S.; Pekel, G. Association of inner retinal reflectivity with qualitative and quantitative changes in retinal layers over time in diabetic eyes without retinopathy. *Eye* **2022**, *36*, 1253–1260. [CrossRef]
66. Hamadneh, T.; Aftab, S.; Sherali, N.; Vetrivel Suresh, R.; Tsouklidis, N.; An, M. Choroidal Changes in Diabetic Patients With Different Stages of Diabetic Retinopathy. *Cureus* **2020**, *12*, e10871. [CrossRef]
67. Endo, H.; Kase, S.; Saito, M.; Yokoi, M.; Takahashi, M.; Ishida, S.; Kase, M. Choroidal Thickness in Diabetic Patients Without Diabetic Retinopathy: A Meta-analysis. *Am. J. Ophthalmol.* **2020**, *218*, 68–77. [CrossRef]
68. Duran, M.; Cevher, S.; Kendirci, H.N.P. Choroidal thickness and choroidal vascularity index changes in children with type 1 diabetes mellitus without retinopathy. *Photodiagnosis Photodyn. Ther.* **2023**, *43*, 103706. [CrossRef]
69. Xu, F.; Li, Z.; Yang, X.; Gao, Y.; Li, Z.; Li, G.; Wang, S.; Ning, X.; Li, J. Assessment of choroidal structural changes in patients with pre- and early-stage clinical diabetic retinopathy using wide-field SS-OCTA. *Front. Endocrinol.* **2022**, *13*, 1036625. [CrossRef]
70. Deng, X.; Li, Z.; Li, Z.; Zhou, Q.; Lan, Y. Changes in the choroid detected by ultrawide-field optical coherence tomography angiography in type 2 diabetes mellitus patients without diabetic retinopathy. *Photodiagnosis Photodyn. Ther.* **2023**, *44*, 103823. [CrossRef]
71. Zhao, Q.; Wang, C.; Meng, L.; Cheng, S.; Gu, X.; Chen, Y.; Zhao, X. Central and peripheral changes in the retina and choroid in patients with diabetes mellitus without clinical diabetic retinopathy assessed by ultra-wide-field optical coherence tomography angiography. *Front. Public Health.* **2023**, *11*, 1194320. [CrossRef]
72. Wijesingha, N.; Tsai, W.S.; Keskin, A.M.; Holmes, C.; Kazantzis, D.; Chandak, S.; Kubravi, H.; Sivaprasad, S. Optical Coherence Tomography Angiography as a Diagnostic Tool for Diabetic Retinopathy. *Diagnostics* **2024**, *14*, 326. [CrossRef] [PubMed]
73. Yu, G.; Aaberg, M.T.; Patel, T.P.; Iyengar, R.S.; Powell, C.; Tran, A.; Miranda, C.; Young, E.; Demetriou, K.; Devisetty, L.; et al. Quantification of Retinal Nonperfusion and Neovascularization With Ultrawidefield Fluorescein Angiography in Patients With Diabetes and Associated Characteristics of Advanced Disease. *JAMA Ophthalmol.* **2020**, *138*, 680–688. [CrossRef] [PubMed]
74. Waheed, N.K.; Rosen, R.B.; Jia, Y.; Munk, M.R.; Huang, D.; Fawzi, A.; Chong, V.; Nguyen, Q.D.; Sepah, Y.; Pearce, E. Optical coherence tomography angiography in diabetic retinopathy. *Prog. Retin. Eye Res.* **2023**, *97*, 101206. [CrossRef] [PubMed]

75. Crincoli, E.; Sacconi, R.; Querques, L.; Querques, G. OCT angiography 2023 update: Focus on diabetic retinopathy. *Acta Diabetol.* **2024**, *61*, 533–541. [CrossRef] [PubMed]
76. Nouri, H.; Abtahi, S.H.; Mazloumi, M.; Samadikhadem, S.; Arevalo, J.F.; Ahmadieh, H. Optical coherence tomography angiography in diabetic retinopathy: A major review. *Surv. Ophthalmol.* **2024**, *35*, 149–161. [CrossRef]
77. Karst, S.G.; Heisler, M.; Lo, J.; Schuck, N.; Safari, A.; Sarunic, M.V.; Maberley, D.A.L.; Navajas, E.V. Evaluating Signs of Microangiopathy Secondary to Diabetes in Different Areas of the Retina with Swept Source OCTA. *Investig. Ophthalmol. Vis. Sci.* **2020**, *61*, 8. [CrossRef]
78. Qi, Z.; Si, Y.; Feng, F.; Zhu, J.; Yang, X.; Wang, W.; Zhang, Y.; Cui, Y. Analysis of retinal and choroidal characteristics in patients with early diabetic retinopathy using WSS-OCTA. *Front. Endocrinol.* **2023**, *14*, 1184717. [CrossRef]
79. Xu, F.; Li, Z.; Gao, Y.; Yang, X.; Huang, Z.; Li, Z.; Zhang, R.; Wang, S.; Guo, X.; Hou, X.; et al. Retinal Microvascular Signs in Pre- and Early-Stage Diabetic Retinopathy Detected Using Wide-Field Swept-Source Optical Coherence Tomographic Angiography. *J. Clin. Med.* **2022**, *11*, 4332. [CrossRef]
80. Wang, W.; Guo, X.; Chen, Y.; Xiong, K.; Gong, X.; Yuan, M.; Liang, X.; Huang, W. Choriocapillaris perfusion assessed using swept source optical coherence tomographic angiography and the severity of diabetic retinopathy. *Br. J. Ophthalmol.* **2023**, *107*, 836–841. [CrossRef]
81. Dai, Y.; Zhou, H.; Chu, Z.; Zhang, Q.; Chao, J.R.; Rezaei, K.A.; Wang, R.K. Microvascular Changes in the Choriocapillaris of Diabetic Patients Without Retinopathy Investigated by Swept-Source OCT Angiography. *Investig. Ophthalmol. Vis. Sci.* **2020**, *61*, 50. [CrossRef]
82. Loria, O.; Kodjikian, L.; Denis, P.; Vartin, C.; Dimassi, S.; Gervolino, L.; Maignan, A.; Kermarrec, R.; Chambard, C.; Pradat, P.; et al. Quantitative Analysis of Choriocapillaris Alterations in Swept-Source Optical Coherence Tomography Angiography in Diabetic Patients. *Retina* **2021**, *41*, 1809–1818. [CrossRef] [PubMed]
83. Zheng, F.; Deng, X.; Zhang, Q.; He, J.; Ye, P.; Liu, S.; Li, P.; Zhou, J.; Fang, X. Advances in swept-source optical coherence tomography and optical coherence tomography angiography. *Adv. Ophthalmol. Pract. Res.* **2023**, *3*, 67–79. [CrossRef]
84. Gao, Y.; Tuokedaerhan, Z.; Zhang, J.; Yang, L.; Zhang, Y.; Cheng, W.; Zhao, Y.; Wang, J. Comparative study of the vascular structures of the retina and choroid in Chinese Han and Uygur populations with proliferative diabetic retinopathy: An OCTA study. *Photodiagnosis Photodyn. Ther.* **2024**, *45*, 103995. [CrossRef] [PubMed]
85. Xia, F.; Hua, R. The Latest Updates in Swept-Source Optical Coherence Tomography Angiography. *Diagnostics* **2023**, *14*, 47. [CrossRef] [PubMed]
86. Zeng, Y.; Liu, M.; Li, M.; Wei, D.; Mao, M.; Liu, X.; Chen, S.; Liu, Y.; Chen, B.; Yang, L.; et al. Early changes to retinal structure in patients with diabetic retinopathy as determined by ultrawide swept-source optical coherence tomography-angiography. *Front. Endocrinol.* **2023**, *14*, 1143535. [CrossRef] [PubMed]
87. Grieshop, J.; Gaffney, M.; Linderman, R.E.; Cooper, R.F.; Carroll, J. The Shape of the Foveal Avascular Zone: When a Circle Isn't Round. *Transl. Vis. Sci. Technol.* **2023**, *12*, 26. [CrossRef] [PubMed]
88. Zhang, Z.; Huang, X.; Meng, X.; Chen, T.; Gu, Y.; Wu, Y.; Wu, Z. In vivo assessment of macula in eyes of healthy children 8 to 16 years old using optical coherence tomography angiography. *Sci. Rep.* **2017**, *7*, 8936. [CrossRef] [PubMed]
89. Eldaly, Z.; Soliman, W.; Sharaf, M.; Reyad, A.N. Morphological Characteristics of Normal Foveal Avascular Zone by Optical Coherence Tomography Angiography. *J. Ophthalmol.* **2020**, *2020*, 8281459. [CrossRef]
90. Custo Greig, E.; Brigell, M.; Cao, F.; Levine, E.S.; Peters, K.; Moult, E.M.; Fujimoto, J.G.; Waheed, N.K. Macular and Peripapillary Optical Coherence Tomography Angiography Metrics Predict Progression in Diabetic Retinopathy: A Sub-analysis of TIME-2b Study Data. *Am. J. Ophthalmol.* **2020**, *219*, 66–76. [CrossRef]
91. Sun, Z.; Tang, F.; Wong, R.; Lok, J.; Szeto, S.K.H.; Chan, J.C.K.; Chan, C.K.M.; Tham, C.C.; Ng, D.S.; Cheung, C.Y. OCT Angiography Metrics Predict Progression of Diabetic Retinopathy and Development of Diabetic Macular Edema: A Prospective Study. *Ophthalmology* **2019**, *126*, 1675–1684. [CrossRef]
92. Kim, K.; Kim, E.S.; Yu, S.Y. Optical coherence tomography angiography analysis of foveal microvascular changes and inner retinal layer thinning in patients with diabetes. *Br. J. Ophthalmol.* **2018**, *102*, 1226–1231. [CrossRef] [PubMed]
93. Linderman, R.E.; Muthiah, M.N.; Omoba, S.B.; Litts, K.; Tarima, S.; Visotcky, A.; Kim, J.E.; Carroll, J. Variability of Foveal Avascular Zone Metrics Derived From Optical Coherence Tomography Angiography Images. *Transl. Vis. Sci. Technol.* **2018**, *7*, 20. [CrossRef] [PubMed]
94. Krawitz, B.D.; Mo, S.; Geyman, L.S.; Agemy, S.A.; Scripsema, N.K.; Garcia, P.M.; Chui, T.Y.P.; Rosen, R.B. Acircularity index and axis ratio of the foveal avascular zone in diabetic eyes and healthy controls measured by optical coherence tomography angiography. *Vis. Res.* **2017**, *139*, 177–186. [CrossRef]
95. Hoffmann, M.B.; Bach, M.; Kondo, M.; Li, S.; Walker, S.; Holopigian, K.; Viswanathan, S.; Robson, A.G. ISCEV standard for clinical multifocal electroretinography (mfERG) (2021 update). *Doc. Ophthalmol.* **2021**, *142*, 5–16. [CrossRef] [PubMed]
96. Jia, Y.; Lin, Q.; Xiao, Y.; Zhou, X.; Zou, H.; Yang, C. Are We Overlooking the Neurodegeneration in the Early Stage of Type 1 Diabetes Mellitus without Visual Impairment or Diabetic Retinopathy: Is It Probably Occurred before Retinal Vasculature Dysfunction? *Curr. Eye Res.* **2023**, *48*, 433–440. [CrossRef] [PubMed]
97. Arias-Alvarez, M.; Tomas-Grasa, C.; Sopena-Pinilla, M.; Orduna-Hospital, E.; Fernandez-Espinosa, G.; Bielsa-Alonso, S.; Acha-Perez, J.; Rodriguez-Mena, D.; Pinilla, I. Electrophysiological findings in long-term type 1 diabetes patients without diabetic retinopathy using different ERG recording systems. *Sci. Rep.* **2024**, *14*, 3520. [CrossRef] [PubMed]

98. Ba-Ali, S.; Larsen, M.; Andersen, H.U.; Lund-Andersen, H. Full-field and multifocal electroretinogram in non-diabetic controls and diabetics with and without retinopathy. *Acta Ophthalmol.* **2022**, *100*, e1719–e1728. [CrossRef] [PubMed]
99. Han, Y.; Bearse, M.A., Jr.; Schneck, M.E.; Barez, S.; Jacobsen, C.H.; Adams, A.J. Multifocal electroretinogram delays predict sites of subsequent diabetic retinopathy. *Investig. Ophthalmol. Vis. Sci.* **2004**, *45*, 948–954. [CrossRef] [PubMed]
100. Srinivasan, S.; Sivaprasad, S.; Rajalakshmi, R.; Anjana, R.M.; Malik, R.A.; Kulothungan, V.; Raman, R.; Bhende, M. Assessment of optical coherence tomography angiography and multifocal electroretinography in eyes with and without nonproliferative diabetic retinopathy. *Indian J. Ophthalmol.* **2021**, *69*, 3235–3240. [CrossRef]
101. Srinivasan, S.; Sivaprasad, S.; Rajalakshmi, R.; Anjana, R.M.; Malik, R.A.; Kulothungan, V.; Natarajan, V.; Raman, R.; Bhende, M. Early retinal functional alteration in relation to diabetes duration in patients with type 2 diabetes without diabetic retinopathy. *Sci. Rep.* **2022**, *12*, 11422. [CrossRef]
102. Li, R.R.; Yang, Y.; Zhang, M.G.; Wang, J.; Chen, H.; Liu, S.; Miao, H.; Wang, Y.C. Abnormalities of retinal function in type 2 diabetes mellitus patients without clinical diabetic retinopathy detected by multifocal electroretinogram. *BMC Ophthalmol.* **2024**, *24*, 71. [CrossRef] [PubMed]
103. Ozawa, G.Y.; Bearse, M.A., Jr.; Bronson-Castain, K.W.; Harrison, W.W.; Schneck, M.E.; Barez, S.; Adams, A.J. Neurodegenerative differences in the retinas of male and female patients with type 2 diabetes. *Investig. Ophthalmol. Vis. Sci.* **2012**, *53*, 3040–3046. [CrossRef] [PubMed]
104. Molina-Martin, A.; Perez-Cambrodi, R.J.; Pinero, D.P. Current Clinical Application of Microperimetry: A Review. *Semin. Ophthalmol.* **2018**, *33*, 620–628. [CrossRef]
105. Baba, T. Detecting Diabetic Retinal Neuropathy Using Fundus Perimetry. *Int. J. Mol. Sci.* **2021**, *22*, 10726. [CrossRef]
106. Sabeti, F.; Nolan, C.J.; James, A.C.; Jenkins, A.; Maddess, T. Multifocal Pupillography Identifies Changes in Visual Sensitivity According to Severity of Diabetic Retinopathy in Type 2 Diabetes. *Investig. Ophthalmol. Vis. Sci.* **2015**, *56*, 4504–4513. [CrossRef]
107. Sabeti, F.; Carle, C.F.; Nolan, C.J.; Jenkins, A.J.; James, A.C.; Baker, L.; Coombes, C.E.; Cheung, V.; Chiou, M.; Maddess, T. Multifocal pupillographic objective perimetry for assessment of early diabetic retinopathy and generalised diabetes-related tissue injury in persons with type 1 diabetes. *BMC Ophthalmol.* **2022**, *22*, 166. [CrossRef] [PubMed]
108. Sabeti, F.; van Kleef, J.P.; Iyer, R.M.; Carle, C.F.; Nolan, C.J.; Chia, R.H.; Maddess, T. Discriminating early-stage diabetic retinopathy with subjective and objective perimetry. *Front. Endocrinol.* **2023**, *14*, 1333826. [CrossRef]
109. Thomas, R.L.; Luzio, S.D.; North, R.V.; Banerjee, S.; Zekite, A.; Bunce, C.; Owens, D.R. Retrospective analysis of newly recorded certifications of visual impairment due to diabetic retinopathy in Wales during 2007–2015. *BMJ Open* **2017**, *7*, e015024. [CrossRef]
110. Silva-Viguera, M.C.; Garcia-Romera, M.C.; Lopez-Izquierdo, I.; De-Hita-Cantalejo, C.; Sanchez-Gonzalez, M.C.; Bautista-Llamas, M.J. Contrast Sensitivity Assessment in Early Diagnosis of Diabetic Retinopathy: A Systematic Review. *Semin. Ophthalmol.* **2023**, *38*, 319–332. [CrossRef]
111. Tang, V.T.S.; Symons, R.C.A.; Fourlanos, S.; Guest, D.; McKendrick, A.M. Contrast Increment and Decrement Processing in Individuals With and Without Diabetes. *Investig. Ophthalmol. Vis. Sci.* **2023**, *64*, 26. [CrossRef]
112. Silva-Viguera, M.C.; Garcia-Romera, M.C.; Bautista-Llamas, M.J. Contrast sensitivity function under three light conditions in patients with type 1 diabetes mellitus without retinopathy: A cross-sectional, case-control study. *Graefes Arch. Clin. Exp. Ophthalmol.* **2023**, *261*, 2497–2505. [CrossRef] [PubMed]
113. Bodduluri, L.; Dain, S.J.; Hameed, S.; Verge, C.F.; Boon, M.Y. Visual function and retinal thickness in children with type 1 diabetes mellitus. *Clin. Exp. Optom.* **2024**, 1–9. [CrossRef]
114. El-Tawab, S.S.; Ibrahim, I.K.; Megallaa, M.H.; Mgeed, R.M.A.; Elemary, W.S. Neutrophil–lymphocyte ratio as a reliable marker to predict pre-clinical retinopathy among type 2 diabetic patients. *Egypt. Rheumatol. Rehabil.* **2023**, *50*, 11. [CrossRef]
115. Vanajarani, C. *Evaluation of Retinal Ganglion Cell Activity by Pattern Visual Evoked Potentials in Type 2 Diabetic Patients*; Chengalpattu Medical College: Chengalpattu, India, 2017.
116. Garhofer, G.; Bek, T.; Boehm, A.G.; Gherghel, D.; Grunwald, J.; Jeppesen, P.; Kergoat, H.; Kotliar, K.; Lanzl, I.; Lovasik, J.V.; et al. Use of the retinal vessel analyzer in ocular blood flow research. *Acta Ophthalmol.* **2010**, *88*, 717–722. [CrossRef] [PubMed]
117. Lott, M.E.; Slocomb, J.E.; Shivkumar, V.; Smith, B.; Quillen, D.; Gabbay, R.A.; Gardner, T.W.; Bettermann, K. Impaired retinal vasodilator responses in prediabetes and type 2 diabetes. *Acta Ophthalmol.* **2013**, *91*, e462–e469. [CrossRef] [PubMed]
118. Lim, L.S.; Ling, L.H.; Ong, P.G.; Foulds, W.; Tai, E.S.; Wong, E.; Lee, S.Y.; Wong, D.; Cheung, C.M.; Wong, T.Y. Dynamic responses in retinal vessel caliber with flicker light stimulation in eyes with diabetic retinopathy. *Investig. Ophthalmol. Vis. Sci.* **2014**, *55*, 5207–5213. [CrossRef]
119. Lim, L.S.; Ling, L.H.; Ong, P.G.; Foulds, W.; Tai, E.S.; Wong, T.Y. Dynamic Responses in Retinal Vessel Caliber With Flicker Light Stimulation and Risk of Diabetic Retinopathy and Its Progression. *Investig. Ophthalmol. Vis Sci.* **2017**, *58*, 2449–2455. [CrossRef] [PubMed]
120. Baier, J.M.; Funck, K.L.; Petersen, L.; Vernstrom, L.; Knudsen, S.T.; Bek, T.; Poulsen, P.L.; Laugesen, E. Retinal vessel reactivity is not attenuated in patients with type 2 diabetes compared with matched controls and is associated with peripheral endothelial function in controls. *J. Diabetes Complicat.* **2019**, *33*, 641–647. [CrossRef]
121. Safi, H.; Nourinia, R.; Safi, S.; Hadian, E.; Kheiri, B.; Ahmadieh, H. Retinal Vascular Response to Hyperoxia in Patients with Diabetes Mellitus without Diabetic Retinopathy. *J. Ophthalmol.* **2021**, *2021*, 9877205. [CrossRef]

122. Chen, Q.; Ma, Q.; Wu, C.; Tan, F.; Chen, F.; Wu, Q.; Zhou, R.; Zhuang, X.; Lu, F.; Qu, J.; et al. Macular Vascular Fractal Dimension in the Deep Capillary Layer as an Early Indicator of Microvascular Loss for Retinopathy in Type 2 Diabetic Patients. *Investig. Ophthalmol. Vis. Sci.* **2017**, *58*, 3785–3794. [CrossRef]
123. Ashimatey, B.S.; Green, K.M.; Chu, Z.; Wang, R.K.; Kashani, A.H. Impaired Retinal Vascular Reactivity in Diabetic Retinopathy as Assessed by Optical Coherence Tomography Angiography. *Investig. Ophthalmol. Vis. Sci.* **2019**, *60*, 2468–2473. [CrossRef] [PubMed]
124. Boned-Murillo, A.; Fernandez-Espinosa, G.; Orduna-Hospital, E.; Diaz-Barreda, M.D.; Sanchez-Cano, A.; Sopena-Pinilla, M.; Bielsa-Alonso, S.; Pinilla, I. Changes in Inner Retina Thickness and Macular Sensitivity in Patients with Type 2 Diabetes with Moderate Diabetic Retinopathy. *Biomedicines* **2023**, *11*, 2972. [CrossRef] [PubMed]
125. Bandello, F.; Borrelli, E.; Trevisi, M.; Lattanzio, R.; Sacconi, R.; Querques, G. Imaging Biomarkers of Mesopic and Dark-Adapted Macular Functions in Eyes With Treatment-Naive Mild Diabetic Retinopathy. *Am. J. Ophthalmol.* **2023**, *253*, 56–64. [CrossRef] [PubMed]
126. Tsai, A.S.H.; Gan, A.T.L.; Ting, D.S.W.; Wong, C.W.; Teo, K.Y.C.; Tan, A.C.S.; Lee, S.Y.; Wong, T.Y.; Tan, G.S.W.; Gemmy Cheung, C.M. Diabetic Macular Ischemia: Correlation of Retinal Vasculature Changes by Optical Coherence Tomography Angiography and Functional Deficit. *Retina* **2020**, *40*, 2184–2190. [CrossRef] [PubMed]
127. Alonso-Plasencia, M.; Abreu-Gonzalez, R.; Gomez-Culebras, M.A. Structure-Function Correlation Using OCT Angiography And Microperimetry In Diabetic Retinopathy. *Clin. Ophthalmol.* **2019**, *13*, 2181–2188. [CrossRef] [PubMed]
128. Levine, E.S.; Moult, E.M.; Greig, E.C.; Zhao, Y.; Pramil, V.; Gendelman, I.; Alibhai, A.Y.; Baumal, C.R.; Witkin, A.J.; Duker, J.S.; et al. Multiscale Correlation of Microvascular Changes on Optical Coherence Tomography Angiography with Retinal Sensitivity in Diabetic Retinopathy. *Retina* **2022**, *42*, 357–368. [CrossRef]
129. Harrison, W.W.; Bearse, M.A., Jr.; Ng, J.S.; Jewell, N.P.; Barez, S.; Burger, D.; Schneck, M.E.; Adams, A.J. Multifocal electroretinograms predict onset of diabetic retinopathy in adult patients with diabetes. *Investig. Ophthalmol. Vis. Sci.* **2011**, *52*, 772–777. [CrossRef]
130. Ng, J.S.; Bearse, M.A., Jr.; Schneck, M.E.; Barez, S.; Adams, A.J. Local diabetic retinopathy prediction by multifocal ERG delays over 3 years. *Investig. Ophthalmol. Vis. Sci.* **2008**, *49*, 1622–1628. [CrossRef]
131. Ratra, D.; Nagarajan, R.; Dalan, D.; Prakash, N.; Kuppan, K.; Thanikachalam, S.; Das, U.; Narayansamy, A. Early structural and functional neurovascular changes in the retina in the prediabetic stage. *Eye* **2021**, *35*, 858–867. [CrossRef]
132. Zagst, A.J.; Smith, J.D.; Wang, R.; Harrison, W.W. Foveal avascular zone size and mfERG metrics in diabetes and prediabetes: A pilot study of the relationship between structure and function. *Doc. Ophthalmol.* **2023**, *147*, 99–107. [CrossRef]
133. Santos, A.R.; Ribeiro, L.; Bandello, F.; Lattanzio, R.; Egan, C.; Frydkjaer-Olsen, U.; Garcia-Arumi, J.; Gibson, J.; Grauslund, J.; Harding, S.P.; et al. Functional and Structural Findings of Neurodegeneration in Early Stages of Diabetic Retinopathy: Cross-sectional Analyses of Baseline Data of the EUROCONDOR Project. *Diabetes* **2017**, *66*, 2503–2510. [CrossRef] [PubMed]
134. Islam, M.M.; Yang, H.C.; Poly, T.N.; Jian, W.S.; Jack Li, Y.C. Deep learning algorithms for detection of diabetic retinopathy in retinal fundus photographs: A systematic review and meta-analysis. *Comput. Methods Programs Biomed.* **2020**, *191*, 105320. [CrossRef]
135. Hai, Z.; Zou, B.; Xiao, X.; Peng, Q.; Yan, J.; Zhang, W.; Yue, K. A novel approach for intelligent diagnosis and grading of diabetic retinopathy. *Comput. Biol. Med.* **2024**, *172*, 108246. [CrossRef] [PubMed]
136. Wang, Z.; Li, Z.; Li, K.; Mu, S.; Zhou, X.; Di, Y. Performance of artificial intelligence in diabetic retinopathy screening: A systematic review and meta-analysis of prospective studies. *Front. Endocrinol.* **2023**, *14*, 1197783. [CrossRef] [PubMed]
137. Salongcay, R.P.; Aquino, L.A.C.; Alog, G.P.; Locaylocay, K.B.; Saunar, A.V.; Peto, T.; Silva, P.S. Accuracy of Integrated Artificial Intelligence Grading Using Handheld Retinal Imaging in a Community Diabetic Eye Screening Program. *Ophthalmol. Sci.* **2024**, *4*, 100457. [CrossRef] [PubMed]
138. Gulshan, V.; Peng, L.; Coram, M.; Stumpe, M.C.; Wu, D.; Narayanaswamy, A.; Venugopalan, S.; Widner, K.; Madams, T.; Cuadros, J.; et al. Development and Validation of a Deep Learning Algorithm for Detection of Diabetic Retinopathy in Retinal Fundus Photographs. *JAMA* **2016**, *316*, 2402–2410. [CrossRef] [PubMed]
139. Gargeya, R.; Leng, T. Automated Identification of Diabetic Retinopathy Using Deep Learning. *Ophthalmology* **2017**, *124*, 962–969. [CrossRef] [PubMed]
140. Abramoff, M.D.; Lavin, P.T.; Birch, M.; Shah, N.; Folk, J.C. Pivotal trial of an autonomous AI-based diagnostic system for detection of diabetic retinopathy in primary care offices. *NPJ Digit Med.* **2018**, *1*, 39. [CrossRef]
141. Ipp, E.; Liljenquist, D.; Bode, B.; Shah, V.N.; Silverstein, S.; Regillo, C.D.; Lim, J.I.; Sadda, S.; Domalpally, A.; Gray, G.; et al. Pivotal Evaluation of an Artificial Intelligence System for Autonomous Detection of Referrable and Vision-Threatening Diabetic Retinopathy. *JAMA Netw. Open.* **2021**, *4*, e2134254. [CrossRef]
142. Grzybowski, A.; Brona, P. Approval and Certification of Ophthalmic AI Devices in the European Union. *Ophthalmol. Ther.* **2023**, *12*, 633–638. [CrossRef]
143. Chou, Y.B.; Kale, A.U.; Lanzetta, P.; Aslam, T.; Barratt, J.; Danese, C.; Eldem, B.; Eter, N.; Gale, R.; Korobelnik, J.F.; et al. Current status and practical considerations of artificial intelligence use in screening and diagnosing retinal diseases: Vision Academy retinal expert consensus. *Curr. Opin. Ophthalmol.* **2023**, *34*, 403–413. [CrossRef] [PubMed]
144. Zang, P.; Hormel, T.T.; Wang, X.; Tsuboi, K.; Huang, D.; Hwang, T.S.; Jia, Y. A Diabetic Retinopathy Classification Framework Based on Deep-Learning Analysis of OCT Angiography. *Transl. Vis. Sci. Technol.* **2022**, *11*, 10. [CrossRef]

145. Zang, P.; Hormel, T.T.; Wang, J.; Guo, Y.; Bailey, S.T.; Flaxel, C.J.; Huang, D.; Hwang, T.S.; Jia, Y. Interpretable Diabetic Retinopathy Diagnosis Based on Biomarker Activation Map. *IEEE Trans. Biomed. Eng.* **2024**, *71*, 14–25. [CrossRef]
146. Niederleithner, M.; de Sisternes, L.; Stino, H.; Sedova, A.; Schlegl, T.; Bagherinia, H.; Britten, A.; Matten, P.; Schmidt-Erfurth, U.; Pollreisz, A.; et al. Ultra-Widefield OCT Angiography. *IEEE Trans. Med. Imaging* **2023**, *42*, 1009–1020. [CrossRef] [PubMed]
147. Ryu, G.; Lee, K.; Park, D.; Park, S.H.; Sagong, M. A deep learning model for identifying diabetic retinopathy using optical coherence tomography angiography. *Sci Rep.* **2021**, *11*, 23024. [CrossRef]
148. Yasser, I.; Khalifa, F.; Abdeltawab, H.; Ghazal, M.; Sandhu, H.S.; El-Baz, A. Automated Diagnosis of Optical Coherence Tomography Angiography (OCTA) Based on Machine Learning Techniques. *Sensors* **2022**, *22*, 2342. [CrossRef]
149. Sandhu, H.S.; Elmogy, M.; Taher Sharafeldeen, A.; Elsharkawy, M.; El-Adawy, N.; Eltanboly, A.; Shalaby, A.; Keynton, R.; El-Baz, A. Automated Diagnosis of Diabetic Retinopathy Using Clinical Biomarkers, Optical Coherence Tomography, and Optical Coherence Tomography Angiography. *Am. J. Ophthalmol.* **2020**, *216*, 201–206. [CrossRef]
150. Zhou, Y.; Chia, M.A.; Wagner, S.K.; Ayhan, M.S.; Williamson, D.J.; Struyven, R.R.; Liu, T.; Xu, M.; Lozano, M.G.; Woodward-Court, P.; et al. A foundation model for generalizable disease detection from retinal images. *Nature* **2023**, *622*, 156–163. [CrossRef] [PubMed]
151. Rajesh, A.E.; Olvera-Barrios, A.; Warwick, A.N.; Wu, Y.; Stuart, K.V.; Biradar, M.; Ung, C.Y.; Khawaja, A.P.; Luben, R.; Foster, P.J.; et al. Ethnicity is not biology: Retinal pigment score to evaluate biological variability from ophthalmic imaging using machine learning. *medRxiv* **2023**, *preprint*. [CrossRef]
152. Xie, Y.; Nguyen, Q.D.; Hamzah, H.; Lim, G.; Bellemo, V.; Gunasekeran, D.V.; Yip, M.Y.T.; Qi Lee, X.; Hsu, W.; Li Lee, M.; et al. Artificial intelligence for teleophthalmology-based diabetic retinopathy screening in a national programme: An economic analysis modelling study. *Lancet Digit Health.* **2020**, *2*, e240–e249. [CrossRef]
153. Huang, X.M.; Yang, B.F.; Zheng, W.L.; Liu, Q.; Xiao, F.; Ouyang, P.W.; Li, M.J.; Li, X.Y.; Meng, J.; Zhang, T.T.; et al. Cost-effectiveness of artificial intelligence screening for diabetic retinopathy in rural China. *BMC Health Serv. Res.* **2022**, *22*, 260. [CrossRef] [PubMed]
154. Fuller, S.D.; Hu, J.; Liu, J.C.; Gibson, E.; Gregory, M.; Kuo, J.; Rajagopal, R. Five-Year Cost-Effectiveness Modeling of Primary Care-Based, Nonmydriatic Automated Retinal Image Analysis Screening Among Low-Income Patients With Diabetes. *J. Diabetes Sci. Technol.* **2022**, *16*, 415–427. [CrossRef] [PubMed]
155. Rajalakshmi, R. The impact of artificial intelligence in screening for diabetic retinopathy in India. *Eye* **2020**, *34*, 420–421. [CrossRef] [PubMed]
156. Tomic, M.; Vrabec, R.; Hendelja, D.; Kolaric, V.; Bulum, T.; Rahelic, D. Diagnostic Accuracy of Hand-Held Fundus Camera and Artificial Intelligence in Diabetic Retinopathy Screening. *Biomedicines* **2023**, *12*, 214–230. [CrossRef] [PubMed]
157. Mertoglu, C.; Gunay, M. Neutrophil-Lymphocyte ratio and Platelet-Lymphocyte ratio as useful predictive markers of prediabetes and diabetes mellitus. *Diabetes Metab. Syndr.* **2017**, *11* (Suppl. S1), S127–S131. [CrossRef] [PubMed]
158. Rajendrakumar, A.L.; Hapca, S.M.; Nair, A.T.N.; Huang, Y.; Chourasia, M.K.; Kwan, R.S.; Nangia, C.; Siddiqui, M.K.; Vijayaraghavan, P.; Matthew, S.Z.; et al. Competing risks analysis for neutrophil to lymphocyte ratio as a predictor of diabetic retinopathy incidence in the Scottish population. *BMC Med.* **2023**, *21*, 304. [CrossRef] [PubMed]
159. Wang, L.; Zhou, X.; Yin, Y.; Mai, Y.; Wang, D.; Zhang, X. Hyperglycemia Induces Neutrophil Extracellular Traps Formation Through an NADPH Oxidase-Dependent Pathway in Diabetic Retinopathy. *Front. Immunol.* **2018**, *9*, 3076. [CrossRef] [PubMed]
160. Lessieur, E.M.; Liu, H.; Saadane, A.; Du, Y.; Tang, J.; Kiser, J.; Kern, T.S. Neutrophil-Derived Proteases Contribute to the Pathogenesis of Early Diabetic Retinopathy. *Investig. Ophthalmol. Vis. Sci.* **2021**, *62*, 7. [CrossRef]
161. Hu, G.; Gu, L.; Wang, R.; Jian, Q.; Lv, K.; Xia, M.; Lai, M.; Shen, T.; Hu, J.; Yang, S.; et al. Ethanolamine as a biomarker and biomarker-based therapy for diabetic retinopathy in glucose-well-controlled diabetic patients. *Sci. Bull.* **2024**, *69*, 1920–1935. [CrossRef]
162. Quek, D.Q.Y.; He, F.; Sultana, R.; Banu, R.; Chee, M.L.; Nusinovici, S.; Thakur, S.; Qian, C.; Cheng, C.Y.; Wong, T.Y.; et al. Novel Serum and Urinary Metabolites Associated with Diabetic Retinopathy in Three Asian Cohorts. *Metabolites* **2021**, *11*, 614. [CrossRef]
163. Oshitari, T. Diabetic retinopathy: Neurovascular disease requiring neuroprotective and regenerative therapies. *Neural Regen. Res.* **2022**, *17*, 795–796. [CrossRef] [PubMed]
164. Simo, R.; Simo-Servat, O.; Bogdanov, P.; Hernandez, C. Neurovascular Unit: A New Target for Treating Early Stages of Diabetic Retinopathy. *Pharmaceutics* **2021**, *13*, 1320. [CrossRef] [PubMed]
165. Nian, S.; Lo, A.C.Y.; Mi, Y.; Ren, K.; Yang, D. Neurovascular unit in diabetic retinopathy: Pathophysiological roles and potential therapeutical targets. *Eye Vis.* **2021**, *8*, 15. [CrossRef] [PubMed]
166. Gardner, T.W.; Davila, J.R. The neurovascular unit and the pathophysiologic basis of diabetic retinopathy. *Graefes Arch. Clin. Exp. Ophthalmol.* **2017**, *255*, 1–6. [CrossRef] [PubMed]
167. Barber, A.J.; Lieth, E.; Khin, S.A.; Antonetti, D.A.; Buchanan, A.G.; Gardner, T.W. Neural apoptosis in the retina during experimental and human diabetes. Early onset and effect of insulin. *J. Clin. Investig.* **1998**, *102*, 783–791. [CrossRef]
168. Yang, Q.; Yasvoina, M.; Olvera-Barrios, A.; Mendes, J.; Zhu, M.; Egan, C.; Tufail, A.; Fruttiger, M. Disconnection Between Microvascular Damage and Neurodegeneration in Early Diabetic Retinopathy. *bioRxiv* **2024**, *preprint*. [CrossRef]
169. Liu, K.; Zhu, T.; Gao, M.; Yin, X.; Zheng, R.; Yan, Y.; Gao, L.; Ding, Z.; Ye, J.; Li, P. Functional OCT angiography reveals early retinal neurovascular dysfunction in diabetes with capillary resolution. *Biomed Opt. Express.* **2023**, *14*, 1670–1684. [CrossRef]

170. Zhang, Y.; Ranaei Pirmardan, E.; Jiang, H.; Barakat, A.; Hafezi-Moghadam, A. VEGFR-2 adhesive nanoprobes reveal early diabetic retinopathy in vivo. *Biosens. Bioelectron.* **2023**, *237*, 115476. [CrossRef]
171. de la Zerda, A.; Paulus, Y.M.; Teed, R.; Bodapati, S.; Dollberg, Y.; Khuri-Yakub, B.T.; Blumenkranz, M.S.; Moshfeghi, D.M.; Gambhir, S.S. Photoacoustic ocular imaging. *Opt. Lett.* **2010**, *35*, 270–272. [CrossRef] [PubMed]
172. Tian, C.; Zhang, W.; Mordovanakis, A.; Wang, X.; Paulus, Y.M. Noninvasive chorioretinal imaging in living rabbits using integrated photoacoustic microscopy and optical coherence tomography. *Opt. Express.* **2017**, *25*, 15947–15955. [CrossRef]
173. Li, Y.; Xia, X.; Paulus, Y.M. Novel Retinal Imaging Technologies. *Int. J. Ophthalmol. Eye Sci.* **2017**, *5*, 329–333.
174. Nguyen, V.P.; Li, Y.; Aaberg, M.; Zhang, W.; Wang, X.; Paulus, Y.M. In Vivo 3D Imaging of Retinal Neovascularization Using Multimodal Photoacoustic Microscopy and Optical Coherence Tomography Imaging. *J. Imaging* **2018**, *4*, 150. [CrossRef]
175. Nguyen, V.P.; Paulus, Y.M. Photoacoustic Ophthalmoscopy: Principle, Application, and Future Directions. *J. Imaging* **2018**, *4*, 149. [CrossRef] [PubMed]
176. Zhang, W.; Li, Y.; Nguyen, V.P.; Huang, Z.; Liu, Z.; Wang, X.; Paulus, Y.M. High-resolution, in vivo multimodal photoacoustic microscopy, optical coherence tomography, and fluorescence microscopy imaging of rabbit retinal neovascularization. *Light Sci. Appl.* **2018**, *7*, 103. [CrossRef] [PubMed]
177. Zhang, W.; Li, Y.; Yu, Y.; Derouin, K.; Qin, Y.; Nguyen, V.P.; Xia, X.; Wang, X.; Paulus, Y.M. Simultaneous photoacoustic microscopy, spectral-domain optical coherence tomography, and fluorescein microscopy multi-modality retinal imaging. *Photoacoustics* **2020**, *20*, 100194. [CrossRef]
178. Nguyen, V.P.; Qian, W.; Wang, X.; Paulus, Y.M. Functionalized contrast agents for multimodality photoacoustic microscopy, optical coherence tomography, and fluorescence microscopy molecular retinal imaging. *Methods Enzymol.* **2021**, *657*, 443–480. [CrossRef]
179. Abou Taha, A.; Dinesen, S.; Vergmann, A.S.; Grauslund, J. Present and future screening programs for diabetic retinopathy: A narrative review. *Int. J. Retina Vitreous.* **2024**, *10*, 14. [CrossRef]

biomedicines

MDPI

Review

The Role of Natural Products in Diabetic Retinopathy

Yuxuan Zhao [1,2], Yi Chen [1] and Naihong Yan [1,*]

1 Research Laboratory of Ophthalmology, West China Hospital, Sichuan University, Chengdu 610041, China; zhaoyx413@163.com (Y.Z.); chenyicycycy0723@gmail.com (Y.C.)
2 Department of Optometry and Visual Science, West China Hospital, Sichuan University, Chengdu 610041, China
* Correspondence: yannaihong@wchscu.cn

Abstract: Diabetic retinopathy (DR) is one of the most severe complications of diabetes mellitus and potentially leads to significant visual impairment and blindness. The complex mechanisms involved in the pathological changes in DR make it challenging to achieve satisfactory outcomes with existing treatments. Diets conducive to glycemic control have been shown to improve outcomes in diabetic patients, thus positioning dietary interventions as promising avenues for DR treatment. Investigations have demonstrated that natural products (NPs) may effectively manage DR. Many types of natural compounds, including saponins, phenols, terpenoids, flavonoids, saccharides, alkaloids, and vitamins, have been shown to exert anti-inflammatory, antioxidant, anti-neovascular, and antiapoptotic effects in vivo and in vitro. Nevertheless, the clinical application of NPs still faces challenges, such as suboptimal specificity, poor bioavailability, and a risk of toxicity. Prospective clinical studies are imperative to validate the therapeutic potential of NPs in delaying or preventing DR.

Keywords: diabetic retinopathy; natural products; mechanism; toxicity

1. Introduction

Diabetes mellitus (DM) is a metabolic disorder characterized by chronic hyperglycemia due to a variety of etiological factors. A survey by the International Diabetes Federation indicated that in 2021, approximately 537 million individuals aged 20–79 years were diagnosed with DM. Diabetic retinopathy (DR) is a severe complication of DM, and persistent hyperglycemia and hypertension can lead to retinal dysfunction, thus ultimately resulting in significant visual impairment and even blindness [1]. Factors such as hyperglycemia, hypertension, dyslipidemia, and duration of DM are associated with increased risks of DR [2,3]. By 2045, DR is expected to affect an estimated 1.6 million people worldwide [4].

DR can be divided into two stages: non-proliferative diabetic retinopathy (NPDR) and advanced proliferative diabetic retinopathy (PDR) [5]. As the early stage of DR, NPDR may present without subjective symptoms, yet the fundus exhibits pathological alterations, such as microaneurysms, hemorrhages, cotton-wool spots, and hard exudates. PDR, which is a progressive stage of NPDR, is mainly associated with persistent hyperglycemia and inadequate glycemic control [6]. This advanced stage is characterized by retinal microvascular damage and pericyte loss, thus manifesting as vitreous or preretinal hemorrhages and neovascularization (Figure 1).

The pathogenesis of DR is very complex because it involves multiple cross-linking mechanisms, which lead to retinal dysfunction [7]. Current treatments for DR include medications to control blood glucose levels, retinal laser photocoagulation, anti-vascular endothelial growth factor (VEGF) injection, and para plana vitrectomy (PPV). Although VEGF inhibitors and other antiangiogenic agents have been widely used in the clinical settings, many patients still do not achieve satisfactory visual recovery [8]. Consequently, the identification of novel therapeutic strategies to ameliorate DR is urgently needed.

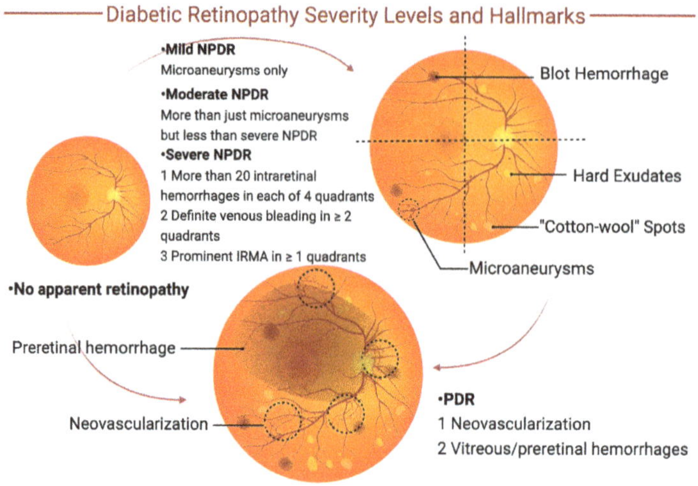

Figure 1. Diabetic retinopathy severity levels and hallmarks. Initially, diabetic patients may exhibit no apparent signs of retinopathy. However, as diabetic retinopathy (DR) progresses, it may evolve into non-proliferative diabetic retinopathy (NPDR) and eventually advance to proliferative diabetic retinopathy (PDR), or it may transition directly to PDR. According to international classifications, NPDR is categorized into mild, moderate, and severe stages. Clinical manifestations of NPDR include blot hemorrhages, hard exudates, "cotton-wool" spots, and microaneurysms. The more advanced stage, PDR, is characterized by the emergence of neovascularization and/or vitreous or preretinal hemorrhages. Abbreviations: IRMA, intraretinal microvascular abnormalities.

Currently, the rapidly developing economic model has changed individuals' lifestyles and dietary patterns. An increased consumption of sugar and fats, as well as diminished physical activity, may exacerbate DM. Diet and lifestyle modifications constitute the foundational strategy for DR management. Natural products (NPs) derived from various fauna and flora have emerged as being dietary drug supplements and have increasingly become a focus of research interest. One study demonstrated that increasing daily fruit consumption may mitigate DR risks, with a notable 50% reduction attributed to the abundant vitamins and nutrients in fruits [9]. The benefits of a wide range of vegetables and fruits reinforce the shift toward dietary-based therapeutic modalities.

This review summarizes and updates the current evidence on the possible role of NPs in DR, ranging from experimental findings to the possible challenges that may be encountered in clinical application; moreover, we expect to introduce a novel therapeutic method for DR patients.

2. Method

The search strategy was based on the Preferred Reporting Items for Systematic Reviews and Meta-Analyses (PRISMA) guidelines [10]. Studies related to diabetic retinopathy and natural products were collected through searches on the Web of Science and PubMed, from January 1974 to January 2024. The keywords "Diabetic Retinopathy", "Biological Products", and "Natural Products" were utilized, combined as Mesh terms and text words. Boolean operators were used to construct the search strategy. Relevant reference lists were also searched, ensuring that all relevant literature was involved.

Inclusion criteria:

1. Natural extracts from plants, animals, or medical herbs were considered.
2. The effectiveness of natural products in treating diabetic retinopathy was validated through in vitro, in vivo, or human clinical trials.
3. The results included effects, therapeutic potentials, signaling mechanisms, etc.

Exclusion criteria:

1. Studies not relevant to natural products were excluded.
2. Natural products lacking clear chemical structures were omitted.
3. Natural products with multiple components that did not specify the active components were excluded.

3. Diabetic Retinopathy

3.1. Pathophysiology of Diabetic Retinopathy

The pathophysiologic changes in DR are associated with chronic hyperglycemia. Persistent elevation of blood glucose is implicated in physiological and biochemical retinal alterations, thus precipitating microvascular injury and retinal dysfunction. Moreover, chronic hyperglycemia is known to induce microaneurysms, hemorrhages, and thickening of the retinal basement membrane, which increase the permeability of the blood–retina barrier (BRB) and cause leakage from retinal vessels. Concurrently, compromised vascular permeability contributes to capillary occlusion and subsequent retinal hypoxia, thus potentially leading to increased VEGF levels [11] and fostering PDR [3]. PDR is pathologically characterized by the emergence of retinal neovascularization and fibrovascular membranes, with potential progression to vitreous hemorrhage and retinal detachment, thus culminating in visual impairment and blindness. Diabetic macular edema (DME) represents another prevalent cause of visual loss in DR and is characterized by disruption of the BRB and subsequent accumulation of fluid in the macula, thus resulting in increased macular thickness and edema [12]. DME may occur at any stage of DR and may cause severe image distortion and vision loss. Additionally, indicators such as inflammation, micro-vasculopathy, oxidative stress, and neurodegeneration have been implicated in DR-related retinal damage.

3.1.1. Inflammation

Inflammation plays a pivotal role in all stages of DR. Inflammatory factors can be consistently detected at low doses in diabetic patients and animal models [13,14]. Adhesion-molecule-mediated leukocyte-endothelial cell adhesion is associated with leukostasis in DR, and it has been proven that leukostasis is correlated with endothelial cell loss and BRB damage in diabetic models [15]. In addition, increased expression of leukocyte adhesion molecules and endothelial cell adhesion molecules has been detected in diabetic patients and animal models [16,17].

Furthermore, chemokines, such as monocyte chemotactic protein-1 (MCP-1), macrophage inflammatory protein-1α (MIP-1α), and MIP-1β, are involved in DR progression [18]. These chemokines can attract and activate leukocytes, thus exacerbating leukostasis. The expression of inflammatory mediators, including tumor necrosis factor-alpha (TNF-α), interleukin 6 (IL-6), IL-10, IL-23, and IL-1β, is also upregulated in DR patients [19].

Microglial activation is involved in the inflammatory response in DR. Under high-glucose conditions, microglia are activated, followed by increased levels of TNF-α, IL-6, MCP-1, and VEGF [20]. Müller cells and astrocytes also contribute to this response, thus releasing large amounts of pro-inflammatory factors that further exacerbate inflammation in the retina [21].

3.1.2. Retinal Micro-Vasculopathy

DR has long been recognized as a microvascular disease [22]. Chronic hyperglycemia is known to induce vasodilatation and hemodynamic changes, which potentially occur as a retinal adaptation to altered metabolic demands [23]. In DR, systemic and ocular hypertension, in addition to hyperglycemia, contribute to the disruption of tight junctions between pericytes and endothelial cells. This disruption leads to pericyte apoptosis, which precipitates the uncontrolled proliferation of vascular endothelial cells and new vessel formation [24]. Due to the fact that pericytes support capillary integrity, their loss is implicated in the pathogenesis of capillary dilation and subsequent microaneurysm development [25]. Moreover, the newly formed vasculature, which tends to be delicate and excessively permeable, can lead to leakage, thus resulting in hemorrhage and swelling in the retina [26].

Retinal ischemia or hypoxia stimulates hypoxia-inducible factor-1 (HIF-1), thus stimulating VEGF upregulation [27]. VEGF has been implicated as a principal factor in the pathogenesis of PDR and DME. VEGF can increase vascular permeability by phosphorylating tight-junction proteins [28]. Furthermore, VEGF facilitates endothelial cell proliferation via mitogen-activated protein (MAP) activation [29]. Elevated VEGF levels have been detected in DR patients and animal models [30–32].

3.1.3. Oxidative Stress

Oxidative stress is a key factor contributing to the diminished capacity of intracellular antioxidant defense systems and fostering pro-inflammatory factor production [33]. The excessive accumulation of reactive oxygen species (ROS) precipitates oxidative stress. Under physiological conditions, organisms resist ROS through the antioxidant defense system, thus maintaining a balance between ROS generation and elimination [34]. However, chronic hyperglycemia leads to decreased antioxidant defenses and increased oxidative stress [35]. Hyperglycemia activates metabolic pathways, stimulates mitochondrial oxidative phosphorylation, and activates nicotinamide adenine dinucleotide phosphate oxidase, all of which contribute to increased ROS levels [36]. Elevated ROS levels may alter cellular homeostasis, thus leading to cellular dysfunction. In addition, the retina is particularly susceptible to oxidative stress, considering its high unsaturated fatty acid content and substantial oxygen consumption for glucose metabolism. In diabetic mouse models, a significant increase in ROS production and concomitant suppression of antioxidant enzyme activity were observed [37].

3.1.4. Retinal Neurodegeneration

Retinal neurodegeneration may occur early in DR, and upregulated expression of pro-apoptotic factors (such as cleaved caspase-3, Bax, and Fas) has been detected in DR patients and animal models [38–40]. Studies have indicated that sustained exposure to high glucose levels is correlated with increased mitochondrial fragmentation and apoptosis in vitro [41]. Observations in diabetic mouse models demonstrated ganglion cell loss and reduced retinal thickness, which precede the onset of retinal micro-vasculopathy [42].

3.2. *Current Therapy for Diabetic Retinopathy*

Current treatment modalities for DR include medications, anti-VEGF injections, laser photocoagulation, and PPV [8]. Nevertheless, the available methods for treating DR remain unsatisfactory. The optimal management of blood glucose and diabetic progression remains of utmost importance [43]. In the stages of normal or mild to moderate NPDR without macular edema, glycemic control is typically achieved through pharmacological methods, which include the use of insulin-promoting agents, such as sulfonylureas, glinides, dipeptidyl peptidase IV inhibitors, and hypoglycemic agents acting through other mechanisms, such as bisphosphonoids, thiazolidinediones, α-glycosidase inhibitors, and sodium-glucose cotransporter protein 2 inhibitors. Concurrently, the risk of diabetic retinopathy onset and progression can be reduced through the use of antihypertensive drugs (angiotensin-converting enzyme inhibitors, angiotensin II receptor antagonists, and calcium channel blockers) and hypolipidemic drugs (stains, fibrates, and nicotinic acid).

Clinically, anti-VEGF agents, such as faricimab-svoa, ranibizumab, aflibercept, and bevacizumab, are also prevalently used to inhibit retinal neovascularization and mitigate macular edema. Nonetheless, intravitreal anti-VEGF injections have several disadvantages, such as high costs and potential side effects [44]. The short half-life of these drugs necessitates frequent, monthly, or bimonthly administration to sustain therapeutic benefits, and long-term intravitreal treatments increase the risk of complications, such as endophthalmitis, uveitis, and subconjunctival hemorrhage [45]. These issues, including long-term treatment necessity, high costs, and associated risks, may render sustained therapy infeasible for a majority of patients.

Laser photocoagulation serves as an efficacious adjunct therapy for DR patients. The Early Treatment Diabetes Retinopathy Study (ETDRS), which lasted for three years, established that focal/grid macular laser photocoagulation was beneficial for individuals with DME, thus significantly reducing the likelihood of vision loss [46]. Pan-retinal photocoagulation (PRP) has been shown to suppress VEGF production by ameliorating retinal microcirculatory hemodynamics and augmenting the oxygenation of the retina. Despite its efficacy, PRP may induce adverse effects, such as slight central visual loss, vitreous hemorrhage, and subsequent neovascularization. The integration of focal laser and anti-VEGF injections in DME patients can lessen the need for frequent anti-VEGF injections, thereby mitigating complication risks, and has become a popular treatment modality for DR patients [47].

In cases of PDR complicated by vitreous hemorrhage or tractional retinal detachment, PPV is employed as the principal intervention. PPV facilitates the removal of intraocular blood and diminishes the vitreous concentrations of VEGF and inflammatory mediators, thus consequently ameliorating disruptions in the retinal microenvironment. Concurrently, excision of the fibrovascular membrane (FVM) during surgery alleviates traction, thus re-establishing the normal structure of the retina. However, PPV possesses a greater risk of hemorrhage during the operation and presents challenges for achieving successful surgical outcomes. Current treatment options for DR and their side effects can be seen in Figure 2.

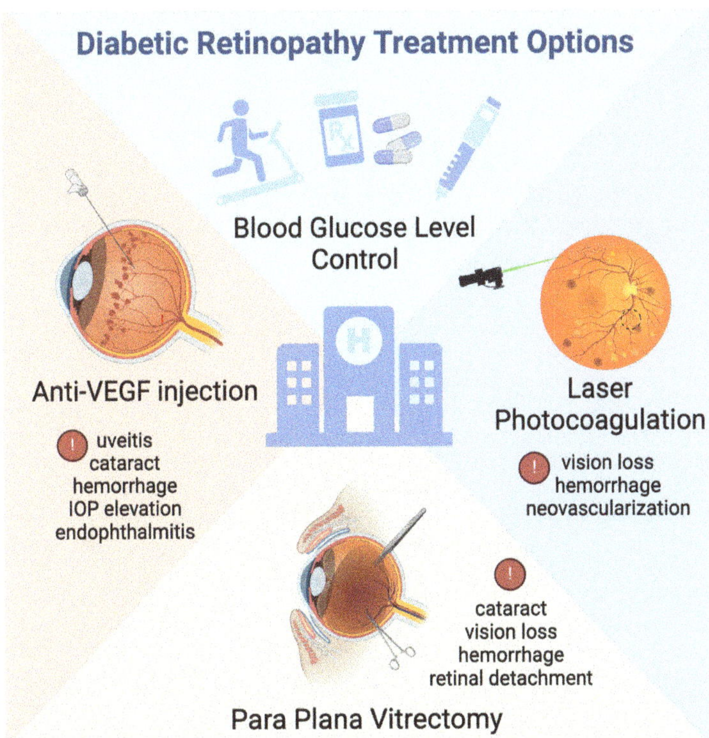

Figure 2. Diabetic retinopathy treatment options. Controlling the blood glucose level is critical, which involves healthy lifestyle, medical management, and insulin injections. Additionally, clinical practices commonly employ anti-vascular endothelial growth factor (VEGF) injections, laser photocoagulation, and pars plana vitrectomy. While these interventions are prevalent, they can present certain adverse effects and complications.

4. Experimental Models for Diabetes Research

4.1. Cell Models

Research utilizing cell models has proven to play an essential role in elucidating the responses of cells in different retinal layers to diabetes-related stimuli, such as high glucose, lipids, shear stress, metabolite imbalance, cytokines, and growth factors [43]. These models facilitate the investigation of the crucial molecular mechanisms that are involved in the interaction between pharmacological agents and DR. In studies of NPs related to DR, endothelial cells and retinal pigment epithelium (RPE) cells are the predominant cell models that are employed, with fewer studies using pericytes, Müller cells, and ganglion cells.

Pathological neovascularization is the leading cause of DR progression, and researchers usually utilize endothelial cells in vitro to stimulate human retinal angiogenesis [48]. NP investigations have employed human retinal endothelial cells (HRECs), rhesus monkey retinal and choroid endothelial cells (RF/6A), human umbilical vein endothelial cells (HUVECs), and human microvascular endothelial cells (HMVECs), the latter two of which serve as non-specific models for angiogenic replication. In vitro, cells are treated with high glucose concentrations to stimulate a diabetic condition. Endothelial cells are commonly utilized to investigate cell proliferation, migration, tube formation, and signaling pathways related to inflammation and apoptosis. Expressions of HIF-1α and VEGF are often assessed in these studies [49–51]. However, differences in the secretory functions of HREC and HUVEC and their modulation by glucose suggest regional specificity of cellular functions. Considering that DR is a microvascular disease and is specifically restricted in the retina, the use of HUVECs, a macrovascular cell type, in in vitro studies may be inadequate for inferring pathophysiologic changes in DR [52].

RPE cells, which are located between the retina and the choroid, are crucial for preserving the integrity of photoreceptors in terms of both structure and function [53]. Nevertheless, studies have indicated that DR can lead to RPE cells' dysfunction and impaired clearance of fluid leakage from choroidal capillaries, thus culminating in retinal edema [54]. Extensive research has demonstrated that high glucose exposure contributes to retinal barrier dysfunction, early apoptosis, and aberrant cytokine expression. NPs have been identified as being protective agents for RPE cells, delivering anti-inflammatory and antioxidant properties [55,56].

Other in vitro studies have utilized specific retinal cells, including glial cells, macrophages, and retinal neuronal cells. The human retina is comprised of three types of glial cells: microglia, astrocytes, and Müller cells. These glial cells are crucial supporters of neuronal tissue, closely associating and interacting with retinal vessels and other structures to maintain the homeostasis of the retinal microenvironment. In vitro studies involving glial cells typically investigate the relationship between DR vasculopathy and neuropathy [57]. The migration of macrophages is closely linked to inflammation and angiogenesis in DR; thus, studies employing macrophages are pivotal in elucidating the underlying mechanisms [58]. Evidence indicates that profound morphological changes and electrophysiologic defects occur in retinal neurons early over the course of DR [59]. Research employing retinal neuronal cells, including photoreceptors and retinal ganglion cells, plays a vital role in understanding the neurodegeneration associated with DR [60].

It must be acknowledged that investigations on the role of NPs in DR through cell models have inherent limitations. The retina is an intricate tissue composed of multiple interrelated cell types, and the isolation of specific cells fails to represent the entirety of retinal microenvironmental alterations [61]. Besides, due to long-term development of diabetic complications, possibly due to the accumulation of epigenetic changes [62], in vitro models with a relatively rapid experimental duration are inferior to animal models. Therefore, animal models are posited to be a more appropriate alternative.

4.2. Animal Models

Diabetic animal models have been instrumental in understanding the molecular pathology underlying DR and assessing NPs as potential alternative treatments. Commonly used models in DR research include mice, rats, cats, dogs, pigs, and non-human primates. Due to their small size, short lifespan, and rapid reproduction rate, mouse and rat models are particularly prevalent [63]. This review focuses on four model types: chemical-induced, genetic, diet-induced, and neovascularization models.

4.2.1. Chemical-Induced Models

Chemical-induced models, which are known for their simple development and distinctive pathological changes, are prevalently utilized in DR research. Initially, alloxan was utilized to induce diabetes: this uric acid derivative selectively impairs pancreatic β-cells, and the death of β-cells leads to insulin release and subsequent hypoglycemia, with diabetes onset occurring within 24 h [64]. However, STZ has superseded alloxan in recent years due to its superior stability and rapid disease induction, thus becoming the gold-standard drug for diabetic research [65]. STZ acts mainly through the destruction of pancreatic islets and the ablation of islet β-cells in Langerhans [66]. Elevated blood glucose levels can be observed at one month after STZ injection, and this hyperglycemic state can be sustained for 22 to 24 months [67]. Early pathological changes, such as BRB disruption, thinning of the retinal inner nuclear layer and outer nuclear layer, reduction of neuronal cell numbers, and increased neuroglial cell apoptosis, appear approximately one month after STZ injection. Subsequent microvascular changes include increased permeability, neovascularization, and capillary basement membrane thickening [68,69]. Additionally, retinal dysfunction can be observed, such as increased retinal oxidative stress markers, pro-inflammatory factor levels, and pro-angiogenic markers [70–72]. In STZ-induced rat and mouse models, retinal morphological changes are almost identical; however, there are some differences in drug dose and disease progression [73].

4.2.2. Genetic Models

The *Ins2*^{Akita} mouse serves as a typical type 1 diabetes model. In this model, the *Insulin 2* gene is mutated, leading to a progressive loss of function in pancreatic islet β-cells. *Ins2*^{Akita} mice develop pronounced hyperglycemia by four weeks. By 12 weeks, DR manifests, characterized by increased vascular permeability and reactive microglia. At 22 weeks post-hyperglycemia onset, there is a decrease in the thickness of the inner plexiform and inner nuclear layers of the retina, accompanied by a reduction in the number of retinal ganglion cells [74].

The NOD mouse is another commonly used type 1 diabetes model, where pancreatic islet β-cells are destroyed by CD4+ and CD8+ T cells through an autoimmune response [75]. Hyperglycemia typically initiates at 12 weeks. Four weeks after the onset of hyperglycemia, increased cell apoptosis, vascular abnormalities, and elevated VEGF levels can be detected in NOD mice [76].

The *db/db* mouse model, which is a spontaneous mutant strain, is a typical type 2 DM model characterized by leptin receptor mutation, which induces obesity and hyperglycemia. Additionally, a decreased number of RGCs and an increased thickness of the central retina can be observed as early as 6 weeks, thus progressing to BRB disruption, pericyte loss, RGC apoptosis, glial cell activation, and increased levels of VEGF, oxidative stress markers, and pro-inflammatory cytokines by 15 months [77]. The *db/db* mouse model is considered a reliable model for studying diabetes-induced optic neuropathy and for exploring the potential capacities of therapeutic agents in DR [78].

The *ob/ob* mouse model serves as another typical type 2 diabetes model, characterized by a mutation in the gene encoding the obese protein, which leads to leptin deficiency. This deficiency prompts hepatic lipogenesis and gluconeogenesis, while hyperglycemia stimulates insulin secretion, creating a negative cycle of insulin resistance. Hyperglycemia is observed at three weeks, and electroretinography reveals early retinal function loss by six weeks. By 20 weeks, a significant reduction in retinal thickness and the number of nuclei in the inner retinal layer are noted. Compared to the *Ins2*^{Akita} and NOS models, DR onset occurs at approximately 8–12 weeks in the *ob/ob* mouse model, making it suitable for early DR research [79].

4.2.3. Diet-Induced Models

Diet-induced models typically involve feeding rodents a high-fat diet to induce insulin resistance. This induction may occur alone or in combination with STZ. Rodents are usually induced with STZ either at the onset of the high-fat diet or 2–8 weeks after feeding on the diet, which reduces the amount of STZ required and thus minimizes its damage to other tissues [80]. However, diet-induced models are usually characterized by a lengthy development time and high experimental costs.

4.2.4. Neovascularization Models

Retinal neovascularization is a major factor contributing to blindness in DR, and the establishment of related animal models is critical for studying the disease mechanism. The oxygen-induced retinopathy (OIR) model is the most commonly used animal model for investigating retinal neovascularization diseases. It offers the advantages of simple construction and high reproducibility.

In the OIR mouse model, mice and their lactating dams are placed in an environment of 75% ± 2% oxygen for five days, starting on day seven. Subsequently, the mice are returned to a standard oxygen environment with a concentration of 21% [81]. The rat model follows a similar protocol, and neovascularization is observed upon return to the normal oxygen environment [26]. The OIR model is characterized by two developmental phases: the immature vascular occlusion phase and the neovascularization pathologic proliferation phase.

Cell and animal experiment workflows are shown in Figure 3. It is well known that cell and animal models offer predictive insights into disease mechanisms and potential therapeutic benefits of drugs. However, due to the complexity and heterogeneity inherent in human pathophysiology, these models may not fully simulate disease progression within the human body [64]. Despite this limitation, such experimental models are foundational to clinical research, thus emphasizing the importance of selecting appropriate models for research. Moreover, the translation of these findings to clinical practice necessitates rigorous validation to confirm drug efficacy in patients.

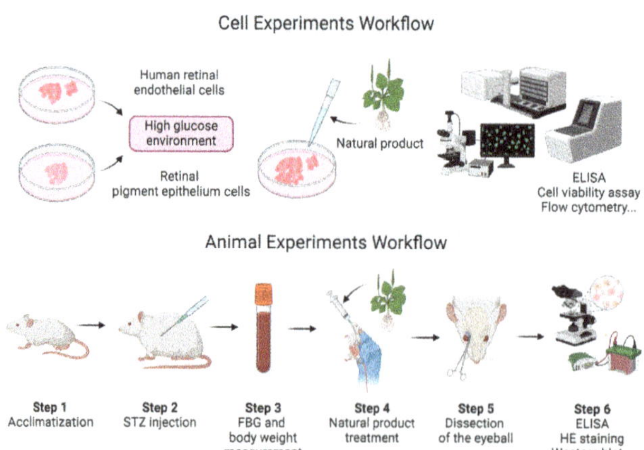

Figure 3. Workflow of cell and animal experiments. In vitro, cells are initially established in a high-glucose environment to simulate hyperglycemic conditions. Subsequently, cells are cultivated with natural product extracts. A series of experiments are then conducted to detect alterations in intracellular markers. In vivo, the experiment begins with the acclimatization of animals to a new environment. Following this, a calculated dose of streptozotocin (STZ) is administered. Throughout the experiment, fasting blood glucose (FBG) and body weight of animals are monitored. Oral treatment with natural product extracts is then administered over a period. Subsequently, the animals are euthanized, and the eyeballs are dissected. Finally, the therapeutic effects of natural products in diabetic retinopathy (DR) are validated through a series of experiments.

5. Natural Products in the Treatment of Diabetic Retinopathy

The use of NPs and their metabolites is expanding in the therapeutic management of various diseases. Currently, there is increasing interest in natural extracts as alternative treatment approaches for DR [82,83]. Each category of NPs is discussed separately with respect to their protective role in DR (Tables 1 and 2; Figures 4 and 5).

Table 1. Current research on the protective effects and mechanisms of natural products in DR.

Category	Compound Name	Natural Product	Cell/ Animal Model	Efficacy	Mechanism	References
Key Natural Products	Astragaloside-IV 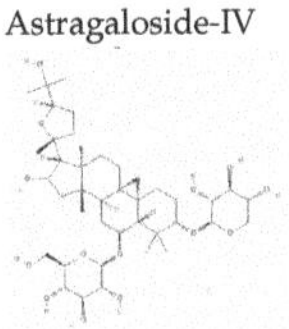	*Astragalus mambranaceus*	Human retinal pigment epithelium cells (ARPE-19 cells)/*db/db* mouse/STZ rats	1. Decreased the rate of ferroptosis by inhibiting expression of miR-138-5p 2. Decreased GSH content, mitochondria size, and ridge 3. Increased expression of glutathione peroxidase 4, glutamate cysteine ligase, and glutamate cysteine ligase catalytic subunit 4. Inhibited aldose reductase (AR) activation and the overexpression of NF-kB and ERK1/2 phosphorylation 5. Improved the amplitude in pattern electroretinogram and reduced apoptosis 6. Increased retinal thickness, alleviated DR-induced histopathological changes, and elevated blood glucose levels 7. Elevated DR-depressed protein levels of PI3K and AKT	1. miR-138-5p/ Sirt1/Nrf2 2. PI3K/Akt	[55,84,85]
	Resveratrol 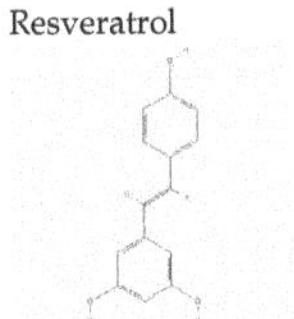	Grape, peanuts, berries	Rat retinal endothelial cells (RRECs)/STZ rats/STZ mice	1. Revocered the insulin level and PON1 expression and activity 2. Regulated retinal vascular permeability and mRNA expression of paraoxonase 1 (PON1), VEGF, bFGF, low-density lipoprotein (LDL), and high-density lipoprotein (HDL) 3. Inhibited retinal apoptosis by regulating Ox-LDL, caspase-3, and PON1 activity 4. Reduced inflammatory factors of IL-1β, IL-6, TNF-α, VEGF, Interferon-γ, and MCP-1 5. Mediated alterations in gene and protein expressions related to apoptosis 6. Enhanced SOD activity and reduced the 8-isoprostane level and GSSG/GSH ratio 7. Improved retinal layer disorganization and attenuated retinal thickness reduction 8. Blocked the increase in CaMKII and phosphor-CaMKII protein levels	1. PON1 2. NF-κB	[86–89]

Table 1. *Cont.*

Category	Compound Name	Natural Product	Cell/ Animal Model	Efficacy	Mechanism	References
Key Natural Products	Astaxanthin (ASX) 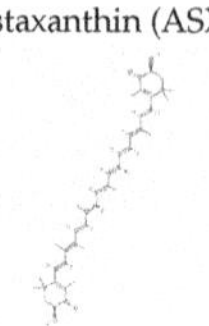	*Haematococcus pluvialis*, shrimps	STZ rats	1. Alleviated the decrease in retinal thickness and ganglion cell layer cell loss 2. Downregulated inflammatory factors of TNF-α, IL-1β, IL-6, MIC-1, and IL-10 3. Exerted antioxidant effects by regulating GSH, GPx, and total antioxidant capacity, malonic dialdehyde (MDA), and ROS levels 4. Fostered the expressions of HO-1 and NQO1 5. Exerted anti-apoptosis effects by regulating caspase-3, Bcl-2, and BAX expressions 6. Decreased the endothelial cell/pericyte ratio and the number of acellular capillaries	Nrf2/Keap 1	[40,90]
	Quercetin 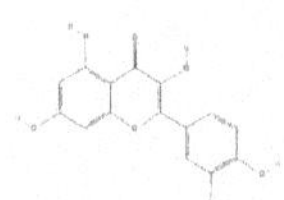	Licorice	STZ rats	1. Decreased the expression of BDNF, NGF, TrkB receptor, synaptophysin, and p-Akt 2. Attenuated apoptosis by decreasing caspase-3 and cytochrome c levels, and increasing Bcl-2 expression 3. Increased GSH levels 4. Decreased pro-inflammatory cytokines of TNF-α and IL-1β 5. Increased retinal thickness and cell count in the ganglion cell layer	BNDF/TrkB/Akt/ synaptophysin	[91,92]
	Berberine 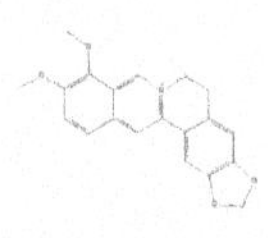	*Rhizoma Coptidis*	HRECs/STZ mice/STZ rats/*db/db* mice	1. Increased retinal layer thickness 2. Suppressed VEGF and HIF-1α expressions 3. Suppressed neovascularization 4. Reduced oxidative stress 5. Inhibited leukocyte-mediated killing of HRECs	1. Akt/mTOR/ HIF-1α/VEGF 2. NF-κB	[31,93,94]
Saponins	Asiaticoside 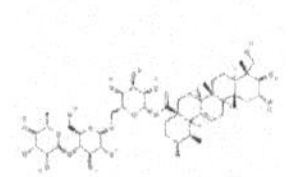	*Centella asiatica*	ARPE-19 cells	1. Restored the cell survival rate 2. Suppressed inflammation cytokines (TNF-α, IL-1β, and IL-6) 3. Regulated apoptosis levels (Bcl-2, Bax, caspase-3, and caspase-9) 4. Activated cAMP and PKA	cAMP/PKA	[95]
	Astragalin 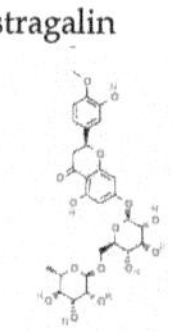	*Astragalus mambranaceus*	Rat retinal Müller cells	1. Decreased VEGF expression	VEGF	[96]

Table 1. *Cont.*

Category	Compound Name	Natural Product	Cell/ Animal Model	Efficacy	Mechanism	References
Phenols	Carnosol 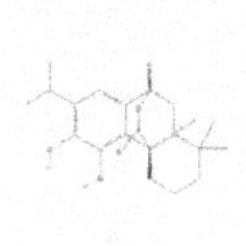	Rosemary	Human retinal endothelial cells (HRECs)	1. Increased cell viability and attenuated apoptosis 2. Induced HO-1 expression via Nrf2 activation	ERK1/2/Nrf2/ HO-1	[97]
	Magnolol 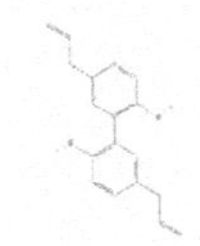	*Magoolia officinalis*	ARPE-19 cells	1. Prevented TGF-β1 and fibronectin expression 2. Inhibited ERK/MAPK/Akt activity	ERK/MAPK/Akt	[56]
Terpenoids	Nimbolide 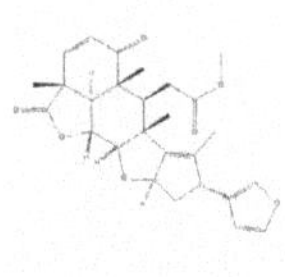	Neem plants	STZ rats	1. Suppressed inflammatory factors (TNF-α, IL-1β, and IL-6) 2. Suppressed MCP-1, VEGF, and MMP-9 levels 3. Improved antioxidant levels (SOD, GSH, SOD/CAT, and GSH/GSSG) 4. Suppressed TLR4 and NF-kB expressions	TLR4/NF-kB	[98]
	Arjunolic acid 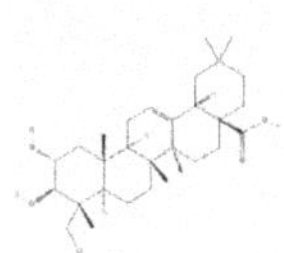	*Cyclocarya paliurus*	ARPE-19 cells/STZ rats	1. Prevented weight loss and increased the retinal thickness and nuclei counts 2. Inhibited oxidative stress, inflammation, and apoptosis 3. Upregulated the HO-1 protein level 4. Activated the AMPK/mTOR/HO-1/autophagy pathway	AMPK/ mTOR/HO-1/ autophagy	[37]
	Palbinone 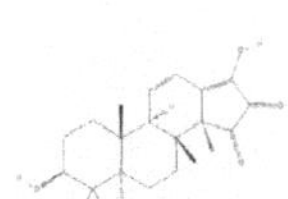	*Paeonia suffruticosa*	STZ rats	1. Improved morphometric and pathological changes of retina tissues 2. Enhanced antioxidant activities (SOD, catalase, and GPx) 3. Alleviated vascular permeability via inhibiting NLRP3 inflammasome formation 4. Reduced pro-inflammatory cytokines (IL-18, and IL-1β)	Nrf2/HO-1	[99]
	Andrographolide 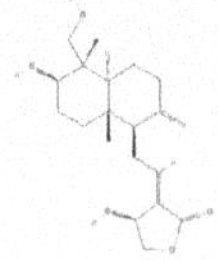	*Andrographis paniculate (Burm. F.) Nees*	STZ rats	1. Halted the sustained hyperglycemia and reversed the body weight and blood glucose level 2. Boosted cellular antioxidant defense by restoring the GSH level 3. Inhibited IDO and consequential changes in Kynurenine metabolites	-	[100]
	Glechomanamide B 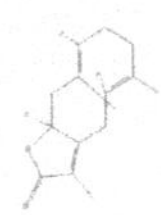	Salvia	Human microvascular endothelial cells (HMVECs)	1. Decreased the expressions of VEGF-R2, GLUT1, HK2, and ANGPT2 2. Inhibited tube formation induced by VEGF and BMP4	VEGF	[49]

Table 1. *Cont.*

Category	Compound Name	Natural Product	Cell/ Animal Model	Efficacy	Mechanism	References
Terpenoids	Tanshinone IIA 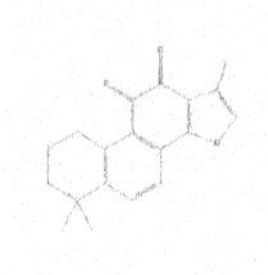	*Salvia miltiorrhiza* bunge	STZ rats	1. Exerted anti-inflammatory and antioxidation effects by regulating IL-1β, IL-6, TNF-α, SOD, GSH-PX, and MDA expressions 2. Regulated cell proliferation, apoptosis, and neovascularization	-	[101]
Flavonoids	Kaempferol 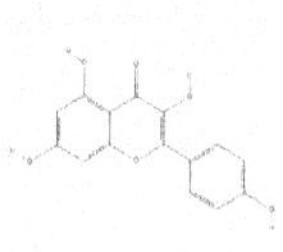	*Kaempferia galanga* L.	Retinal ganglion cells (RGCs)/HRECs	1. Attenuated apoptosis, caspase-3 activity, and LDH leakage 2. Promoted cell viability and decreased ROS levels 3. Inhibited cell proliferation, migration, and tube formation 4. Suppressed the expression of VEGF and PGF 5. Suppressed PI3L expression and ERK1/2, Src, and Akt1 activation	1. ERK/VASH1 2. Src/Akt1/ ERK1/2	[102,103]
	Tilianin 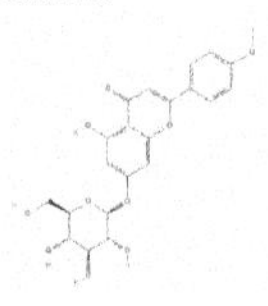	*Traversia baccharoides Hook.f.*	STZ rats	1. Reduced fasting glucose status, HbA1c levels, and augmented serum insulin status 2. Increased Nrf2 and HO-1 expressions and decreased MDA levels 3. Increased SOD, CAT, and GPx levels 4. Decreased expression of TXNIP, NLRP3, ASC, caspase-1, and IL-1β 5. Ameliorated retinal morphological and morphometric changes	Nrf2/TXNIP/ NLRP3	[104]
	Chrysin 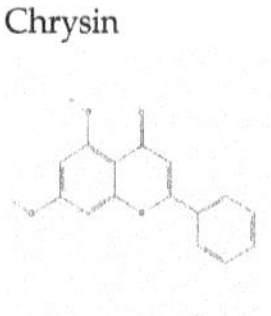	*Oroxylum indicum (Linn.) Bentham ex Kurz*	Choroid endothelial cells (RF/6A cells)	1. Inhibited cell migration via inhibiting AKT and ERK phosphorylation 2. Decreased MMP-2 expression 3. Inhibited HIF-1α and VEGF expressions	VEGF	[50]
	Morin 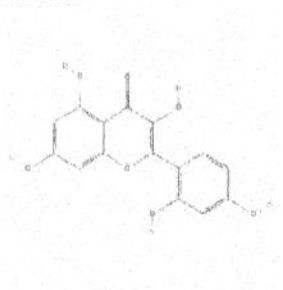	Moraceae family plants	STZ rats	1. Decreased blood glucose levels 2. Improved endogenous antioxidant enzymes' activity (GPx, CAT, and SOD) 3. Reduced TNF-α, IL-β, and VEGF expressions 4. Increased retina thickness and cell count in the ganglion cell layer	-	[105]
	Gambogic acid 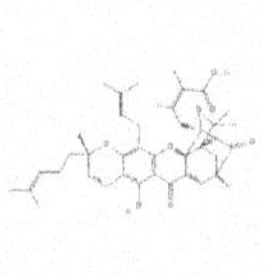	Gamboges resin	RF/6A cells/STZ mice	1. Suppressed cell proliferation, migration, and tube formation 2. Decreased HIF-1α and VEGF expressions 3. Attenuated retinal neovascularization	1. HIF-1α/VEGF 2. PI3K/Akt	[51]

Table 1. *Cont.*

Category	Compound Name	Natural Product	Cell/ Animal Model	Efficacy	Mechanism	References
Flavonoids	7,8-Dihydroxyflavone 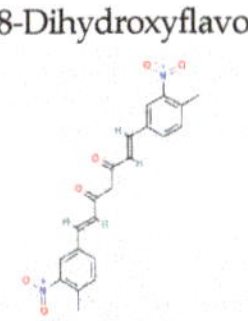	Citrus, grains, tea	ARPE-19 cells	1. Ameliorated apoptosis by inhibiting caspase-9 activity and phosphorylating TrkB protein	TrkB	[106]
	Nobiletin 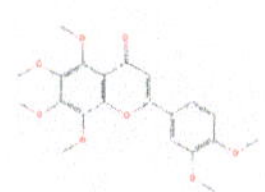	Citrus plants	Human retinal Müller cells (MIO-M1 cells)	1. Attenuated MMP-9 enzymatic activity 2. Regulated MMP-9 and tissue inhibitor of metalloproteinase-1 expression	PI3K/Akt	[107]
	Isoflavones 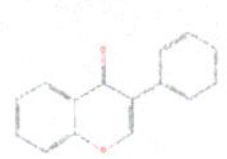	*Caesalpinia pulcherrima*	STZ rats	1. Inhibited AR activity 2. Decreased thiobarbituric acid-reactive substances and protein carbonyl levels 3. Restored GSH levels 4. Increased antioxidant enzymes' activities (SOD, GPx, and catalase)	-	[108]
	Epicatechin 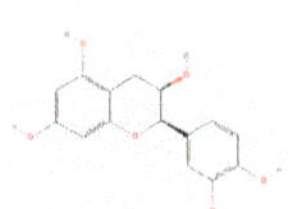	Green tea, coconut	AGE-injected rats/glycated bovine serum albumin	1. Reduced AGEs accumulation 2. Inhibited retinal apoptosis	-	[109]
Saccharides	Fucoidan 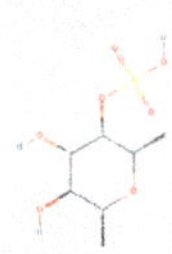	Brown algae	ARPE-19 cells/brain microvascular endothelial cells/STZ mice	1. Inhibited apoptosis and ROS generation 2. Inhibited high-glucose-mediated Ca^{2+} influx 3. Inhibited ERK phosphorylation 4. Inhibited cell proliferation, angiogenic vessels, and VEGF expression 5. Inhibited HIF-1α expression	1. Ca^{2+}-dependent ERK 2. HIF-1α/VEGF	[110,111]
Quinones	Aloe-emodin 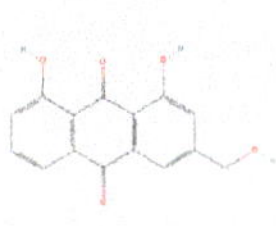	Radix et Rhizoma Rhei	ARPE-19 cells/ OIR rats	1. Inhibited the secretion of VEGFA in the ARPE-19 cells under hypoxia conditions 2. Decreased the mRNA and protein expressions of VEGFA and PHD-2 in the ARPE-19 cells 3. Inhibited hypoxia-induced retinal neovascularization in vivo	HIF-a/VEGF	[112]

Table 1. *Cont.*

Category	Compound Name	Natural Product	Cell/ Animal Model	Efficacy	Mechanism	References
Steroids	Diosgenin 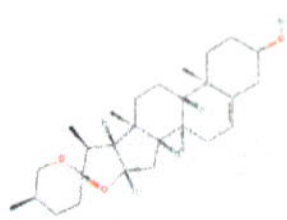	Fenugreek seeds, Wild yam roots	ARPE-19 cells/ *db/db* mice	1. Increased the viability of ARPE-19 cells 2. Inhibited apoptosis of ARPE-19 cells 3. Reduced the inflammatory response and oxidative stress of ARPE-19 cells 4. Activated the AMPK/Nrf2/HO-1 pathway 5. Increased HDL levels and decreased LDL levels 6. Improved the thickness of the retinal layer 7. Decreased retinal cell apoptosis	AMPK/Nrf2/ HO-1	[113,114]
Multiple Bioactive Agents	Ginsenoside Rg1, Ginsenoside Rb1 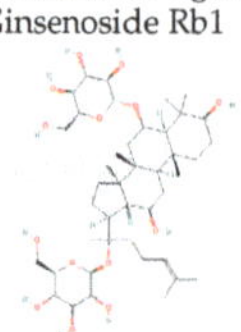 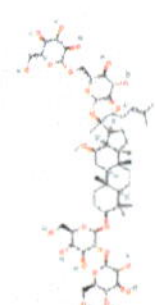	*Panax notoginseng sponins*	MIO-M1 cells/STZ rats	1. Increased retinal inner nuclear layer thickness, reduced acellular capillaries, and attenuated BRB disruption by upregulated claudin-1 and occluding 2. Abrogated microglial cell activation, and reversed leukocyte adhesion by downregulated intercellular molecule-1 and vascular cell adhesion molecule-1 3. Reduced pro-inflammatory factors (TNF-α, IL-6, and IL-1β), and inhibited expressions of p-IKK, p-IκB, p-p65, and nuclear translocation of p65	NF-κB	[14]
	60% Edible ethanolic extract of U. davidiana, catechin 7-O-β-D-apiofuranoside 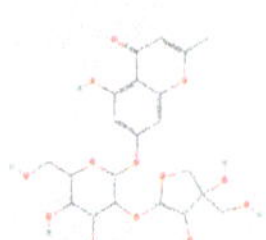	*Ulmus dacidiana*	Human placental pericytes/ HMVECs	1. Prevented pericyte apoptosis by blocking the activities of p38 and JNK 2. Increased ZO-1 expression and reduced endothelial permeability by preventing pericyte apoptosis	-	[115]

Table 2. Protective effects of natural products in the treatment of DR.

Target	Effects	Compound Name	Natural Product	Category	Reference
Inflammation	Reduced inflammatory factors (IL-1β, IL-6, TNF-α, Interferon-γ, and MCP-1)	Resveratrol	Grape, peanuts, berries	Phenols	[86–89]
	1. Downregulated inflammatory factors (TNF-α, IL-1β, IL-6, MIC-1, and IL-10) 2. Downregulated NF- kB level	Astaxanthin	*Haematococcus pluvialis*, shrimps	Terpenoids	[40,90]
	Suppressed inflammatory cytokines (TNF-α and IL-1β)	Quercetin	Licorice	Flavonoids	[91,92]
	Suppressed inflammatory cytokines (TNF-α, IL-1β, and IL-6)	Asiaticoside	*Centella asiatica*	Saponins	[95]
	1. Suppressed inflammatory factors (TNF-α, IL-1β, and IL-6) 2. Suppressed TLR4 and NF-kB expressions	Nimbolide	Neem plants	Terpenoids	[98]

Table 2. *Cont.*

Target	Effects	Compound Name	Natural Product	Category	Reference
Inflammation	Suppressed inflammatory cytokines (TNF-α, IL-1β, and IL-6)	Argunolic acid	*Cyclocarya paliurus*	Terpenoids	[37]
	1. Reduced pro-inflammatory cytokines (IL-18 and IL-1β) 2. Inhibited NLRP3 inflammasome formation	Palbinone	*Paeonia suffruticosa*	Terpenoids	[99]
	Suppressed inflammatory cytokines (TNF-α, IL-1β, and IL-6)	Tanshinone IIA	*Salvia miltiorrhiza* bunge	Terpenoids	[101]
	Downregulated the expression of inflammasome components (NLRP3 and ASC) along with their downstream targets (caspase-1 and IL-1β)	Tilianin	*Traversia baccharoides Hook.f.*	Flavonoids	[104]
	Suppressed inflammatory cytokines (TNF-α and IL-1β)	Morin	Moraceae family plants	Flavonoids	[105]
	1. Suppressed inflammatory cytokines (TNF-α, IL-1β, and IL-6) 2. Downregulated the expressions of COX-2 and p65	Diosgenin	Fenugreek seeds, wild yam roots	Steroids	[113,114]
	1. Suppressed pro-inflammatory factors (TNF-α, IL-6, and IL-1β) 2. Inhibited the activation of the NF-kB signaling pathway	Ginsenoside Rg1, Ginsenoside Rb1	*Panax notoginseng sponins*	-	[14]
Neovascularization/ VEGF	1. Suppressed VEGF and HIF-1α expressions 2. Suppressed neovascularization by inactivation of cell proliferation and migration	Berberine	*Rhizoma Coptidis*	Alkaloids	[31,93,94]
	Reduced VEGF expression	Astragalin	*Astragalus mambranaceus*	Saponins	[96]
	Inhibited tube formation induced by VEGFR2 and BMP4	Glechomanamides B	Salvia	Terpenoids	[49]
	Reduced VEGF expression	Tanshinone IIA	*Salvia miltiorrhiza* bunge	Terpenoids	[101]
	1. Inhibited cell proliferation, migration, and tube formation 2. Suppressed the expressions of VEGF and PGF	Kaempferol	*Kaempferia galanga* L.	Flavonoids	[102,103]
	1. Inhibited cell migration 2. Inhibited HIF-1α and VEGF expressions	Chrysin	*Oroxylum indicum (Linn.) Bentham ex Kurz*	Flavonoids	[50]
	1. Suppressed cell proliferation, migration, and tube formation 2. Inhibited HIF-1α and VEGF expressions 3. Decreased angiogenesis-related expressions of FGF2 and PAI-1	Gambogic acid	Gamboges resin	Flavonoids	[51]
	1. Inhibited cell proliferation 2. Inhibited HIF-1α and VEGF expressions	Fucoidan	Brown algae	Saccharides	[110,111]
	1. Inhibited the secretion of VEGFA 2. Decreased the mRNA expressions of VEGFA and PHD-2 3. Inhibited hypoxia-induced retinal neovascularization	Aloe-emodin	Radix et Rhizoma Rhei	Quinones	[112]
Oxidative stress	Reduced lipid peroxidation level and ROS content	Astragaloside-IV	*Astragalus mambranaceus*	Saponins	[55,84,85]
	1. Enhanced SOD activity and reduced the 8-isoprostane level and GSSG/GSH ratio in both blood and retina tissue 2. Decreased oxidative stress marker 4-HNE	Resveratrol	Grape, peanuts, berries	Phenols	[86–89]

Table 2. *Cont.*

Target	Effects	Compound Name	Natural Product	Category	Reference
Oxidative stress	1. Regulated GSH, GPx, MDA, and ROS levels 2. Fostered the expressions of HO-1, NQO1, and IL-10 and restrained the expression of NF-kB	Astaxanthin	*Haematococcus pluvialis*, shrimps	Terpenoids	[40,90]
	Increased GSH and antioxidant enzymes' activities (SOD and CAT)	Quercetin	Licorice	Flavonoids	[91,92]
	Reduced oxidative stress	Berberine	*Rhizoma Coptidis*	Alkaloids	[31,93,94]
	1. Decreased ROS production 2. Increased HO-1 activity	Carnosol	Rosemary	Phenols	[97]
	Decreased MDA and lipid peroxidation levels	Magnolol	*Magoolia officinalis*	Phenols	[56]
	Improved antioxidants' status by regulating SOD, GSH, SOD/CAT ratio, and GSH/GSSG ratio	Nimbolide	Neem plants	Terpenoids	[98]
	1. Upregulated the HO-1 protein level 2. Downregulated ROS and MDA levels	Argunolic acid	*Cyclocarya paliurus*	Terpenoids	[37]
	1. Enhanced antioxidant activities (SOD, CAT, and GPx) 2. Enhanced the HO-1 expression	Palbinone	*Paeonia suffruticosa*	Terpenoids	[99]
	1. Restored the GSH level 2. Inhibited IDO and consequential changes in Kynurenine metabolites	Andrographolide	*Andrographis paniculate (Burm. F.) Nees*	Terpenoids	[100]
	Decreased ROS levels	Kaempferol	*Hippophae rhamnoides* L.	Flavonoids	[102,103]
	1. Increased Nrf2 and HO-1 expressions and decreased MDA levels 2. Increased SOD, CAT, and GPX levels and decreased MDA levels	Tilianin	*Traversia baccharoides Hook.f.*	Flavonoids	[104]
	1. Improved endogenous antioxidant enzymes' activity (GPx, CAT, and SOD) 2. Decreased lipid peroxidase levels	Morin	Moraceae family plants	Flavonoids	[105]
	1. Restored GSH activity 2. Decreased thiobarbituric acid-reactive substances and protein carbonyl levels 3. Inhibited AR activity 4. Increased antioxidant enzymes' activities (SOD, GPx, and CAT)	Isoflavones	*Caesalpinia pulcherrima*	Flavonoids	[108]
	Inhibited ROS generation through Ca^{2+}-dependent ERK1/2 signaling pathway	Fucoidan	Brown algae	Saccharides	[110,111]
	Increased SOD and GPX levels and decreased MDA levels	Diosgenin	Fenugreek seeds, wild yam roots	Steroids	[112]
Apoptosis	Decreased cell apoptosis	Astragaloside-IV	*Astragalus mambranaceus*	Saponins	[55,84,85]
	1. Mediated alternations in gene and protein expressions related to apoptosis (p53, Bax, Bcl-2, caspase-3, caspase-9, p38aMAPK, c-Jun N-terminal kinase-1, and extracellular signal-regulated kinase-1) 2. Blocked the increase in CaMKII and phosphor-CaMKII protein levels	Resveratrol	Grape, peanuts, berries	Phenol	[86–89]
	1. Inhibited retinal pericytes apoptosis 2. Regulated apoptosis-related proteins (Bcl-2, BAX, and caspase-3)	Astaxanthin	*Haematococcus pluvialis*, shrimps	Terpenoids	[40,90]

Table 2. *Cont.*

Target	Effects	Compound Name	Natural Product	Category	Reference
Apoptosis	1. Attenuated apoptosis by decreasing caspase-3 and cytochrome c levels, and increasing Bcl-2 expression 2. Decreased the expression of BDNF, NGF, TrkB receptor, synaptophysin, and p-Akt 3. Suppressed NF-kB activity	Quercetin	Licorice	Flavonoids	[91,92]
	regulated apoptosis-related proteins (Bcl-2, Bax, caspase-3, and caspase-9)	Asiaticoside	*Centella asiatica*	Saponins	[95]
	Attenuated cell apoptosis and caspase-3 activity	Kaempferol	*Kaempferia galanga* L.	Flavonoids	[102,103]
	Ameliorated apoptosis by inhibiting caspase-9 activity	7,8-Dihydroxyflavone	Citrus, grains, tea	Flavonoids	[106]
	Inhibited retinal cell apoptosis	Epicatechin	Green tea, coconut	Flavonoids	[109]
	1. Suppressed cell apoptosis 2. Regulated apoptosis-related proteins (Bcl-2, BAX, and caspase-3)	Diosgenin	Fenugreek seeds, wild yam roots	Steroids	[113,114]
	1. Prevented pericyte apoptosis by blocking the activities of p38 and JNK 2. Prevented apoptosis-associated protein (capsase-3)	U60E, C7A	*Ulmus dacidiana*	-	[115]
Ferroptosis	Decreased the rate of ferroptosis by inhibiting the expression of miR-138-5p	Astragaloside-IV	*Astragalus mambranaceus*	Saponins	[55,84,85]
Cell phosphorylation	Regulated ERK1/2 phosphorylation	Astragaloside-IV	*Astragalus mambranaceus*	Saponins	[55,84,85]
	Regulated ERK1/2 phosphorylation	Kaempferol	*Kaempferia galanga* L.	Flavonoids	[102,103]
	Regulated AKT and ERK phosphorylation	Chrysin	*Oroxylum indicum (Linn.) Bentham ex Kurz*	Flavonoids	[50]
AGEs accumulation	Decreased AGEs production	Resveratrol	Grape, peanuts, berries	Phenols	[86–89]
	Decreased AGEs production	Astaxanthin	*Haematococcus pluvialis*, shrimps	Terpenoids	[40,90]
	Reduced AGEs burden	Epicatechin	Green tea	Flavonoids	[109]
MMP	Decreased MMP-2 expression	Chrysin	*Oroxylum indicum (Linn.) Bentham ex Kurz*	Flavonoids	[50]
	Attenuated MMP-9 enzymatic activity	Nobiletin	Citrus plants	Flavonoids	[107]
Autophagy	Activated the AMPK/mTOR/HO-1-regulated autophagy pathway	Arjunolic acid	*Cyclocarya paliurus*	Terpenoids	[37]
Leukocyte adhesion	Inhibited leukocyte adhesion and decreased ICAM-1 expression	Berberine	*Rhizoma Coptidis*	Alkaloids	[31,93,94]
	Downregulated the protein expression of ICAM-1 and VCAM-1	Ginsenoside Rg1, Ginsenoside Rb1	*Panax notoginseng sponins*	-	[14]

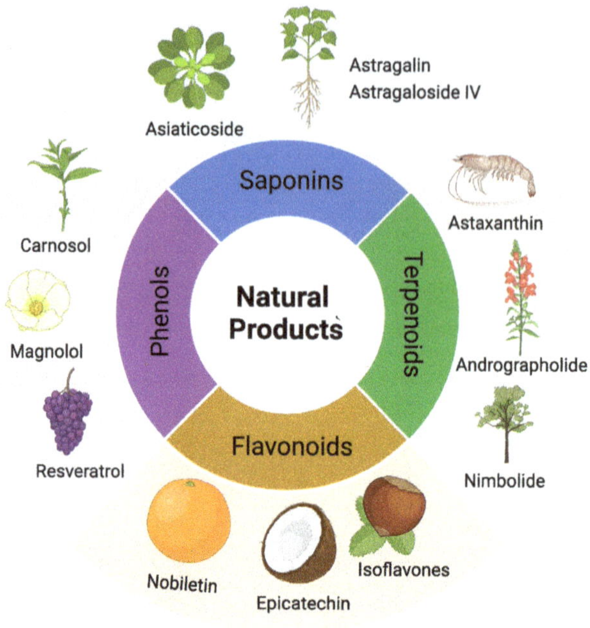

Figure 4. Classifications and natural sources of natural products.

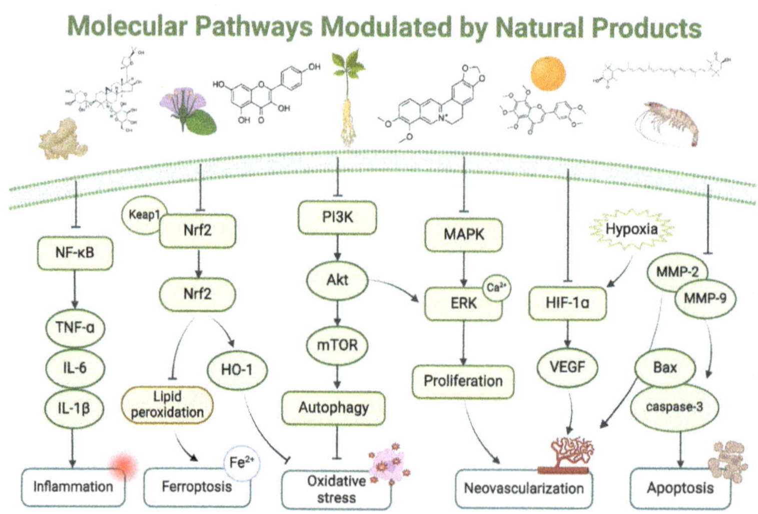

Figure 5. Molecular pathways modulated by natural products in diabetic retinopathy. Various natural products play regulatory roles in inflammation, ferroptosis, oxidative stress, neovascularization, and apoptosis-related signaling pathways in diabetic retinopathy. Abbreviations: NF-κB, nuclear factor kappa-B; TNF-α, tumor necrosis factor-alpha; IL-6, interleukin 6; Keap1, Kelch-like ECH-associated protein 1; Nrf2, nuclear factor erythroid-2-related factor 2; HO-1, heme oxygenase-1; PI3K, phosphoinositide 3-kinase; mTOR, mammalian target of rapamycin; MAPK, mitogen-activated protein kinases; ERK, extracellular signal-regulated kinase; HIF-1α, hypoxia-inducible factor-1 alpha; VEGF, vascular endothelial growth factor; MMP 2, matrix metalloproteinase 2.

5.1. Key Natural Products in DR Treatment

5.1.1. Astragaloside-IV

Astragaloside-IV (AS-IV) is the main bioactive agent of *Astragalus membranaceus* and has excellent antioxidant capacity. Tang et al. [55] found that high-glucose conditions promoted ferroptosis in RPE cells. Moreover, AS-IV inhibited miR-138-5p expression, augmented Sirt1/Nrf2 pathway activity, and enhanced cellular antioxidant defense, thus leading to a reduction in ferroptosis in RPE cells. Ting et al. [84] noted that AS-IV significantly repressed aldose reductase (AR) activation, NF-κB overexpression, and ERK1/2 phosphorylation in a *db/db* mouse model, thus exerting anti-inflammatory and neuroprotective effects. Additionally, AS-IV was found to decrease apoptosis and dysfunction in RGCs. Zhao et al. [85] reported that AS-IV administration increased retinal thickness, alleviated DR-induced histopathological changes, and moderated elevated blood glucose levels in diabetic rats. AS-IV may exert an anti-inflammatory effect through the PI3K/AKT pathway.

5.1.2. Resveratrol

Resveratrol is a polyphenolic compound that has been shown to have favorable ROS-scavenging efficacy across multiple pathways. In age-related macular degeneration, some studies have demonstrated that resveratrol has a beneficial impact on the retina [116,117]. In the STZ-induced diabetic rat model, resveratrol diminished the inflammatory response and retinal damage through the PON1 pathway, thus elevating PON1 expression while reducing Ox-DLD, advanced glycosylated end products (AGEs), and inflammatory factors (IL-1β, IL-6, TNF-α, Interferon-γ, MCP-1, and VEGF). Additionally, resveratrol reduced caspase-3 activity and Ox-LDL expression in rat retinal endothelial cells [86]. Hussaini found that resveratrol regulated the expression of multiple genes and proteins related to apoptotic pathways in RPE cells. It was observed that the transcript levels of the pro-apoptotic genes, *tumor suppressor protein 53 (p53)*, *BAX*, *caspase-3*, and *caspase-9*, and the anti-apoptotic gene *Bcl-2*, were increased, which consequently led to G2/M arrest and thus reduced apoptosis. Therefore, one of the protective pathways of resveratrol against diabetes-induced damage in RPE cells was through the inhibition of endogenous apoptotic pathway-related proteins [87]. Soufi found that long-term treatment with resveratrol reduced hyperglycemia and HbA1c levels, while improving energy metabolism and attenuating weight loss. Additionally, four months of oral resveratrol treatment decreased retinal oxidative stress and NF-κB activity, thereby reducing apoptosis rates in the retina of diabetic rats [88]. Ca^{2+}/calmodulin-dependent protein kinase II (CaMKII), a serine-threonine protein kinase involved in neuronal cell death, was also found to be effectively inhibited by resveratrol, which prevented diabetes-induced apoptosis and upregulated CaMKII expression in RGCs. Kim et al. hypothesized that resveratrol may modulate CaMKII expression by interfering with calcium- and voltage-gated calcium channel-regulated processes, ultimately exerting neuroprotective effects in DR [89]. Furthermore, some clinical trials have shown that resveratrol is well tolerated, has relatively few side effects, and there is no clear evidence of serious adverse events directly attributable to resveratrol [118]. In conclusion, resveratrol may be a promising drug for the treatment of DR.

5.1.3. Astaxanthin

Astaxanthin (ASX), which is a natural compound prevalent in a variety of plants and animals, is known for its anticancer and antioxidant functions. In the STZ-induced diabetic rat model, ASX increased retinal thickness and ganglion cell numbers. Furthermore, ASX suppressed Keap1 expression, facilitated Nrf2 translocation into the nucleus, and enhanced the expression of heme oxygenase-1 (HO-1), quinone oxidoreductase 1 (NQO1), γ-glutamylcysteine synthetase, and glutathione (GSH) peroxidase (GPx) [40]. Additionally, ASX mitigated DR-related damage by decreasing AGEs production and reducing pericyte apoptosis and inflammation. Although ASX did not lower elevated blood glucose levels in a rat model, its anti-inflammatory, antioxidant, and antiapoptotic effects also contributed to attenuating DR pathology [90].

5.1.4. Quercetin

Quercetin is a major representative of the flavonoid family that can be found in various vegetables and fruits. Quercetin plays an important role in treating numerous diseases by exerting anti-inflammatory, antioxidant, anti-neovascular, and neuroprotective effects [119–121]. In diabetic rats, quercetin supplementation increased neurotrophic factors and inhibited cytochrome c and caspase-3, thereby protecting the retina from oxidative stress and apoptosis. Hence, quercetin was deemed to protect retinal neurons against DR via the BDNF/TrkB/Akt/synaptophysin pathway [91]. Additionally, quercetin modulated the activities of SOD and CAT, increased GSH levels, and prevented the release of TNF-α and IL-1β, thus suppressing NF-kB and caspase-3 activity. It also prevents retinal edema by inhibiting glial fibrillary acidic protein and aquaporin-4 elevation [92].

5.1.5. Berberine

Berberine (BBR), which is a bioactive alkaloid isolated from the traditional Chinese medicine *Rhizoma Coptidis* [122], is known for its extensive medical value, including its anticancer, antiviral, and antibacterial effects [123,124]. Insulin injection is one of the most important treatment modalities for patients with type 1 DM and advanced type 2 DM. However, some studies have shown that insulin treatment may accelerate the progression of DR [125]. Wang et al. [31] reported on the role of BBR in suppressing DR progression in insulin-treated type 1 and type 2 diabetic mice. Insulin treatment activated retinal endothelial cells, which led to increased expressions of HIF-1α and VEGF, whereas BBR reversed these effects by inhibiting the Akt/mTOR signaling pathway. BBR improved retinopathy and reduced neovascularization and neuronal injury, thus complementing the effect of insulin therapy. Tian et al. [93] found that BBR attenuated interleukin-induced damage to retinal endothelial cells and suppressed the expression of inflammatory and oxidative stress markers under hyperglycemic conditions, which is likely partially through inhibition of the NF-κB signaling pathway. To further investigate the core mechanism by which BBR ameliorates DR, Na et al. [94] used four-dimensional independent data acquisition proteomics combined with bioinformatics analysis and experimental validation. These approaches further confirmed the therapeutic potential of BBR and highlighted its regulatory influence on molecular networks, particularly considering the significance of carbonic anhydrase 1.

5.2. Other Potential Natural Products in DR Treatment

5.2.1. Saponins

Asiaticoside, which is a major active compound isolated from *Centella asiatica*, is known for its anxiolytic, scar healing, analgesic, antibacterial, anti-inflammatory, and antioxidant effects [126,127]. In high-glucose-cultured RPE cells, asiaticoside reduced the levels of inflammatory cytokines, including TNF-α, IL-6, and IL-1β, and reversed the upregulated expression of apoptosis-related proteins. Moreover, the protective effects of asiaticoside were abolished when the cAMP inhibitor SQ22536 was introduced. Consequently, asiaticoside may ameliorate the inflammatory response and apoptosis in DR by activating the cAMP/PKA signaling pathway [95].

Astragalin is another bioactive compound that is produced by *Astragalus membranaceus* and has beneficial effects on hyperglycemia [128–130]. In Müller cells, astragalin significantly reduced VEGF expression, thereby diminishing retinal neovascularization [96].

5.2.2. Phenols

Carnosol, which is a phenolic extract from the herb rosemary, is known for its antioxidant properties. In HRECs cultured under high-glucose conditions, carnosol at concentrations of 10 μM or 20 μM facilitated cellular rejuvenation. It also attenuated cell apoptosis and ROS accumulation. Consequently, carnosol activated Nrf2/HO-1 signaling via the modulation of the ERK1/2 pathway, thereby mitigating high-glucose-induced damage in HRECs [97].

Magnolol, which is extracted from Magnolia officinalis, has potent anti-inflammatory, antioxidative, and anticancer effects [131–133]. In high-glucose- or S100b-induced (a specific receptor for AGEs ligand) RPE cells, magnolol inhibited the ERK/MAPK/Akt signaling pathway, thereby preventing the upregulated expression of transforming growth factor-β1 (TGF-β1) and fibronectin. It also curtailed lipid peroxidation triggered by S100b, thus decelerating the pathologic development of DR [56].

5.2.3. Terpenoids

Nimbolide, which is a terpenoid found in neem plants, has been reported to be advantageous for cancer therapy [134,135]. This research demonstrated that nimbolide decreased inflammatory markers, alleviated oxidative stress, enhanced antioxidant defenses, and suppressed the TLR4/NF-κB pathway in diabetic rats. Moreover, its effect was similar to that of metformin, thus demonstrating its potential as a complementary DR therapy [98].

Cyclocarya paliurus is a traditional Chinese herbal medicine, and arjunolic acid (AA) is the major active compound that has significant protective effects against a variety of metabolic diseases. AA attenuated weight loss and increased retinal thickness and nucleus numbers in diabetic rats. Moreover, the protein expression of HO-1 was upregulated. In addition, AA modulated autophagy via the AMPK/mTOR pathway, thereby attenuating retinal cell damage and apoptosis. This study demonstrated that AA could treat DR by attenuating retinal cell damage and reducing oxidative stress, inflammation, and apoptosis through the AMPK/mTOR/HO-1/autophagy pathway [37].

Palbinone (PB), which is a triterpenoid isolated from *Paeonia suffruticosa*, decreased the levels of pro-inflammatory cytokines (IL-18 and IL-1β) and enhanced the activities of antioxidant enzymes, including superoxide dismutase (SOD), catalase (CAT), and GSH peroxidase (GPx) in STZ-induced diabetic rats. Furthermore, PB activated the Nrf2 pathway, elevated HO-1 expression, and inhibited NLRP3 inflammasome formation, thereby attenuating retinal inflammation and oxidative stress in DR [99].

The natural compound andrographolide is derived from the medicinal herb *Andrographis paniculate Nees*. Overproduction of indoleamine 2,3-dioxygenase (IDO), which is a pivotal enzyme in the kynurenine pathway, leads to oxidative stress in DR [136]. Andrographolide notably curbed IDO production and consequential changes in kynurenine metabolites, thereby attenuating the oxidative stress level in DR. In addition, it reduced oxidative stress markers, thus suggesting that it is a promising antioxidative therapeutic agent [100].

Wang et al. [49] isolated six compounds from Salvia and elucidated their structures via spectroscopy and X-ray diffraction. In particular, glechomanamide B hindered VEGF-induced tube formation in HUVECs by affecting the VEGF2 signaling pathway, thus potentially inhibiting DR-related neovascularization.

Tanshinone IIA is sourced from the traditional Chinese herb *Salvia miltiorrhiza* and is known to have cardiovascular benefits [137,138]. In recent years, tanshinone IIA has been found to have specific effects on DR. The molecular mechanism, pharmacodynamic target, and protein interaction network of tanshinone IIA were analyzed by using integrated pharmacology and verified by animal experiments. Tanshinone IIA restored the retinal structure of the rats, decreased the mRNA expressions of VEGF, IL-1β, IL-6, TNF-α, and caspase-3, and modulated the protein expression of Bcl-2, Bax, and VEGFA. These results suggested that tanshinone IIA could alleviate hyperglycemia-induced retinal damage, thus offering anti-inflammatory and antiangiogenic benefits in DR [101].

5.2.4. Flavonoids

Flavonoids are heterocyclic compounds that can be widely found in various vegetables and fruits, such as tomatoes, grapes, and nuts. Flavonoids are known for their significant antioxidant properties, which can potentially mitigate oxidative stress and neurodegeneration in DR [83].

Kaempferol is a medicinal flavonol that can be found in numerous fruits and vegetables. It has been shown to inhibit lactate dehydrogenase release, apoptosis, caspase-3 activity, and ROS levels in RGCs. Moreover, kaempferol potentially protected RGCs from retinopathy induced by high glucose by modulating the ERK/VASH1 signaling pathway [102]. In HRECs cultured under high-glucose conditions, kaempferol decreased VEGF and placental growth factor (PGF) levels and inhibited cell proliferation and migration. Kaempferol may inhibit the Src/Akt1/Erk1/2 signaling pathway, thus decreasing retinal neovascularization [103].

Tilianin (TN) is a natural polyphenolic flavonoid. Oral administration of TN to diabetic rats markedly decreased their food consumption, blood glucose level, and serum insulin status. TN increased the expression of nuclear factor erythroid-2-related factor 2 (Nrf2) and its target gene HO-1, while decreasing thioredoxin-interacting protein (TXNIP), NOD-like receptor protein 3 (NLRP3), apoptosis-associated speck-like protein containing a CARD, caspase-1, and IL-1β protein levels. TN thereby manifests potent antioxidant and anti-inflammatory effects in DR, potentially by modulating the Nrf2/TXNIP/NLRP3 inflammasome pathways [104].

Chrysin is a member of the flavonoid family, and the structure of chrysin can modulate the immune system [139]. In addition, chrysin notably decreased the phosphorylation of AKT, ERK, and MMP-2 in RF/6A cells cultured in a high-glucose environment, thus reducing the influence of VEGF and its receptor VEGFR, and thereby curbing RE/6A cell migration [50].

Morin is a dietary bioflavonoid from the Moraceae family of plants. Moreover, morin has been shown to reduce lipid peroxidase activity and enhance the levels of endogenous antioxidants (GPx, CAT, and SOD) in the retina. Further, morin can decrease the concentrations of TNF-α, IL-1β, and VEGF, and contribute to increases in retinal thickness and ganglion cell numbers. Thus, morin may attenuate retinal damage by exerting antioxidant effects in STZ-induced diabetic rat models [105].

Gambogic acid (GA) is a flavonoid natural product extracted from the traditional Chinese medicine gamboges resin. GA can suppress proliferation, migration, and tube formation in high-glucose-cultured RF/6A cells. GA can also ameliorate retinal morphology in diabetic mice by suppressing neovascularization via the inhibition of HIF-1α and VEGF. Furthermore, the PI3K/AKT signaling pathway has been implicated in the inhibitory effects of GA on DR [51].

DHF (7,8-dihydroxyflavone) is a natural extract from non-mammalian animals or plants, such as citrus plants, grains, tea, vegetables, and fruits. In high-glucose-injured RPE cells, DHF significantly reduced the expression of the apoptotic factor caspase-9 at both the RNA and protein levels. DHF also attenuated apoptosis by activating the TrkB signaling pathway, whereas the TrkB antagonist K252a inhibited the protective effect of DHF by dephosphorylating TrkB signaling [106].

Nobiletin is the major polymethoxylated flavone isolated from citrus fruits. Matrix metalloproteinases (MMPs) play a promoting role in the development of PDR; however, the clinical application of many MMP inhibitors is restricted due to their non-specificity, low bioavailability, and adverse effects. This study demonstrated that nobiletin can reduce the enzymatic activity of MMP-9 by inhibiting its gene transcription and by augmenting the production of tissue inhibitor of metalloproteinase-1 in Müller cells. Moreover, the metabolite of nobiletin, 4′-demethylated nobiletin, can ensure its efficacy in the body. A further understanding of the bioavailability of nobiletin is needed to assess its bioactivity within target tissues [107].

Isoflavones are a member of the flavonoid family that have strong antioxidant effects. In STZ-induced diabetic rats, isoflavones exerted potent antioxidative effects, thus reducing retinal sorbitol accumulation by decreasing AR enzyme activity, thereby slowing DR progression. Additionally, isoflavones decrease thiobarbituric acid-reactive substances and protein carbonyl levels in a dose-dependent manner while enhancing GSH, thus diminishing oxidative stress in the retina [108].

Epicatechin, which is a prevalent flavonoid found in human dietary sources, is recognized for its role in enhancing insulin responsiveness and managing blood glucose levels [140,141]. Increases in AGEs are strongly associated with diabetic retinopathy [142]. Epicatechin disrupted AGE antigen formation and mitigated AGE accumulation in a dose-dependent manner in the retina. Moreover, in diabetic rats exogenously injected with AGEs, epicatechin can also ameliorate retinal vascular cell apoptosis and reduce the AGEs burden [109].

5.2.5. Saccharide

Fucoidan is a polysaccharide compound extracted from brown seaweeds that can be found in the sea and on land. In high-glucose-cultured RPE cells, fucoidan prevented ROS production by inhibiting the Ca^{2+}-dependent ERK1/2 signaling pathway, thereby attenuating the retinal damage attributed to high glucose [110]. In addition, in high-glucose-induced microvascular endothelial cells, fucoidan inhibited vascular endothelial cell proliferation and VEGF expression, thus demonstrating antiangiogenic effects. In conclusion, fucoidan exerted similar effects as calcium dobesilate in alleviating retinal pathological changes and blocking neovascularization in a *db/db* type 1 diabetic mouse model [111].

5.2.6. Quinone

Aloe-emodin (AE), a natural compound derived from the traditional Chinese medicine Radix et Rhizoma Rhei, has been known to possess antiangiogenic, antioxidant, and anti-tumor properties [143]. Wu et al. discovered that AE inhibited hypoxia-induced retinal neovascularization via the HIF-1α/VEGF signaling pathway, utilizing both an in vitro model of $CoCl_2$-induced VEGF secretion and an in vivo model of oxygen-induced neovascularization. In vitro, the mRNA expressions of VEGFA and prolyl hydroxylase-2 (PHD-2) were downregulated, and the protein levels of VEGFA, HIF-1α, and PHD-2 decreased. In vivo, AE inhibited retinal neovascularization in the OIR rat model. This study suggests that AE may potentially treat DR by inhibiting retinal neovascularization [112].

5.2.7. Steroid

Trigonella foenum-graceum Linn. (Fenugreek) is an annual herb that was initially used as a vegetable and spice in India. Fenugreek seeds contain various saponins, including 4-hydroxyisoleucine, trigonelline, and diosgenin. Gupta et al. discovered that fenugreek played a crucial role in attenuating oxidative stress and inhibiting inflammatory and angiogenic molecular biomarkers in diabetic rats. Additionally, fenugreek was found to inhibit basement membrane thickening and BRB destruction [144]. Diosgenin, an important natural compound extracted from fenugreek seeds, was found to enhance cell viability in RPE cells under high-glucose conditions, and reduce inflammation, oxidative stress, and apoptosis levels through the activation of the AMPK/Nrf2/HO-1 signaling pathway. Moreover, the protective effects of diosgenin on high-glucose-induced RPE cells were reversed by dorsomorphin (an AMPK inhibitor) [113]. Liao et al. demonstrated that diosgenin increased the total retinal thickness, photoreceptor layer, and outer nuclear layer thickness, and ameliorated ganglion cell loss in the *db/db* mouse model. Additionally, diosgenin was shown to increase Bcl-2 expression while reducing caspase-3 expression, suggesting its potential as an anti-apoptosis agent in vivo [114]. These studies suggest that fenugreek and its extracts may serve as a new modality for DR treatment.

5.2.8. Vitamin D

Vitamin D is one of the essential nutrients for the body to maintain normal physiological functions, and it is extensively employed as a dietary supplement for health preservation [145]. Most of the studies have aimed to investigate whether individual vitamin D serum levels are associated with DR, yet the conclusions have remained inconclusive.

A cross-sectional study by Long et al. assessed the relationship between vitamin D deficiency and DR severity in 842 individuals stratified according to glycemic control, and they demonstrated that vitamin D deficiency may be associated with severe DR only in those individuals with well-controlled blood glucose levels [146].

The findings of Alcubierre et al. suggested that vitamin D deficiency may be associated with DR severity; however, vitamin D consumption did not significantly differ between DR patients and healthy individuals [147]. Moreover, a longitudinal investigation by Millen et al. over three years also did not observe a connection between vitamin D and DR [148].

In conclusion, vitamin D supplementation may be advantageous for treating DR, but additional large-scale randomized controlled trials are needed.

5.2.9. Natural Products with Various Bioactive Agents

Panax notoginseng saponins (PNS), which are the primary constituents of *Panax notoginseng*, exhibit a variety of anti-inflammatory, antioxidant, and neuroprotective properties. Investigations have demonstrated that ginsenoside Rg1 (GRg1) and GRb1, which are key components of the PNS, exerted anti-inflammatory effects in DR. GRg1 and GRb1 increased the retinal inner nuclear layer thickness, decreased retinal acellular capillaries, alleviated BRB destruction, eliminated microglial activation, reversed leukocyte adhesion, and suppressed elevated inflammatory factor levels in the serum. In conclusion, GRg1 and GRb1 decreased retinal damage, attributable to high glucose through the NF-κB signaling pathway [14].

The deciduous plant *Ulmus davidiana*, which is extensively cultivated in China, South Korea, and many other countries, serves as a traditional herbal remedy because its roots and stems are used to alleviate numerous ailments, such as cancer and asthma [149–152]. The primary active bioactive compounds that have been identified in *Ulmus davidiana* are a 60% edible ethanolic extract (U60E) and the catechin 7-O-β-D-apiofuranoside (C7A). In high-glucose- and TNF-α-stimulated cells, U60E and C7A inhibited pericyte apoptosis by suppressing p38 and JNK activities. Additionally, when pericytes and endothelial cells were co-cultured, U60E and C7A were found to restore the suppressed expression of connexin ZO-1 and reduce the increased vascular permeability [115].

6. Mechanisms of Action, Toxicity, and Drug–Drug Interactions of Natural Products

6.1. Bioavailability and Ocular Metabolic Pathways of Natural Products

The main methods of drug delivery into the ocular system include intravitreal injections and systemic, periocular, subretinal, suprachoroidal, or topical administration [153]. Specifically, for DR, the inhibition of neovascularization is often achieved through the intravitreal injection of VEGF antibodies. NP supplements offer the unique advantage of efficiently reaching the retina through oral systemic administration. Within the body, NPs are metabolized, assimilated into the bloodstream, traverse the BRB, and subsequently nourish retinal cells. RPE cells have the capacity to take up vitamins and nutrients from the blood circulation and deliver them to RGCs [154].

However, some current NPs are limited by their low efficiency in drug delivery. Therefore, more research has focused on improving drug delivery systems through nanotechnology. Nano-synthetic drugs potentially improve the safety of systemic delivery and ensure drug targeting. Currently, an increasing number of new nanomaterials are emerging for DR treatment, thus offering non-invasive and safe drug delivery or modification strategies [155]. Although quercetin is a promising therapeutic drug for DR, its high oral dose requirement and limited bioavailability have limited its clinical use [156–158]. Gui et al. reported that ultrasmall Fe-Quer nanozymes (NZs), which are synthesized by binding quercetin with low-toxicity ions, showed increased delivery efficacy, robust ROS scavenging, and vascular protection in both in vivo and in vitro experiments. Histologic examination further confirmed the low toxicity of Fe-Quer NZs, thus suggesting a safe and effective drug delivery system [159]. Moreover, Toragall et al. designed a lutein-loaded chitosan-sodium alginate nanocarrier comprising an oleic acid core (LNC) for improving the solubility, instability, and bioavailability of lutein. Studies have indicated that LNCs with a smaller size and smooth spherical morphology do not affect normal cell viability at a concentration of 20 μM, and LNCs exhibit a high cellular uptake rate, even under H_2O_2-induced oxidative stress conditions [160]. These observations provide avenues for the use of nanomaterials encapsulating NPs as a new therapeutic strategy for DR management.

Ocular drug clearance mainly occurs through the anterior chamber with aqueous humor circulation or through the BRB, with subsequent systemic circulation to the liver. The efficiency of ocular drug clearance depends on drug permeability, molecular size, and lipophilicity. Low-molecular-weight drugs permeate the BRB more efficiently than high-molecular-weight drugs [161], and protein clearance mainly occurs through BRB metabolism [162]. Furthermore, hydrophilic drugs tend to be primarily cleared by passive diffusion through the anterior chamber pathway, whereas lipophilic drugs are mainly cleared through the BRB. The progression of ocular diseases may induce changes in the pathophysiological environment of the eyes, which can correspondingly influence the drug's metabolic profile [153]. Inappropriate metabolic processing of drugs may cause adverse reactions.

6.2. Toxicity and Side Effects

Safety remains the foremost concern in the utilization of pharmaceuticals. Currently, there has been a growing interest in natural compounds, some of which have been formulated as dietary supplements. NPs are generally considered to have lower toxicity and fewer side effects; therefore, they are currently widely used. However, rigorous clinical trial validation of the safety of many dietary supplements or herbal medicines is lacking, and indiscriminate supplementation with NPs may be harmful.

Many NPs are administered orally; additionally, due to their natural connotations, their potential toxicity may be underestimated. The significance of dosage for medical efficacy is well established. Overconsumption can disrupt normal metabolic pathways, thus leading to drug accumulation in certain organs and resulting in cytotoxicity [163,164]. Furthermore, drugs may be harmful due to overdose, metabolic processes, and drug-drug interactions (DDIs). For example, although moderate vitamin D supplementation helps to improve the body's absorption of calcium and phosphorus, excessive supplementation can induce toxic side effects, such as hypercalcemia, vomiting, and dehydration [165–167].

The liver and kidneys serve as pivotal organs for metabolic processes, thus necessitating vigilant monitoring for potential hepatoxicity and nephrotoxicity when administering medications. BBR may suppress hepatic gluconeogenesis and potentially induce hepatoxicity by inhibiting energy metabolism and pyruvate carboxylation [168]. Pyrrolizidine alkaloids, which are toxic compounds found in numerous Chinese medicinal herbs and a small percentage of flowering plants, are known to cause hepatoxicity via metabolic activation by CYP450s to form toxic intermediates in the liver [169]. Teucirum chamaedrys is a traditional food and medicinal plant that has also been reported to have hepatoxicity [170]. In Latin America, there is an increasing incidence of hepatoxicity due to the use of herbal medicines and dietary supplements, and these patients have a higher rate of mortality or need for liver transplantation than those treated with traditional medications [171].

In this review, NPs did not show notable toxic effects in either in vivo or in vitro experiments. For example, polysaccharide compounds from algae were shown to be non-toxic at concentrations ranging from 100 μg/mL to the minimal effective dose of 0.1 μg/mL [172]. Furthermore, a meta-analysis by Li et al. reported of the safety of Chinese herbal compounds for the treatment of DR, with a significantly lower probability of adverse risks than in the conventional treatment group [173]. However, cellular and animal models may not fully predict human toxicological outcomes. Therefore, more research is needed to explore the possible adverse effects of NPs on the human body and provide more evidence for the future application of NPs.

6.3. Drug–Drug Interactions

DDIs are combined effects that manifest when multiple drugs are administered consecutively. These effects may enhance or diminish drug efficacy and, in some cases, lead to toxicity. DDIs are more likely to occur in those who suffer from chronic diseases or those undergoing treatment with a combination of traditional medicines and NPs [174]. Currently, NPs are often used in combination with conventional medicines, which certainly raises concerns regarding the potential for toxicity due to DDIs [175]. Studies have indicated that NPs can exert bidirectional influences on pharmacological agents; for example, BBR displays differential modulatory effects on the uptake of nimodipine by cerebral microvascular endothelial cells, with an inhibitory effect at high concentrations and an enhancing effect at low concentrations [176]. Enzymes involved in metabolism and transport proteins are also instrumental in the modulation of DDIs [177]. Co-administration of multiple compounds can cause competitive metabolic processes, which may alter drug bioavailability and pharmacokinetics, thus modifying therapeutic outcomes and possibly inducing adverse reactions [178,179]. For example, the co-administration of metformin and BBR has been shown to promote drug accumulation in hepatic and renal tissues, which is attributed to inhibited multidrug and toxin extrusion-1-mediated urinary and biliary excretion [180].

DDIs may also enhance therapeutic outcomes. Oh et al. explored the antioxidant effects of ascorbic acid in conjunction with ASX in RPE cells subjected to oxidative stress via H_2O_2 or UVB exposure. The results indicated an increase in cell viability and a concomitant decrease in intracellular ROS levels. Ultimately, the combination of ascorbic acid and ASX has been shown to amplify antioxidant effects [181]. In traditional Chinese medicine (TCM), several herbs are usually mixed in specific proportions to form a single formula, in which the therapeutic effects may be attributed to the synergistic, additive, and antagonistic effects of several different ingredients, thus ultimately enhancing its efficacy and reducing its toxicity. For example, LDD, which is a classical TCM formula, consists of six herbs. Its efficacy in DR treatment may be attributable to the synergistic effects of multiple active ingredients engaging in different biological targets and pathways [182]. Furthermore, a meta-analysis by Li et al., comparing the effects of combining traditional Chinese medicine and conventional Western medicine treatment for DR, showed that combining therapies could lower blood glucose levels, improve fundus hemorrhage, and restore visual function in DR patients [183].

7. Limitations and Perspectives

It is generally acknowledged that cell cultures and animal models cannot entirely mimic the entire process of disease progression. Any new therapeutic intervention must be based on rigorous basic research and clinical trials to determine the exact mechanisms and targets of the drug and validate its efficacy in large population cohorts. Most of the studies that were included in this review involved only cell and/or animal experiments, thus indicating the need for additional preclinical and clinical trials to confirm the effectiveness of these methods in populations. Additionally, it is critical to investigate whether the process of absorption, distribution, metabolism, and excretion of NPs in the human body will potentially cause toxicity or adverse effects and how to avoid the risks associated with the use and overdose of multiple drugs. NPs may interact through myriad mechanisms and targets, the complete mechanisms of which remain to be fully understood. By leveraging advancements in technology and bioinformatics, such as high-throughput screening, high-content screening, and virtual screening, we hope to facilitate our understanding of the definitive action of NPs.

8. Conclusions

DR is one of the most severe complications of DM, and its pathological changes include inflammation, retinal micro-vasculopathy, oxidative stress, and retinal neurodegeneration. The complexity of the multiple mechanisms underlying these pathologic changes in DR makes achieving satisfactory outcomes with current treatments challenging. Considering the pivotal role of dietary and lifestyle habits in diabetes management, therapeutic strategies based on diet present a promising frontier for DR treatment.

We noted that research predominantly concentrates on preclinical studies involving supplementation with one or more natural compounds that are administered either through cell culture or animal diets. In vitro studies usually employ cellular models, such as endothelial cells and RPE cells, whereas in vivo experiments frequently utilize STZ-induced diabetic rats or mice, as well as *db/db* mouse models.

This review summarizes current investigations on the potential impacts of NPs on DR. NPs still face some challenges, such as poor bioavailability, rapid breakdown, low targeting, and inconsistent distribution within the human body [184]. They are widely available and easily accessible, thus presenting advantages over small-molecule drugs. Moreover, NPs have demonstrated anti-inflammatory, antioxidative, antiangiogenic, and neuroprotective effects in diabetic models, and the associated signaling pathways include NF-kB, Nrf2/Keap1, cAMP/PKA, AMPK/mTOR/HO-1, and miR-138-5p/Sirt1/Nrf2. Future research incorporating nanomaterial-encapsulated NPs and employing bioinformatics-based NPs may lead to significant advances.

In conclusion, NPs are a non-invasive treatment with high therapeutic potential and are expected to be used either alone or in combination with other traditional Western medications in the future for the prevention of DR. We anticipate more preclinical and clinical research to validate the effects of NPs on DR.

Author Contributions: Writing—original draft preparation, Y.Z.; writing—review and editing, Y.C. and N.Y.; supervision, N.Y.; funding acquisition, N.Y. All authors have read and agreed to the published version of the manuscript.

Funding: This research was funded by The Aier Eye-Sichuan University Research Foundation, grant number "23JZH046".

Conflicts of Interest: The authors declare no conflicts of interest.

References

1. Zhu, J.; Huang, J.; Sun, Y.; Xu, W.; Qian, H. Emerging Role of Extracellular Vesicles in Diabetic Retinopathy. *Theranostics* **2024**, *14*, 1631–1646. [CrossRef] [PubMed]
2. Bryl, A.; Mrugacz, M.; Falkowski, M.; Zorena, K. The Effect of Hyperlipidemia on the Course of Diabetic Retinopathy-Literature Review. *J. Clin. Med.* **2022**, *11*, 2761. [CrossRef] [PubMed]
3. Mao, Y.; Zhong, W. HbA1c Variability as an Independent Risk Factor for Microvascular Complications in Type 1 Diabetes. *J. Diabetes Sci. Technol.* **2024**, *18*, 380–388. [CrossRef] [PubMed]
4. Teo, Z.L.; Tham, Y.-C.; Yu, M.; Chee, M.L.; Rim, T.H.; Cheung, N.; Bikbov, M.M.; Wang, Y.X.; Tang, Y.; Lu, Y.; et al. Global Prevalence of Diabetic Retinopathy and Projection of Burden through 2045: Systematic Review and Meta-Analysis. *Ophthalmology* **2021**, *128*, 1580–1591. [CrossRef] [PubMed]
5. Mrowicka, M.; Mrowicki, J.; Majsterek, I. Relationship between Biochemical Pathways and Non-Coding RNAs Involved in the Progression of Diabetic Retinopathy. *J. Clin. Med.* **2024**, *13*, 292. [CrossRef] [PubMed]
6. Gangwani, R.A.; Lian, J.X.; McGhee, S.M.; Wong, D.; Li, K.K. Diabetic Retinopathy Screening: Global and Local Perspective. *Hong Kong Med. J.* **2016**, *22*, 486–495. [CrossRef] [PubMed]
7. Semeraro, F.; Cancarini, A.; dell'Omo, R.; Rezzola, S.; Romano, M.R.; Costagliola, C. Diabetic Retinopathy: Vascular and Inflammatory Disease. *J. Diabetes Res.* **2015**, *2015*, 582060. [CrossRef] [PubMed]
8. Flaxel, C.J.; Adelman, R.A.; Bailey, S.T.; Fawzi, A.; Lim, J.I.; Vemulakonda, G.A.; Ying, G.-S. Diabetic Retinopathy Preferred Practice Pattern®. *Ophthalmology* **2020**, *127*, P66–P145. [CrossRef] [PubMed]
9. Tanaka, S.; Yoshimura, Y.; Kawasaki, R.; Kamada, C.; Tanaka, S.; Horikawa, C.; Ohashi, Y.; Araki, A.; Ito, H.; Akanuma, Y.; et al. Fruit Intake and Incident Diabetic Retinopathy with Type 2 Diabetes. *Epidemiology* **2013**, *24*, 204–211. [CrossRef] [PubMed]
10. Hutton, B.; Salanti, G.; Caldwell, D.M.; Chaimani, A.; Schmid, C.H.; Cameron, C.; Ioannidis, J.P.A.; Straus, S.; Thorlund, K.; Jansen, J.P.; et al. The PRISMA Extension Statement for Reporting of Systematic Reviews Incorporating Network Meta-Analyses of Health Care Interventions: Checklist and Explanations. *Ann. Intern. Med.* **2015**, *162*, 777–784. [CrossRef] [PubMed]
11. Cheung, N.; Mitchell, P.; Wong, T.Y. Diabetic Retinopathy. *Lancet* **2010**, *376*, 124–136. [CrossRef] [PubMed]

12. Marques, I.P.; Madeira, M.H.; Messias, A.L.; Martinho, A.C.-V.; Santos, T.; Sousa, D.C.; Figueira, J.; Cunha-Vaz, J. Different Retinopathy Phenotypes in Type 2 Diabetes Predict Retinopathy Progression. *Acta Diabetol.* **2021**, *58*, 197–205. [CrossRef] [PubMed]
13. Tang, L.; Xu, G.-T.; Zhang, J.-F. Inflammation in Diabetic Retinopathy: Possible Roles in Pathogenesis and Potential Implications for Therapy. *Neural Regen. Res.* **2023**, *18*, 976–982. [CrossRef] [PubMed]
14. Wang, Y.; Sun, X.; Xie, Y.; Du, A.; Chen, M.; Lai, S.; Wei, X.; Ji, L.; Wang, C. Panax Notoginseng Saponins Alleviate Diabetic Retinopathy by Inhibiting Retinal Inflammation: Association with the NF-κB Signaling Pathway. *J. Ethnopharmacol.* **2024**, *319*, 117135. [CrossRef] [PubMed]
15. Herdade, A.S.; Silva, I.M.; Calado, Â.; Saldanha, C.; Nguyen, N.-H.; Hou, I.; Castanho, M.; Roy, S. Effects of Diabetes on Microcirculation and Leukostasis in Retinal and Non-Ocular Tissues: Implications for Diabetic Retinopathy. *Biomolecules* **2020**, *10*, 1583. [CrossRef] [PubMed]
16. Rangasamy, S.; McGuire, P.G.; Franco Nitta, C.; Monickaraj, F.; Oruganti, S.R.; Das, A. Chemokine Mediated Monocyte Trafficking into the Retina: Role of Inflammation in Alteration of the Blood-Retinal Barrier in Diabetic Retinopathy. *PLoS ONE* **2014**, *9*, e108508. [CrossRef]
17. Sun, W.-J.; An, X.-D.; Zhang, Y.-H.; Zhao, X.-F.; Sun, Y.-T.; Yang, C.-Q.; Kang, X.-M.; Jiang, L.-L.; Ji, H.-Y.; Lian, F.-M. The Ideal Treatment Timing for Diabetic Retinopathy: The Molecular Pathological Mechanisms Underlying Early-Stage Diabetic Retinopathy Are a Matter of Concern. *Front. Endocrinol.* **2023**, *14*, 1270145. [CrossRef] [PubMed]
18. Kaštelan, S.; Orešković, I.; Bišćan, F.; Kaštelan, H.; Gverović Antunica, A. Inflammatory and Angiogenic Biomarkers in Diabetic Retinopathy. *Biochem. Med.* **2020**, *30*, 030502. [CrossRef] [PubMed]
19. Zhang, H.; Liang, L.; Huang, R.; Wu, P.; He, L. Comparison of Inflammatory Cytokines Levels in the Aqueous Humor with Diabetic Retinopathy. *Int. Ophthalmol.* **2020**, *40*, 2763–2769. [CrossRef] [PubMed]
20. Zhang, W.; Yao, J.; Chen, C.; Wang, J.; Zhou, A. Fetuin-B Overexpression Promotes Inflammation in Diabetic Retinopathy Through Activating Microglia and the NF-κB Signaling Pathway. *Curr. Eye Res.* **2024**, *49*, 168–179. [CrossRef] [PubMed]
21. Augustine, J.; Pavlou, S.; Harkin, K.; Stitt, A.W.; Xu, H.; Chen, M. IL-33 Regulates Müller Cell-Mediated Retinal Inflammation and Neurodegeneration in Diabetic Retinopathy. *Dis. Models Mech.* **2023**, *16*, dmm050174. [CrossRef] [PubMed]
22. Wang, W.; Lo, A. Diabetic Retinopathy: Pathophysiology and Treatments. *Int. J. Mol. Sci.* **2018**, *19*, 1816. [CrossRef] [PubMed]
23. Bek, T. Diameter Changes of Retinal Vessels in Diabetic Retinopathy. *Curr. Diabetes Rep.* **2017**, *17*, 82. [CrossRef] [PubMed]
24. Rangasamy, S.; Monickaraj, F.; Legendre, C.; Cabrera, A.P.; Llaci, L.; Bilagody, C.; McGuire, P.; Das, A. Transcriptomics Analysis of Pericytes from Retinas of Diabetic Animals Reveals Novel Genes and Molecular Pathways Relevant to Blood-Retinal Barrier Alterations in Diabetic Retinopathy. *Exp. Eye Res.* **2020**, *195*, 108043. [CrossRef] [PubMed]
25. An, D.; Tan, B.; Yu, D.-Y.; Balaratnasingam, C. Differentiating Microaneurysm Pathophysiology in Diabetic Retinopathy Through Objective Analysis of Capillary Nonperfusion, Inflammation, and Pericytes. *Diabetes* **2022**, *71*, 733–746. [CrossRef] [PubMed]
26. Vähätupa, M.; Järvinen, T.A.H.; Uusitalo-Järvinen, H. Exploration of Oxygen-Induced Retinopathy Model to Discover New Therapeutic Drug Targets in Retinopathies. *Front. Pharmacol.* **2020**, *11*, 873. [CrossRef] [PubMed]
27. Gu, L.; Xu, H.; Zhang, C.; Yang, Q.; Zhang, L.; Zhang, J. Time-Dependent Changes in Hypoxia- and Gliosis-Related Factors in Experimental Diabetic Retinopathy. *Eye* **2019**, *33*, 600–609. [CrossRef] [PubMed]
28. Yang, Y.; Liu, Y.; Li, Y.; Chen, Z.; Xiong, Y.; Zhou, T.; Tao, W.; Xu, F.; Yang, H.; Ylä-Herttuala, S.; et al. MicroRNA-15b Targets VEGF and Inhibits Angiogenesis in Proliferative Diabetic Retinopathy. *J. Clin. Endocrinol. Metab.* **2020**, *105*, 3404–3415. [CrossRef] [PubMed]
29. Rousseau, S.; Houle, F.; Landry, J.; Huot, J. P38 MAP Kinase Activation by Vascular Endothelial Growth Factor Mediates Actin Reorganization and Cell Migration in Human Endothelial Cells. *Oncogene* **1997**, *15*, 2169–2177. [CrossRef] [PubMed]
30. Sozen-Delil, F.I.; Cekic, O.; Haklar, G. Serum and Vitreous Vascular Endothelial Growth Factor Levels in Diabetic Retinopathy. *Int. Ophthalmol.* **2023**, *43*, 2247–2255. [CrossRef] [PubMed]
31. Ning, W.; Cheng, Z.; Yu, X.; HorYue, T.; Haiyong, C.; Yibin, F. Berberine Improves Insulin-Induced Diabetic Retinopathy through Exclusively Suppressing Akt/mTOR-Mediated HIF-1α/VEGF Activation in Retina Endothelial Cells. *Int. J. Biol. Sci.* **2021**, *17*, 4316.
32. Wang, L.; Li, S.; Wang, L.; Lin, K.; Du, J.; Miao, W.; Zhang, L. Uncovering the Protective Mechanism of Taohong Siwu Decoction against Diabetic Retinopathy via HIF-1 Signaling Pathway Based on Network Analysis and Experimental Validation. *BMC Complement. Med. Ther.* **2020**, *20*, 298. [CrossRef] [PubMed]
33. Fu, S.; Zheng, Y.; Sun, Y.; Lai, M.; Qiu, J.; Gui, F.; Zeng, Q.; Liu, F. Suppressing Long Noncoding RNA OGRU Ameliorates Diabetic Retinopathy by Inhibition of Oxidative Stress and Inflammation via miR-320/USP14 Axis. *Free Radic. Biol. Med.* **2021**, *169*, 361–381. [CrossRef] [PubMed]
34. Guzman, D.C.; Olguín, H.J.; García, E.H.; Peraza, A.V.; de la Cruz, D.Z.; Soto, M.P. Mechanisms Involved in the Development of Diabetic Retinopathy Induced by Oxidative Stress. *Redox Rep.* **2017**, *22*, 10–16. [CrossRef] [PubMed]
35. Hirsch, G.E.; Heck, T.G. Inflammation, Oxidative Stress and Altered Heat Shock Response in Type 2 Diabetes: The Basis for New Pharmacological and Non-Pharmacological Interventions. *Arch. Physiol. Biochem.* **2022**, *128*, 411–425. [CrossRef]
36. Satari, M.; Aghadavod, E.; Mobini, M.; Asemi, Z. Association between miRNAs Expression and Signaling Pathways of Oxidative Stress in Diabetic Retinopathy. *J. Cell Physiol.* **2019**, *234*, 8522–8532. [CrossRef] [PubMed]

37. Zhang, X.; Ji, Y.; Zhu, L.; Wang, Z.; Fang, C.; Jiang, C.; Pan, K.; Zhang, J.; Yin, Z. Arjunolic Acid from *Cyclocarya paliurus* Ameliorates Diabetic Retinopathy through AMPK/mTOR/HO-1 Regulated Autophagy Pathway. *J. Ethnopharmacol.* **2022**, *284*, 114772. [CrossRef] [PubMed]
38. Karam-Palos, S.; Andrés-Blasco, I.; Campos-Borges, C.; Zanón-Moreno, V.; Gallego-Martínez, A.; Alegre-Ituarte, V.; García-Medina, J.J.; Pastor-Idoate, S.; Sellés-Navarro, I.; Vila-Arteaga, J.; et al. Oxidative Stress Mediates Epigenetic Modifications and the Expression of miRNAs and Genes Related to Apoptosis in Diabetic Retinopathy Patients. *J. Clin. Med.* **2023**, *13*, 74. [CrossRef] [PubMed]
39. Andrés-Blasco, I.; Gallego-Martínez, A.; Machado, X.; Cruz-Espinosa, J.; Di Lauro, S.; Casaroli-Marano, R.; Alegre-Ituarte, V.; Arévalo, J.F.; Pinazo-Durán, M.D. Oxidative Stress, Inflammatory, Angiogenic, and Apoptotic Molecules in Proliferative Diabetic Retinopathy and Diabetic Macular Edema Patients. *Int. J. Mol. Sci.* **2023**, *24*, 8227. [CrossRef] [PubMed]
40. Fang, J.; Bai, W.; Yang, L. Astaxanthin Inhibits Oxidative Stress and Apoptosis in Diabetic Retinopathy. *Acta Histochem.* **2023**, *125*, 152069. [CrossRef] [PubMed]
41. Nonarath, H.J.; Hall, A.E.; SenthilKumar, G.; Abroe, B.; Eells, J.T.; Liedhegner, E.S. 670nm Photobiomodulation Modulates Bioenergetics and Oxidative Stress, in Rat Müller Cells Challenged with High Glucose. *PLoS ONE* **2021**, *16*, e0260968. [CrossRef]
42. Sohn, E.H.; van Dijk, H.W.; Jiao, C.; Kok, P.H.B.; Jeong, W.; Demirkaya, N.; Garmager, A.; Wit, F.; Kucukevcilioglu, M.; van Velthoven, M.E.J.; et al. Retinal Neurodegeneration May Precede Microvascular Changes Characteristic of Diabetic Retinopathy in Diabetes Mellitus. *Proc. Natl. Acad. Sci. USA* **2016**, *113*, E2655–E2664. [CrossRef] [PubMed]
43. Stitt, A.W.; Curtis, T.M.; Chen, M.; Medina, R.J.; McKay, G.J.; Jenkins, A.; Gardiner, T.A.; Lyons, T.J.; Hammes, H.-P.; Simó, R.; et al. The Progress in Understanding and Treatment of Diabetic Retinopathy. *Prog. Retin Eye Res.* **2016**, *51*, 156–186. [CrossRef] [PubMed]
44. Lee, H.-J.; Cho, S.; Park, J.; Jin, Y.; Kim, H.M.; Jee, D. Cost-Effectiveness of the Anti-Vascular Endothelial Growth Factor Intravitreal Injection and Panretinal Photocoagulation for Patients with Proliferative Diabetic Retinopathy in South Korea. *BMC Health Serv. Res.* **2023**, *23*, 1388. [CrossRef] [PubMed]
45. Zehden, J.A.; Mortensen, X.M.; Reddy, A.; Zhang, A.Y. Systemic and Ocular Adverse Events with Intravitreal Anti-VEGF Therapy Used in the Treatment of Diabetic Retinopathy: A Review. *Curr. Diabetes Rep.* **2022**, *22*, 525–536. [CrossRef] [PubMed]
46. Early Treatment Diabetic Retinopathy Study Research Group. Treatment Techniques and Clinical Guidelines for Photocoagulation of Diabetic Macular Edema. Early Treatment Diabetic Retinopathy Study Report Number 2. *Ophthalmology* **1987**, *94*, 761–774. [CrossRef] [PubMed]
47. Fallico, M.; Maugeri, A.; Lotery, A.; Longo, A.; Bonfiglio, V.; Russo, A.; Avitabile, T.; Pulvirenti, A.; Furino, C.; Cennamo, G.; et al. Intravitreal Anti-Vascular Endothelial Growth Factors, Panretinal Photocoagulation and Combined Treatment for Proliferative Diabetic Retinopathy: A Systematic Review and Network Meta-Analysis. *Acta Ophthalmol.* **2021**, *99*, e795–e805. [CrossRef] [PubMed]
48. Kim, M.-K.; Kim, S.-G.; Lee, S.K. 4-Hexylresorcinol-in Duced Angiogenesis Potential in Human Endothelial Cells. *Maxillofac. Plast. Reconstr. Surg.* **2020**, *42*, 23. [CrossRef] [PubMed]
49. Wang, C.Y.; Kim, D.; Zhu, Y.K.; Oh, D.-C.; Huang, R.Z.; Wang, H.-S.; Liang, D.; Lee, S.K. Glechomanamides A–C, Germacrane Sesquiterpenoids with an Unusual Δ^8-7,12-Lactam Moiety from *Salvia scapiformis* and Their Antiangiogenic Activity. *J. Nat. Prod.* **2019**, *82*, 3056–3064. [CrossRef]
50. Liao, Z.-Y.; Liang, I.-C.; Li, H.-J.; Wu, C.-C.; Lo, H.-M.; Chang, D.-C.; Hung, C.-F. Chrysin Inhibits High Glucose-Induced Migration on Chorioretinal Endothelial Cells via VEGF and VEGFR Down-Regulation. *Int. J. Mol. Sci.* **2020**, *21*, 5541. [CrossRef] [PubMed]
51. Cui, J.; Gong, R.; Hu, S.; Cai, L.; Chen, L. Gambogic Acid Ameliorates Diabetes-Induced Proliferative Retinopathy through Inhibition of the HIF-1α/VEGF Expression via Targeting PI3K/AKT Pathway. *Life Sci.* **2018**, *192*, 293–303. [CrossRef]
52. Rymaszewski, Z.; Abplanalpl, M.A. Human Retinal Vascular Cells Differ from Umbilical Cells in Synthetic Functions and Their Response to Glucose. *Proc. Soc. Exp. Biol. Med.* **1992**, *199*, 183–191. [CrossRef] [PubMed]
53. Zhang, S.-M.; Fan, B.; Li, Y.-L.; Zuo, Z.-Y.; Li, G.-Y. Oxidative Stress-Involved Mitophagy of Retinal Pigment Epithelium and Retinal Degenerative Diseases. *Cell Mol. Neurobiol.* **2023**, *43*, 3265–3276. [CrossRef] [PubMed]
54. Li, M.; Tian, M.; Wang, Y.; Ma, H.; Zhou, Y.; Jiang, X.; Liu, Y. Updates on RPE Cell Damage in Diabetic Retinopathy (Review). *Mol. Med. Rep.* **2023**, *28*, 185. [CrossRef] [PubMed]
55. Tang, X.; Li, X.; Zhang, D.; Han, W. Astragaloside-IV Alleviates High Glucose-Induced Ferroptosis in Retinal Pigment Epithelial Cells by Disrupting the Expression of miR-138-5p/Sirt1/Nrf2. *Bioengineered* **2022**, *13*, 8238–8253. [CrossRef] [PubMed]
56. Kim, Y.S.; Jung, D.H.; Kim, N.H.; Lee, Y.M.; Kim, J.S. Effect of Magnolol on TGF-B1 and Fibronectin Expression in Human Retinal Pigment Epithelial Cells under Diabetic Conditions. *Eur. J. Pharmacol.* **2007**, *562*, 12–19. [CrossRef] [PubMed]
57. Rungger-Brändle, E.; Dosso, A.A.; Leuenberger, P.M. Glial Reactivity, an Early Feature of Diabetic Retinopathy. *Investig. Ophthalmol. Vis. Sci.* **2000**, *41*, 1971–1980.
58. Abu El-Asrar, A.M.; Ahmad, A.; Siddiquei, M.M.; De Zutter, A.; Allegaert, E.; Gikandi, P.W.; De Hertogh, G.; Van Damme, J.; Opdenakker, G.; Struyf, S. The Proinflammatory and Proangiogenic Macrophage Migration Inhibitory Factor Is a Potential Regulator in Proliferative Diabetic Retinopathy. *Front. Immunol.* **2019**, *10*, 2752. [CrossRef]

59. Sergeys, J.; Etienne, I.; Van Hove, I.; Lefevere, E.; Stalmans, I.; Feyen, J.H.M.; Moons, L.; Van Bergen, T. Longitudinal In Vivo Characterization of the Streptozotocin-Induced Diabetic Mouse Model: Focus on Early Inner Retinal Responses. *Investig. Ophthalmol. Vis. Sci.* **2019**, *60*, 807–822. [CrossRef] [PubMed]
60. Catalani, E.; Cervia, D. Diabetic Retinopathy: A Matter of Retinal Ganglion Cell Homeostasis. *Neural Regen. Res.* **2020**, *15*, 1253–1254. [CrossRef] [PubMed]
61. Moleiro, A.F.; Conceição, G.; Leite-Moreira, A.F.; Rocha-Sousa, A. A Critical Analysis of the Available In Vitro and Ex Vivo Methods to Study Retinal Angiogenesis. *J. Ophthalmol.* **2017**, *2017*, 3034953. [CrossRef] [PubMed]
62. Liu, D.-D.; Zhang, C.-Y.; Zhang, J.-T.; Gu, L.-M.; Xu, G.-T.; Zhang, J.-F. Epigenetic Modifications and Metabolic Memory in Diabetic Retinopathy: Beyond the Surface. *Neural Regen. Res.* **2023**, *18*, 1441–1449. [CrossRef] [PubMed]
63. Quiroz, J.; Yazdanyar, A. Animal Models of Diabetic Retinopathy. *Ann. Transl. Med.* **2021**, *9*, 1272. [CrossRef] [PubMed]
64. McLetchie, N.G. Alloxan Diabetes: A Discovery, Albeit a Minor One. *J. R. Coll. Physicians Edinb.* **2002**, *32*, 134–142. [PubMed]
65. Sadikan, M.Z.; Abdul Nasir, N.A.; Lambuk, L.; Mohamud, R.; Reshidan, N.H.; Low, E.; Singar, S.A.; Mohmad Sabere, A.S.; Iezhitsa, I.; Agarwal, R. Diabetic Retinopathy: A Comprehensive Update on in Vivo, in Vitro and Ex Vivo Experimental Models. *BMC Ophthalmol.* **2023**, *23*, 421. [CrossRef] [PubMed]
66. Polewik, K.; Kosek, M.; Jamrozik, D.; Matuszek, I.; Smędowski, A.; Lewin-Kowalik, J.; Pietrucha-Dutczak, M. Rodent Models of Diabetic Retinopathy as a Useful Research Tool to Study Neurovascular Cross-Talk. *Biology* **2023**, *12*, 262. [CrossRef] [PubMed]
67. Feit-Leichman, R.A.; Kinouchi, R.; Takeda, M.; Fan, Z.; Mohr, S.; Kern, T.S.; Chen, D.F. Vascular Damage in a Mouse Model of Diabetic Retinopathy: Relation to Neuronal and Glial Changes. *Investig. Ophthalmol. Vis. Sci.* **2005**, *46*, 4281–4287. [CrossRef] [PubMed]
68. Su, L.; Ji, J.; Bian, J.; Fu, Y.; Ge, Y.; Yuan, Z. Tacrolimus (FK506) Prevents Early Retinal Neovascularization in Streptozotocin-Induced Diabetic Mice. *Int. Immunopharmacol.* **2012**, *14*, 606–612. [CrossRef]
69. Zhu, M.; Gao, S.; Gao, S.; Wang, Y.; Li, N.; Shen, X. Interleukin-17A Attenuates Photoreceptor Cell Apoptosis in Streptozotocin-Induced Diabetic Mouse Model. *Bioengineered* **2022**, *13*, 14175–14187. [CrossRef] [PubMed]
70. Sadikan, M.Z.; Nasir, N.A.A.; Iezhitsa, I.; Agarwal, R. Antioxidant and Anti-Apoptotic Effects of Tocotrienol-Rich Fraction against Streptozotocin-Induced Diabetic Retinopathy in Rats. *Biomed. Pharmacother.* **2022**, *153*, 113533. [CrossRef] [PubMed]
71. Sadikan, M.Z.; Abdul Nasir, N.A.; Bakar, N.S.; Iezhitsa, I.; Agarwal, R. Tocotrienol-Rich Fraction Reduces Retinal Inflammation and Angiogenesis in Rats with Streptozotocin-Induced Diabetes. *BMC Complement. Med. Ther.* **2023**, *23*, 179. [CrossRef] [PubMed]
72. Abdul Ghani, N.A.; Abdul Nasir, N.A.; Lambuk, L.; Sadikan, M.Z.; Agarwal, R.; Ramli, N. The Effect of Palm Oil-Derived Tocotrienol-Rich Fraction in Preserving Normal Retinal Vascular Diameter in Streptozotocin-Induced Diabetic Rats. *Graefe's Arch. Clin. Exp. Ophthalmol.* **2023**, *261*, 1587–1596. [CrossRef] [PubMed]
73. Furman, B.L. Streptozotocin-Induced Diabetic Models in Mice and Rats. *Curr. Protoc.* **2021**, *1*, e78. [CrossRef] [PubMed]
74. Barber, A.J.; Antonetti, D.A.; Kern, T.S.; Reiter, C.E.N.; Soans, R.S.; Krady, J.K.; Levison, S.W.; Gardner, T.W.; Bronson, S.K. The *Ins2Akita* Mouse as a Model of Early Retinal Complications in Diabetes. *Investig. Ophthalmol. Vis. Sci.* **2005**, *46*, 2210–2218. [CrossRef] [PubMed]
75. Leiter, E.H. The NOD Mouse: A Model for Analyzing the Interplay Between Heredity and Environment in Development of Autoimmune Disease. *ILAR J.* **1993**, *35*, 4–14. [CrossRef]
76. Li, C.-R.; Sun, S.-G. VEGF Expression and Cell Apoptosis in NOD Mouse Retina. *Int. J. Ophthalmol.* **2010**, *3*, 224–227. [CrossRef]
77. Olivares, A.M.; Althoff, K.; Chen, G.F.; Wu, S.; Morrisson, M.A.; DeAngelis, M.M.; Haider, N. Animal Models of Diabetic Retinopathy. *Curr. Diab. Rep.* **2017**, *17*, 93. [CrossRef]
78. Bogdanov, P.; Corraliza, L.; Villena, J.A.; Carvalho, A.R.; Garcia-Arumí, J.; Ramos, D.; Ruberte, J.; Simó, R.; Hernández, C. The *Db/Db* Mouse: A Useful Model for the Study of Diabetic Retinal Neurodegeneration. *PLoS ONE* **2014**, *9*, e97302. [CrossRef] [PubMed]
79. Lee, V.K. BTBR *Ob/Ob* Mouse Model of Type 2 Diabetes Exhibits Early Loss of Retinal Function and Retinal Inflammation Followed by Late Vascular Changes. *Diabetologia* **2018**, *61*, 2422–2432. [CrossRef] [PubMed]
80. Kowluru, R.A. Retinopathy in a Diet-Induced Type 2 Diabetic Rat Model and Role of Epigenetic Modifications. *Diabetes* **2020**, *69*, 689–698. [CrossRef] [PubMed]
81. Connor, K.M.; Krah, N.M.; Dennison, R.J.; Aderman, C.M.; Chen, J.; Guerin, K.I.; Sapieha, P.; Stahl, A.; Willett, K.L.; Smith, L.E.H. Quantification of Oxygen-Induced Retinopathy in the Mouse: A Model of Vessel Loss, Vessel Regrowth and Pathological Angiogenesis. *Nat. Protoc.* **2009**, *4*, 1565–1573. [CrossRef] [PubMed]
82. Rodríguez, M.L.; Pérez, S.; Mena-Mollá, S.; Desco, M.C.; Ortega, Á.L. Oxidative Stress and Microvascular Alterations in Diabetic Retinopathy: Future Therapies. *Oxid. Med. Cell. Longev.* **2019**, *2019*, 4940825. [CrossRef] [PubMed]
83. Rossino, M.G.; Casini, G. Nutraceuticals for the Treatment of Diabetic Retinopathy. *Nutrients* **2019**, *11*, 771. [CrossRef] [PubMed]
84. Ding, Y.; Yuan, S.; Liu, X.; Mao, P.; Zhao, C.; Huang, Q.; Zhang, R.; Fang, Y.; Song, Q.; Yuan, D.; et al. Protective Effects of Astragaloside IV on Db/Db Mice with Diabetic Retinopathy. *PLoS ONE* **2014**, *9*, e112207. [CrossRef]
85. Zhao, Z.-H.; Xu, M.; Fu, C.; Huang, Y.; Wang, T.-H.; Zuo, Z.-F.; Liu, X.-Z. A Mechanistic Exploratory Study on the Therapeutic Efficacy of Astragaloside IV Against Diabetic Retinopathy Revealed by Network Pharmacology. *Front. Pharmacol.* **2022**, *13*, 903485. [CrossRef] [PubMed]
86. Chen, Y.; Meng, J.; Li, H.; Wei, H.; Bi, F.; Liu, S.; Tang, K.; Guo, H.; Liu, W. Resveratrol Exhibits an Effect on Attenuating Retina Inflammatory Condition and Damage of Diabetic Retinopathy via PON1. *Exp. Eye Res.* **2019**, *181*, 356–366. [CrossRef] [PubMed]

87. Al-Hussaini, H. Effects of Trans-Resveratrol on Type 1 Diabetes-Induced up-Regulation of Apoptosis and Mitogen-Activated Protein Kinase Signaling in Retinal Pigment Epithelium of Dark Agouti Rats. *Eur. J. Pharmacol.* **2021**, *904*, 174167. [CrossRef] [PubMed]
88. Soufi, F.G.; Mohammad-Nejad, D.; Ahmadieh, H. Resveratrol Improves Diabetic Retinopathy Possibly through Oxidative Stress—Nuclear Factor κB—Apoptosis Pathway. *Pharmacol. Rep.* **2012**, *64*, 1505–1514. [CrossRef] [PubMed]
89. Kim, Y.-H.; Kim, Y.-S.; Kang, S.-S.; Cho, G.-J.; Choi, W.-S. Resveratrol Inhibits Neuronal Apoptosis and Elevated Ca^{2+}/Calmodulin-Dependent Protein Kinase II Activity in Diabetic Mouse Retina. *Diabetes* **2010**, *59*, 1825–1835. [CrossRef] [PubMed]
90. Yang, M.; Zhao, T.; Deng, T.; Wang, Z. Protective Effects of Astaxanthin against Diabetic Retinal Vessels and Pro-Inflammatory Cytokine Synthesis. *Int. J. Clin. Exp. Med.* **2019**, *12*, 4725–4734.
91. Ola, M.S.; Ahmed, M.M.; Shams, S.; Al-Rejaie, S.S. Neuroprotective Effects of Quercetin in Diabetic Rat Retina. *Saudi J. Biol. Sci.* **2017**, *24*, 1186–1194. [CrossRef] [PubMed]
92. Kumar, B.; Gupta, S.K.; Nag, T.C.; Srivastava, S.; Saxena, R.; Jha, K.A.; Srinivasan, B.P. Retinal Neuroprotective Effects of Quercetin in Streptozotocin-Induced Diabetic Rats. *Exp. Eye Res.* **2014**, *125*, 193–202. [CrossRef] [PubMed]
93. Tian, P.; Ge, H.; Liu, H.; Kern, T.S.; Du, L.; Guan, L.; Su, S.; Liu, P. Leukocytes from Diabetic Patients Kill Retinal Endothelial Cells: Effects of Berberine. *Mol. Vis.* **2013**, *19*, 2092. [PubMed]
94. Na, L.; Xu, M.; Chen, J.-L.; Chen, G.-J.; Sun, J.; Zhang, Q.; Li, J.-Q.; Guo, X.-L.; Zuo, Z.-F.; Liu, X.-Z.; et al. 4D-DIA Quantitative Proteomics Revealed the Core Mechanism of Diabetic Retinopathy after Berberine Treatment. *Eur. J. Pharmacol.* **2023**, *958*, 175947. [CrossRef] [PubMed]
95. Zhang, Y.; Meng, X.; Liu, K. The Modulation of cAMP/PKA Pathway by Asiaticoside Ameliorates High Glucose-Induced Inflammation and Apoptosis of Retinal Pigment Epithelial Cells. *J. Bioenerg. Biomembr.* **2022**, *54*, 9–16. [CrossRef] [PubMed]
96. Ke, M.; Hu, X.-Q.; Ouyang, J.; Dai, B.; Xu, Y. The Effect of Astragalin on the VEGF Production of Cultured Müller Cells under High Glucose Conditions. *Bio-Med. Mater. Eng.* **2012**, *22*, 113–119. [CrossRef] [PubMed]
97. D'Agata, V.; D'Amico, A.G.; Maugeri, G.; Bucolo, C.; Rossi, S.; Giunta, S. Carnosol Attenuates High Glucose Damage in Human Retinal Endothelial Cells through Regulation of ERK/Nrf2/HO-1 Pathway. *J. Asian Nat. Prod. Res.* **2023**, *25*, 783–795. [CrossRef] [PubMed]
98. Shu, X.; Hu, Y.; Huang, C.; Wei, N. Nimbolide Ameliorates the Streptozotocin-Induced Diabetic Retinopathy in Rats through the Inhibition of TLR4/NF-κB Signaling Pathway. *Saudi J. Biol. Sci.* **2021**, *28*, 4255–4262. [CrossRef] [PubMed]
99. Shi, Q.; Wang, J.; Cheng, Y.; Dong, X.; Zhang, M.; Pei, C. Palbinone Alleviates Diabetic Retinopathy in STZ-induced Rats by Inhibiting NLRP3 Inflammatory Activity. *J. Biochem. Mol. Toxicol.* **2020**, *34*, e22489. [CrossRef] [PubMed]
100. Kumar, M.P.; Mamidala, E.; Al-Ghanim, K.A.; Al-Misned, F.; Mahboob, S. Evaluation of the Andrographolides Role and Its Indoleamine 2,3-Dioxygenase Inhibitory Potential and Attendant Molecular Mechanism against STZ-Induced Diabetic Rats. *Saudi J. Biol. Sci.* **2020**, *27*, 713–719. [CrossRef]
101. Zeng, X.; Deng, Y.; Yuan, M.; He, Q.; Wu, Y.; Li, S. Study on the Antioxidant Effect of Tanshinone IIA on Diabetic Retinopathy and Its Mechanism Based on Integrated Pharmacology. *Evid.-Based Complement. Altern. Med.* **2022**, *2022*, 9990937. [CrossRef] [PubMed]
102. Zhao, L.; Sun, J.; Shi, S.; Qin, X.; Zhang, K.; Xu, J. Kaempferol Protects Retinal Ganglion Ceils from High-Glucose-Induced Injury by Regulating Vasohibin-1. *Neurosci. Lett.* **2020**, *716*, 134633. [CrossRef] [PubMed]
103. Xu, X.H.; Zhao, C.; Peng, Q.; Xie, P.; Liu, Q.H. Kaempferol Inhibited VEGF and PGF Expression and in Vitro Angiogenesis of HRECs under Diabetic-like Environment. *Braz. J. Med. Biol. Res.* **2017**, *50*, e5396. [CrossRef] [PubMed]
104. Zhang, Y.; Gao, Z.; Gao, X.; Yuan, Z.; Ma, T.; Li, G.; Zhang, X. Tilianin Protects Diabetic Retina through the Modulation of Nrf2/TXNIP/NLRP3 Inflammasome Pathways. *J. Environ. Pathol. Toxicol. Oncol.* **2020**, *39*, 89–99. [CrossRef] [PubMed]
105. Jiang, B.; Geng, Q.; Li, T.; Mohammad Firdous, S.; Zhou, X. Morin Attenuates STZ-Induced Diabetic Retinopathy in Experimental Animals. *Saudi J. Biol. Sci.* **2020**, *27*, 2139–2142. [CrossRef] [PubMed]
106. Yu, X.; Liu, Q.; Wang, X.; Liu, H.; Wang, Y. 7,8-Dihydroxyflavone Ameliorates High-Glucose Induced Diabetic Apoptosis in Human Retinal Pigment Epithelial Cells by Activating TrkB. *Biochem. Biophys. Res. Commun.* **2018**, *495*, 922–927. [CrossRef] [PubMed]
107. Miyata, Y.; Nagase, T.; Katsura, Y.; Takahashi, H.; Natsugari, H.; Oshitari, T.; Kosano, H. In Vitro Studies on Nobiletin Isolated from Citrus Plants and the Bioactive Metabolites, Inhibitory Action against Gelatinase Enzymatic Activity and the Molecular Mechanisms in Human Retinal Müller Cell Line. *Biomed. Pharmacother.* **2017**, *93*, 70–80. [CrossRef] [PubMed]
108. Kumar, M.P.; Sankeshi, V.; Naik, R.R.; Thirupathi, P.; Das, B.; Raju, T.N. The Inhibitory Effect of Isoflavones Isolated from *Caesalpinia pulcherrima* on Aldose Reductase in STZ Induced Diabetic Rats. *Chem.-Biol. Interact.* **2015**, *237*, 18–24. [CrossRef] [PubMed]
109. Kim, J.; Kim, C.-S.; Moon, M.K.; Kim, J.S. Epicatechin Breaks Preformed Glycated Serum Albumin and Reverses the Retinal Accumulation of Advanced Glycation End Products. *Eur. J. Pharmacol.* **2015**, *748*, 108–114. [CrossRef] [PubMed]
110. Li, X.; Zhao, H.; Wang, Q.; Liang, H.; Jiang, X. Fucoidan Protects ARPE-19 Cells from Oxidative Stress via Normalization of Reactive Oxygen Species Generation through the Ca^{2+}-Dependent ERK Signaling Pathway. *Mol. Med. Rep.* **2015**, *11*, 3746–3752. [CrossRef]

111. Yang, W.; Yu, X.; Zhang, Q.; Lu, Q.; Wang, J.; Cui, W.; Zheng, Y.; Wang, X.; Luo, D. Attenuation of Streptozotocin-Induced Diabetic Retinopathy with Low Molecular Weight Fucoidan via Inhibition of Vascular Endothelial Growth Factor. *Exp. Eye Res.* **2013**, *115*, 96–105. [CrossRef] [PubMed]
112. Wu, J.; Ke, X.; Wang, W.; Zhang, H.; Ma, N.; Fu, W.; Zhao, M.; Gao, X.; Hao, X.; Zhang, Z. Aloe-Emodin Suppresses Hypoxia-Induced Retinal Angiogenesis via Inhibition of HIF-1α/VEGF Pathway. *Int. J. Biol. Sci.* **2016**, *12*, 1363–1371. [CrossRef] [PubMed]
113. Hao, Y.; Gao, X. Diosgenin Protects Retinal Pigment Epithelial Cells from Inflammatory Damage and Oxidative Stress Induced by High Glucose by Activating *AMPK/Nrf2/HO-1* Pathway. *Immun. Inflam. Dis.* **2022**, *10*, e698. [CrossRef]
114. Liao, W.-L.; Huang, C.-P.; Wang, H.-P.; Lei, Y.-J.; Lin, H.-J.; Huang, Y.-C. Diosgenin, a Natural Steroidal Sapogenin, Alleviates the Progression of Diabetic Retinopathy in Diabetic Mice. *In Vivo* **2023**, *37*, 661–666. [CrossRef] [PubMed]
115. Kim, I.; Seo, J.; Lee, D.H.; Kim, Y.-H.; Kim, J.-H.; Wie, M.-B.; Byun, J.-K.; Yun, J.-H. Ulmus Davidiana 60% Edible Ethanolic Extract for Prevention of Pericyte Apoptosis in Diabetic Retinopathy. *Front. Endocrinol.* **2023**, *14*, 1138676. [CrossRef] [PubMed]
116. Abu-Amero, K.K.; Kondkar, A.A.; Chalam, K.V. Resveratrol and Ophthalmic Diseases. *Nutrients* **2016**, *8*, 200. [CrossRef] [PubMed]
117. Kang, J.-H.; Choung, S.-Y. Protective Effects of Resveratrol and Its Analogs on Age-Related Macular Degeneration In Vitro. *Arch. Pharm. Res.* **2016**, *39*, 1703–1715. [CrossRef] [PubMed]
118. Brown, K.; Theofanous, D.; Britton, R.G.; Aburido, G.; Pepper, C.; Sri Undru, S.; Howells, L. Resveratrol for the Management of Human Health: How Far Have We Come? A Systematic Review of Resveratrol Clinical Trials to Highlight Gaps and Opportunities. *Int. J. Mol. Sci.* **2024**, *25*, 747. [CrossRef] [PubMed]
119. Wang, T.; Lv, L.; Feng, H.; Gu, W. Unlocking the Potential: Quercetin and Its Natural Derivatives as Promising Therapeutics for Sepsis. *Biomedicines* **2024**, *12*, 444. [CrossRef] [PubMed]
120. Carrillo-Martinez, E.J.; Flores-Hernández, F.Y.; Salazar-Montes, A.M.; Nario-Chaidez, H.F.; Hernández-Ortega, L.D. Quercetin, a Flavonoid with Great Pharmacological Capacity. *Molecules* **2024**, *29*, 1000. [CrossRef]
121. Laky, M.; Arslan, M.; Zhu, X.; Rausch-Fan, X.; Moritz, A.; Sculean, A.; Laky, B.; Ramseier, C.A.; Stähli, A.; Eick, S. Quercetin in the Prevention of Induced Periodontal Disease in Animal Models: A Systematic Review and Meta-Analysis. *Nutrients* **2024**, *16*, 735. [CrossRef]
122. Wang, K.; Feng, X.; Chai, L.; Cao, S.; Qiu, F. The Metabolism of Berberine and Its Contribution to the Pharmacological Effects. *Drug Metab. Rev.* **2017**, *49*, 139–157. [CrossRef] [PubMed]
123. Stoyanova, N.; Ignatova, M.; Manolova, N.; Rashkov, I.; Toshkova, R.; Georgieva, A. Nanoparticles Based on Complex of Berberine Chloride and Polymethacrylic or Polyacrylic Acid with Antioxidant and in Vitro Antitumor Activities. *Int. J. Pharm.* **2020**, *584*, 119426. [CrossRef] [PubMed]
124. Ratanakomol, T.; Roytrakul, S.; Wikan, N.; Smith, D.R. Berberine Inhibits Dengue Virus through Dual Mechanisms. *Molecules* **2021**, *26*, 5501. [CrossRef]
125. Wat, N.; Wong, R.L.; Wong, I.Y. Associations between Diabetic Retinopathy and Systemic Risk Factors. *Hong Kong Med. J.* **2016**, *22*, 589–599. [CrossRef]
126. He, Z.; Hu, Y.; Niu, Z.; Zhong, K.; Liu, T.; Yang, M.; Ji, L.; Hu, W. A Review of Pharmacokinetic and Pharmacological Properties of Asiaticoside, a Major Active Constituent of *Centella asiatica* (L.) Urb. *J. Ethnopharmacol.* **2023**, *302*, 115865. [CrossRef] [PubMed]
127. Liu, Y.; Zhao, J.; Mu, X.; Deng, J.; Wu, X.; He, W.; Liu, Y.; Gu, R.; Han, F.; Nie, X. Asiaticoside-Nitric Oxide Promoting Diabetic Wound Healing through the miRNA-21-5p/TGF-B1/SMAD7/TIMP3 Signaling Pathway. *J. Ethnopharmacol.* **2024**, *319*, 117266. [CrossRef] [PubMed]
128. Mao, X.; Wu, Y.; Wu, K.; Liu, M.; Zhang, J.; Zou, F.; Ou-Yang, J. *Astragalus* Polysaccharide Reduces Hepatic Endoplasmic Reticulum Stress and Restores Glucose Homeostasis in a Diabetic KKAy Mouse Model. *Acta Pharmacol. Sin.* **2007**, *28*, 1947–1956. [CrossRef] [PubMed]
129. Liu, M.; Wu, K.; Mao, X.; Wu, Y.; Ouyang, J. Astragalus Polysaccharide Improves Insulin Sensitivity in KKAy Mice: Regulation of PKB/GLUT4 Signaling in Skeletal Muscle. *J. Ethnopharmacol.* **2010**, *127*, 32–37. [CrossRef] [PubMed]
130. Mao, X.; Yu, F.; Wang, N.; Wu, Y.; Zou, F.; Wu, K.; Liu, M.; Ouyang, J. Hypoglycemic Effect of Polysaccharide Enriched Extract of *Astragalus membranaceus* in Diet Induced Insulin Resistant C57BL/6J Mice and Its Potential Mechanism. *Phytomedicine* **2009**, *16*, 416–425. [CrossRef] [PubMed]
131. Liu, Y.; Lu, M.; Sun, Q.; Guo, Z.; Lin, Y.; Li, S.; Huang, Y.; Li, Y.; Fu, Q. Magnolol Attenuates Macrophage Pyroptosis Triggered by *Streptococcus equi* Subsp. *zooepidemicus*. *Int. Immunopharmacol.* **2024**, *131*, 111922. [CrossRef] [PubMed]
132. Szałabska-Rąpała, K.; Zych, M.; Borymska, W.; Londzin, P.; Dudek, S.; Kaczmarczyk-Żebrowska, I. Beneficial Effect of Honokiol and Magnolol on Polyol Pathway and Oxidative Stress Parameters in the Testes of Diabetic Rats. *Biomed. Pharmacother.* **2024**, *172*, 116265. [CrossRef] [PubMed]
133. Zhang, H.; Zhang, Y.; Hu, Y.; Wei, S.; Adu-Frimpong, M.; Sun, C.; Qi, G. Improving Cellular Uptake and Synergetic Anti-Tumor Effects of Magnolol and *Brucea javanica* Oil through Self-Microemulsion. *Drug Dev. Ind. Pharm.* **2024**, 1–9. [CrossRef] [PubMed]
134. Lin, H.; Qiu, S.; Xie, L.; Liu, C.; Sun, S. Nimbolide Suppresses Non-Small Cell Lung Cancer Cell Invasion and Migration via Manipulation of DUSP4 Expression and ERK1/2 Signaling. *Biomed. Pharmacother.* **2017**, *92*, 340–346. [CrossRef] [PubMed]
135. Nagini, S.; Nivetha, R.; Palrasu, M.; Mishra, R. Nimbolide, a Neem Limonoid, Is a Promising Candidate for the Anticancer Drug Arsenal. *J. Med. Chem.* **2021**, *64*, 3560–3577. [CrossRef]

136. Munipally, P.K.; Agraharm, S.G.; Valavala, V.K.; Gundae, S.; Turlapati, N.R. Evaluation of Indoleamine 2,3-Dioxygenase Expression and Kynurenine Pathway Metabolites Levels in Serum Samples of Diabetic Retinopathy Patients. *Arch. Physiol. Biochem.* **2011**, *117*, 254–258. [CrossRef] [PubMed]
137. Wu, S.; Lu, D.; Gajendran, B.; Hu, Q.; Zhang, J.; Wang, S.; Han, M.; Xu, Y.; Shen, X. Tanshinone IIA Ameliorates Experimental Diabetic Cardiomyopathy by Inhibiting Endoplasmic Reticulum Stress in Cardiomyocytes via SIRT1. *Phytother. Res.* **2023**, *37*, 3543–3558. [CrossRef] [PubMed]
138. Zhai, P.; Chen, Q.; Wang, X.; Ouyang, X.; Yang, M.; Dong, Y.; Li, J.; Li, Y.; Luo, S.; Liu, Y.; et al. The Combination of Tanshinone IIA and Astragaloside IV Attenuates Myocardial Ischemia-Reperfusion Injury by Inhibiting the STING Pathway. *Chin. Med.* **2024**, *19*, 34. [CrossRef] [PubMed]
139. Wang, J.; Wang, Z.; Liu, J.; Zhou, M.; Wang, H.; Zhu, H.; Jiang, M.; Bo, Q.; Sun, X. Chrysin Alleviates DNA Damage to Improve Disturbed Immune Homeostasis and Pro-Angiogenic Environment in Laser-Induced Choroidal Neovascularization. *Biochim. Biophys. Acta Mol. Cell Res.* **2024**, *1871*, 119657. [CrossRef] [PubMed]
140. Zeng, H.; Liu, C.; Wan, L.; Peng, L.; Wen, S.; Fang, W.; Chen, H.; Wang, K.; Yang, X.; Huang, J.; et al. (-)-Epicatechin Ameliorates Type 2 Diabetes Mellitus by Reshaping the Gut Microbiota and Gut-Liver Axis in GK Rats. *Food Chem.* **2024**, *447*, 138916. [CrossRef] [PubMed]
141. Qu, Z.; Liu, A.; Li, P.; Liu, C.; Xiao, W.; Huang, J.; Liu, Z.; Zhang, S. Advances in Physiological Functions and Mechanisms of (-)-Epicatechin. *Crit. Rev. Food Sci. Nutr.* **2021**, *61*, 211–233. [CrossRef] [PubMed]
142. Kang, Q.; Dai, H.; Jiang, S.; Yu, L. Advanced Glycation End Products in Diabetic Retinopathy and Phytochemical Therapy. *Front. Nutr.* **2022**, *9*, 1037186. [CrossRef] [PubMed]
143. Luoa, H.; Jia, X.; Zhanga, M.; Renb, Y.; Tana, R.; Jianga, H.; Wua, X. Aloe-Emodin: Progress in Pharmacological Activity, Safety, and Pharmaceutical Formulation Applications. *Mini Rev. Med. Chem.* **2024**. [CrossRef] [PubMed]
144. Gupta, S.K.; Kumar, B.; Nag, T.C.; Srinivasan, B.P.; Srivastava, S.; Gaur, S.; Saxena, R. Effects of *Trigonella foenum-graecum* (L.) on Retinal Oxidative Stress, and Proinflammatory and Angiogenic Molecular Biomarkers in Streptozotocin-Induced Diabetic Rats. *Mol. Cell Biochem.* **2014**, *388*, 1–9. [CrossRef] [PubMed]
145. Fortmann, S.P.; Burda, B.U.; Senger, C.A.; Lin, J.S.; Whitlock, E.P. Vitamin and Mineral Supplements in the Primary Prevention of Cardiovascular Disease and Cancer: An Updated Systematic Evidence Review for the U.S. Preventive Services Task Force. *Ann. Intern. Med.* **2013**, *159*, 824–834. [CrossRef] [PubMed]
146. Long, M.; Wang, C.; Liu, D. Glycated Hemoglobin A1C and Vitamin D and Their Association with Diabetic Retinopathy Severity. *Nutr. Diabetes* **2017**, *7*, e281. [CrossRef] [PubMed]
147. Kaur, H.; Donaghue, K.C.; Chan, A.K.; Benitez-Aguirre, P.; Hing, S.; Lloyd, M.; Cusumano, J.; Pryke, A.; Craig, M.E. Vitamin D Deficiency Is Associated with Retinopathy in Children and Adolescents with Type 1 Diabetes. *Diabetes Care* **2011**, *34*, 1400–1402. [CrossRef] [PubMed]
148. Millen, A.E.; Sahli, M.W.; Nie, J.; LaMonte, M.J.; Lutsey, P.L.; Klein, B.E.K.; Mares, J.A.; Meyers, K.J.; Andrews, C.A.; Klein, R. Adequate Vitamin D Status Is Associated with the Reduced Odds of Prevalent Diabetic Retinopathy in African Americans and Caucasians. *Cardiovasc. Diabetol.* **2016**, *15*, 128. [CrossRef]
149. Lee, M.-Y.; Seo, C.-S.; Ha, H.; Jung, D.; Lee, H.; Lee, N.-H.; Lee, J.-A.; Kim, J.-H.; Lee, Y.-K.; Son, J.-K.; et al. Protective Effects of Ulmus Davidiana Var. Japonica against OVA-Induced Murine Asthma Model via Upregulation of Heme Oxygenase-1. *J. Ethnopharmacol.* **2010**, *130*, 61–69. [CrossRef] [PubMed]
150. Choi, H.G.; Park, Y.M.; Lu, Y.; Chang, H.W.; Na, M.; Lee, S.H. Inhibition of Prostaglandin D_2 Production by Trihydroxy Fatty Acids Isolated from Ulmus Davidiana Var. Japonica. *Phytother. Res.* **2013**, *27*, 1376–1380. [CrossRef] [PubMed]
151. Pan, J.H.; Lim, Y.; Kim, J.H.; Heo, W.; Lee, K.Y.; Shin, H.J.; Kim, J.K.; Lee, J.H.; Kim, Y.J. Root Bark of Ulmus Davidiana Var. Japonica Restrains Acute Alcohol-Induced Hepatic Steatosis Onset in Mice by Inhibiting ROS Accumulation. *PLoS ONE* **2017**, *12*, e0188381. [CrossRef] [PubMed]
152. Lee, D.-E.; Jang, E.H.; Bang, C.; Kim, G.L.; Yoon, S.Y.; Lee, D.H.; Koo, J.; Na, J.H.; Lee, S.; Kim, J.-H. Bakuchiol, Main Component of Root Bark of Ulmus Davidiana Var. Japonica, Inhibits TGF-β-Induced in Vitro EMT and In Vivo Metastasis. *Arch. Biochem. Biophys.* **2021**, *709*, 108969. [CrossRef] [PubMed]
153. Del Amo, E.M.; Rimpelä, A.-K.; Heikkinen, E.; Kari, O.K.; Ramsay, E.; Lajunen, T.; Schmitt, M.; Pelkonen, L.; Bhattacharya, M.; Richardson, D.; et al. Pharmacokinetic Aspects of Retinal Drug Delivery. *Prog. Retin. Eye Res.* **2017**, *57*, 134–185. [CrossRef] [PubMed]
154. Thomas, S.E.; Harrison, E.H. Mechanisms of Selective Delivery of Xanthophylls to Retinal Pigment Epithelial Cells by Human Lipoproteins. *J. Lipid Res.* **2016**, *57*, 1865–1878. [CrossRef] [PubMed]
155. Silva, M.; Peng, T.; Zhao, X.; Li, S.; Farhan, M.; Zheng, W. Recent Trends in Drug-Delivery Systems for the Treatment of Diabetic Retinopathy and Associated Fibrosis. *Adv. Drug Deliv. Rev.* **2021**, *173*, 439–460. [CrossRef] [PubMed]
156. Rezvan, N.; Moini, A.; Janani, L.; Mohammad, K.; Saedisomeolia, A.; Nourbakhsh, M.; Gorgani-Firuzjaee, S.; Mazaherioun, M.; Hosseinzadeh-Attar, M.J. Effects of Quercetin on Adiponectin-Mediated Insulin Sensitivity in Polycystic Ovary Syndrome: A Randomized Placebo-Controlled Double-Blind Clinical Trial. *Horm. Metab. Res.* **2017**, *49*, 115–121. [CrossRef]
157. Edwards, R.L.; Lyon, T.; Litwin, S.E.; Rabovsky, A.; Symons, J.D.; Jalili, T. Quercetin Reduces Blood Pressure in Hypertensive Subjects. *J. Nutr.* **2007**, *137*, 2405–2411. [CrossRef]

158. Brüll, V.; Burak, C.; Stoffel-Wagner, B.; Wolffram, S.; Nickenig, G.; Müller, C.; Langguth, P.; Alteheld, B.; Fimmers, R.; Stehle, P.; et al. No Effects of Quercetin from Onion Skin Extract on Serum Leptin and Adiponectin Concentrations in Overweight-to-Obese Patients with (Pre-)Hypertension: A Randomized Double-Blinded, Placebo-Controlled Crossover Trial. *Eur. J. Nutr.* **2017**, *56*, 2265–2275. [CrossRef] [PubMed]
159. Gui, S.; Tang, W.; Huang, Z.; Wang, X.; Gui, S.; Gao, X.; Xiao, D.; Tao, L.; Jiang, Z.; Wang, X. Ultrasmall Coordination Polymer Nanodots Fe-Quer Nanozymes for Preventing and Delaying the Development and Progression of Diabetic Retinopathy. *Adv. Funct. Mater.* **2023**, *33*, 2300261. [CrossRef]
160. Toragall, V.; Muzaffar, J.C.; Baskaran, V. Lutein Loaded Double-Layered Polymer Nanocarrier Modulate H_2O_2 and $CoCl_2$ Induced Oxidative and Hypoxia Damage and Angiogenic Markers in ARPE-19 Cells. *Int. J. Biol. Macromol.* **2023**, *240*, 124378. [CrossRef]
161. Ramsay, E.; Hagström, M.; Vellonen, K.-S.; Boman, S.; Toropainen, E.; Del Amo, E.M.; Kidron, H.; Urtti, A.; Ruponen, M. Role of Retinal Pigment Epithelium Permeability in Drug Transfer between Posterior Eye Segment and Systemic Blood Circulation. *Eur. J. Pharm. Biopharm.* **2019**, *143*, 18–23. [CrossRef]
162. Del Amo, E.M.; Urtti, A. Rabbit as an Animal Model for Intravitreal Pharmacokinetics: Clinical Predictability and Quality of the Published Data. *Exp. Eye Res.* **2015**, *137*, 111–124. [CrossRef] [PubMed]
163. Mandal, S.K.; Maji, A.K.; Mishra, S.K.; Ishfaq, P.M.; Devkota, H.P.; Silva, A.S.; Das, N. Goldenseal (*Hydrastis canadensis* L.) and Its Active Constituents: A Critical Review of Their Efficacy and Toxicological Issues. *Pharmacol. Res.* **2020**, *160*, 105085. [CrossRef] [PubMed]
164. Yarmohammadi, F.; Hayes, A.W.; Karimi, G. The Therapeutic Effects of Berberine against Different Diseases: A Review on the Involvement of the Endoplasmic Reticulum Stress. *Phytother. Res.* **2022**, *36*, 3215–3231. [CrossRef] [PubMed]
165. Kaur, P.; Mishra, S.K.; Mithal, A. Vitamin D Toxicity Resulting from Overzealous Correction of Vitamin D Deficiency. *Clin. Endocrinol.* **2015**, *83*, 327–331. [CrossRef] [PubMed]
166. Taylor, P.N.; Davies, J.S. A Review of the Growing Risk of Vitamin D Toxicity from Inappropriate Practice. *Br. J. Clin. Pharmacol.* **2018**, *84*, 1121–1127. [CrossRef] [PubMed]
167. Galior, K.; Grebe, S.; Singh, R. Development of Vitamin D Toxicity from Overcorrection of Vitamin D Deficiency: A Review of Case Reports. *Nutrients* **2018**, *10*, 953. [CrossRef] [PubMed]
168. Moreira, E.S.; Ames-Sibin, A.P.; Bonetti, C.I.; Leal, L.E.; Peralta, R.M.; de Sá-Nakanishi, A.B.; Comar, J.F.; Bracht, A.; Bracht, L. The Short-Term Effects of Berberine in the Liver: Narrow Margins between Benefits and Toxicity. *Toxicol. Lett.* **2022**, *368*, 56–65. [CrossRef] [PubMed]
169. Wang, Y.-K.; Li, W.Q.; Xia, S.; Guo, L.; Miao, Y.; Zhang, B.-K. Metabolic Activation of the Toxic Natural Products From Herbal and Dietary Supplements Leading to Toxicities. *Front. Pharmacol.* **2021**, *12*, 758468. [CrossRef]
170. Nencini, C.; Galluzzi, P.; Pippi, F.; Menchiari, A.; Micheli, L. Hepatotoxicity of *Teucrium chamaedrys* L. Decoction: Role of Difference in the Harvesting Area and Preparation Method. *Indian J. Pharmacol.* **2014**, *46*, 181–184. [CrossRef] [PubMed]
171. Bessone, F.; García-Cortés, M.; Medina-Caliz, I.; Hernandez, N.; Parana, R.; Mendizabal, M.; Schinoni, M.I.; Ridruejo, E.; Nunes, V.; Peralta, M.; et al. Herbal and Dietary Supplements-Induced Liver Injury in Latin America: Experience From the LATINDILI Network. *Clin. Gastroenterol. Hepatol.* **2022**, *20*, e548–e563. [CrossRef] [PubMed]
172. Xie, P.; Fujii, I.; Zhao, J.; Shinohara, M.; Matsukura, M. A Novel Polysaccharide Compound Derived from Algae Extracts Protects Retinal Pigment Epithelial Cells from High Glucose-Induced Oxidative Damage In Vitro. *Biol. Pharm. Bull.* **2012**, *35*, 1447–1453. [CrossRef] [PubMed]
173. Li, X.; Zhang, J.; He, R.; Su, X.; Li, Z.; Xie, X. Effect of Chinese Herbal Compounds on Ocular Fundus Signs and Vision in Conventional Treated-Persons with Non-Proliferative Diabetic Retinopathy: A Systematic Review and Meta-Analysis. *Front. Endocrinol.* **2022**, *13*, 977971. [CrossRef] [PubMed]
174. Wang, X.; Zhu, H.-J.; Munoz, J.; Gurley, B.J.; Markowitz, J.S. An Ex Vivo Approach to Botanical-Drug Interactions: A Proof of Concept Study. *J. Ethnopharmacol.* **2015**, *163*, 149–156. [CrossRef] [PubMed]
175. Li, L.; Sun, S.; Weng, Y.; Song, F.; Zhou, S.; Bai, M.; Zhou, H.; Zeng, S.; Jiang, H. Interaction of Six Protoberberine Alkaloids with Human Organic Cation Transporters 1, 2 and 3. *Xenobiotica* **2016**, *46*, 175–183. [CrossRef] [PubMed]
176. Zhang, D.; Liu, H.; Xie, L.; Liu, X. Effect of Baicalin and Berberine on Transport of Nimodipine on Primary-Cultured, Rat Brain Microvascular Endothelial Cells. *Acta Pharmacol. Sin.* **2007**, *28*, 573–578. [CrossRef] [PubMed]
177. Xiang, Z.-D.; Guan, H.-D.; Zhao, X.; Xie, Q.; Cai, F.-J.; Xie, Z.-J.; Dang, R.; Li, M.-L.; Wang, C.-H. Protoberberine Alkaloids: A Review of the Gastroprotective Effects, Pharmacokinetics, and Toxicity. *Phytomedicine* **2024**, *126*, 155444. [CrossRef] [PubMed]
178. Patil, D.; Gautam, M.; Gairola, S.; Jadhav, S.; Patwardhan, B. Effect of Botanical Immunomodulators on Human CYP3A4 Inhibition: Implications for Concurrent Use as Adjuvants in Cancer Therapy. *Integr. Cancer Ther.* **2014**, *13*, 167–175. [CrossRef]
179. Singh, A.; Zhao, K.; Bell, C.; Shah, A.J. Effect of Berberine on in Vitro Metabolism of Sulfonylureas: A Herb-Drug Interactions Study. *Rapid Commun. Mass Spectrom.* **2020**, *34* (Suppl. S4), e8651. [CrossRef] [PubMed]
180. Shi, R.; Xu, Z.; Xu, X.; Jin, J.; Zhao, Y.; Wang, T.; Li, Y.; Ma, Y. Organic Cation Transporter and Multidrug and Toxin Extrusion 1 Co-Mediated Interaction between Metformin and Berberine. *Eur. J. Pharm. Sci.* **2019**, *127*, 282–290. [CrossRef]
181. Oh, S.; Kim, Y.J.; Lee, E.K.; Park, S.W.; Yu, H.G. Antioxidative Effects of Ascorbic Acid and Astaxanthin on ARPE-19 Cells in an Oxidative Stress Model. *Antioxidants* **2020**, *9*, 833. [CrossRef] [PubMed]

182. Yuan, M.; He, Q.; Long, Z.; Zhu, X.; Xiang, W.; Wu, Y.; Lin, S. Exploring the Pharmacological Mechanism of Liuwei Dihuang Decoction for Diabetic Retinopathy: A Systematic Biological Strategy-Based Research. *Evid. -Based Complement. Altern. Med.* **2021**, *2021*, 5544518. [CrossRef] [PubMed]
183. Li, H.-D.; Li, M.-X.; Zhang, W.-H.; Zhang, S.-W.; Gong, Y.-B. Effectiveness and Safety of Traditional Chinese Medicine for Diabetic Retinopathy: A Systematic Review and Network Meta-Analysis of Randomized Clinical Trials. *World J. Diabetes* **2023**, *14*, 1422–1449. [CrossRef] [PubMed]
184. Yao, H.; Liu, J.; Xu, S.; Zhu, Z.; Xu, J. The Structural Modification of Natural Products for Novel Drug Discovery. *Expert Opin. Drug Discov.* **2017**, *12*, 121–140. [CrossRef]

biomedicines

MDPI

Review

Aldose Reductase as a Key Target in the Prevention and Treatment of Diabetic Retinopathy: A Comprehensive Review

Alexandra-Ioana Dănilă [1], Laura Andreea Ghenciu [2,*], Emil Robert Stoicescu [3,4,5,6], Sorin Lucian Bolintineanu [1], Roxana Iacob [1,3,4], Mihai-Alexandru Săndesc [7] and Alexandra Corina Faur [1]

1 Department of Anatomy and Embriology, 'Victor Babes' University of Medicine and Pharmacy Timisoara, Eftimie Murgu Square No. 2, 300041 Timisoara, Romania; alexandra.danila@umft.ro (A.-I.D.); s.bolintineanu@umft.ro (S.L.B.); roxana.iacob@umft.ro (R.I.); faur.alexandra@umft.ro (A.C.F.)
2 Department of Functional Sciences, 'Victor Babes' University of Medicine and Pharmacy Timisoara, Eftimie Murgu Square No. 2, 300041 Timisoara, Romania
3 Doctoral School, 'Victor Babes' University of Medicine and Pharmacy Timisoara, Eftimie Murgu Square No. 2, 300041 Timisoara, Romania; stoicescu.emil@umft.ro
4 Field of Applied Engineering Sciences, Specialization Statistical Methods and Techniques in Health and Clinical Research, Faculty of Mechanics, 'Politehnica' University Timisoara, Mihai Viteazul Boulevard No. 1, 300222 Timisoara, Romania
5 Department of Radiology and Medical Imaging, 'Victor Babes' University of Medicine and Pharmacy Timisoara, Eftimie Murgu Square No. 2, 300041 Timisoara, Romania
6 Research Center for Pharmaco-Toxicological Evaluations, 'Victor Babes' University of Medicine and Pharmacy Timisoara, Eftimie Murgu Square No. 2, 300041 Timisoara, Romania
7 Department of Orthopedics and Traumatology, 'Victor Babes' University of Medicine and Pharmacy Timisoara, Eftimie Murgu Square No. 2, 300041 Timisoara, Romania; sandesc.mihai@umft.ro
* Correspondence: bolintineanu.laura@umft.ro

Abstract: The escalating global prevalence of diabetes mellitus (DM) over the past two decades has led to a persistent high incidence of diabetic retinopathy (DR), necessitating screening for early symptoms and proper treatment. Effective management of DR aims to decrease vision impairment by controlling modifiable risk factors including hypertension, obesity, and dyslipidemia. Moreover, systemic medications and plant-based therapy show promise in advancing DR treatment. One of the key mechanisms related to DR pathogenesis is the polyol pathway, through which aldose reductase (AR) catalyzes the conversion of glucose to sorbitol within various tissues, including the retina, lens, ciliary body and iris. Elevated glucose levels activate AR, leading to osmotic stress, advanced glycation end-product formation, and oxidative damage. This further implies chronic inflammation, vascular permeability, and angiogenesis. Our comprehensive narrative review describes the therapeutic potential of aldose reductase inhibitors in treating DR, where both synthetic and natural inhibitors have been studied in recent decades. Our synthesis aims to guide future research and clinical interventions in DR management.

Keywords: diabetic retinopathy; aldose reductase; polyol pathway; aldose reductase inhibitor

1. Introduction

Diabetes mellitus (DM) is a multifactorial metabolic disorder characterized by dysregulation of glucose metabolism, originating from inadequate insulin secretion by pancreatic beta cells and/or impaired insulin sensitivity, leading to persistent hyperglycemia and several important complications. The most common complications of diabetes include neuropathy, retinopathy, nephropathy, and cardiovascular disease [1,2]. Approximately 12% of all new cases of severe visual impairment in the United States are caused by diabetic retinopathy (DR), which is the most common cause of blindness in adult patients [1,3]. Moreover, DR is the most common diagnosis for 80% of people who have had DM for more than 20 years. However, it was demonstrated that when effective therapies were given, at least 90% of new patients had their retinal structure and function restored [4]. Since there is currently insufficient effectiveness in screening for DR, the condition can advance unnoticed until irreversible ocular changes have occurred [5]. The pathophysiology of DR is characterized by a cascade of events including vascular endothelial dysfunction, breakdown of the blood–retinal barrier, microvascular occlusion, and ultimately retinal ischemia and neovascularization [6–8]. These changes result in a spectrum of clinical manifestations ranging from mild non-proliferative diabetic retinopathy (NPDR) to severe proliferative diabetic retinopathy (PDR), with the latter being associated with the highest risk of vision loss [6]. Several risk factors contribute to the development and progression of DR. Prolonged duration of diabetes, poor glycemic control, hypertension (both systemic and ocular), dyslipidemia, cigarette smoking, and genetic susceptibility are among the most significant factors [7]. Additionally, pregnancy can exacerbate DR, particularly in women with pre-existing diabetes; therefore, pre-conceptional care is needed [9].

Given the dramatic rise in the global prevalence of DM in the past 20 years and the ongoing high incidence of DR in patients with both type I and type II diabetes, screening is essential for prompt detection of patients who are showing symptoms of chronic hyperglycemia-related vision impairment and who need a thorough fundoscopy and proper treatment [10]. Management of DR aims to prevent vision loss by controlling modifiable risk factors, such as hypertension, obesity and dyslipidemia, and treating sight-threatening complications. Tight glycemic control, blood pressure management, and lipid-lowering therapy are essential components of DR management [7]. Additionally, systemic medications—hypoglycemic, hypolipidemic, and antihypertensive drugs—as well as plant-based pharmaceuticals have shown encouraging treatment in the advancement of DR [5,6,10]. Advances in the science of pluripotent stem cells have made it possible to restore retinal functions when these cells are transplanted into animals that have retinal degeneration [11]. In cases of advanced disease, laser photocoagulation, intravitreal injections containing antivascular endothelial growth factor (anti-VEGF) agents, and vitrectomy surgery may be indicated to stabilize or potentially improve vision [12].

Aldose reductase (AR), the first enzyme involved in the polyol pathway, plays an important role in the pathogenesis of DR. Elevated glucose levels in DM lead to increased activity of AR, resulting in the conversion of glucose to sorbitol within retinal cells. Sorbitol accumulation contributes to osmotic stress, formation of advanced glycation end (AGE) products, and depletion of NADPH, exacerbating oxidative damage and cellular dysfunction. Additionally, aldose reductase-derived fructose metabolism leads to the generation of diacylglycerol and activation of protein kinase C (PKC), further promoting low-grade inflammation, vascular permeability, and angiogenesis [13–15].

Our purpose was to conduct a comprehensive review focusing on the potential therapeutic efficacy of aldose reductase inhibitors in the treatment of diabetic retinopathy. Through our review, we aimed to critically evaluate the preclinical and clinical evidence supporting the use of synthetic and natural aldose reductase inhibitors as a therapeutic strategy for DR, with the ultimate goal of informing future research directions and clinical practice in the management of DR.

2. Pathophysiology

2.1. Hyperglycemia, Retinal Microvasculopathy and Metabolic Pathways

Based on its tissue-damaging effects, chronic hyperglycemia is the primary cause of disease development and progression in DR, as reported in the UKPDS [16] and DCCT [17] studies. Individual sensitivity to those effects, however, may be influenced by genetics, and other clinical variables, such as pregnancy, hypertension, and dyslipidemia, have also been linked [3,6,18]. The most important risk factors linked to the onset and progression of DR are described in Table 1.

Table 1. Risk factors for the onset and progression of diabetic retinopathy.

Risk Factor	Description
Duration of diabetes [17]	well-known risk factor for the development and progression of DR
Glycemic control [16,17]	poor glycemic control (high HbA1C) is linked to increased risk of DR
Intraocular/systemic blood pressure [16,19]	systemic hypertension might lead to progression of DR through increased vascular permeability and microvascular damage
Dyslipidemia [20]	elevated levels of triglycerides, low-density lipoprotein cholesterol (LDL-C), and reduced levels of high-density lipoprotein cholesterol (HDL-C) managed through diet modification and lipid-lowering drugs
Obesity [21]	elevated body mass index (BMI) and abdominal adiposity leads to the release of cytokines, adipokines and to insulin-resistance (which is thought to be an independent risk factor) weight management is essential
Cigarette smoking [22]	a modifiable risk factor can compromise retinal microvascular integrity and function
Genetic predisposition [23]	an important number of genetic variants have been studied can be managed by targeted therapy in high-risk patients

DR is known worldwide as a microvascular disease. It is believed that hyperglycemia is a key factor in the pathophysiology of retinal microvascular injury, which may lead to irreversible intra- and extracellular changes if untreated [24]. Numerous metabolic processes, such as the polyol path, the formation of AGEs, the PKC pathway, and the hexosamine pathway, have been linked to hyperglycemia-induced vascular injury. These pathways, in conjunction with genetic risk factors, ultimately lead to the activation of growth factors, cytokines and chemokines, which in consequence cause increased vascular permeability, microvascular occlusion, and malfunction of the vascular endothelium [18,25–27]. Following microvascular occlusion, retinal ischemia stimulates neovascularization and the development of intraretinal microvascular abnormalities [25].

2.1.1. The Polyol Pathway

Excess glucose is metabolized via overactivity of the polyol route causing irreversible cell damage. Nicotinamide adenine dinucleotide phosphate (NADPH) is used as a cofactor by the retinal enzyme AR to convert glucose to sorbitol. Sorbitol dehydrogenase (SDH), the second enzyme of the pathway, then transforms sorbitol into fructose. [13,14]. Osmotic injury is one of the many negative consequences of sorbitol accumulation in retinal cells [15]. There is insufficient NADPH available for use by glutathione reductase, which is essential for the production of reduced glutathione, as a result of NADPH being used as a cofactor in the first step of the polyol pathway. Subsequently, increased flux in the polyol pathway will cause oxidative stress and ultimately leading to damage of the retinal cells [13].

Early research on the pathophysiology of DR using the polyol pathway was carried out in diabetic animals [28,29]. These investigations demonstrated that the incidence and severity of diabetic retinal lesions in the galactose-fed rats might be decreased by treatment with synthetic aldose reductase inhibitors (ARIs).

Further study has shown that raised AR is localized in many retinal cells, such as glial cells [30], pericytes [31], retinal pigment epithelial cells [32], retinal endothelial cells [32], ganglion cells [30,33], and neurons [33]. These investigations also show that retinal cell degeneration correlates with elevated AR activity. Cell vitality decreased when capillary pericytes or endothelial cells were exposed to higher amounts of glucose or galactose. However, a few articles have emphasized that careful utilization of ARIs prevented cell death and inhibited specific DR changes [34,35].

2.1.2. Advanced Glycation End-Product (AGE) Formation

Although the exact mechanism is still uncertain, increased levels of AGEs in the bloodstream are typically associated with pathologies such as DR, leading to microvascular damage and blood-barrier disfunction. AGEs are heterogeneous compounds formed through non-enzymatic glycation reactions between reducing glucose and macromolecules, such as proteins, lipids, or nucleic acids [36]. In the context of DR, chronic exposure to high glucose levels fosters an accelerated formation and accumulation of AGEs within retinal tissues, making them a key therapeutic target in the potential treatment of DR. AGEs induce structural alterations in retinal proteins through protein cross-linking, thereby perturbing their normal function. Moreover, AGEs trigger a state of increased oxidative stress by generating reactive oxygen species (ROS), which in turn exacerbate pro-inflammatory signaling, microvascular abnormalities and cell death [37]. Furthermore, AGEs modulate the composition of the retinal extracellular matrix (ECM) by directly promoting the synthesis of fibronectin, collagen, and other ECM components. Aberrant ECM remodeling disrupts the structural integrity of retinal blood vessels, fostering fibrosis and exacerbating microvascular dysfunction [38].

Only a small percentage of AGEs that arise in vivo have received thorough characterization and structural definition to date [36]. The rate at which proteins are broken down for glycoxidation, the intensity of hyperglycemia, and the level of oxidative stress in the surroundings are critical elements that determine the development of AGEs [39]. Apart from the endogenous pathway of AGEs, another source is the exogenous path, through smoking and diet [40].

Microvascular alterations, including capillary dropout, microaneurysm formation, and increased vascular permeability, lead to retinal ischemia, vitreous hemorrhage, exudative retinal detachment, and diabetic macular edema. Chronic low-grade inflammation and oxidative stress further exacerbate retinal damage, promoting neurodegeneration, including retinal ganglion cell loss, thinning of the retinal nerve fiber layer, and disruption of the neurovascular unit [25,36].

2.1.3. Protein Kinase C (PKC) Activation

In response to prolonged hyperglycemia, PKC isoforms, particularly PKC-β, are activated within endothelial cells, pericytes, and Müller cells. PKC activation mediates multiple pathological processes, including increased microvascular permeability, endothelial dysfunction, leukostasis (which is believed to be of utmost importance in the beginning of DR), retinal microvascular constriction, and chronic inflammation [24,25]. Furthermore, PKC signaling pathways contribute to the upregulation of VEGF, a key mediator of abnormal angiogenesis and vascular leakage in DR, which can ultimately lead to vitreous hemorrhage and exudative retinal detachment. Consequently, PKC activation exacerbates retinal microvascular abnormalities, promotes prolonged retinal inflammation, and contributes to the progression and complications of DR [24].

2.1.4. The Hexosamine Pathway

In DR, increased flux through the hexosamine pathway occurs due to elevated intracellular glucose levels. This pathway diverts excess glucose metabolites, particularly fructose-6-phosphate, into the production of uridine diphosphate N-acetylglucosamine (UDP-GlcNAc). Elevated UDP-GlcNAc levels lead to hyperglycosylation of proteins, altering their structure and function, and to altered gene expression, ultimately leading to cell apoptosis [24]. This process contributes to the pathogenesis of DR by promoting exaggerated inflammation, oxidative stress, and vascular endothelial dysfunction, exacerbating vascular abnormalities and retinal damage [24,41].

2.2. Oxidative Stress

Oxidative stress in DR arises from an imbalance between the production ROS and the antioxidant defense system. Sustained hyperglycemia leads to excess ROS generation within retinal cells, overwhelming antioxidant mechanisms and causing cellular damage. Chronic oxidative stress contributes to damage to macromolecules (DNA, lipids, proteins), vascular dysfunction, inflammation, neurodegeneration, and ultimately vision impairment in diabetic retinopathy. Research on animals has shown that oxidative stress has a role in the development of DR, as well as the metabolic memory phenomenon, which is the resistance of DR changes after adequate glucose levels restored [37].

2.3. *Inflammation*

Inflammation in DR involves the activation of inflammatory pathways due to low-grade chronic hyperglycemia. This triggers the release of pro-inflammatory cytokines-tumor necrosis factor-alpha (TNF-α), interleukin-1β (IL-1β), and interleukin-6 (IL-6) and adhesion molecule intercellular adhesion molecule-1 (ICAM-1) and vascular cell adhesion molecule-1 (VCAM-1), in diabetic animal models and patients, leading to leukostasis, vascular lesions, and recruitment of monocytes and granulocytes into the retina [42]. Inflammatory processes contribute to vascular abnormalities, neurodegeneration, and vision impairment.

2.4. *Vascular Endothelial Growth Factor (VEGF)*

VEGF plays an important role in DR, leading to abnormal angiogenesis and vascular leakage; additionally, it is one of the factors implicated in the development of DME. Hyperglycemia stimulates VEGF production, promoting vascular endothelial cell proliferation, increased vasopermeability and cell migration [40,43,44]. It is currently believed that VEGF functions as an NPDR modulator, and also as a primary PDR initiator. Studies have indicated an association between blood VEGF concentrations and the severity of vascular and retinal changes, as well as the incidence of DR [8]. Nineteen patients with NPDR and twenty patients with PDR had their VEGF concentrations tested in the study of Jain et al. The results were compared to those of nineteen diabetics without ocular disease and nineteen healthy controls. With VEGF, the degree of retinopathy significantly increased [45].

2.5. *Retinal Neurodegeneration*

Retinal neurodegeneration is one of the first phenomena in the development of DR and involves progressive damage to ganglion cells, amacrine cells, and photoreceptors, due to chronic hyperglycemia and associated metabolic disturbances. This event manifests as thinning of the retinal nerve fiber layer (RNFL), loss of neuronal function, and cell apoptosis [44,46]. Contributing factors include oxidative stress, inflammation, altered neurotrophic support, and impaired neurotransmission. Retinal neurodegeneration in DR contributes to vision loss and other visual impairments independent of vascular changes, highlighting that this process may be an independent risk factor [46].

3. Biology and Characterization of Aldose Reductase

Aldose reductase, a cytosolic enzyme, is present in various tissues throughout the body, including the retina and presents important substrate specificity [40]. It is particularly abundant in tissues exposed to high glucose concentrations, such as the kidneys, lens, and myelin sheath tissues, and a key factor in developing several of the most important DM complications. In the retina, aldose reductase is found in various cell types, including retinal endothelial cells, retinal capillary wall pericytes, retinal glial cells (Müller cells), and neuronal cells. The enzyme is encoded by the *AKR1B1* gene, and its expression and activity can be mediated by variable factors such as glucose levels, oxidative stress, and several inflammatory cytokines (such as IL-8, IL-6, TNF-alpha) [44,45].

Aldose reductase is a monomeric protein composed of a single polypeptide chain, which folds into a globular structure with multiple alpha-helices and beta-sheets. Aldose reductase also contains a substrate-binding site, where aldose substrates, such as glucose, bind for enzymatic conversion to their corresponding sugar alcohols (sorbitol) [47]. Additionally, the enzyme may have active allosteric-binding sites that modulate its activity in response to regulatory molecules [48]. The first stage of the two-step polyol cycle of glucose metabolism is the reduction of glucose to sorbitol (catalyzed by AR and requires NADPH), which is then transformed into fructose. Several tissues, such as the kidneys, Schwann cells, and retina, lack the enzyme SDH, which raises concerns about the sorbitol pathway. Because of this, sorbitol builds up to dangerous amounts in diabetics or people with exceptionally high glucose levels. Both SDH and AR activities must be strictly controlled at optimal level [49]. With chronic high glucose levels, the antioxidant capacity of cells is diminished by increased AR activity. These processes can increase the production of ROS, which will induce oxidative stress and are thought to be the primary initiating factor of diabetes complications [50] (Figure 1).

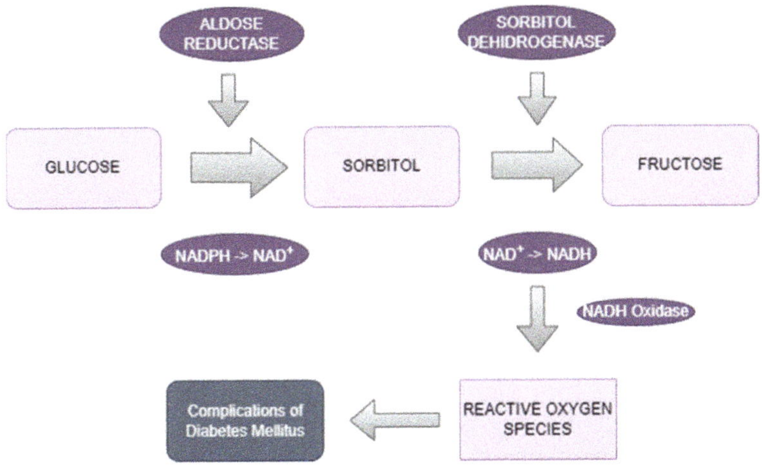

Figure 1. The polyol pathway.

4. Measurement of Aldose Reductase

Measurement of aldose reductase in DR involves various techniques aimed at assessing its activity and expression levels within retinal tissues or biological solutions obtained from patients. Enzymatic assays represent a direct method for quantifying AR activity, typically involving the detection of the conversion of glucose to sorbitol, by the increased activity of aldose reductase in DM patients [9,51]. Immunohistochemical staining techniques [52,53] and spectrophotometric tests may allow quantification of aldose reductase expression [54]. Gerhardinger et al. have studied the mechanism of action and effects of sorbinil and aspirin using immunohistochemistry and real-time PCR (RT-PCR) [55]. A large study has also used spectrophotometry in detecting AR inhibition of medicinal plants in the potential treatment of DR [56].

Many studies have used cultures of human RPE cells for the detection of AR activity [57,58]. Results have shown that AR activity was highest when RPE cells were cultured in pathophysiological levels of glucose. Additionally, Western blot test allows for the quantification of aldose reductase protein levels in human ocular tissues treated with lysis buffer, providing information about its expression levels [52]. There have been a few studies using Western blot for the determination of AR in various tissues before and after treatment with an ARI [53]. Quantitative real-time PCR (qRT-PCR) is a accurate and efficient molecular investigation [59], which can be utilized to measure aldose reductase mRNA levels in the retina, as well as in the cornea, ciliary body, iris and lens [60]. RNA sequencing analysis can also demonstrate the downregulation of cytokine and inflammatory-related genes following AR inhibition [54,61]. An uniquely developed immunoassay technique that uses a particular antibody directed against AR can measure the enzyme's concentration [58]. In a study it was shown to strongly correspond with the activity of AR that was extracted from the same people's erythrocytes [62].

These measurement techniques contribute to the understanding of the role of AR in diabetic retinopathy pathogenesis. Elevated AR activity and expression have been implicated in the development and progression of retinal complications associated with DM, leading to visual impairment [13,31]. By measuring AR levels, researchers can gain insights into the molecular mechanisms underlying DR, including the polyol pathway-mediated osmotic stress, oxidative damage, and cellular dysfunction. Furthermore, assessing AR levels may aid in identifying potential therapeutic targets for intervention in DR [52,57].

5. Treatment Targeting Aldose Reductase

Inhibition of AR represents a therapeutic strategy for DR aimed at inhibiting the consequences of elevated polyol pathway activity. Pharmacological inhibition or inactivation of the AR gene lowers AR activity and protects the retina from retinal barrier leakage and neovascularization [63,64]. Furthermore, hyperglycemia increases the flux of glucose metabolism via the polyol pathway, which raises the risk of inflammation and oxidative stress. Retinal inflammation and glucose-induced oxidative stress are avoided when AR inhibitors block the polyol pathway [63,65]. Several potential approaches have been explored to inhibit aldose reductase activity in the context of DR (Figure 2).

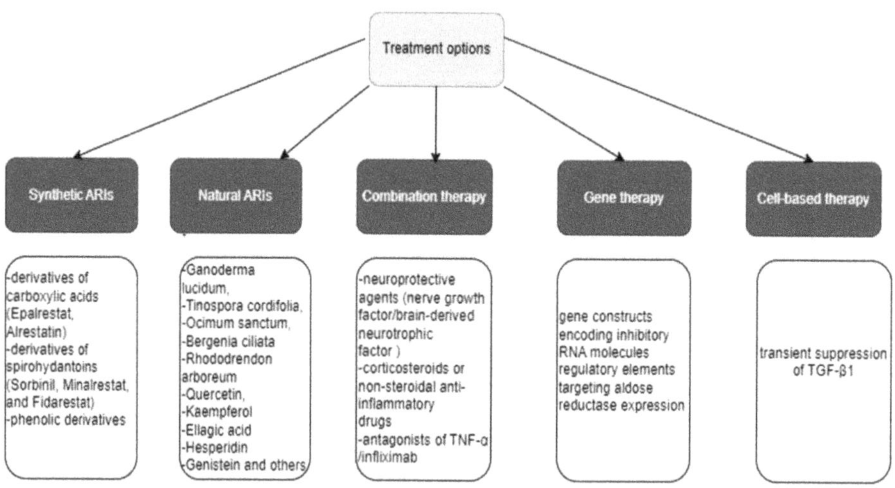

Figure 2. Treatment options targeting aldose reductase inhibition.

5.1. Aldose Reductase Inhibitors

Small-molecule inhibitors targeting AR have been developed and investigated as potential therapeutic agents for DR. These ARIs competitively inhibit the enzymatic activity of aldose reductase, thereby reducing the conversion of glucose to sorbitol and attenuating downstream polyol pathway-mediated complications. Clinical studies on ARIs show that a therapeutic response can be induced by partially inhibiting ALR2 [66].

A variety of structural classes of ARIs have been developed: (1) derivatives of carboxylic acids (e.g., Epalrestat and Alrestatin); (2) derivatives of spirohydantoins and other cyclic amides (e.g., Sorbinil, Minalrestat, and Fidarestat); and (3) phenolic derivatives (e.g., related to Benzopyran-4-one and Chalcone). Epalrestat is the sole inhibitor among these that is now marketed for sale. Furthermore, several additional ARIs, including Ranirestat and Sorbinil, had progressed to the late stages of clinical testing and were determined to be safe for use in humans [67,68]. Reducing the variables that contribute to DR's progression is the most important step in managing the condition. Effective AR inhibition requires potent ARIs because AR inhibition may regulate the factors involved [65]. Historically, there were two types of ARIs that were widely used: spirosuccinimide and carboxylic acids. Subsequently, it was discovered that oral active pyridazinones exhibited more AR selectivity than other drugs [69]. There has been some evidence that administering ARIs to an animal model of diabetes at the beginning of the disease can help avoid diabetic retinopathy [35,70–72].

Treatment with ARIs may also inhibit the basement membrane from thickening, as demonstrated in diabetic rat models studies [73]. A study by Hattori et al. showed that leukocyte adherence to endothelial cells mediated by adhesion molecules may be inhibited by adding an ARI to a diabetic rat model [35]. Administration of ARIs has been demonstrated to inhibit two hallmark processes of diabetic retinopathy: an increase in vascular permeability and a breakdown of the blood–retinal barrier [68,74–76]. According to recent research, sorbitol and fructose inhibition are both necessary to provide positive outcomes in diabetic retinopathy [68].

Based on long-term studies, Epalrestat was an effective medication in preventing the development of diabetic retinopathy in its early stages [77]. Cunha-Vaz et al. also showed that, when compared to a placebo group, treatment with ARIs for six months significantly decreased the rapid penetration of fluorescein in individuals with early stages of diabetic retinopathy [78].

The studies of Kakehashi et al. have demonstrated inhibition of the polyol pathway in the course of DR in SDT rats by Fidarestat, an ARI [79]. Fidarestat inhibited the amount of VEGF in the ocular fluid and stopped significant fluorescein leakage around the optic disc. They also studied the effect of Ranirestat in the development of fundus changes in DR and observed the inhibitory effect on VEGF levels [80]. Other ocular and non-ocular DM complications, such as cataract and diabetic neuropathy were also studied, confirming that patients under treatment with Ranirestat had a more positive outcome [81]. Other study considered the possibility that ranirestat decreases the retinal thickness in SDT rats. Considering all present and past results, they highlighted that ranirestat might inhibit vascular permeability and minimize the posibility of DME [82]. Other research regarding Fidarestat has observed that the treatment reduced the amount of pericytes, basement membrane thickness, and number of microaneurysms; at a higher dose, it even supressed fundus changes. Fidarestat also prevented the build-up of sorbitol in the retina in a dose-dependent manner [70].

Over a relatively long period, Epalrestat was demonstrated to supress the onset or to diminish the progression of diabetic neuropathy, retinopathy, and nephropathy. However, it was uncertain if Epalrestat's inhibition of AR, the maintenance of diabetic neuropathy, or a combination of the two is responsible for the prevention of the advancement of diabetic retinopathy/nephropathy [83]. Diabetic neuropathy may act as a potential trigger for the onset or advancement of diabetic retinopathy, diabetic nephropathy, and other microvascular complications, demonstrating intrincacies between these three vascular complicationd of DM. An ARI prevented upregulation of genes in the transforming growth factor (TGF)-β pathway and apoptosis in the retinal vasculature of diabetic rats, as demonstrated by Gerhardinger et al. [55].

A highly selective ARI of a new structural class, pyridazinones, demonstrated efficacy in preventing or reversing early retinal abnormalities in experimental diabetic retinopathy. ARI-809 showed promising results in inhibiting retinal polyol accumulation, improving survival, inhibiting cataract development, normalizing retinal sorbitol and fructose levels, and protecting the retina from abnormalities associated with DM [68]. Another relatively new topical ARI inhibitor, Kinostat, has been studied with the purpose of inhibiting diabetic cataract formation in diabetic animals. Although effective in animals, further studies are still needed for human use [84].

Another study has identified small-molecule ARIs that may be employed in the synthesis of diabetic treatment medications. By choosing specific inhibitors, they suggested that compared to ALR1 and AKR1B10, these may be more potent against the ALR2 protein [81].

5.2. Phytocompounds

Several phytocompounds have been investigated for their potential therapeutic effects in DR. These compounds, derived from different plants, possess various bioactive properties that may help inhibit retinal damage and prevent vision loss. Research has demonstrated that phytochemicals' antiangiogenic, antioxidant, and anti-inflammatory properties may inhibit the advancement of DR [50,85]. Numerous plants have been shown to have AR inhibiting effect and to be employed in the management of diabetic complications, representing a safer option that synthetic compounds [56,70]. A phytocompound that possesses both antioxidative and AR inhibitory activity may be more efficient than one that only possesses only one of these characteristics [86]. Numerous AR inhibitors and antioxidants are derived from plants, including *G. lucidum, A. indica, T. cordifolia, O. sanctum, B. ciliata* and *R. arboreum* [56]. When *Ocimum Sanctum* is used in combination with vitamin E, it protects against DR [87].

Julius et al. explored the potential of using natural phytocompounds such as quercetin, kaempferol, and ellagic acid as aldose reductase inhibitors for the treatment of DR. The research suggests that these novel ARIs derived from natural sources could offer a promising and alternative approach to managing DR, showing even higher potency than Epalrestat [66]. Quercetin has been reported to attenuate retinal inflammation and vascular leakage in diabetic animals, potentially through inhibition of the NF-κB signaling pathway [88].

When hesperidin, a flavonoid derived from citrus fruits, was delivered to STZ-induced rats, superoxide dismutase (SOD) expression was elevated and aldose reductase activity and malondialdehyde were decreased [89]. Genistein, a naturally occuring compound belonging to the isoflavones, could inhibit the increased level of aldose reductase caused by hyperglycemic conditions in ARPE-19 cells, from the retinal pigment epithelial cell line [90]. Quercitin and Genistein have also been found to delay the development of diabetic cataract, another major ocular complication [91,92]. Isoflavones derived from Caesalpinia pulcherrima have been demonstrated to lower oxidative stress and inhibit AR activity in DR [93].

5.3. Combination Therapy

Given the multifactorial nature of DR, combination therapies targeting multiple pathways involved in its pathogenesis, including AR inhibition, have been investigated. Combining ARI with other pharmacological agents targeting oxidative stress, inflammation, vascular dysfunction, or neuroprotection may offer synergistic effects and improved therapeutic outcomes in DR. Combining ARIs with neuroprotective agents, such as nerve growth factor (NGF) or brain-derived neurotrophic factor (BDNF), addresses both aldose reductase-mediated neurodegeneration and other previously mentioned neurotoxic pathways in the early stages of DR [94].

Anti-inflammatory drugs, such as corticosteroids or non-steroidal anti-inflammatory drugs (NSAIDs), targets both aldose reductase-mediated inflammation and other inflammatory pathways implicated in DR. Aspirin [95], Meloxicam (COX-2 inhibitor) [96], Nepafenac (COX-1 and COX-2 inhibitor) and Etanercept (receptor of TNF-α) [97] have all been studied and have been known to protect against DR microangiopathy and damage to retinal vascularization. Combination therapy might reduce retinal inflammation and suppress vascular dysfunction and neurodegeneration. Antivascular endothelial growth factor (VEGF) agents, such as ranibizumab or aflibercept, addresses both aldose reductase-mediated vascular abnormalities and VEGF-induced neovascularization and vascular leakage in DR; therefore, dual administration of ARI and anti-VEGF substances might inhibit retinal complications, preventing PDR, macular edema and DR evolution [98].

A clinical investigation recently evaluated the role of the angiotensin II antagonist candesartan in both type 1 and type 2 DM with or without early DR, based on promising preclinical studies [99]. Overall, this medication showed promise in slowing the course of DR and, in some cases, reversing it as determined by the ETDRS scale [100,101].

The chemokine ligand CCL2.279 is a powerful mediator of inflammation and the deterioration of the blood retinal barrier. A CCR2/5 receptor antagonist was studied on DR patients [102]. In patients with persistent diabetic macular edema (DME), a clinical trial using infliximab, a monoclonal antibody antagonist of TNF-α, showed a significant improvement in VA and a general reduction in retinal thickness [103]. Since TNF-α stimulates the expression of AR [104], combined therapy with antagonists of TNF-α and ARIs, might be of important value in the treatment of DR.

In addition to the current end-stage strategies for treating DR, cell-based therapy may offer an exciting new approach. In order to improve vascular repair, reverse ischemia, lessen hypoxic/inflammatory stimuli, and stop the advancement of these diseases to their late, sight-threatening phases, this strategy is intended to target the early/intermediate stages of vasodegeneration [105]. In diabetic CD34+ cells, transient suppression of TGF-β1 may be a promising therapeutic approach to restore vascular reparative activity and may improve the chances of effective cellular therapy [106]. As ARIs may prevent upregulation of genes in the TGF-β pathway and apoptosis of retinal cells [55], more detailed studies regarding a combination therapy might be of use.

5.4. Gene Therapy

Gene therapy approaches aimed at modulating aldose reductase expression or activity within the (*AKR1B1*) genetic variant was revealed to be the most strongly related with DR in a recent meta-analysis of over 160 candidate gene studies reported for DR [96]. However, many of the studies have not taken into account risk factors in the development of DR. By delivering gene constructs encoding inhibitory RNA molecules or regulatory elements targeting aldose reductase expression, it may be possible to achieve sustained inhibition of aldose reductase activity and ameliorate retinal damage associated with DM. A few promising articles showed that gene therapy combined with AR inhibitors may sustain retinal ganglionar cell survival and even axon regeneration; however, there is no reported data on visual restoration [53]. Polymorphisms in the AR gene have been connected with susceptibility to DR as well as other pathologies linked to DM [107,108]. These connections have been studied in DM type I and II and in several ethnic groups [108]. The recognition of the susceptibility genes may aid in the development of future treatment.

Preclinical studies utilizing gene therapy to inhibit aldose reductase expression or activity have shown promising results in animal models of diabetic retinopathy. These studies have demonstrated improvements in retinal function, preservation of retinal structure, and attenuation of vascular abnormalities following gene-based aldose reductase inhibition [59]. While these preclinical findings are encouraging, translating gene therapy approaches targeting aldose reductase inhibition into clinical practice for DR requires further investigation. Challenges such as optimizing vector delivery, ensuring target specificity, and assessing long-term safety and efficacy in human subjects need to be addressed. RNA sequencing analysis demonstrated that, following AR inhibition, cytokine and inflammatory associated genes are downregulated, which is in line with studies showing TNF-α downregulation and linking AR inhibition to TNF-α driven signaling. Through anti-inflammatory reactions, AR inhibition temporarily protects the retina and optic nerve by postponing retinal ganglionar cells death and axon degeneration. Axon regrowth cannot be aided by AR inhibition alone. Combining an AR inhibitor with the well-known axon regeneration promoters shKLF9/Sox11 may have a synergistic effect on axon regeneration [56].

6. Benefits and Limitations

Many studies highlight the long-term etiology of DR and the significantly lower success rate of pharmaceutical interventions that inhibit fundus changes once they are already present, compared to preventative treatment before early and potentially irreversible retinal alterations occur [109]. Therefore, if the clinical research design does not take into consideration known risk factors for DR, efficacy for a certain treatment may not be able to be established, even if the therapeutic premise for AR inhibition is valid. A few studies have investigated treatment with ARI as a tool in the prevention, reversal or delay in the onset and progression of DM complications [110]. Since achieving generalized glycemic control is extremely challenging, more research into developing effective, selective, and non-toxic ARIs is warranted. Safe medications are necessary for long-term DM complications. Since these medications would prevent rather than cure diabetes, they have to be given to all individuals with the condition. Since vitamin C has been shown to normalize the level of sorbitol in red blood cells, regardless of changes in diabetes management, it has been suggested that an ARI may be associated with ascorbic acid for the prevetion and treatment of diabetic complications. Several three-component associations (ascorbic acid, ARIs, and unsaturated fatty acids) have been patented for the treatment of DM complications due to a synergistic mechanism [111]. There is also a belief that a diet with ARIs from natural sources might have the same potency in the prevention of DM complications [111]. While this is convenient and has also shown a promising effect against AR, further studies are needed to evaluate the quantities of dietary ARIs at which we could expect these effects.

Overall, while ARIs offer a targeted approach for reducing polyol pathway-mediated damage in diabetic retinopathy with many potential benefits (Table 2) [13,15,40,69,73,112], their use is associated with certain disadvantages, including limited efficacy, systemic side effects, cataract formation, hypoglycemia risk, and the lack of long-term data [113,114]. Despite the promising results seen in laboratory settings, clinical trials have had mixed success in demonstrating long-term efficacy and safety of ARIs for the treatment of diabetic retinopathy [82]. Despite these challenges, novel ARIs with higher selectivity and fewer side effects, such as ARI-809 [68], have shown promising results in preclinical studies. Continued research and development of new ARIs with enhanced selectivity and safety profiles remain vital to advancing the field of diabetic retinopathy treatment [115]. Moreover, several studies have emphasized the effects of natural compounds against AR, paving a new way into DR treatment.

Table 2. Potential benefits of using aldose reductase inhibitors (ARIs) for treating diabetic retinopathy.

Decreased production of sorbitol and fructose, which reduces oxidative stress and preserves the antioxidant defense system within the retina
Protection against neuronal apoptosis, glial reactivity, and complement deposition, all of which contribute to retinal damage
Reduction in microaneurysms, basement membrane thickness, and vascular permeability
Blockage of the expression of various pro-inflammatory cytokines and growth factors
Potential prevention of initial focal laser therapy, especially in cases of DME
Prevention of cataract development
Promising outcomes with novel ARIs, which demonstrate higher selectivity and fewer side effects compared to earlier generations of ARIs

7. Conclusions

AR's pathogenic role in diabetes mellitus has been established through many intensive investigations. Several ARIs have been used in the treatment of diabetes mellitus and its complications. However, since the majority of studied ARIs were withdrawn due to unfavorable side effects, primarily from the ARIs' non-specific binding to the aldo–keto reductase family of proteins, which shares a high degree of structural similarity with AR, the identification of novel ARIs has become increasingly important in research. Moreover, research has shown that many natural compounds possess AR inhibitory effects, paving the way to a guided treatment using both lifestyle/diet changes and pharmacologic therapies.

Author Contributions: Conceptualization, A.-I.D. and A.C.F.; methodology, E.R.S. investigation, R.I.; resources, L.A.G.; writing—original draft preparation, L.A.G. and A.-I.D.; writing—review and editing, S.L.B. and M.-A.S.; visualization, R.I.; supervision, A.C.F. All authors have read and agreed to the published version of the manuscript.

Funding: This research received no external funding.

Acknowledgments: We would like to acknowledge Victor Babes University of Medicine and Pharmacy Timisoara for their support in covering the costs of publication for this research paper.

Conflicts of Interest: The authors declare no conflict of interest.

References

1. Bourne, R.R.A.; Jonas, J.B.; Bron, A.M.; Cicinelli, M.V.; Das, A.; Flaxman, S.R.; Friedman, D.S.; Keeffe, J.E.; Kempen, J.H.; Leasher, J.; et al. Prevalence and Causes of Vision Loss in High-Income Countries and in Eastern and Central Europe in 2015: Magnitude, Temporal Trends and Projections. *Br. J. Ophthalmol.* **2018**, *102*, 575–585. [CrossRef] [PubMed]
2. Avogaro, A.; Fadini, G.P. Microvascular Complications in Diabetes: A Growing Concern for Cardiologists. *Int. J. Cardiol.* **2019**, *291*, 29–35. [CrossRef]
3. Hoerger, T.J.; Harris, R.; Hicks, K.A.; Donahue, K.; Sorensen, S.; Engelgau, M. Screening for Type 2 Diabetes Mellitus: A Cost-Effectiveness Analysis. *Ann. Intern. Med.* **2004**, *140*, 689. [CrossRef] [PubMed]
4. Tapp, R.J.; Shaw, J.E.; Harper, C.A.; De Courten, M.P.; Balkau, B.; McCarty, D.J.; Taylor, H.R.; Welborn, T.A.; Zimmet, P.Z.; on behalf of the AusDiab Study Group. The Prevalence of and Factors Associated with Diabetic Retinopathy in the Australian Population. *Diabetes Care* **2003**, *26*, 1731–1737. [CrossRef] [PubMed]
5. Bebu, I.; Lachin, J.M. Optimal screening schedules for disease progression with application to diabetic retinopathy. *Biostatistics* **2018**, *19*, 1–13. [CrossRef] [PubMed]
6. Hendrick, A.M.; Gibson, M.V.; Kulshreshtha, A. Diabetic retinopathy. *Prim. Care* **2015**, *42*, 451–464. [CrossRef] [PubMed]
7. Song, S.J.; Wong, T.Y. Current Concepts in Diabetic Retinopathy. *Diabetes Metab. J.* **2014**, *38*, 416–425. [CrossRef]
8. Borțea, C.I.; Stoica, F.; Boia, M.; Iacob, E.R.; Dinu, M.; Iacob, R.; Iacob, D. Risk Factors Associated with Retinopathy of Prematurity in Very and Extremely Preterm Infants. *Medicina* **2021**, *57*, 420. [CrossRef]
9. Rosu, L.M.; Prodan-Bărbulescu, C.; Maghiari, A.L.; Bernad, E.S.; Bernad, R.L.; Iacob, R.; Stoicescu, E.R.; Borozan, F.; Ghenciu, L.A. Current Trends in Diagnosis and Treatment Approach of Diabetic Retinopathy during Pregnancy: A Narrative Review. *Diagnostics* **2024**, *14*, 369. [CrossRef]
10. Vujosevic, S.; Aldington, S.J.; Silva, P.; Hernández, C.; Scanlon, P.; Peto, T.; Simó, R. Screening for Diabetic Retinopathy: New Perspectives and Challenges. *Lancet Diabetes Endocrinol.* **2020**, *8*, 337–347. [CrossRef]
11. Sharma, A.; Jaganathan, B.G. Stem Cell Therapy for Retinal Degeneration: The Evidence to Date. *Biol. Targets Ther.* **2021**, *15*, 299–306. [CrossRef] [PubMed]
12. Tomita, Y.; Lee, D.; Tsubota, K.; Negishi, K.; Kurihara, T. Updates on the Current Treatments for Diabetic Retinopathy and Possibility of Future Oral Therapy. *J. Clin. Med.* **2021**, *10*, 4666. [CrossRef] [PubMed]
13. Gabbay, K.H. Hyperglycemia, polyol metabolism, and complications of diabetes mellitus. *Annu. Rev. Med.* **1975**, *26*, 521–536. [CrossRef] [PubMed]
14. Kinoshita, J.H. A Thirty Year Journey in the Polyol Pathway. *Exp. Eye Res.* **1990**, *50*, 567–573. [CrossRef] [PubMed]
15. Steinmetz, P.R.; Balko, C.; Gabbay, K.H. The Sorbitol Pathway and the Complications of Diabetes. *N. Engl. J. Med.* **1973**, *288*, 831–836. [CrossRef] [PubMed]
16. UK Prospective Diabetes Study (UKPDS) Group. Intensive Blood-Glucose Control with Sulphonylureas or Insulin Compared with Conventional Treatment and Risk of Complications in Patients with Type 2 Diabetes (UKPDS 33). *Lancet* **1998**, *352*, 837–853. [CrossRef]
17. The Diabetes Control and Complications Trial Research Group. The Effect of Intensive Treatment of Diabetes on the Development and Progression of Long-Term Complications in Insulin-Dependent Diabetes Mellitus. *N. Engl. J. Med.* **1993**, *329*, 977–986. [CrossRef] [PubMed]
18. Sharma, A.; Valle, M.L.; Beveridge, C.; Liu, Y.; Sharma, S. Unraveling the Role of Genetics in the Pathogenesis of Diabetic Retinopathy. *Eye* **2019**, *33*, 534–541. [CrossRef] [PubMed]
19. Abikoye, T.M.; Oluleye, T.S.; Aribaba, O.T.; Musa, K.O.; Idowu, O.O.; Onakoya, A.O. Is Primary Open-Angle Glaucoma a Risk Factor for Diabetic Retinopathy? *Int. Ophthalmol.* **2020**, *40*, 3233–3240. [CrossRef]
20. Buse, J.B. Action to Control Cardiovascular Risk in Diabetes (ACCORD) Trial: Design and Methods. *Am. J. Cardiol.* **2007**, *99*, S21–S33. [CrossRef]
21. Klein, R.; Knudtson, M.D.; Lee, K.E.; Gangnon, R.; Klein, B.E.K. The Wisconsin Epidemiologic Study of Diabetic Retinopathy XXII. *Ophthalmology* **2008**, *115*, 1859–1868. [CrossRef] [PubMed]
22. Cai, X.; Chen, Y.; Yang, W.; Gao, X.; Han, X.; Ji, L. The Association of Smoking and Risk of Diabetic Retinopathy in Patients with Type 1 and Type 2 Diabetes: A Meta-Analysis. *Endocrine* **2018**, *62*, 299–306. [CrossRef] [PubMed]
23. Kuo, J.Z.; Gao, X.; Guo, X.; Taylor, K.D.; Klein, R.; Klein, B.E.; Ipp, E.; Chen, Y.-D.I.; Varma, R.; Rotter, J.I. A Candidate-Wide Association Study of Diabetic Retinopathy in Latinos Implicates TNF Receptor Pathophysiology: Genetics of Latino Diabetic Retinopathy (GOLDR) and Los Angeles Latino Eye (LALES) studies. *Investig. Ophthalmol. Vis. Sci.* **2014**, *55*, 4509.
24. Mathebula, S.D. Biochemical Changes in Diabetic Retinopathy Triggered by Hyperglycaemia: A Review. *Afr. Vis. Eye Health* **2018**, *77*, a439. [CrossRef]
25. Shukla, U.V.; Tripathy, K. *Diabetic Retinopathy*; StatPearls Publishing: Treasure Island, FL, USA, 2021.

26. Pan, D.; Xu, L.; Guo, M. The Role of Protein Kinase C in Diabetic Microvascular Complications. *Front. Endocrinol.* **2022**, *13*, 973058. [CrossRef] [PubMed]
27. Rübsam, A.; Parikh, S.; Fort, P. Role of Inflammation in Diabetic Retinopathy. *Int. J. Mol. Sci.* **2018**, *19*, 942. [CrossRef] [PubMed]
28. Frank, R.N.; Keirn, R.J.; Kennedy, A.; Frank, K.W. Galactose-Induced Retinal Capillary Basement Membrane Thickening: Prevention by Sorbinil. *Investig. Ophthalmol. Vis. Sci.* **1983**, *24*, 1519–1524.
29. Chakrabarti, S.; Sima, A.A.F.; Nakajima, T.; Yagihashi, S.; Greene, D.A. Aldose Reductase in the BB Rat: Isolation, Immunological Identification and Localization in the Retina and Peripheral Nerve. *Diabetologia* **1987**, *30*, 244–251. [CrossRef] [PubMed]
30. Hohman, T.C.; Nishimura, C.; Robison, W.G. Aldose Reductase and Polyol in Cultured Pericytes of Human Retinal Capillaries. *Exp. Eye Res.* **1989**, *48*, 55–60. [CrossRef]
31. Dagher, Z.; Park, Y.S.; Asnaghi, V.; Hoehn, T.; Gerhardinger, C.; Lorenzi, M. Studies of Rat and Human Retinas Predict a Role for the Polyol Pathway in Human Diabetic Retinopathy. *Diabetes* **2004**, *53*, 2404–2411. [CrossRef]
32. Cheung, A.K.H.; Fung, M.K.L.; Lo, A.C.Y.; Lam, T.T.L.; So, K.F.; Chung, S.S.M.; Chung, S.K. Aldose Reductase Deficiency Prevents Diabetes-Induced Blood-Retinal Barrier Breakdown, Apoptosis, and Glial Reactivation in the Retina of *Db/Db* Mice. *Diabetes* **2005**, *54*, 3119–3125. [CrossRef] [PubMed]
33. Miwa, K.; Nakamura, J.; Hamada, Y.; Naruse, K.; Nakashima, E.; Kato, K.; Kasuya, Y.; Yasuda, Y.; Kamiya, H.; Hotta, N. The Role of Polyol Pathway in Glucose-Induced Apoptosis of Cultured Retinal Pericytes. *Diabetes Res. Clin. Pract.* **2003**, *60*, 1–9. [CrossRef] [PubMed]
34. Beltramo, E.; Berrone, E.; Buttiglieri, S.; Porta, M. Thiamine and Benfotiamine Prevent Increased Apoptosis in Endothelial Cells and Pericytes Cultured in High Glucose. *Diabetes Metab. Res.* **2004**, *20*, 330–336. [CrossRef] [PubMed]
35. Hattori, T.; Matsubara, A.; Taniguchi, K.; Ogura, Y. Aldose Reductase Inhibitor Fidarestat Attenuates Leukocyte-Endothelial Interactions in Experimental Diabetic Rat Retina In Vivo. *Curr. Eye Res.* **2010**, *35*, 146–154. [CrossRef] [PubMed]
36. Schmidt, A.M.; Yan, S.D.; Wautier, J.-L.; Stern, D. Activation of Receptor for Advanced Glycation End Products: A Mechanism for Chronic Vascular Dysfunction in Diabetic Vasculopathy and Atherosclerosis. *Circ. Res.* **1999**, *84*, 489–497. [CrossRef] [PubMed]
37. Oshitari, T. Advanced Glycation End-Products and Diabetic Neuropathy of the Retina. *Int. J. Mol. Sci.* **2023**, *24*, 2927. [CrossRef] [PubMed]
38. Strieder-Barboza, C.; Baker, N.A.; Flesher, C.G.; Karmakar, M.; Neeley, C.K.; Polsinelli, D.; Dimick, J.B.; Finks, J.F.; Ghaferi, A.A.; Varban, O.A.; et al. Advanced Glycation End-Products Regulate Extracellular Matrix-Adipocyte Metabolic Crosstalk in Diabetes. *Sci. Rep.* **2019**, *9*, 19748. [CrossRef] [PubMed]
39. Kang, Q.; Dai, H.; Jiang, S.; Yu, L. Advanced Glycation End Products in Diabetic Retinopathy and Phytochemical Therapy. *Front. Nutr.* **2022**, *9*, 1037186. [CrossRef] [PubMed]
40. Sharma, Y.; Saxena, S.; Mishra, A.; Saxena, A.; Natu, S.M. Advanced Glycation End Products and Diabetic Retinopathy. *J. Ocul. Biol. Dis. Inform.* **2012**, *5*, 63–69. [CrossRef]
41. Wang, W.; Lo, A.C.Y. Diabetic Retinopathy: Pathophysiology and Treatments. *Int. J. Mol. Sci.* **2018**, *19*, 1816. [CrossRef]
42. Yue, T.; Shi, Y.; Luo, S.; Weng, J.; Wu, Y.; Zheng, X. The Role of Inflammation in Immune System of Diabetic Retinopathy: Molecular Mechanisms, Pathogenetic Role and Therapeutic Implications. *Front. Immunol.* **2022**, *13*, 1055087. [CrossRef]
43. Gupta, N.; Mansoor, S.; Sharma, A.; Sapkal, A.; Sheth, J.; Falatoonzadeh, P.; Kuppermann, B.; Kenney, M. Diabetic Retinopathy and VEGF. *Open Ophthalmol. J.* **2013**, *7*, 4–10. [CrossRef] [PubMed]
44. Kowluru, R.A.; Chan, P.-S. Oxidative Stress and Diabetic Retinopathy. *Exp. Diabetes Res.* **2007**, *2007*, 043603. [CrossRef] [PubMed]
45. Jain, A.; Saxena, S.; Khanna, V.K.; Shukla, R.K.; Meyer, C.H. Status of Serum VEGF and ICAM-1 and Its Association with External Limiting Membrane and Inner Segment-Outer Segment Junction Disruption in Type 2 Diabetes Mellitus. *Mol. Vis.* **2013**, *19*, 1760–1768. [PubMed]
46. Sohn, E.H.; van Dijk, H.W.; Jiao, C.; Kok, P.H.; Jeong, W.; Demirkaya, N.; Garmager, A.; Wit, F.; Kucukevcilioglu, M.; van Velthoven, M.E.; et al. Retinal neurodegeneration may precede microvascular changes characteristic of diabetic retinopathy in diabetes mellitus. *Proc. Natl. Acad. Sci. USA* **2016**, *113*, E2655–E2664. [CrossRef]
47. Wermuth, B.; Bürgisser, H.; Bohren, K.; Von Wartburg, J. Purification and Characterization of Human-Brain Aldose Reductase. *Eur. J. Biochem.* **1982**, *127*, 279–284. [CrossRef]
48. Ward, W.H.J.; Cook, P.N.; Mirrlees, D.J.; Brittain, D.R.; Preston, J.; Carey, F.; Tuffin, D.P.; Howe, R. (2,6-Dimethylphenylsulphonyl) Nitromethane: A New Structural Type of Aldose Reductase Inhibitor Which Follows Biphasic Kinetics and Uses an Allosteric Binding Site. *Biochem. Pharmacol.* **1991**, *42*, 2115–2123. [CrossRef]
49. Li, W.; Chen, S.; Mei, Z.; Zhao, F.; Xiang, Y. Polymorphisms in Sorbitol-Aldose Reductase (Polyol) Pathway Genes and Their Influence on Risk of Diabetic Retinopathy Among Han Chinese. *Med. Sci. Monit.* **2019**, *25*, 7073–7078. [CrossRef]
50. Singh Grewal, A.; Bhardwaj, S.; Pandita, D.; Lather, V.; Singh Sekhon, B. Updates on Aldose Reductase Inhibitors for Management of Diabetic Complications and Non-Diabetic Diseases. *Mini-Rev. Med. Chem.* **2015**, *16*, 120–162. [CrossRef]
51. Patel, D.; Kumar, R.; Kumar, M.; Sairam, K.; Hemalatha, S. Evaluation of in Vitro Aldose Reductase Inhibitory Potential of Different Fraction of *Hybanthus enneaspermus* Linn F. Muell. *Asian Pac. J. Trop. Biomed.* **2012**, *2*, 134–139. [CrossRef]
52. Rao, M.; Huang, Y.-K.; Liu, C.-C.; Meadows, C.; Cheng, H.-C.; Zhou, M.; Chen, Y.-C.; Xia, X.; Goldberg, J.L.; Williams, A.M.; et al. Aldose Reductase Inhibition Decelerates Optic Nerve Degeneration by Alleviating Retinal Microglia Activation. *Sci. Rep.* **2023**, *13*, 5592. [CrossRef] [PubMed]

53. Chang, K.-C.; Shieh, B.; Petrash, J.M. Influence of Aldose Reductase on Epithelial-to-Mesenchymal Transition Signaling in Lens Epithelial Cells. *Chem.-Biol. Interact.* **2017**, *276*, 149–154. [CrossRef] [PubMed]
54. Reddy, G.B.; Satyanarayana, A.; Balakrishna, N.; Ayyagari, R.; Padma, M.; Viswanath, K.; Petrash, J.M. Erythrocyte Aldose Reductase Activity and Sorbitol Levels in Diabetic Retinopathy. *Mol. Vis.* **2008**, *14*, 593–601. [PubMed]
55. Gerhardinger, C.; Dagher, Z.; Sebastiani, P.; Park, Y.S.; Lorenzi, M. The Transforming Growth Factor-β Pathway Is a Common Target of Drugs That Prevent Experimental Diabetic Retinopathy. *Diabetes* **2009**, *58*, 1659–1667. [CrossRef] [PubMed]
56. Upadhyaya, S.R.; Magar, L.B.; Thapa, R.; Joshi, S.; Khadayat, K.; Marasini, B.P.; Parajuli, N. Biochemical Analysis and Human Aldose Reductase Inhibition Activity of Selected Medicinal Plants of Nepal. *J. Chem.* **2023**, *2023*, 9614164. [CrossRef]
57. Henry, D.N.; Frank, R.N.; Hootman, S.R.; Rood, S.E.; Heilig, C.W.; Busik, J.V. Glucose-Specific Regulation of Aldose Reductase in Human Retinal Pigment Epithelial Cells in Vitro. *Investig. Ophthalmol. Vis. Sci.* **2000**, *41*, 1554–1560.
58. Sato, S.; Lin, L.-R.; Reddy, V.N.; Kador, P.F. Aldose Reductase in Human Retinal Pigment Epithelial Cells. *Exp. Eye Res.* **1993**, *57*, 235–241. [CrossRef] [PubMed]
59. Ghenciu, L.A.; Faur, A.C.; Bolintineanu, S.L.; Salavat, M.C.; Maghiari, A.L. Recent Advances in Diagnosis and Treatment Approaches in Fungal Keratitis: A Narrative Review. *Microorganisms* **2024**, *12*, 161. [CrossRef]
60. Petrash, J.; Huang, S.-P. Elevation of Aldose Reductase in the Diabetic Eye. *Investig. Ophthalmol. Vis. Sci.* **2007**, *48*, 2029.
61. Wang, Y.; Yang, X.; Zhang, Y.; Hong, L.; Xie, Z.; Jiang, W.; Chen, L.; Xiong, K.; Yang, S.; Lin, M.; et al. Single-Cell RNA Sequencing Reveals Roles of Unique Retinal Microglia Types in Early Diabetic Retinopathy. *Diabetol. Metab. Syndr.* **2024**, *16*, 49. [CrossRef]
62. Nishimura, C.; Hamada, Y.; Tachikawa, T.; Ishikawa, T.; Gui, T.; Tsubouchi, J.; Hotta, N.; Tanimoto, T.; Urakami, T. Enzyme Immunoassay for Erythrocyte Aldose Reductase. *Clin. Chem.* **1994**, *40*, 889–894. [CrossRef]
63. Tang, J.; Du, Y.; Petrash, J.M.; Sheibani, N.; Kern, T.S. Deletion of Aldose Reductase from Mice Inhibits Diabetes-Induced Retinal Capillary Degeneration and Superoxide Generation. *PLoS ONE* **2013**, *8*, e62081. [CrossRef] [PubMed]
64. Ramana, K.V.; Friedrich, B.; Srivastava, S.; Bhatnagar, A.; Srivastava, S.K. Activation of Nulcear Factor-κB by Hyperglycemia in Vascular Smooth Muscle Cells Is Regulated by Aldose Reductase. *Diabetes* **2004**, *53*, 2910–2920. [CrossRef]
65. Kakehashi, A. Aldose Reductase Inhibitor Fidarestat Prevents Diabetic Ocular Complications in Spontaneously Diabetic Torii Rats. *Open Diabetes J.* **2011**, *4*, 101–107. [CrossRef]
66. Julius, A.; Renuka, R.R.; Hopper, W.; Babu Raghu, P.; Rajendran, S.; Srinivasan, S.; Dharmalingam, K.; Alanazi, A.M.; Arokiyaraj, S.; Prasath, S. Inhibition of Aldose Reductase by Novel Phytocompounds: A Heuristic Approach to Treating Diabetic Retinopathy. *Evid.-Based Complement. Altern. Med.* **2022**, *2022*, 9624118. [CrossRef] [PubMed]
67. Oka, M.; Kato, N. Aldose Reductase Inhibitors. *J. Enzym. Inhib.* **2001**, *16*, 465–473. [CrossRef]
68. Sun, W.; Oates, P.J.; Coutcher, J.B.; Gerhardinger, C.; Lorenzi, M. A Selective Aldose Reductase Inhibitor of a New Structural Class Prevents or Reverses Early Retinal Abnormalities in Experimental Diabetic Retinopathy. *Diabetes* **2006**, *55*, 2757–2762. [CrossRef] [PubMed]
69. Ola, M.S. Novel Drugs and Their Targets in the Potential Treatment of Diabetic Retinopathy. *Med. Sci. Monit.* **2013**, *19*, 300–308. [CrossRef] [PubMed]
70. Kato, N.; Yashima, S.; Suzuki, T.; Nakayama, Y.; Jomori, T. Long-Term Treatment with Fidarestat Suppresses the Development of Diabetic Retinopathy in STZ-Induced Diabetic Rats. *J. Diabetes Its Complicat.* **2003**, *17*, 374–379. [CrossRef]
71. Obrosova, I.G.; Minchenko, A.G.; Vasupuram, R.; White, L.; Abatan, O.I.; Kumagai, A.K.; Frank, R.N.; Stevens, M.J. Aldose Reductase Inhibitor Fidarestat Prevents Retinal Oxidative Stress and Vascular Endothelial Growth Factor Overexpression in Streptozotocin-Diabetic Rats. *Diabetes* **2003**, *52*, 864–871. [CrossRef]
72. Cusick, M. Effects of Aldose Reductase Inhibitors and Galactose Withdrawal on Fluorescein Angiographic Lesions in Galactose-Fed Dogs. *Arch. Ophthalmol.* **2003**, *121*, 1745. [CrossRef] [PubMed]
73. Wells-Knecht, K.J.; Brinkmann, E.; Wells-Knecht, M.C.; Litchfield, J.E.; Ahmed, M.U.; Reddy, S.; Zyzak, D.V.; Thorpe, S.R.; Baynes, J.W. New Biomarkers of Maillard Reaction Damage to Proteins. *Nephrol. Dial. Transplant.* **1996**, *11*, 41–47. [CrossRef] [PubMed]
74. Park, K.; Chen, Y.; Hu, Y.; Mayo, A.S.; Kompella, U.B.; Longeras, R.; Ma, J. Nanoparticle-Mediated Expression of an Angiogenic Inhibitor Ameliorates Ischemia-Induced Retinal Neovascularization and Diabetes-Induced Retinal Vascular Leakage. *Diabetes* **2009**, *58*, 1902–1913. [CrossRef] [PubMed]
75. Kim, J.-H.; Kim, J.H.; Jun, H.-O.; Yu, Y.S.; Kim, K.-W. Inhibition of Protein Kinase C δ Attenuates Blood-Retinal Barrier Breakdown in Diabetic Retinopathy. *Am. J. Pathol.* **2010**, *176*, 1517–1524. [CrossRef] [PubMed]
76. Lightman, S.; Rechthand, E.; Terubayashi, H.; Palestine, A.; Rapoport, S.; Kador, P. Permeability Changes in Blood-Retinal Barrier of Galactosemic Rats Are Prevented by Aldose Reductase Inhibitors. *Diabetes* **1987**, *36*, 1271–1275. [CrossRef] [PubMed]
77. Oates, P.J. Aldose Reductase, Still a Compelling Target for Diabetic Neuropathy. *Curr. Drug Targets* **2008**, *9*, 14–36. [CrossRef] [PubMed]
78. Cunha-Vaz, J.G.; Mota, C.C.; Leite, E.C.; Abreu, J.R.; Ruas, M.A. Effect of Sorbinil on Blood-Retinal Barrier in Early Diabetic Retinopathy. *Diabetes* **1986**, *35*, 574–578. [CrossRef]
79. Kakehashi, A.; Ota, A.; Toyoda, F.; Kinoshita, N.; Yamagami, H.; Obata, H.; Matsumoto, T.; Tsuji, J.; Dobashi, Y.; Fujimoto, W.Y.; et al. Prophylactic Medical Treatment of Diabetic Retinopathy. In *Diabetic Retinopathy*; Ola, M.S., Ed.; InTech: London, UK, 2012; ISBN 9789535100447.

80. Ota, A.; Kakehashi, A.; Toyoda, F.; Kinoshita, N.; Shinmura, M.; Takano, H.; Obata, H.; Matsumoto, T.; Tsuji, J.; Dobashi, Y.; et al. Effects of Long-Term Treatment with Ranirestat, a Potent Aldose Reductase Inhibitor, on Diabetic Cataract and Neuropathy in Spontaneously Diabetic Torii Rats. *J. Diabetes Res.* **2013**, *2013*, 175901. [CrossRef] [PubMed]
81. Shahab, M.; Zheng, G.; Alshabrmi, F.M.; Bourhia, M.; Wondmie, G.F.; Mohammad Salamatullah, A. Exploring Potent Aldose Reductase Inhibitors for Anti-Diabetic (Anti-Hyperglycemic) Therapy: Integrating Structure-Based Drug Design, and MMGBSA Approaches. *Front. Mol. Biosci.* **2023**, *10*, 1271569. [CrossRef] [PubMed]
82. Toyoda, F.; Tanaka, Y.; Ota, A.; Shimmura, M.; Kinoshita, N.; Takano, H.; Matsumoto, T.; Tsuji, J.; Kakehashi, A. Effect of Ranirestat, a New Aldose Reductase Inhibitor, on Diabetic Retinopathy in SDT Rats. *J. Diabetes Res.* **2014**, *2014*, 672590. [CrossRef]
83. Hotta, N.; Akanuma, Y.; Kawamori, R.; Matsuoka, K.; Oka, Y.; Shichiri, M.; Toyota, T.; Nakashima, M.; Yoshimura, I.; Sakamoto, N.; et al. Long-Term Clinical Effects of Epalrestat, an Aldose Reductase Inhibitor, on Diabetic Peripheral Neuropathy. *Diabetes Care* **2006**, *29*, 1538–1544. [CrossRef]
84. Kador, P.F.; Wyman, M.; Oates, P.J. Aldose Reductase, Ocular Diabetic Complications and the Development of Topical Kinostat®. *Prog. Retin. Eye Res.* **2016**, *54*, 1–29. [CrossRef] [PubMed]
85. Lupo, G.; Cambria, M.T.; Olivieri, M.; Rocco, C.; Caporarello, N.; Longo, A.; Zanghì, G.; Salmeri, M.; Foti, M.C.; Anfuso, C.D. Anti-angiogenic Effect of Quercetin and Its 8-methyl Pentamethyl Ether Derivative in Human Microvascular Endothelial Cells. *J. Cell. Mol. Med.* **2019**, *23*, 6565–6577. [CrossRef]
86. Dodda, D.; Ciddi, V. Plants Used in the Management of Diabetic Complications. *Indian J. Pharm. Sci.* **2014**, *76*, 97–106. [PubMed]
87. Halim, E.M.; Mukhopadhyay, A.K. Effect of *Ocimum sanctum* (Tulsi) and Vitamin E on Biochemical Parameters and Retinopathy in Streptozotocin Induced Diabetic Rats. *Indian J. Clin. Biochem.* **2006**, *21*, 181–188. [CrossRef]
88. Chai, G.-R.; Liu, S.; Yang, H.-W.; Chen, X.-L. Quercetin Protects against Diabetic Retinopathy in Rats by Inducing Heme Oxygenase-1 Expression. *Neural Regen. Res.* **2021**, *16*, 1344. [CrossRef] [PubMed]
89. Shi, X.; Liao, S.; Mi, H.; Guo, C.; Qi, D.; Li, F.; Zhang, C.; Yang, Z. Hesperidin Prevents Retinal and Plasma Abnormalities in Streptozotocin-Induced Diabetic Rats. *Molecules* **2012**, *17*, 12868–12881. [CrossRef]
90. Dongare, S.H.; Rajendran, S.H.; Senthilkumari, S.; Gupta, S.K.; Mathur, R.; Saxena, R.; Srivastava, R. Genistein alleviates high glucose induced toxicity and angiogenesis in cultured human RPE cells. *Int. J. Pharm. Pharm. Sci.* **2015**, *7*, 294–298.
91. Varma, S.D.; Shocket, S.S.; Richards, R.D. Implications of aldose reductase in cataracts in human diabetes. *Investig. Ophthalmol. Vis. Sci.* **1979**, *18*, 237–241.
92. Stefek, M. Natural Flavonoids as Potential Multifunctional Agents in Prevention of Diabetic Cataract. *Interdiscip. Toxicol.* **2011**, *4*, 69–77. [CrossRef]
93. Kumar, M.P.; Sankeshi, V.; Naik, R.R.; Thirupathi, P.; Das, B.; Raju, T.N. The Inhibitory Effect of Isoflavones Isolated from Caesalpinia Pulcherrima on Aldose Reductase in STZ Induced Diabetic Rats. *Chem.-Biol. Interact.* **2015**, *237*, 18–24. [CrossRef] [PubMed]
94. Hernández, C.; Simó, R. Neurodegeneration in Diabetic Retinopathy: Current Concepts and Therapeutic Implications. *Av. Diabetol.* **2014**, *30*, 72–79. [CrossRef]
95. Sun, W.; Gerhardinger, C.; Dagher, Z.; Hoehn, T.; Lorenzi, M. Aspirin at Low-Intermediate Concentrations Protects Retinal Vessels in Experimental Diabetic Retinopathy through Non–Platelet-Mediated Effects. *Diabetes* **2005**, *54*, 3418–3426. [CrossRef] [PubMed]
96. Zheng, L.; Howell, S.J.; Hatala, D.A.; Huang, K.; Kern, T.S. Salicylate-Based Anti-Inflammatory Drugs Inhibit the Early Lesion of Diabetic Retinopathy. *Diabetes* **2007**, *56*, 337–345. [CrossRef] [PubMed]
97. Kern, T.S.; Miller, C.M.; Du, Y.; Zheng, L.; Mohr, S.; Ball, S.L.; Kim, M.; Jamison, J.A.; Bingaman, D.P. Topical Administration of Nepafenac Inhibits Diabetes-Induced Retinal Microvascular Disease and Underlying Abnormalities of Retinal Metabolism and Physiology. *Diabetes* **2007**, *56*, 373–379. [CrossRef] [PubMed]
98. Bahr, T.A.; Bakri, S.J. Update on the Management of Diabetic Retinopathy: Anti-VEGF Agents for the Prevention of Complications and Progression of Nonproliferative and Proliferative Retinopathy. *Life* **2023**, *13*, 1098. [CrossRef] [PubMed]
99. Abhary, S.; Hewitt, A.W.; Burdon, K.P.; Craig, J.E. A Systematic Meta-Analysis of Genetic Association Studies for Diabetic Retinopathy. *Diabetes* **2009**, *58*, 2137–2147. [CrossRef] [PubMed]
100. Moravski, C.J.; Skinner, S.L.; Stubbs, A.J.; Sarlos, S.; Kelly, D.J.; Cooper, M.E.; Gilbert, R.E.; Wilkinson-Berka, J.L. The Renin-Angiotensin System Influences Ocular Endothelial Cell Proliferation in Diabetes. *Am. J. Pathol.* **2003**, *162*, 151–160. [CrossRef] [PubMed]
101. Chaturvedi, N.; Porta, M.; Klein, R.; Orchard, T.; Fuller, J.; Parving, H.H.; Bilous, R.; Sjølie, A.K. Effect of Candesartan on Prevention (DIRECT-Prevent 1) and Progression (DIRECT-Protect 1) of Retinopathy in Type 1 Diabetes: Randomised, Placebo-Controlled Trials. *Lancet* **2008**, *372*, 1394–1402. [CrossRef]
102. Sfikakis, P.P.; Grigoropoulos, V.; Emfietzoglou, I.; Theodossiadis, G.; Tentolouris, N.; Delicha, E.; Katsiari, C.; Alexiadou, K.; Hatziagelaki, E.; Theodossiadis, P.G. Infliximab for Diabetic Macular Edema Refractory to Laser Photocoagulation. *Diabetes Care* **2010**, *33*, 1523–1528. [CrossRef]
103. Campochiaro, P.A.; Sophie, R.; Tolentino, M.; Miller, D.M.; Browning, D.; Boyer, D.S.; Heier, J.S.; Gambino, L.; Withers, B.; Brigell, M.; et al. Treatment of Diabetic Macular Edema with an Inhibitor of Vascular Endothelial-Protein Tyrosine Phosphatase That Activates Tie2. *Ophthalmology* **2015**, *122*, 545–554. [CrossRef] [PubMed]

104. Iwata, T.; Sato, S.; Jimenez, J.; McGowan, M.; Moroni, M.; Dey, A.; Ibaraki, N.; Reddy, V.N.; Carper, D. Osmotic Response Element Is Required for the Induction of Aldose Reductase by Tumor Necrosis Factor-α. *J. Biol. Chem.* **1999**, *274*, 7993–8001. [CrossRef] [PubMed]
105. Shaw, L.C.; Neu, M.B.; Grant, M.B. Cell-Based Therapies for Diabetic Retinopathy. *Curr. Diabetes Rep.* **2011**, *11*, 265–274. [CrossRef] [PubMed]
106. Bhatwadekar, A.D.; Guerin, E.P.; Jarajapu, Y.P.R.; Caballero, S.; Sheridan, C.; Kent, D.; Kennedy, L.; Lansang, M.C.; Ruscetti, F.W.; Pepine, C.J.; et al. Transient Inhibition of Transforming Growth Factor-B1 in Human Diabetic CD34+ Cells Enhances Vascular Reparative Functions. *Diabetes* **2010**, *59*, 2010–2019. [CrossRef]
107. Demaine, A.G. Polymorphisms of the Aldose Reductase Gene and Susceptibility to Diabetic Microvascular Complications. *Curr. Med. Chem.* **2003**, *10*, 1389–1398. [CrossRef] [PubMed]
108. Ereqat, S.; Abdelhafez, M.; Iriqat, S.; Ghaleb, Q.; Abu Shams, A.; Abd Aldayem, O.; Ghattas, M.; Nasereddin, A. Aldose Reductase (−106) C/T Gene Polymorphism and Associated Risk Factors with Proliferative Diabetic Retinopathy in Palestine: A Cross Sectional Study. *Health Sci. Rep.* **2023**, *6*, e1605. [CrossRef] [PubMed]
109. Mansour, M.A. Aldose Reductase in the Retina. *Curr. Enzym. Inhib.* **2007**, *3*, 49–60. [CrossRef]
110. Costantino, L.; Rastelli, G.; Cignarella, G.; Vianello, P.; Barlocco, D. New Aldose Reductase Inhibitors as Potential Agents for the Prevention of Long-Term Diabetic Complications. *Expert Opin. Ther. Pat.* **1997**, *7*, 843–858. [CrossRef]
111. Anjum, A.; Sreeja, J.; Swapna, Y.; Bolleddu, R.; Venkatesh, S. Dietary Aldose Reductase Inhibitors and Prevention of Diabetic Complications. *Indian. J. Health Sci. Biomed. Res.* **2021**, *14*, 194. [CrossRef]
112. Donaldson, M.; Dodson, P.M. Medical Treatment of Diabetic Retinopathy. *Eye* **2003**, *17*, 550–562. [CrossRef]
113. Balestri, F.; Moschini, R.; Mura, U.; Cappiello, M.; Del Corso, A. In Search of Differential Inhibitors of Aldose Reductase. *Biomolecules* **2022**, *12*, 485. [CrossRef] [PubMed]
114. Jannapureddy, S.; Sharma, M.; Yepuri, G.; Schmidt, A.M.; Ramasamy, R. Aldose Reductase: An Emerging Target for Development of Interventions for Diabetic Cardiovascular. *Front. Endocrinol.* **2021**, *12*, 636267. [CrossRef] [PubMed]
115. Wang, L.; Gu, Q.; Zheng, X.; Ye, J.; Liu, Z.; Li, J.; Hu, X.; Hagler, A.; Xu, J. Discovery of New Selective Human Aldose Reductase Inhibitors through Virtual Screening Multiple Binding Pocket Conformations. *J. Chem. Inf. Model.* **2013**, *53*, 2409–2422. [CrossRef] [PubMed]

biomedicines

MDPI

Review

The Impact of Modern Anti-Diabetic Treatment on Endothelial Progenitor Cells

Velimir Altabas [1,2], Jelena Marinković Radošević [1], Lucija Špoljarec [1], Stella Uremović [3] and Tomislav Bulum [1,4,*]

1 Department of Endocrinology, Diabetes and Metabolic Diseases, Sestre Milosrdnice University Clinical Hospital, 10000 Zagreb, Croatia
2 School of Medicine, University of Zagreb, 10000 Zagreb, Croatia
3 Srebrnjak Children's Hospital, 10000 Zagreb, Croatia
4 Vuk Vrhovac University Clinic for Diabetes, Endocrinology and Metabolic Diseases, Merkur University Hospital, 10000 Zagreb, Croatia
* Correspondence: tomobulum@gmail.com

Abstract: Diabetes is one of the leading chronic diseases globally with a significant impact on mortality. This condition is associated with chronic microvascular and macrovascular complications caused by vascular damage. Recently, endothelial progenitor cells (EPCs) raised interest due to their regenerative properties. EPCs are mononuclear cells that are derived from different tissues. Circulating EPCs contribute to regenerating the vessel's intima and restoring vascular function. The ability of EPCs to repair vascular damage depends on their number and functionality. Diabetic patients have a decreased circulating EPC count and impaired EPC function. This may at least partially explain the increased risk of diabetic complications, including the increased cardiovascular risk in these patients. Recent studies have confirmed that many currently available drugs with proven cardiovascular benefits have beneficial effects on EPC count and function. Among these drugs are also medications used to treat different types of diabetes. This manuscript aims to critically review currently available evidence about the ways anti-diabetic treatment affects EPC biology and to provide a broader context considering cardiovascular complications. The therapies that will be discussed include lifestyle adjustments, metformin, sulphonylureas, gut glucosidase inhibitors, thiazolidinediones, dipeptidyl peptidase 4 inhibitors, glucagon-like peptide 1 receptor analogs, sodium-glucose transporter 2 inhibitors, and insulin.

Keywords: endothelial progenitor cells; diabetes; diabetes complications; diabetes treatment

1. Introduction

The endothelium is the innermost cell layer of the blood vessel wall, with distinct metabolic features that are critical in maintaining vascular integrity, regulating vascular tone, blood flow, and preventing thrombosis [1]. Under certain conditions, the endothelium may become damaged and dysfunctional, resulting in inappropriate vasomotion, inflammation, and atherosclerotic plaque build-up [2]. Atherosclerotic plaques compromise the blood supply to downstream tissues, either by vessel narrowing or by total vessel obstruction. Consequently, ischemia or infarction may occur leading to end-organ dysfunction and failure. If vital organs are affected, the most dramatic outcome is death. From the epidemiological viewpoint, atherosclerosis and its complications are the leading cause of death worldwide and represent a global burden to human health [3].

Numerous risk factors related to atherosclerosis have been identified so far; the most important include age, gender and genetics, lifestyle factors (such as smoking and diet), and underlying medical conditions, like arterial hypertension, dyslipidemia, diabetes, and obesity [4,5]. Over time, complex strategies to treat atherosclerosis and vascular events have been developed, mainly targeting already-mentioned risk factors, blood clotting, and end-organ protection [3]. Among various approaches to treat atherosclerosis and its deleterious outcomes, none of them were able to restore vascular function completely and reverse atherosclerosis. The progressive nature of this disease and the limitations of currently available treatment options lead to the general opinion that atherosclerosis is an irreversible process, strongly linked to aging [6,7].

Endothelial progenitor cells (EPCs) have recently raised significant interest since these cells can aid in regenerating the damaged vessels' endothelium and, therefore, restore vascular function. Discovered at the end of the 20th century, they gave new insight into the pathology of atherosclerosis and offered new prospects in curative medicine [8]. EPCs are usually defined as multipotent stem cells with angiogenic potential. These cells are commonly quantified from blood by flow cytometry as mononuclear cells expressing CD34 and VEGFR2+. CD133+ and CD45−/dim are proposed as additional markers for circulating EPCs [9]. The population of EPCs is rather small, with a proportion of up to 0.05% of mononuclear blood cells [10]. Since the proportion of EPCs in blood cells is very low, some technical considerations need to be highlighted. The analysis of rare cells may be compromised with background noise. Therefore, special attention needs to be given to several preanalytical and analytical steps. These include appropriate blood sampling, collection tube choice and handling temperature, the choice of appropriate flow cytometers, erythrocyte depletion and wash/no wash protocols, background control, etc. [9]. However, to determine the proliferation capacity and the ability to form blood vessel-like forms, it is crucial to cultivate EPCs. In cultures, it became apparent that the phenotype and function of EPCs are heterogeneous, and that the cell markers differ from those in EPCs detected by flow cytometry. Originally, these subpopulations were named after the time they appeared in cultures as early and late outgrowth endothelial cells. These cells express distinct cell markers and behave diversely in cultures. They have different abilities to act as paracrine producers or to proliferate and differentiate into mature endothelial cells, contributing to the formation of new blood vessels or repairing the damaged ones. Therefore, the cells were renamed into myeloid angiogenic cells (MACs) and endothelial colony-forming cells (ECFCs). These EPC subpopulations act synergistically in vivo [11–13]. It is noteworthy, that there are also technical challenges in stem cell cultivation in general that may have an impact on EPC cultivation, like sample preparation, cell isolation and purification, seeding density, choice of culture media, etc. [14]. The main characteristics of these EPC subtypes isolated in culture are shown in Table 1.

Table 1. Characteristics of distinct EPC subtypes in cultures [13].

Lineage	Myeloid Angiogenic Cells	Endothelial Colony-Forming Cells
positive cell markers	CD45, CD31, CD14	CD31, CD105, CD 146 VE-cadherin, von Willebrand factor, VEGFR2 CD34+/−
negative cell markers	CD146, CD34	CD45, CD14
in vitro effects	conditioned media necessary for the endothelial formation	intrinsic tube forming capacity
function	provide paracrine angiogenic factors	provide cells as building blocks release of paracrine factors
time of appearance in culture	early	late

Due to their unique angiogenic features, EPCs seem to be a promising tool to treat conditions like atherosclerosis and atherosclerosis-related conditions such as ischemic heart disease, peripheral artery disease, and diabetic vascular complications [15–17]. In various research, improved parameters of EPC biology (e.g., increased EPC blood count quantified by flow cytometry or improved EPC function in cultures) could be correlated with improved flow-mediated dilation, brachial ankle index, or intima media thickness [18–20]. Furthermore, EPC biology was found to correlate with clinical outcomes like limb amputation, stroke, myocardial infarction, or death [21–24].

EPC-based therapies aim to enhance vascular repair and promote the growth of new blood vessels, ultimately improving blood flow to ischemic tissues, but there are challenges to be addressed. These include improving methods for EPC isolation and expansion, enhancing their engraftment and survival in target tissues, and optimizing the timing and delivery of EPC-based therapies [25,26].

It is noteworthy that many currently prescribed drugs have proven beneficial effects on EPC biology, like several antihypertensive drugs, statins, various classes of anti-diabetic medications, some hormones, bisphosphonates, and others [27]. Since at least some of these drugs are proven to decrease the incidence of cardiovascular incidents and mortality, it may be assumed that improved EPC biology may contribute to this effect [28]. In addition, the EPC count in the bloodstream assessed by flow cytometry or altered behavior of EPCs detected in culture can also serve as biomarkers for cardiovascular health. Reduced EPC numbers or impaired EPC function are associated with various cardiovascular diseases, correlating with advanced disease stage and response to treatment [22]. Understanding the biology of EPCs, and the way they react to currently available pharmacologic interventions is essential for unlocking their full potential in clinical practice [29].

The aim of this review is to discuss the impact of modern anti-diabetic treatment on EPC-mediated vascular repair, correlate it to proven clinical effects on vascular health, and discuss the potential effect of EPCs on recent cardiovascular outcome trial results.

2. Endothelial Progenitor Cells in Health and Disease

There are established regenerative cell responses identified that can diminish and even heal vascular injury and re-establish endothelial integrity and function. A prominent role in vascular repair in adult humans is had by resident endothelial progenitor cells, located in the blood vessel wall. These cells may replicate and differentiate into mature endothelial cells in response to vascular injury. In contrast to resident endothelial progenitor cells present in blood vessels' walls, another type of endothelial progenitor cells may be found in distant tissues like bone marrow, fat tissue, and the spleen. EPCs from distant locations may be mobilized into the bloodstream under certain conditions like ischemia and hypoxia. Under conditions with limited oxygen supply, hypoxia-induced factor 1 (HIF-1) is released, thus inducing stromal-derived factor 1 (SDF-1) production and release. SDF-1 is the key regulator of EPC mobilization. SDF-1 interacts with other mobilizing factors like VEGF and E-selectin, and the PI3K/Akt/eNOS-dependent signal transduction pathway, leading to mobilization of progenitor cells into the blood flow. In addition, there are certain enzymes involved in this EPC mobilization like matrix metalloproteinase 8 and 9 (MMP-9) that inactivate retention factors at the site of EPCs' origin [30,31]. Blood glucose, erythropoietin, thyroid hormones, and estrogen may modulate EPC mobilization [11,27,32].

EPCs enter the blood circulation, migrate to the place of vessel injury, embed there in a process named homing, and produce various paracrine substances like SDF-1, nitric oxide (NO), vascular endothelial growth factor (VEGF), fibroblast growth factor (FGF), insulin-like growth factor (IGF), and others. SDF-1 leads to upregulation of its specific chemokine receptor type 4 (CXCR-4 receptor) on the EPC surface, resulting in enhanced homing of these cells to the injured blood vessel. Other adhesion molecules, like E-selectin, integrins, intercellular adhesion molecule (ICAM), and vascular cell adhesion molecule (VCAM) are also included in this process [30]. Responding to paracrine factors secreted by embedded circulatory EPCs like VEGF, IGF-1, and gasotransmitters, resident endothelial progenitor cells proliferate and differentiate in situ resulting in vascular repair [11,30,32]. The AMPK/Akt/eNOS and AMPK/eNOS signaling pathways with their activators (adipokines, prostaglandins) have an important role in enhancing further EPC differentiation and vessel formation [33,34].

As mentioned earlier, circulating EPCs represent a heterogeneous cell population with varying characteristics. Two types of EPCs could be detected in the circulation and characterized after in vitro cultivation: MACs or early-onset EPCs, and ECFCs, known also as late-onset EPCs. MACs form colonies in cultures under special conditions only, and ECFCs are better differentiated and provide mature endothelial cells as building blocks important for physical endothelial integrity and function. Both progenitor cell types can produce paracrine substances like nitric oxide (NO) and express receptors for growth factors like the vascular endothelial growth factor receptor 2 (VEGF-R2) [35–37].

In healthy individuals, both resident and circulating EPCs contribute to the maintenance of vascular health by continuously replenishing and repairing the endothelial lining [38]. Considering the impact of circulating EPCs on vascular repair, it seems that their paracrine function is more important since the resident progenitor cells provide the majority of newly differentiated cells necessary for vascular repair [11,39].

It has to be noticed that the turnover of healthy human endothelial cells is rather low in regions with laminar blood flow, with a cell lifespan of many years [40]. However, in regions with turbulent blood flow, like vessel curvatures and branching points, the lifespan of endothelial cells may be shortened and cell turnover increased. In humans, the endothelial turnover is within the range from 47 to 23,000 days [41,42]. Endothelial damage may occur over time due to various mechanical and chemical stimuli. Mechanical factors like increased blood pressure may directly harm the endothelium, while chemical factors like hyperglycemia or smoking may trigger premature endothelial cell apoptosis. All these mentioned factors disrupt endothelial integrity, resulting in an elevated mature endothelial cell count in peripheral blood, as a marker of endothelial damage. Without the functional innermost layer, NO production is compromised, and vascular tone and blood flow become dysregulated, resulting in endothelial dysfunction and downstream tissue ischemia. In addition, a cascade of inflammatory processes on the site of injury triggers cholesterol accumulation and oxidation promoting further growth of atherosclerotic plaques. Furthermore, cytokines secreted by the damaged tissue attract smooth muscle cells that migrate from the artery's muscle layer into the vascular intima. These cells further proliferate leading to plaque build-up. Oxidized cholesterol attracts macrophages, further contributing to a pro-inflammatory environment. The plaque surface is covered by a fibrous cap that may become unstable in a pro-inflammatory environment and finally rupture, leading to activation of the clotting cascade, resulting in vessel obstruction and infarction of related tissues [43,44].

In conditions where blood flow is compromised, such as in ischemic diseases (e.g., peripheral artery disease or myocardial infarction), repairing mechanisms are activated: EPCs from distant tissues enter the circulation, providing paracrine factors from myeloid angiogenic cells to stimulate both embedded late outgrowth endothelial progenitor cells and resident endothelial progenitor cells, leading to vascular repair [11,36]. In that way, the presence of EPCs helps restore blood flow by contributing to the formation of collateral vessels, which bypass blocked or narrowed arteries.

Functional EPCs decrease the risks of thrombotic events. This occurs either by replacing aged and injured endothelial cells with EPCs or by releasing substances that inhibit blood clot formation from EPCs to an extent that is still under debate [45,46]. The number and function of EPCs decline with age, which can contribute to the development of age-related vascular diseases, such as atherosclerosis. Gender-specific differences with a protective higher estrogen-dependent EPC count in fertile women during the ovulatory phase compared to age-matched men have been found [47]. EPC dysfunction is also implicated in various other related pathologies, including diabetes, dyslipidemia, and arterial hypertension, highlighting their significance in vascular disease progression [46,48].

3. Diabetes and Endothelial Progenitor Cells Biology

Diabetes mellitus is a metabolic disorder characterized by chronically elevated blood glucose levels. Depending on the diabetes type, deficient insulin action and insulin resistance may additionally contribute to the occurrence of other metabolic abnormalities like dyslipidemia and abnormal protein metabolism, resulting in inflammation and oxidative stress [49]. These metabolic alterations result in endothelial dysfunction, a key initiating event in vascular complications. Furthermore, diabetes is often accompanied by other conditions affecting endothelial function and vascular health like obesity, arterial hypertension, and dyslipidemia [50]. In addition, diabetes is associated with changes in the coagulation cascade, platelet function, and fibrinolysis, creating a prothrombotic state and increasing the risks of thrombotic events [51]. Over time, chronic diabetic complications may develop. These conditions are linked to vascular dysfunction and structural damage, affecting both large and small blood vessels in the body [52].

An important pathophysiological mechanism linking diabetes and its complications seems to be related to both MACs and ECFCs. Namely, hyperglycemia, hypoglycemia, and increased glucose variability occurring in diabetic patients, regardless of diabetes type, have detrimental effects on EPC biology [53]. Patients with both type 1 and type 2 diabetes have reduced numbers of circulating EPCs. This decrease can be noticed early after the diagnosis of type 1 and type 2 diabetes, regardless of patients' age [54,55]. Additional studies have shown that in individuals with diabetes, EPCs often exhibit reduced mobilization capacity, shortened survival, and impaired ability to differentiate into mature endothelial cells [37,53,56–58].

Aside from the specific metabolic environment determined primarily by blood glucose abnormalities, possible mechanisms involved in the deterioration of EPCs abilities for vascular repair include disruptions in NO pathways, impaired intracellular signaling in other pathways (MAPK/ERK, SDF-1/CXCR-4) and the p53/sirtuin1 (SIRT1)/p66Shc axis, inflammation, reactive oxygen species, accumulation of advanced glycation end products (AGE), low levels of gasotransmitters, imbalance in adipokine production, and direct effects of insulin and IGF-1, as shown in Figure 1 [27,53,59–61]. In particular, MAPK causes NF-κB-dependent inflammatory stress response in the bone marrow, disrupting hematopoietic progenitor activity and enhancing inflammation-induced hypoxic injury [62], while p53/sirtuin/p66Shc disruption promotes EPC senescence [63]. Reactive oxidative species impair EPCs viability, increase apoptosis, and negatively impact tube formation, and AGE accumulation disrupts NO production and significantly decreases anti-oxidant enzymes, thus increasing oxidative stress [64]. Impaired gasotransmitter function, including decreased NO, CO, and H_2S signaling, may alter extracellular matrix properties, affecting metalloproteinase function [65].

EPC dysfunction results in compromised function of both large and small blood vessels and contributes to the development and progression of diabetes-related vascular complications [53,66,67]. It has been shown that EPC dysfunction is closely linked to the occurrence of diabetic microvascular complications, such as retinopathy, nephropathy, and neuropathy [66,68,69]. These complications may lead over time to vision impairment and blindness, kidney function decline and end-stage renal disease, altered or loss of sensation in the extremities, and delayed wound healing, and are therefore leading causes of invalidity in developed countries [70,71]. In other words, enhanced EPC-mediated angiogenesis and endothelial repair in the renal, retinal, and peripheral vasculature could contribute to better outcomes in diabetic individuals.

EPC dysfunction is also implicated in macrovascular diabetic complications, including coronary artery disease, cerebrovascular disease, and peripheral artery disease. Diminished EPC count and function contribute to impaired endothelial repair mechanisms, leading to endothelial dysfunction and accelerated plaque formation, which increase the risk of major cardiovascular events (MACEs) in diabetic individuals. Even more serious, a decreased EPC function is linked to premature mortality [18,72]. It has been proposed that EPC levels and function could serve as valuable biomarkers for diabetes-related complications. Monitoring EPC parameters may help identify individuals at higher risk of developing vascular complications, allowing early intervention and personalized treatment strategies [22]. However, it is important to note that individual patient factors, including age and the presence of comorbidities, can influence the response of EPCs to treatment and modify their effect on the endothelium [6,46]. Therefore, personalized medicine approaches that consider these factors may be necessary to optimize diabetes management.

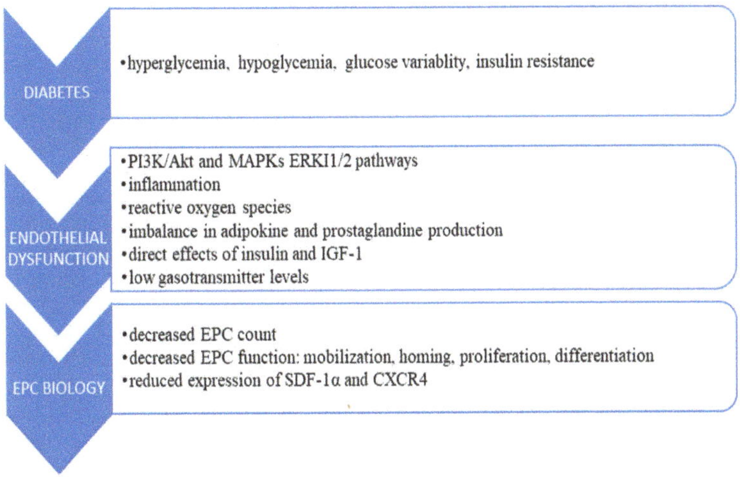

Figure 1. Mechanisms of endothelial dysfunction in diabetes [27,53–55,57,59–61,64,65,72–84].

Several landmark studies have shown that good blood glucose control decreases the risk of developing chronic diabetic complications and mortality [73,74]. Achieving good blood glucose control requires, in general, both non-pharmacological interventions and drug therapy. Recently, some anti-diabetic medications like sodium–glucose transporter-2 inhibitors and glucagon-like peptide-1 (GLP-1) receptor agonists have proven to have better cardiovascular outcomes in patients with type 2 diabetes, and these medications were highlighted in modern international guidelines [75].

4. Currently Available Diabetes Treatments Affecting EPC Count and Function

4.1. Lifestyle Modification

Lifestyle modifications are integral components of diabetes management. Most importantly, evidence-based strategies encompass dietary adjustments, appropriate exercise programs, body weight optimization, smoking cessation, and prudent alcohol choices. A healthy lifestyle has been proven to benefit blood glucose control and, thus, help to reduce diabetic complications in patients with diabetes [76,77]. Nutrition therapy is an umbrella term used for dietary modifications in diabetes therapy. Quality nutrition choices have been shown to improve blood glucose control and, thus, help to reduce diabetic complications [78–82]. At the time, to our best knowledge, there is a single published paper on a trial regarding EPCs in diabetic patients with a focus on nutrition. The authors found a beneficial effect of a Mediterranean diet compared to a low-fat diet on EPC count (CD34+VEGFR2+ and CD34+VEGFR2+CD133+) and carotid intima-media thickness in patients with type 2 diabetes. The increased EPC count correlated with improvements in blood glucose control, insulin sensitivity, total cholesterol, high-density lipoprotein cholesterol, and systolic blood pressure, decreasing the risk for chronic diabetic complications [83].

Several other studies focused on non-diabetic study populations with risk factors for cardiovascular events or on healthy volunteers. However, because of the complex interplay of diabetes, other risk factors, and cardiovascular disease, these trials are also relevant for diabetic macrovascular complications. Adding vegetables to the diet improved EPC counts in a randomized small study in Japan involving healthy volunteers. From a contemporary viewpoint, a serious limitation of the study is the lack of a precise EPC definition [84].

Better EPC (CD34+/VEGFR2+) counts and improved vasomotor function measured by flow-mediated vasodilation on the brachial artery were detected when flavanols were added to the diet of patients with coronary artery disease [85]. The Mediterranean diet, rich in vegetables and unsaturated fats also increased EPC (CD34+/VEGFR2+/CD133+) counts and reduced endothelial cell microparticles related to mature EC apoptosis in a small group of elderly people with a clinical correlate of improved ischemic reactive hyperemia, indicating reduced endothelial damage and improved endothelial regenerative capacity [86]. Similar results, like improved EPC (CD34+/VEGFR+/CD133+) counts, a decreased level of circulating microparticles, an improved anti-inflammatory profile, and increased flow-mediated vasodilation were found in the larger CORDIOPREV trial involving patients with already diagnosed coronary artery disease who were put on the Mediterranean diet. A simplified dietary approach with fat restriction was statistically inferior in this trial [87]. Calorie restriction in combination with the Mediterranean diet and exercise also had beneficial effects on EPC (CD34+/VEGFR2+) count in patients with metabolic syndrome after three months of intervention. Insulin sensitivity and blood pressure were also improved and body weight loss was promoted. However, endothelial function was improved only in subjects randomized to exercise [88]. Adding polyunsaturated fat from fish was also shown to improve both circulatory EPC (CD34+/VEGFR+; CD133+) count and tube-formation function after a 6-week intervention, but this effect ceased in the following 6 weeks after the intervention was stopped. An improvement in several inflammatory substances like TNF α, interleukin 8 (IL-8), and an improvement in adhesion molecule profile was also detected [89]. In another randomized trial, replacing saturated with monounsaturated and polyunsaturated dietary fats in a larger sample of people at moderate risk for cardiovascular disease increased EPC (CD34+/VEGFR2+) and decreased microparticle numbers, suggesting beneficial effects on endothelial repair and maintenance [90]. Intriguingly, excluding meat and fish from nutrition showed less favorable effects on EPC (CD34+/CD133+/CD45−/dim) than adhering to the full Mediterranean diet in the CARDIVEG study [91]. An ancient type of grain also showed an increase in EPCs (defined as CD34+ or CD133+ cells) in comparison to modern grain varieties after an intervention of 8 weeks. At the same time, significantly better blood glucose control and cholesterol levels were achieved [92].

Besides the approach with the Mediterranean diet, green tea may improve the EPC count (CD34+/VEGFR2+/CD45−/dim) even over the short term in a population of chronic smokers. In the same period, an improvement of vascular function assessed by flow-mediated dilation was detected. However, since there was no control group in the study, definitive conclusions cannot be made [93]. Wise alcohol choices may also benefit EPC biology. In a trial with a cross-over design, the effect of beer and non-alcoholic beer on circulating EPC (CD34+/VEGFR2+/CD133+) levels was tested in patients with high cardiovascular risk, compared to gin. The beer and non-alcoholic beer increased the circulating EPC count and SDF-1 in the peripheral blood. On the other hand, while the same subjects were drinking gin during the control period, there was a decrease in EPC count. A major study limitation is the lack of a control group drinking water [94]. Considering other types of alcohol, red wine has been shown to increase circulating EPC (CD34+/VEGFR2+/CD133+) levels and to improve EPC function (attenuated senescence and improved adhesion, migration, and tube formation) by modifying nitric oxide bioavailability, at least in healthy volunteers who were randomized either on red wine, vodka, beer, or water. Clinically, improved FMD vasodilation was seen in patients drinking red wine [95]. White wine also increases the EPC (CD34+/VEGFR2+, CD133+) count and decreases concentrations of several pro-inflammatory markers in a population with increased cardiovascular risk, but there was also no control group on water [96]. It is unclear if alcohol is the key effect mediator since grape seeds have been shown to also improve CD34+ cell counts. A more precise EPC characterization would be necessary to confirm this result [97].

Essentially, dietary adjustments recommended for patients with diabetes do not only improve blood glucose control but reduce the need for pharmacotherapy. It seems that they may improve vascular health by benefitting several aspects of EPC biology like EPC count, modifying NO production, and reducing the number of endothelial microparticles in circulation. However, the best dietary approach for diabetic patients needs still to be established since there is only one study performed in this population. This study showed the benefits of the Mediterranean diet. Other approaches like adding unsaturated fat, vegetarian diet, caloric restriction, and others still need to be evaluated in diabetic patients. Correlating EPC findings with clinical tests like FMD would enhance the predictive value of such research. However, eating more vegetables, adding more unsaturated fat to the diet, and caloric restriction could positively impact EPCs in non-diabetic persons, but in some parts of these studies, there was no correlate with other clinical findings. The exact mechanisms by which food influences EPC biology remain to be elucidated, but improved insulin sensitivity, decreased inflammatory parameters, and prostaglandins could play a significant role [98–101]. Intriguingly, alcohol could not show benefits on EPC parameters, with the exception of red wine, and there could not be a definitive conclusion drawn on green tea. In addition, EPCs are not equally defined in these studies, making comparations between studies difficult.

Exercise is another lifestyle factor that affects blood glucose control, but also cardiovascular morbidity and mortality in patients with diabetes. There are several trials dealing with the effect of exercise on EPC biology in diabetic patients. Acute exercise loads promptly increased the EPC (CD34+/CD133+) count in patients with type 2 diabetes with and without nephropathy [102]. In patients with type 2 diabetes and diagnosed coronary artery disease, an elevated level of microparticles and EPC could be detected. In contrast, patients with type 1 diabetes have shown a blunted EPC response to both aerobic and resistance exercise. The authors concluded that these findings may suggest a low reserve of EPC (CD34+/CD45dim and CD34+/VEGFR2+/CD45dim) in the bone marrow in patients with type 1 diabetes [103]. These findings have been confirmed by another trial by an independent group of authors, testing CD34+/VEGFR+ and CD34+/VEGFR2*/CD45dim EPC count [104]. More studies have shown the impact of exercise in non-diabetic populations, with or without other cardiovascular risk factors. Studied populations include healthy volunteers, obese adolescents, patients with renal failure, patients with heart failure, and patients with coronary artery disease [105–109]. In general, moderate exercise increases the EPC count, improves their migratory capacity, and reduces EPC apoptosis, with beneficial effects on vascular healing. Exercise may influence EPC counts and EPC function by several mechanisms that include increased NO production, improved insulin sensitivity, decreased inflammation, and improved hormonal and cytokine signaling [110,111]. However, EPCs are not universally equally defined in these research, making direct comparison hard.

Finally, an important lifestyle factor affecting diabetic and vascular outcomes is smoking. While nicotine is responsible for tobacco addiction, cigarette smoke contains many substances resulting from tobacco combustion. Oxidizing chemicals, carbon monoxide, particulates, heavy metals, nitrosamines, and polycyclic aromatic hydrocarbon carcinogens are drivers of tobacco toxicity and may affect EPC biology. One important mechanism responsible for endothelial damage is compromised tetrahydrobiopterin depletion leading to decreased NO availability, endothelial dysfunction, increased inflammation, and activation of platelets, resulting in accelerated atherogenesis [112]. Smokers are shown to have decreased EPC (CD34+/VEGFR2+) counts and impaired endothelial-dependent vasodilatation compared to non-smokers. The survival of EPC is also shortened [113]. Both active and passive smoking impact EPC biology negatively. Smoking cessation increases EPC (CD34+/VEGFR2+/CD133+) count and function by reducing hypoxia, reactive oxygen species (ROS) generation, and inflammation [113]. Intriguingly, consuming electronic cigarettes increases acutely the count of CD34+/CD309+ cells in regular smokers, maybe indicating an acute bone marrow response to vascular injury. Still, there is not enough evidence to draw definitive conclusions about electronic cigarettes [114]. Important to note, these studies are not consistent in EPC characterization, and there are no studies involving diabetic patients performed up to the present time, making conclusions on this topic elusive.

4.2. Anti-Diabetic Agents

Many different anti-diabetic agents are currently used to treat diabetes. Better glucose control itself is associated with improved endothelial function and a decreased risk of microvascular and macrovascular diabetic complications. There is mounting evidence about the impact of currently available anti-diabetic drugs on cardiovascular health. Furthermore, since 2008, every new anti-diabetic drug needs to be tested in a cardiovascular outcome trial if seeking approval from the Food and Drug Agency (FDA). In these trials, new agents are compared to standard treatment, and must at least prove non-inferiority considering cardiovascular outcomes. Cardiovascular outcomes of interest typically include cardiovascular death, non-fatal myocardial infarction, and stroke. Optional other outcomes may be additionally considered, like total mortality, hospitalizations for heart failure, lower limb amputations, albuminuria, etc. A brief overview on anti-diabetic medications, their mode of action, cardiovascular safety/superiority, and clinical trials involving EPC biology is shown in Table 2.

Table 2. Currently available anti-diabetic medications, their main mode of action, cardiovascular effects, and effects on EPCs.

Drug Class	Mode of Action	Cardiovascular Effects	Effects on EPCs	Reference
Biguanides: Metformin	reduces hepatic glucose production facilitates peripheral glucose uptake and utilization, in part by increasing insulin action reduces basal hyperinsulinemia alters glucose turnover in the gut increases glucose uptake from circulation and decreases absorption from food increases the release of glucagon-like peptide-1 (GLP-1) alters the gut microbiome activates adenosine monophosphate-protein-kinase (AMPK) activator and increases the transport capacity of all types of membrane glucose transporters (GLUTs)	beneficial effects not proven in CVOTs	↑EPC (CD34+/VEGFR2+/CD45-/dim) count assessed by flow cytometry ↑FMD	[115]
			↑EPC (CD34+/VEGFR2+/CD45-/dim) count assessed by flow cytometry ↑ECFC colonies number ↑adhesion capability of proangiogenic cells using fibronectin adhesion assay	[116] *
			↑EPC (CD34+/VEGFR2+/CD45-/dim) count assessed by flow cytometry	[117]
1Sulphonylureas: Gliclazide Glimepiride Gliquidon	stimulates insulin secretion from the β-cells of the islets of Langerhans increases insulin and C-peptide secretion	second generation sulphonylureas are superior to first generation finding not proven in CVOTs	gliclazide only: ↑EPC (CD34+/VEGFR2+/CD45-/dim) count assessed by flow cytometry ↑FMD	[118]
			no proven effects for other sulphonylureas	[119,120]

Table 2. *Cont.*

Drug Class	Mode of Action	Cardiovascular Effects	Effects on EPCs	Reference
Thiazolidinediones: Pioglitazone Rosiglitazone	reduces insulin resistance and reduces insulin concentrations activates peroxisome proliferator-activated receptor gamma increases insulin sensitivity of liver, fat, and skeletal muscle cells reduces hepatic glucose output increases peripheral glucose disposal	improves some MACEs not proven in CVOTs increased risk of heart failure	pioglitazone: ↑EPC (CD34+/VEGFR2+) count assessed by flow cytometry	[121]
			pioglitazone: ↑ circulating CD34+ cell count	[122]
			pioglitazone: ↑EPC (CD34+) count assessed by flow cytometry ↑increased migratory response and adhesion capacity to fibronectin and collagen in culture	[123]
			pioglitazone: ↑EPC (CD34+/VEGFR2+) count assessed by flow cytometry ↑ SDF1 induced migratory capacity ↑ ECFC in cultures	[124]
			pioglitazone: no effect on EPC count	[125]
DPP-4 inhibitors Sitagliptin Linagliptin Alogliptin Saxagliptin Vildagliptin Teneligliptin	inhibits dipeptidyl peptidase 4 (DPP-4) enhances the levels of glucagon-like peptide-1 (GLP-1) and glucose-dependent insulinotropic polypeptide (GIP) in a glucose-dependent manner improves beta cell responsiveness to glucose and stimulates insulin biosynthesis and release lowers glucagon secretion reduces hepatic glucose production	non-inferiority to standard treatment/class effect proven in CVOTs except for vildagliptin and teneligliptin increased risk for heart failure for saxagliptin	sitagliptin: ↑EPC (CD34+/VEGFR2+) count assessed by flow cytometry ↑ SDF1 blood concentrations	[126]
			sitagliptin: ↑EPC (CD34+/CXCR4+) count assessed by flow cytometry ↓ SDF1 blood concentrations	[120]
			sitagliptin: ↑EPC (CD34+/VEGFR2+ and CD34+/VEGFR2+/CD133+) count assessed by flow cytometry ↑GLP-1, NO and SDF-1 blood concentrations	[127]
			sitagliptin: ↑EPC (CD34+) count assessed by flow cytometry ↑FMD	[128]
			linagliptin: ↑EPC (CD34+/VEGFR2+ and CD34+/CD133+) count ↑GLP-1, and SDF-1 blood concentrations	[129]
			linalgiptin no effect on EPCs ↑SDF-1 blood concentrations	[130]

Table 2. *Cont.*

Drug Class	Mode of Action	Cardiovascular Effects	Effects on EPCs	Reference
DPP-4 inhibitors Sitagliptin Linagliptin Alogliptin Saxagliptin Vildagliptin Teneligliptin	inhibits dipeptidyl peptidase 4 (DPP-4) enhances the levels of glucagon-like peptide-1 (GLP-1) and glucose-dependent insulinotropic polypeptide (GIP) in a glucose-dependent manner improves beta cell responsiveness to glucose and stimulates insulin biosynthesis and release lowers glucagon secretion reduces hepatic glucose production	non-inferiority to standard treatment/class effect proven in CVOTs except for vildagliptin and teneligliptin increased risk for heart failure for saxagliptin	linagliptin↑CD34+/CD184+ EPC improved arterial stiffness and pulse wave velocity	[131]
			vildagliptin: ↑EPC (CD34+/VEGFR2 +/CD133+) count assessed by flow cytometry ↓SDF1 blood concentrations	[119]
			alogliptin: ↑EPC (CD34+/VEGFR2 +/CD45-/dim) count assessed by flow cytometry	[132]
			saxagliptin: ↑EPC (CD34+/VEGFR +/CD133+) count assessed by flow cytometry ↑FMD	[133]
			saxagliptin: no effect on EPC if added to metformin improved migratory capacity	[134]
			teneligliptin: no significant effect on EPC ↑FMD	[135]
GLP-1 receptor agonists Exenatide Lixisenatide Liraglutide Dulaglutide Semaglutide	activates the GLP-1 receptor stimulates insulin secretion and lowers glucagon secretion in a glucose-dependent manner delays gastric emptying in the early postprandial phase.	liraglutide, dulaglutide, and semaglutide showed cardiovascular superiority in CVOTs or equivalent studies	exenatide in full dose superior to medium dosed liraglutide in ↑EPC (CD34+/VEGFR2 +)	[136]
			liraglutide superior to sitagliptin in ↑VEGF and SDF-1	[137]
			dulaglutide: ↑EPC (CD34+/VEGFR2 +/CD133+) enhanced EPC proliferation, adhesion, migration, and tubule formation abilities improved brachial-ankle pulse wave velocity	[138]
SGLT-2 inhibitors Empagliflozin Dapagliflozin Canagliflozin	inhibits the sodium-glucose cotransporter-2 by dapagliflozin in the proximal renal tubule improves both fasting and postprandial plasma glucose levels	cardiovascular superiority proven in CVOTs beneficial in heart failure and renal failure black box warning for lower limb amputations	dapagliflozin lead to a late increase in EPC count (CD34+/VEGFR2+) no change in EPCs in the empagliflozin group	[139]
			dapagliflozin treatment activated AMPK signaling in EPCs	[140]
			empagliflozin increases CD133+EPC count	[141]
			canagliflozin improved CXCR receptors on EPCs, improving their migratory capacity	[142]

Table 2. *Cont.*

Drug Class	Mode of Action	Cardiovascular Effects	Effects on EPCs	Reference
Insulin and insulin analogs	binds to insulin receptors	proven non-inferiority to standard therapy in CVOTs for newer insulin analogs	detemir and glargin both increased EPC count (CD34+/VEGFR2+ and CD34+/VEGFR2+/CD133+) decreased adhesion molecules	[143]
			no difference in CD34*/VEGFR2+ EPCs between groups receiving NPH insulin, insulin glargin, or oral therapy improved ECFC growth with NPH insulin and glargin decrease in intima media thickness	[144]
			intensive insulin therapy increased EPC count (CD34+/VEGFR2+) no effect on clinical outcomes	[145]
			reduced glucovariability by using insulin pumps increased the EPC count (CD34+/VEGFR+) compared to intensified insulin therapy	[58] *

* indicates studies of patients with type 1 diabetes, ↑ increased, ↓ reduced.

Possible mechanisms of cardiovascular benefits include beneficial effects on EPC health. EPCs may benefit from improved glycemia and insulin sensitivity, enhanced nitric oxide production, reduced oxidative stress, and decreased inflammatory parameters. Some drugs improve EPC homing by other mechanisms, including altered expression of adhesion molecules. Specific effects on EPC may vary according to differences among various classes of anti-diabetic drugs.

Among the drugs with favorable cardiovascular effects is metformin. For many years considered the first-line anti-diabetic therapy for patients with type 2 diabetes, metformin has shown cardiovascular benefits in the landmark UKPDS study [146]. Considering EPC biology, one study found that circulating EPC counts increased after metformin initiation in patients with type 2 diabetes, correlating with increased FMD [115]. Later, an increase in EPCs was proven also in patients with type 1 diabetes, when metformin was given as a supportive treatment in the MERIT trial [116]. Regarding the EPC increase with metformin in patients with type 2 diabetes, this effect could be enhanced when gliclazide, a sulphonylurea, was added [117]. It seems that the most important mechanism affecting EPC biology in metformin-treated patients is increased phosphorylated-eNOS expression and NO production in cultures, as well as altered AMPK function [147].

In general, the effect on EPCs of most other anti-diabetic drugs was tested when these drugs were added to metformin, with few exceptions.

Gliclazide alone was also able to improve EPC biology, correlating with flow-mediated vessel dilatation and improvements in markers of oxidative stress as the key mechanism of action on EPCs [118]. It seems so far that gliclazide is the only sulphonylurea with a proven effect on EPCs. Glibenclamide did not show any increase in EPCs in a trial when it was compared to vildagliptin [119]. The same was shown for glimepiride when compared to sitagliptin [120]. Although hampered by methodological limitations in EPC characterization and the absence of clinical assessment of endothelial function, this finding fits perfectly into the context of better cardiovascular outcomes in patients treated with gliclazide compared to other sulphonylureas after myocardial infarction [148,149].

Another class of oral anti-diabetic drugs are thiazolidinediones, or peroxisome proliferator-activated receptors gamma (PPAR γ) agonists. Although they are used to improve blood glucose control, they have also been shown to affect other cardiovascular risk factors, like dyslipidemia and albuminuria [150,151]. Since these drugs may cause water retention, heart failure may occur [152,153]. Pioglitazone was shown to reduce the incidence of some major adverse cardiovascular events in patients with type 2 diabetes [154,155]. Two members of this class, rosiglitazone and pioglitazone, have been proven to impact EPCs. In patients with type 2 diabetes, rosiglitazone improved EPC re-endothelialization impaired by NADPH oxidase activity, diminishing the effects of oxidative stress [156]. Human studies with pioglitazone have demonstrated increased EPC counts and proliferative ability, decreased EPC apoptosis, and improvements in some metabolic parameters and inflammatory markers [121–124]. Improved adipokine profile and anti-inflammatory properties were also proposed mechanisms to obtain EPC biology improvement [122]. In some studies, CD34+/VEGFR2+ EPCs were investigated, and these studies showed favorable results on EPC health, but the clinical response on endothelial function remains unknown since it was not tested. It has to be mentioned that in one study, pioglitazone showed no impact on EPC counts, but in this study there is no evidence about the method used for EPC determination [125]. These results justify the need for future research regarding the impact of thiazolidindiones on EPCs and clinically assessed endothelial function.

Incretin-based therapies emerged recently as interesting add-ons to diabetic pharmacotherapy. There are two classes of incretin-modulating drugs. The first one contains inhibitors of dipeptidyl peptidase-4 (DPP-4 inhibitors). The main mode of action is inhibiting the breakdown of endogenous incretins, mainly GLP-1, thus maintaining the concentration of this substance within a physiological range. This incretin then enhances food-triggered insulin secretion. The majority of them like sitagliptin, linagliptin, saxagliptin, and alogliptin were tested in cardiovascular outcome trials and were proved to be non-inferior to standard treatment [157–160]. In other words, these drugs were as good as standard treatment at that time, like metformin, gliclazide, thiazolidindiones, or insulin. The impacts of vildagliptin and teneligliptin on cardiovascular outcomes were not tested in large, randomized trials.

Considering the effect of DPP-4 inhibitors on EPCs, there are some results published showing the favorable impact of these drugs. Improved glucoregulation, improved oxidative parameters, increased NO and SDF-1 production, and decreased inflammation are the proposed mechanisms for these effects [127,128,131]. Sitagliptin increased EPCs and SDF-1 during 4 weeks as add-on treatment compared to standard treatment involving metformin and/or insulin secretagogues in a small sample of people with type 2 diabetes [126]. Similar results considering EPC count, but with a decrease in SDF-1α during a 12-week trial in patients with type 2 diabetes, were detected when sitagliptin was added to metformin [120]. These results on SDF-1 fit less well into the proposed mechanism of action of DPP-4 inhibitors since DPP-4 degrades SDF-1 [161]. More recently, sitagliptin was tested against metformin in a short trial for three days. The drug increased EPCs, but also SDF-1α and NO concentration, with the most profound impact on patients receiving both drugs [127]. In another trial, in which voglibose was used as the comparator drug, sitagliptin was shown to increase EPCs and improve flow-mediated vasodilation, while voglibose showed no effect [128]. Linagliptin also increased the EPC count acutely in patients with type 2 diabetes during a 4-day trial, with increased concentrations of SDF-1α. Intriguingly, DPP-4 activity was abated by more than 50%, indicating other mechanisms responsible for an increase in SDF-1α [129]. An increase in SDF-1 with linagliptin has been observed even after 6 months of treatment. The effect on EPCs was not statistically significant [130]. However, in patients with chronic kidney disease, linagliptin improved EPC count, the antioxidant level was enhanced, and clinical parameters like augmentation index and pulse wave parameter were improved during a 12-week trial [131].

As mentioned before, vildagliptin also increases the number of EPCs, but with a reduction in SDF-1α levels after 12 months, in comparison to glibenclamide [119]. Alogliptin showed the same effect as gliclazide on the EPC count. The authors concluded that the observed increase in EPCs seemed to be due to the glucose-lowering effect of both drugs [132].

Furthermore, saxagliptin failed to be superior to metformin in two 12-week trials. Although there was an increase in EPC count and improvement in flow-mediated dilation, metformin showed similar effects when these drugs were given as monotherapy, with no add-on effect on EPCs in dual treatment [133,134]. Finally, teneligliptin showed an increasing trend in the number of EPCs, albeit this did not reach statistical significance. However, flow-mediated vasodilatation improved in the study group, suggesting a mechanism different than EPC [135]. In conclusion, there is some evidence that DDP-4 inhibitors improve certain aspects of EPC health; the main limitation is the absence of clinical endothelial assessment in the majority of research, and a short study duration in some of the trials.

In contrast to DPP-4 inhibitors, GLP-1 receptor agonists override the physiological effects of endogenous GLP-1 and exert a stronger effect on GLP-1 receptors. These are potent anti-diabetic drugs with the main mechanism of action that stimulates insulin secretion after an oral glucose load via the incretin effect. Other medical benefits may include delaying gastric emptying, inhibiting glucagon production, decreasing pancreatic beta-cell apoptosis, promoting weight loss, lowering arterial blood pressure and total cholesterol, improving left ventricular ejection fraction, myocardial contractility, coronary blood flow, cardiac output, and endothelial function while reducing infarction size. Some of them like liraglutide, semaglutide, and dulaglutide are proven to be superior to standard anti-diabetic treatment in secondary cardiovascular prevention [162–164]. Interestingly, there are limited data about their effects on human EPCs. In a small trial, liraglutide was inferior to exenatide considering EPC counts, but liraglutide was not given in the full dose of 1.8 mg daily. The authors speculated about antioxidative/anti-inflammatory effects as mediators on EPC biology [136]. In a head-to-head trial, comparing liraglutide in the full dose of 1.8 mg daily and sitagliptin, there was a similar effect on EPC count, with a more favorable effect of liraglutide on VEGF and SDF-1α after 26 weeks. However, in this trial, CD 34+/VEGFR2+ EPCs were not investigated [137]. So far, dulaglutide is the single GLP-1 receptor agonist that showed an increase in EPC count and function resulting in improved clinical parameters like brachial-ankle pulse wave velocity. Lower grades of inflammation and increased NO production were the supposed mechanisms for these effects [138]. No data on humans for semaglutide have yet been published. Putting all these data into the context of previously published cardiovascular outcome trials which stated superiority for the majority of these drugs [162–164], and borderline significance (p = 0.06) for exenatide [165], it seems that further investigations are justified to prove the beneficial impact of GLP-1 receptor agonists on EPCs.

Sodium-glucose transporter-2 inhibitors (SGLT2i) are the latest introduced class of anti-diabetic treatment. Their main mode of action involves the inhibition of the sodium/glucose co-transporter-2 (SGLT-2) in the kidneys' proximal tubule, causing glycosuria and lowering blood glucose levels independent of insulin action. Empagliflozin was the first anti-diabetic drug to show cardiovascular superiority over standard anti-diabetic treatment [166]. Later it was recognized that the benefit of the entire drug class goes beyond the glucose-lowering effects, from reducing the risk of MACEs, hospitalization for heart failure, and worsening of chronic kidney disease (CKD) in diabetic patients, to reducing the rate of cardiovascular death and hospitalization for heart failure in nondiabetic patients [167]. There is a limited number of clinical research studies considering the impact of SGLT2i on EPC biology. In the first randomized controlled trial of dapagliflozin vs. placebo with an open-label extension and an open-label observational study of empagliflozin treatment on levels of circulating stem cells (CSCs) and EPCs, results showed a non-significant increase in CSC and EPC after short-term treatment with SGLT-2is. After 1.5 years of dapagliflozin treatment, the EPC count significantly increased. The authors concluded that cardiovascular protection cannot be directly correlated with EPC counts, suggesting protection is dominantly attributable to other factors [139]. In another trial, empagliflozin increased the subpopulations of circulating cells expressing CD133+ following 6 months of treatment, while improving inflammation parameters [141]. In addition, dapagliflozin was shown to improve the vasculogenic capacity of EPCs via activating AMPK-mediated inhibition of inflammation and oxidative stress in a study comparing patients with type 2 diabetes with healthy controls over 3 months [140]. Similarly, a significant better expression of the CXCR4 receptor with an increase in the migratory function of CD34+ cells and an increase in the expression of antioxidants (superoxide dismutase 2, catalase, and glutathione peroxidase) in canagliflozin-treated patients as compared to the placebo group was shown [142]. These results suggest that the action of SGLT-2i may also be in part mediated through the effect on EPCs with consequently beneficial effects that go beyond the glucose-lowering effect, but it is still too early to deduce on the effect of this drug class on EPCs. Although there are only a few studies exploring these issues, they showed new directions in explaining and understanding the beneficial effects of SGLT-2i. Future research would surely benefit from better EPC definition.

The effect of insulin analogs on EPCs has also been investigated. In vitro, insulin can mobilize EPCs. In patients suffering from type 2 diabetes, both insulin glargine and detemir raised EPC counts, with no difference between the two drugs over 6 months [143]. However, it seems that long-acting insulin analogs increased the EPC count to a greater extent in comparison to intermediate-acting human insulin and oral drugs with a trend towards improved intima-media thickness [144]. Intensive insulin therapy enhanced EPC counts over 6 months compared to basal–oral therapy (metformin and/or sulphonylureas) in patients with type 2 diabetes and peripheral artery disease undergoing peripheral angiography and subsequent angioplasty procedure. However, the cumulative incidence of restenosis/amputation/limb salvage procedures/death in patients with type 2 diabetes and chronic limb ischemia patients did not differ between groups at the study end, but there was a significant effect on eNOS gene variants [145]. In addition, hypoglycemia during insulin therapy may negatively impact EPC biology and clinical outcomes [56]. Since there was no inherent effect of both NPH insulin and insulin glargine on EPC count compared to escalated oral therapy, it may be concluded that there is no specific effect of insulin beyond better glucose control. These findings fit into the general accepted fact that novel insulins are not superior to standard treatment in terms of reducing MACEs. Other factors, like eNOS genetic polymorphism and eventual hypoglycemic events, may easily overshadow the beneficial effects of insulin therapy.

Finally, it has to be mentioned that trials involving patients with type 1 diabetes are few. The majority of treatment discussed previously is registered for patients with type 2 diabetes. In an interesting trial involving patients with type 1 diabetes, reducing glucose variability with new technologies like insulin pumps showed beneficial effects on EPC count in a 6-month trial [58]. As mentioned before, adding metformin to insulin treatment in type 1 diabetes may improve EPC count and function [116].

5. Conclusions

EPCs are a captivating and vital component of the vascular system. Their roles in vascular repair, regeneration, and potential therapeutic applications make them a subject of ongoing research and hold promise for improving cardiovascular health and advancing regenerative medicine. Vessel regeneration and repairment are both altered in diabetes mellitus. Consequently, micro and macroangiopathic complications may develop. Therefore, EPCs have become the target of interest for many scientists who are putting an effort into discovering treatment options that can affect their count and function. Many available anti-diabetic drugs like metformin, sulphonylureas, PPAR γ agonists, DPP-4 inhibitors, and insulin are proven to improve, under certain conditions, the low number and functional impairment of EPCs. SGLT-2i and GLP-1 receptor agonists are the newest anti-diabetic drugs with limited evidence of beneficial effects on EPC biology. Future research will likely focus on untangling the complexity of EPC biology and developing innovative approaches to harness their full potential both in type 2 and type 1 diabetes.

To conclude, current data suggest that the low number and dysfunction of EPCs can be improved by treatment of diabetes with currently available drugs, either through drugs' specific mechanisms or through improving blood glucose control.

Author Contributions: Conceptualization, V.A. and T.B.; formal analysis, V.A., T.B., J.M.R., L.Š. and S.U.; writing—original draft, V.A., J.M.R. and L.Š.; writing—review and editing, V.A. and T.B. All authors have read and agreed to the published version of the manuscript.

Funding: This research received no external funding.

Conflicts of Interest: The authors declare no conflict of interest.

References

1. Chang, X.; Lochner, A.; Wang, H.-H.; Wang, S.; Zhu, H.; Ren, J.; Zhou, H. Coronary Microvascular Injury in Myocardial Infarction: Perception and Knowledge for Mitochondrial Quality Control. *Theranostics* **2021**, *11*, 6766. [CrossRef] [PubMed]
2. Cavieres, V.; Valdes, K.; Moreno, B.; Moore-Carrasco, R.; Gonzalez, D.R. Vascular Hypercontractility and Endothelial Dysfunction before Development of Atherosclerosis in Moderate Dyslipidemia: Role for Nitric Oxide and Interleukin-6. *Am. J. Cardiovasc. Dis.* **2014**, *4*, 114. [PubMed]
3. Hetherington, I.; Totary-Jain, H. Anti-Atherosclerotic Therapies: Milestones, Challenges, and Emerging Innovations. *Mol. Ther.* **2022**, *30*, 3106–3117. [CrossRef] [PubMed]
4. Prasad, K. Current Status of Primary, Secondary, and Tertiary Prevention of Coronary Artery Disease. *Int. J. Angiol.* **2021**, *30*, 177–186. [CrossRef] [PubMed]
5. Flora, G.D.; Nayak, M.K. A Brief Review of Cardiovascular Diseases, Associated Risk Factors and Current Treatment Regimes. *Curr. Pharm. Des.* **2019**, *25*, 4063–4084. [CrossRef]
6. Pacinella, G.; Ciaccio, A.M.; Tuttolomondo, A. Endothelial Dysfunction and Chronic Inflammation: The Cornerstones of Vascular Alterations in Age-Related Diseases. *Int. J. Mol. Sci.* **2022**, *23*, 15722. [CrossRef]
7. Chen, M.S.; Lee, R.T.; Garbern, J.C. Senescence Mechanisms and Targets in the Heart. *Cardiovasc. Res.* **2022**, *118*, 1173–1187. [CrossRef] [PubMed]
8. Haybar, H.; Shahrabi, S.; Rezaeeyan, H.; Shirzad, R.; Saki, N. Endothelial Cells: From Dysfunction Mechanism to Pharmacological Effect in Cardiovascular Disease. *Cardiovasc. Toxicol.* **2019**, *19*, 13–22. [CrossRef]
9. Van Craenenbroeck, E.M.; Van Craenenbroeck, A.H.; Van Ierssel, S.; Bruyndonckx, L.; Hoymans, V.Y.; Vrints, C.J.; Conraads, V.M. Quantification of Circulating CD34+/KDR+/CD45dim Endothelial Progenitor Cells: Analytical Considerations. *Int. J. Cardiol.* **2013**, *167*, 1688–1695. [CrossRef]
10. Patel, R.S.; Li, Q.; Ghasemzadeh, N.; Eapen, D.J.; Moss, L.D.; Janjua, A.U.; Manocha, P.; Al Kassem, H.; Veledar, E.; Samady, H.; et al. Circulating CD34+ Progenitor Cells and Risk of Mortality in a Population with Coronary Artery Disease. *Circ. Res.* **2015**, *116*, 289–297. [CrossRef]
11. Aquino, J.B.; Sierra, R.; Montaldo, L.A. Diverse Cellular Origins of Adult Blood Vascular Endothelial Cells. *Dev. Biol.* **2021**, *477*, 117–132. [CrossRef] [PubMed]
12. Yan, F.; Li, J.; Zhang, W. Transplantation of Endothelial Progenitor Cells: Summary and Prospect. *Acta Histochem.* **2023**, *125*, 151990. [CrossRef] [PubMed]
13. Medina, R.J.; Barber, C.L.; Sabatier, F.; Dignat-George, F.; Melero-Martin, J.M.; Khosrotehrani, K.; Ohneda, O.; Randi, A.M.; Chan, J.K.; Yamaguchi, T.; et al. Endothelial Progenitors: A Consensus Statement on Nomenclature. *Stem Cells Transl. Med.* **2017**, *6*, 1316–1320. [CrossRef]
14. Mastrolia, I.; Foppiani, E.M.; Murgia, A.; Candini, O.; Samarelli, A.V.; Grisendi, G.; Veronesi, E.; Horwitz, E.M.; Dominici, M. Challenges in Clinical Development of Mesenchymal Stromal/Stem Cells: Concise Review. *Stem Cells Transl. Med.* **2019**, *8*, 1135–1148. [CrossRef] [PubMed]
15. Fujita, Y.; Kawamoto, A. Stem Cell-Based Peripheral Vascular Regeneration. *Adv. Drug Deliv. Rev.* **2017**, *120*, 25–40. [CrossRef] [PubMed]
16. Xiao, S.-T.; Kuang, C.-Y. Endothelial Progenitor Cells and Coronary Artery Disease: Current Concepts and Future Research Directions. *World J. Clin. Cases* **2021**, *9*, 8953. [CrossRef]
17. Rajasekar, P.; O'Neill, C.L.; Eeles, L.; Stitt, A.W.; Medina, R.J. Epigenetic Changes in Endothelial Progenitors as a Possible Cellular Basis for Glycemic Memory in Diabetic Vascular Complications. *J. Diabetes Res.* **2015**, *2015*, 436879. [CrossRef]
18. Cassano, V.; Tripepi, G.; Perticone, M.; Miceli, S.; Scopacasa, I.; Armentaro, G.; Greco, M.; Maio, R.; Hribal, M.L.; Sesti, G.; et al. Endothelial Progenitor Cells Predict Vascular Damage Progression in Naive Hypertensive Patients According to Sex. *Hypertens. Res.* **2021**, *44*, 1451–1461. [CrossRef]
19. Kumawat, R.; Gulati, S.; Ahluwalia, C.; Bahamania, K.; Varshney, P. Relation of Endothelial Progenitor Cells and Carotid Intima Media Thickness in Indian Rheumatoid Arthritis Patients-A Cross Sectional Study. *J. Assoc. Phys. India* **2022**, *70*, 11–12.
20. Wu, W.-Z.; Hu, D.-J.; Wang, Z.-Y.; Liao, L.-S.; Li, C.-C. Endothelial Progenitor Cell Impairment Mediated Vasodilation Dysfunction via Diminishing Nitric Oxide Production in Postmenopausal Females. *Mol. Med. Rep.* **2019**, *19*, 2449–2457. [CrossRef]
21. Santillán-Cortez, D.; Vera-Gómez, E.; Hernández-Patricio, A.; Ruíz-Hernández, A.S.; Gutiérrez-Buendía, J.A.; De la Vega-Moreno, K.; Rizo-García, Y.A.; Loman-Zuñiga, O.A.; Escotto-Sánchez, I.; Rodríguez-Trejo, J.M.; et al. Endothelial Progenitor Cells May Be Related to Major Amputation after Angioplasty in Patients with Critical Limb Ischemia. *Cells* **2023**, *12*, 584. [CrossRef] [PubMed]
22. Heinisch, P.P.; Bello, C.; Emmert, M.Y.; Carrel, T.; Dreßen, M.; Hörer, J.; Winkler, B.; Luedi, M.M. Endothelial Progenitor Cells as Biomarkers of Cardiovascular Pathologies: A Narrative Review. *Cells* **2022**, *11*, 1678. [CrossRef] [PubMed]

23. Pyšná, A.; Bém, R.; Němcová, A.; Fejfarová, V.; Jirkovská, A.; Hazdrová, J.; Jude, E.B.; Dubský, M. Endothelial Progenitor Cells Biology in Diabetes Mellitus and Peripheral Arterial Disease and Their Therapeutic Potential. *Stem Cell Rev. Rep.* **2019**, *15*, 157–165. [CrossRef] [PubMed]
24. Kukumberg, M.; Zaw, A.M.; Wong, D.H.; Toh, C.M.; Chan, B.P.; Seet, R.C.; Wong, P.T.; Yim, E.K. Characterization and Functional Assessment of Endothelial Progenitor Cells in Ischemic Stroke Patients. *Stem Cell Rev. Rep.* **2021**, *17*, 952–967. [CrossRef] [PubMed]
25. Salybekov, A.A.; Kobayashi, S.; Asahara, T. Characterization of Endothelial Progenitor Cell: Past, Present, and Future. *Int. J. Mol. Sci.* **2022**, *23*, 7697. [CrossRef]
26. Chambers, S.E.; Pathak, V.; Pedrini, E.; Soret, L.; Gendron, N.; Guerin, C.L.; Stitt, A.W.; Smadja, D.M.; Medina, R.J. Current Concepts on Endothelial Stem Cells Definition, Location, and Markers. *Stem Cells Transl. Med.* **2021**, *10*, S54–S61. [CrossRef] [PubMed]
27. Altabas, V. Diabetes, Endothelial Dysfunction, and Vascular Repair: What Should a Diabetologist Keep His Eye On? *Int. J. Endocrinol.* **2015**, *2015*, 848272. [CrossRef]
28. Altabas, V.; Biloš, L.S.K. The Role of Endothelial Progenitor Cells in Atherosclerosis and Impact of Anti-Lipemic Treatments on Endothelial Repair. *Int. J. Mol. Sci.* **2022**, *23*, 2663. [CrossRef]
29. Ross, M.D. Endothelial Regenerative Capacity and Aging: Influence of Diet, Exercise and Obesity. *Curr. Cardiol. Rev.* **2018**, *14*, 233–244. [CrossRef]
30. Li, J.-H.; Li, Y.; Huang, D.; Yao, M. Role of Stromal Cell-Derived Factor-1 in Endothelial Progenitor Cell-Mediated Vascular Repair and Regeneration. *Tissue Eng. Regen. Med.* **2021**, *18*, 747–758. [CrossRef]
31. Klein, G.; Schmal, O.; Aicher, W.K. Matrix Metalloproteinases in Stem Cell Mobilization. *Matrix Biol.* **2015**, *44*, 175–183. [CrossRef] [PubMed]
32. Tao, J.; Cao, X.; Yu, B.; Qu, A. Vascular Stem/Progenitor Cells in Vessel Injury and Repair. *Front. Cardiovasc. Med.* **2022**, *9*, 845070. [CrossRef] [PubMed]
33. Wang, S.; Miao, J.; Qu, M.; Yang, G.-Y.; Shen, L. Adiponectin Modulates the Function of Endothelial Progenitor Cells via AMPK/eNOS Signaling Pathway. *Biochem. Biophys. Res. Commun.* **2017**, *493*, 64–70. [CrossRef] [PubMed]
34. Zhu, Z.; Fu, C.; Li, X.; Song, Y.; Li, C.; Zou, M.; Guan, Y.; Zhu, Y. Prostaglandin E2 Promotes Endothelial Differentiation from Bone Marrow-Derived Cells through AMPK Activation. *PLoS ONE* **2011**, *6*, e23554. [CrossRef]
35. Chopra, H.; Hung, M.K.; Kwong, D.L.; Zhang, C.F.; Pow, E.H.N. Insights into Endothelial Progenitor Cells: Origin, Classification, Potentials, and Prospects. *Stem Cells Int.* **2018**, *2018*, 9847015. [CrossRef]
36. Yang, J.-X.; Pan, Y.-Y.; Wang, X.-X.; Qiu, Y.-G.; Mao, W. Endothelial Progenitor Cells in Age-Related Vascular Remodeling. *Cell Transpl.* **2018**, *27*, 786–795. [CrossRef]
37. Morrone, D.; Picoi, M.E.L.; Felice, F.; De Martino, A.; Scatena, C.; Spontoni, P.; Naccarato, A.G.; Di Stefano, R.; Bortolotti, U.; Dal Monte, M. Endothelial Progenitor Cells: An Appraisal of Relevant Data from Bench to Bedside. *Int. J. Mol. Sci.* **2021**, *22*, 12874. [CrossRef]
38. Fadini, G.P.; Mehta, A.; Dhindsa, D.S.; Bonora, B.M.; Sreejit, G.; Nagareddy, P.; Quyyumi, A.A. Circulating Stem Cells and Cardiovascular Outcomes: From Basic Science to the Clinic. *Eur. Heart J.* **2020**, *41*, 4271–4282. [CrossRef]
39. Evans, C.E.; Iruela-Arispe, M.L.; Zhao, Y.-Y. Mechanisms of Endothelial Regeneration and Vascular Repair and Their Application to Regenerative Medicine. *Am. J. Pathol.* **2021**, *191*, 52–65. [CrossRef]
40. Pearson, J.D. Plasticity of Adult Endothelium: How Frequent and to What Extent? *Cardiovasc. Res.* **2015**, *108*, 319–320. [CrossRef]
41. Kliche, K.; Jeggle, P.; Pavenstädt, H.; Oberleithner, H. Role of Cellular Mechanics in the Function and Life Span of Vascular Endothelium. *Pflügers Arch. Eur. J. Physiol.* **2011**, *462*, 209–217. [CrossRef] [PubMed]
42. Hobson, B.; Denekamp, J. Endothelial Proliferation in Tumours and Normal Tissues: Continuous Labelling Studies. *Br. J. Cancer* **1984**, *49*, 405–413. [CrossRef] [PubMed]
43. Milutinović, A.; Šuput, D.; Zorc-Pleskovič, R. Pathogenesis of Atherosclerosis in the Tunica Intima, Media, and Adventitia of Coronary Arteries: An Updated Review. *Bosn. J. Basic Med. Sci.* **2020**, *20*, 21–30. [CrossRef]
44. Beck-Joseph, J.; Lehoux, S. Molecular Interactions between Vascular Smooth Muscle Cells and Macrophages in Atherosclerosis. *Front. Cardiovasc. Med.* **2021**, *8*, 737934. [CrossRef]
45. Murad, H.A.; Rafeeq, M.M.; Alqurashi, T.M. Role and Implications of the CXCL12/CXCR4/CXCR7 Axis in Atherosclerosis: Still a Debate. *Ann. Med.* **2021**, *53*, 1598–1612. [CrossRef] [PubMed]
46. Bochenek, M.L.; Schütz, E.; Schäfer, K. Endothelial Cell Senescence and Thrombosis: Ageing Clots. *Thromb. Res.* **2016**, *147*, 36–45. [CrossRef]
47. Fadini, G.P.; de Kreutzenberg, S.; Albiero, M.; Coracina, A.; Pagnin, E.; Baesso, I.; Cignarella, A.; Bolego, C.; Plebani, M.; Nardelli, G.B.; et al. Gender Differences in Endothelial Progenitor Cells and Cardiovascular Risk Profile: The Role of Female Estrogens. *Arterioscler. Thromb. Vasc. Biol.* **2008**, *28*, 997–1004. [CrossRef]
48. Tripolt, N.J.; Narath, S.H.; Eder, M.; Pieber, T.R.; Wascher, T.C.; Sourij, H. Multiple Risk Factor Intervention Reduces Carotid Atherosclerosis in Patients with Type 2 Diabetes. *Cardiovasc. Diabetol.* **2014**, *13*, 95. [CrossRef]
49. ElSayed, N.A.; Aleppo, G.; Aroda, V.R.; Bannuru, R.R.; Brown, F.M.; Bruemmer, D.; Collins, B.S.; Hilliard, M.E.; Isaacs, D.; Johnson, E.L.; et al. 2. Classification and Diagnosis of Diabetes: Standards of Care in Diabetes—2023. *Diabetes Care* **2023**, *46*, S19–S40. [CrossRef]

50. Jyotsna, F.; Ahmed, A.; Kumar, K.; Kaur, P.; Chaudhary, M.H.; Kumar, S.; Khan, E.; Khanam, B.; Shah, S.U.; Varrassi, G.; et al. Exploring the Complex Connection between Diabetes and Cardiovascular Disease: Analyzing Approaches to Mitigate Cardiovascular Risk in Patients with Diabetes. *Cureus* **2023**, *15*, e43882. [CrossRef]
51. Schneider, D.J. Diabetes and Thrombosis. In *Diabetes and Cardiovascular Disease*; Springer: Berlin/Heidelberg, Germany, 2023; pp. 99–127.
52. Sartore, G.; Ragazzi, E.; Caprino, R.; Lapolla, A. Long-Term HbA1c Variability and Macro-/Micro-Vascular Complications in Type 2 Diabetes Mellitus: A Meta-Analysis Update. *Acta Diabetol.* **2023**, *60*, 721–738. [CrossRef] [PubMed]
53. Wils, J.; Favre, J.; Bellien, J. Modulating Putative Endothelial Progenitor Cells for the Treatment of Endothelial Dysfunction and Cardiovascular Complications in Diabetes. *Pharmacol. Ther.* **2017**, *170*, 98–115. [CrossRef] [PubMed]
54. Fadini, G.P.; Boscaro, E.; De Kreutzenberg, S.; Agostini, C.; Seeger, F.; Dimmeler, S.; Zeiher, A.; Tiengo, A.; Avogaro, A. Time Course and Mechanisms of Circulating Progenitor Cell Reduction in the Natural History of Type 2 Diabetes. *Diabetes Care* **2010**, *33*, 1097–1102. [CrossRef] [PubMed]
55. Hörtenhuber, T.; Rami-Mehar, B.; Satler, M.; Nagl, K.; Höbaus, C.; Höllerl, F.; Koppensteiner, R.; Schernthaner, G.; Schober, E.; Schernthaner, G.-H. Endothelial Progenitor Cells Are Related to Glycemic Control in Children with Type 1 Diabetes over Time. *Diabetes Care* **2013**, *36*, 1647–1653. [CrossRef] [PubMed]
56. Fadini, G.; Albiero, M.; Vigili de Kreutzenberg, S.; Avogaro, A. Hypoglycemia Affects the Changes in Endothelial Progenitor Cell Levels during Insulin Therapy in Type 2 Diabetic Patients. *J. Endocrinol. Investig.* **2015**, *38*, 733–738. [CrossRef]
57. Fadini, G.P.; Boscari, F.; Cappellari, R.; Galasso, S.; Rigato, M.; Bonora, B.M.; D'Anna, M.; Bruttomesso, D.; Avogaro, A. Effects of Hypoglycemia on Circulating Stem and Progenitor Cells in Diabetic Patients. *J. Clin. Endocrinol. Metab.* **2018**, *103*, 1048–1055. [CrossRef]
58. Maiorino, M.I.; Casciano, O.; Volpe, E.D.; Bellastella, G.; Giugliano, D.; Esposito, K. Reducing Glucose Variability with Continuous Subcutaneous Insulin Infusion Increases Endothelial Progenitor Cells in Type 1 Diabetes: An Observational Study. *Endocrine* **2016**, *52*, 244–252. [CrossRef]
59. Qiu, C.; Xie, Q.; Zhang, D.; Chen, Q.; Hu, J.; Xu, L. GM-CSF Induces Cyclin D1 Expression and Proliferation of Endothelial Progenitor Cells via PI3K and MAPK Signaling. *Cell. Physiol. Biochem.* **2014**, *33*, 784–795. [CrossRef]
60. Zhou, Y.; Yan, H.; Guo, M.; Zhu, J.; Xiao, Q.; Zhang, L. Reactive Oxygen Species in Vascular Formation and Development. *Oxidative Med. Cell. Longev.* **2013**, *2013*, 374963. [CrossRef]
61. Toda, N.; Okamura, T. Obesity Impairs Vasodilatation and Blood Flow Increase Mediated by Endothelial Nitric Oxide: An Overview. *J. Clin. Pharmacol.* **2013**, *53*, 1228–1239. [CrossRef]
62. Ramalingam, P.; Poulos, M.G.; Lazzari, E.; Gutkin, M.C.; Lopez, D.; Kloss, C.C.; Crowley, M.J.; Katsnelson, L.; Freire, A.G.; Greenblatt, M.B.; et al. Chronic Activation of Endothelial MAPK Disrupts Hematopoiesis via NFKB Dependent Inflammatory Stress Reversible by SCGF. *Nat. Commun.* **2020**, *11*, 666. [CrossRef] [PubMed]
63. Goligorsky, M.; Hirschi, K. Stress-Induced Premature Senescence of Endothelial and Endothelial Progenitor Cells. *Adv. Pharmacol.* **2016**, *77*, 281–306. [PubMed]
64. Saad, M.I.; Abdelkhalek, T.M.; Saleh, M.M.; Kamel, M.A.; Youssef, M.; Tawfik, S.H.; Dominguez, H. Insights into the Molecular Mechanisms of Diabetes-Induced Endothelial Dysfunction: Focus on Oxidative Stress and Endothelial Progenitor Cells. *Endocrine* **2015**, *50*, 537–567. [CrossRef] [PubMed]
65. Juin, S.K.; Ouseph, R.; Gondim, D.D.; Jala, V.R.; Sen, U. Diabetic Nephropathy and Gaseous Modulators. *Antioxidants* **2023**, *12*, 1088. [CrossRef]
66. Rigato, M.; Bittante, C.; Albiero, M.; Avogaro, A.; Fadini, G.P. Circulating Progenitor Cell Count Predicts Microvascular Outcomes in Type 2 Diabetic Patients. *J. Clin. Endocrinol. Metab.* **2015**, *100*, 2666–2672. [CrossRef]
67. Makino, H.; Miyamoto, Y.; Kikuchi-Taura, A.; Soma, T.; Taguchi, A.; Kishimoto, I. Decreased Levels of Circulating CD 34+ Cells Are Associated with Coronary Heart Disease in Japanese Patients with Type 2 Diabetes. *J. Diabetes Investig.* **2015**, *6*, 473–478. [CrossRef]
68. Yu, C.-G.; Zhang, N.; Yuan, S.-S.; Ma, Y.; Yang, L.-Y.; Feng, Y.-M.; Zhao, D. Endothelial Progenitor Cells in Diabetic Microvascular Complications: Friends or Foes? *Stem Cells Int.* **2016**, *2016*, 1803989. [CrossRef]
69. Das, S.K.; Yuan, Y.F.; Li, M.Q. An Overview on Current Issues and Challenges of Endothelial Progenitor Cell-Based Neovascularization in Patients with Diabetic Foot Ulcer. *Cell. Reprogramming* **2017**, *19*, 75–87. [CrossRef]
70. Naaman, S.C.; Bakris, G.L. Diabetic Nephropathy: Update on Pillars of Therapy Slowing Progression. *Diabetes Care* **2023**, *46*, 1574–1586. [CrossRef]
71. American Diabetes Association. Retinopathy, Neuropathy, and Foot Care: Standards of Care in Diabetes—2023. *Diabetes Care* **2023**, *46*, S203–S215. [CrossRef]
72. Berezin, A.E. Endothelial Progenitor Cells Dysfunction and Impaired Tissue Reparation: The Missed Link in Diabetes Mellitus Development. *Diabetes Metab. Syndr. Clin. Res. Rev.* **2017**, *11*, 215–220. [CrossRef] [PubMed]
73. Holman, R.R.; Paul, S.K.; Bethel, M.A.; Neil, H.A.W.; Matthews, D.R. Long-Term Follow-up after Tight Control of Blood Pressure in Type 2 Diabetes. *N. Engl. J. Med.* **2008**, *359*, 1565–1576. [CrossRef] [PubMed]
74. Fullerton, B.; Jeitler, K.; Seitz, M.; Horvath, K.; Berghold, A.; Siebenhofer, A. Intensive Glucose Control versus Conventional Glucose Control for Type 1 Diabetes Mellitus. *Cochrane Database Syst. Rev.* **2014**, *2016*, CD009122. [CrossRef] [PubMed]

75. ElSayed, N.A.; Aleppo, G.; Aroda, V.R.; Bannuru, R.R.; Brown, F.M.; Bruemmer, D.; Collins, B.S.; Hilliard, M.E.; Isaacs, D.; Johnson, E.L.; et al. 9. Pharmacologic Approaches to Glycemic Treatment: Standards of Care in Diabetes—2023. *Diabetes Care* **2023**, *46*, S140–S157. [CrossRef] [PubMed]
76. Liu, G.; Li, Y.; Pan, A.; Hu, Y.; Chen, S.; Qian, F.; Rimm, E.B.; Manson, J.E.; Stampfer, M.J.; Giatsidis, G.; et al. Adherence to a Healthy Lifestyle in Association with Microvascular Complications Among Adults with Type 2 Diabetes. *JAMA Netw. Open* **2023**, *6*, e2252239. [CrossRef]
77. Monaghan, M.; Helgeson, V.; Wiebe, D. Type 1 Diabetes in Young Adulthood. *Curr. Diabetes Rev.* **2015**, *11*, 239–250. [CrossRef]
78. Mottalib, A.; Salsberg, V.; Mohd-Yusof, B.-N.; Mohamed, W.; Carolan, P.; Pober, D.M.; Mitri, J.; Hamdy, O. Effects of Nutrition Therapy on HbA1c and Cardiovascular Disease Risk Factors in Overweight and Obese Patients with Type 2 Diabetes. *Nutr. J.* **2018**, *17*, 42. [CrossRef]
79. ElSayed, N.A.; Aleppo, G.; Aroda, V.R.; Bannuru, R.R.; Brown, F.M.; Bruemmer, D.; Collins, B.S.; Hilliard, M.E.; Isaacs, D.; Johnson, E.L.; et al. 5. Facilitating Positive Health Behaviors and Well-Being to Improve Health Outcomes: Standards of Care in Diabetes—2023. *Diabetes Care* **2023**, *46*, S68–S96. [CrossRef]
80. Dunkler, D.; Kohl, M.; Heinze, G.; Teo, K.K.; Rosengren, A.; Pogue, J.; Gao, P.; Gerstein, H.; Yusuf, S.; Oberbauer, R.; et al. Modifiable Lifestyle and Social Factors Affect Chronic Kidney Disease in High-Risk Individuals with Type 2 Diabetes Mellitus. *Kidney Int.* **2015**, *87*, 784–791. [CrossRef]
81. Sala-Vila, A.; Díaz-López, A.; Valls-Pedret, C.; Cofán, M.; García-Layana, A.; Lamuela-Raventós, R.-M.; Castañer, O.; Zanon-Moreno, V.; Martinez-Gonzalez, M.A.; Toledo, E.; et al. Dietary Marine Ømega-3 Fatty Acids and Incident Sight-Threatening Retinopathy in Middle-Aged and Older Individuals with Type 2 Diabetes: Prospective Investigation from the PREDIMED Trial. *JAMA Ophthalmol.* **2016**, *134*, 1142–1149. [CrossRef]
82. Storz, M.A.; Küster, O. Plant-Based Diets and Diabetic Neuropathy: A Systematic Review. *Lifestyle Med.* **2020**, *1*, e6. [CrossRef]
83. Maiorino, M.I.; Bellastella, G.; Petrizzo, M.; Gicchino, M.; Caputo, M.; Giugliano, D.; Esposito, K. Effect of a Mediterranean Diet on Endothelial Progenitor Cells and Carotid Intima-Media Thickness in Type 2 Diabetes: Follow-up of a Randomized Trial. *Eur. J. Prev. Cardiol.* **2017**, *24*, 399–408. [CrossRef] [PubMed]
84. Mano, R.; Ishida, A.; Ohya, Y.; Todoriki, H.; Takishita, S. Dietary Intervention with Okinawan Vegetables Increased Circulating Endothelial Progenitor Cells in Healthy Young Women. *Atherosclerosis* **2009**, *204*, 544–548. [CrossRef] [PubMed]
85. Heiss, C.; Jahn, S.; Taylor, M.; Real, W.M.; Angeli, F.S.; Wong, M.L.; Amabile, N.; Prasad, M.; Rassaf, T.; Ottaviani, J.I.; et al. Improvement of Endothelial Function with Dietary Flavanols Is Associated with Mobilization of Circulating Angiogenic Cells in Patients with Coronary Artery Disease. *J. Am. Coll. Cardiol.* **2010**, *56*, 218–224. [CrossRef] [PubMed]
86. Marin, C.; Ramirez, R.; Delgado-Lista, J.; Yubero-Serrano, E.M.; Perez-Martinez, P.; Carracedo, J.; Garcia-Rios, A.; Rodriguez, F.; Gutierrez-Mariscal, F.M.; Gomez, P.; et al. Mediterranean Diet Reduces Endothelial Damage and Improves the Regenerative Capacity of Endothelium. *Am. J. Clin. Nutr.* **2011**, *93*, 267–274. [CrossRef]
87. Yubero-Serrano, E.M.; Fernandez-Gandara, C.; Garcia-Rios, A.; Rangel-Zuñiga, O.A.; Gutierrez-Mariscal, F.M.; Torres-Peña, J.D.; Marin, C.; Lopez-Moreno, J.; Castaño, J.P.; Delgado-Lista, J.; et al. Mediterranean Diet and Endothelial Function in Patients with Coronary Heart Disease: An Analysis of the CORDIOPREV Randomized Controlled Trial. *PLoS Med.* **2020**, *17*, e1003282. [CrossRef]
88. Fernández, J.M.; Rosado-Álvarez, D.; Da Silva Grigoletto, M.E.; Rangel-Zúñiga, O.A.; Landaeta-Díaz, L.L.; Caballero-Villarraso, J.; López-Miranda, J.; Pérez-Jiménez, F.; Fuentes-Jiménez, F. Moderate-to-High-Intensity Training and a Hypocaloric Mediterranean Diet Enhance Endothelial Progenitor Cells and Fitness in Subjects with the Metabolic Syndrome. *Clin. Sci.* **2012**, *123*, 361–373. [CrossRef]
89. Spigoni, V.; Lombardi, C.; Cito, M.; Picconi, A.; Ridolfi, V.; Andreoli, R.; Anelli, N.; Gnudi, L.; Goldoni, M.; Zavaroni, I.; et al. N-3 PUFA Increase Bioavailability and Function of Endothelial Progenitor Cells. *Food Funct.* **2014**, *5*, 1881–1890. [CrossRef]
90. Weech, M.; Altowaijri, H.; Mayneris-Perxachs, J.; Vafeiadou, K.; Madden, J.; Todd, S.; Jackson, K.G.; Lovegrove, J.A.; Yaqoob, P. Replacement of Dietary Saturated Fat with Unsaturated Fats Increases Numbers of Circulating Endothelial Progenitor Cells and Decreases Numbers of Microparticles: Findings from the Randomized, Controlled Dietary Intervention and VAScular Function (DIVAS) Study. *Am. J. Clin. Nutr.* **2018**, *107*, 876–882.
91. Cesari, F.; Dinu, M.; Pagliai, G.; Rogolino, A.; Giusti, B.; Gori, A.M.; Casini, A.; Marcucci, R.; Sofi, F. Mediterranean, but Not Lacto-Ovo-Vegetarian, Diet Positively Influence Circulating Progenitor Cells for Cardiovascular Prevention: The CARDIVEG Study. *Nutr. Metab. Cardiovasc. Dis.* **2019**, *29*, 604–610. [CrossRef]
92. Sereni, A.; Cesari, F.; Gori, A.M.; Maggini, N.; Marcucci, R.; Casini, A.; Sofi, F. Cardiovascular Benefits from Ancient Grain Bread Consumption: Findings from a Double-Blinded Randomized Crossover Intervention Trial. *Int. J. Food Sci. Nutr.* **2017**, *68*, 97–103. [CrossRef] [PubMed]
93. Kim, W.; Jeong, M.H.; Cho, S.H.; Yun, J.H.; Chae, H.J.; Ahn, Y.K.; Lee, M.C.; Cheng, X.; Kondo, T.; Murohara, T.; et al. Effect of Green Tea Consumption on Endothelial Function and Circulating Endothelial Progenitor Cells in Chronic Smokers. *Circ. J.* **2006**, *70*, 1052–1057. [CrossRef] [PubMed]
94. Chiva-Blanch, G.; Condines, X.; Magraner, E.; Roth, I.; Valderas-Martínez, P.; Arranz, S.; Casas, R.; Martínez-Huélamo, M.; Vallverdú-Queralt, A.; Quifer-Rada, P.; et al. The Non-Alcoholic Fraction of Beer Increases Stromal Cell Derived Factor 1 and the Number of Circulating Endothelial Progenitor Cells in High Cardiovascular Risk Subjects: A Randomized Clinical Trial. *Atherosclerosis* **2014**, *233*, 518–524. [CrossRef] [PubMed]

95. Huang, P.-H.; Chen, Y.-H.; Tsai, H.-Y.; Chen, J.-S.; Wu, T.-C.; Lin, F.-Y.; Sata, M.; Chen, J.-W.; Lin, S.-J. Intake of Red Wine Increases the Number and Functional Capacity of Circulating Endothelial Progenitor Cells by Enhancing Nitric Oxide Bioavailability. *Arterioscler. Thromb. Vasc. Biol.* **2010**, *30*, 869–877. [CrossRef] [PubMed]
96. Roth, I.; Casas, R.; Medina-Remón, A.; Lamuela-Raventós, R.M.; Estruch, R. Consumption of Aged White Wine Modulates Cardiovascular Risk Factors via Circulating Endothelial Progenitor Cells and Inflammatory Biomarkers. *Clin. Nutr.* **2019**, *38*, 1036–1044. [CrossRef]
97. Corban, M.T.; Widmer, R.J.; Cilluffo, R.; Kazeck, M.A.; Lennon, R.J.; Lerman, L.O.; Lerman, A. The Effect of Polyphenol-Rich Chardonnay Seed Supplements on Peripheral Endothelial Function. *Eur. J. Nutr.* **2020**, *59*, 3723–3734. [CrossRef]
98. Shannon, O.M.; Stephan, B.C.; Minihane, A.-M.; Mathers, J.C.; Siervo, M. Nitric Oxide Boosting Effects of the Mediterranean Diet: A Potential Mechanism of Action. *J. Gerontol. Ser. A* **2018**, *73*, 902–904. [CrossRef]
99. Medina-Remón, A.; Tresserra-Rimbau, A.; Pons, A.; Tur, J.A.; Martorell, M.; Ros, E.; Buil-Cosiales, P.; Sacanella, E.; Covas, M.I.; Corella, D.; et al. Effects of Total Dietary Polyphenols on Plasma Nitric Oxide and Blood Pressure in a High Cardiovascular Risk Cohort. The PREDIMED Randomized Trial. *Nutr. Metab. Cardiovasc. Dis.* **2015**, *25*, 60–67. [CrossRef]
100. Shah, R.; Makarem, N.; Emin, M.; Liao, M.; Jelic, S.; Aggarwal, B. Mediterranean Diet Components Are Linked to Greater Endothelial Function and Lower Inflammation in a Pilot Study of Ethnically Diverse Women. *Nutr. Res.* **2020**, *75*, 77–84. [CrossRef]
101. Galié, S.; García-Gavilán, J.; Papandreou, C.; Camacho-Barcía, L.; Arcelin, P.; Palau-Galindo, A.; Rabassa, A.; Bulló, M. Effects of Mediterranean Diet on Plasma Metabolites and Their Relationship with Insulin Resistance and Gut Microbiota Composition in a Crossover Randomized Clinical Trial. *Clin. Nutr.* **2021**, *40*, 3798–3806. [CrossRef]
102. Aoki, A.; Murata, M.; Asano, T.; Ikoma, A.; Sasaki, M.; Saito, T.; Otani, T.; Jinbo, S.; Ikeda, N.; Kawakami, M.; et al. Prompt Increases in Retinol-Binding Protein 4 and Endothelial Progenitor Cells during Acute Exercise Load in Diabetic Subjects. *Endocr. J.* **2012**, *59*, 1085–1091. [CrossRef] [PubMed]
103. Waclawovsky, G.; Umpierre, D.; Figueira, F.R.; De Lima, E.S.; Alegretti, A.P.; Schneider, L.; Matte, U.S.; Rodrigues, T.C.; Schaan, B.D. Exercise on Progenitor Cells in Healthy Subjects and Patients with Type 1 Diabetes. *Med. Sci. Sports Exerc.* **2016**, *48*, 190–199. [CrossRef] [PubMed]
104. Taylor, G.S.; Shaw, A.; Smith, K.; Capper, T.E.; Scragg, J.H.; Cronin, M.; Bashir, A.; Flatt, A.; Campbell, M.D.; Stevenson, E.J.; et al. Type 1 Diabetes Patients Increase CXCR4+ and CXCR7+ Haematopoietic and Endothelial Progenitor Cells with Exercise, but the Response Is Attenuated. *Sci. Rep.* **2021**, *11*, 14502. [CrossRef] [PubMed]
105. Bruyndonckx, L.; Hoymans, V.Y.; De Guchtenaere, A.; Van Helvoirt, M.; Van Craenenbroeck, E.M.; Frederix, G.; Lemmens, K.; Vissers, D.K.; Vrints, C.J.; Ramet, J.; et al. Diet, Exercise, and Endothelial Function in Obese Adolescents. *Pediatrics* **2015**, *135*, e653–e661. [CrossRef] [PubMed]
106. Eleuteri, E.; Mezzani, A.; Di Stefano, A.; Vallese, D.; Gnemmi, I.; Delle Donne, L.; Taddeo, A.; Della Bella, S.; Giannuzzi, P. Aerobic Training and Angiogenesis Activation in Patients with Stable Chronic Heart Failure: A Preliminary Report. *Biomarkers* **2013**, *18*, 418–424. [CrossRef]
107. Möbius-Winkler, S.; Hilberg, T.; Menzel, K.; Golla, E.; Burman, A.; Schuler, G.; Adams, V. Time-Dependent Mobilization of Circulating Progenitor Cells during Strenuous Exercise in Healthy Individuals. *J. Appl. Physiol.* **2009**, *107*, 1943–1950. [CrossRef]
108. Manfredini, F.; Rigolin, G.; Malagoni, A.; Catizone, L.; Mandini, S.; Sofritti, O.; Mauro, E.; Soffritti, S.; Boari, B.; Cuneo, A.; et al. Exercise Training and Endothelial Progenitor Cells in Haemodialysis Patients. *J. Int. Med. Res.* **2009**, *37*, 534–540. [CrossRef]
109. Kaźmierski, M.; Wojakowski, W.; Michalewska-W\ludarczyk, A.; Podolecka, E.; Kotowski, M.; Machaliński, B.; Tendera, M. Exercise-Induced Mobilisation of Endothelial Progenitor Cells in Patients with Premature Coronary Heart Disease. *Kardiol. Pol. Pol. Heart J.* **2015**, *73*, 411–418. [CrossRef]
110. Bajer, B.; Vlcek, M.; Galusova, A.; Imrich, R.; Penesova, A. Exercise Associated Hormonal Signals as Powerful Determinants of an Effective Fat Mass Loss. *Endocr. Regul.* **2015**, *49*, 151–163. [CrossRef]
111. Dyakova, E.Y.; Kapilevich, L.V.; Shylko, V.G.; Popov, S.V.; Anfinogenova, Y. Physical Exercise Associated with NO Production: Signaling Pathways and Significance in Health and Disease. *Front. Cell Dev. Biol.* **2015**, *3*, 19. [CrossRef]
112. Benowitz, N.L.; Burbank, A.D. Cardiovascular Toxicity of Nicotine: Implications for Electronic Cigarette Use. *Trends Cardiovasc. Med.* **2016**, *26*, 515–523. [CrossRef] [PubMed]
113. Kondo, T.; Nakano, Y.; Adachi, S.; Murohara, T. Effects of Tobacco Smoking on Cardiovascular Disease. *Circ. J.* **2019**, *83*, 1980–1985. [CrossRef] [PubMed]
114. Antoniewicz, L.; Bosson, J.A.; Kuhl, J.; Abdel-Halim, S.M.; Kiessling, A.; Mobarrez, F.; Lundbäck, M. Electronic Cigarettes Increase Endothelial Progenitor Cells in the Blood of Healthy Volunteers. *Atherosclerosis* **2016**, *255*, 179–185. [CrossRef] [PubMed]
115. Liao, Y.; Chen, L.-L.; Zeng, T.; Li, Y.; Yu, F.; Hu, L.; Yue, L. Number of Circulating Endothelial Progenitor Cells as a Marker of Vascular Endothelial Function for Type 2 Diabetes. *Vasc. Med.* **2010**, *15*, 279–285. [CrossRef] [PubMed]
116. Ahmed, F.W.; Rider, R.; Glanville, M.; Narayanan, K.; Razvi, S.; Weaver, J.U. Metformin Improves Circulating Endothelial Cells and Endothelial Progenitor Cells in Type 1 Diabetes: MERIT Study. *Cardiovasc. Diabetol.* **2016**, *15*, 116. [CrossRef] [PubMed]
117. Chen, L.; Liao, Y.; Zeng, T.; Yu, F.; Li, H.; Feng, Y. Effects of Metformin plus Gliclazide Compared with Metformin Alone on Circulating Endothelial Progenitor Cell in Type 2 Diabetic Patients. *Endocrine* **2010**, *38*, 266–275. [CrossRef] [PubMed]
118. Chen, L.-L.; Yu, F.; Zeng, T.; Liao, Y.; Li, Y.; Ding, H. Effects of Gliclazide on Endothelial Function in Patients with Newly Diagnosed Type 2 Diabetes. *Eur. J. Pharmacol.* **2011**, *659*, 296–301. [CrossRef]

119. Dei Cas, A.; Spigoni, V.; Cito, M.; Aldigeri, R.; Ridolfi, V.; Marchesi, E.; Marina, M.; Derlindati, E.; Aloe, R.; Bonadonna, R.C.; et al. Vildagliptin, but Not Glibenclamide, Increases Circulating Endothelial Progenitor Cell Number: A 12-Month Randomized Controlled Trial in Patients with Type 2 Diabetes. *Cardiovasc. Diabetol.* **2017**, *16*, 27. [CrossRef]
120. Aso, Y.; Jojima, T.; Iijima, T.; Suzuki, K.; Terasawa, T.; Fukushima, M.; Momobayashi, A.; Hara, K.; Takebayashi, K.; Kasai, K.; et al. Sitagliptin, a Dipeptidyl Peptidase-4 Inhibitor, Increases the Number of Circulating CD34+ CXCR4+ Cells in Patients with Type 2 Diabetes. *Endocrine* **2015**, *50*, 659–664. [CrossRef]
121. Esposito, K.; Maiorino, M.; Di Palo, C.; Gicchino, M.; Petrizzo, M.; Bellastella, G.; Saccomanno, F.; Giugliano, D. Effects of Pioglitazone versus Metformin on Circulating Endothelial Microparticles and Progenitor Cells in Patients with Newly Diagnosed Type 2 Diabetes—A Randomized Controlled Trial. *Diabetes Obes. Metab.* **2011**, *13*, 439–445. [CrossRef]
122. Makino, H.; Okada, S.; Nagumo, A.; Sugisawa, T.; Miyamoto, Y.; Kishimoto, I.; Akie, T.K.; Soma, T.; Taguchi, A.; Yoshimasa, Y. Pioglitazone Treatment Stimulates Circulating CD34-Positive Cells in Type 2 Diabetes Patients. *Diabetes Res. Clin. Pract.* **2008**, *81*, 327–330. [CrossRef] [PubMed]
123. Wang, C.-H.; Ting, M.-K.; Verma, S.; Kuo, L.-T.; Yang, N.-I.; Hsieh, I.-C.; Wang, S.-Y.; Hung, A.; Cherng, W.-J. Pioglitazone Increases the Numbers and Improves the Functional Capacity of Endothelial Progenitor Cells in Patients with Diabetes Mellitus. *Am. Heart J.* **2006**, *152*, 1051.e1–1051.e8. [CrossRef] [PubMed]
124. Werner, C.; Kamani, C.H.; Gensch, C.; Bohm, M.; Laufs, U. The Peroxisome Proliferator–Activated Receptor-γ Agonist Pioglitazone Increases Number and Function of Endothelial Progenitor Cells in Patients with Coronary Artery Disease and Normal Glucose Tolerance. *Diabetes* **2007**, *56*, 2609–2615. [CrossRef] [PubMed]
125. Kampoli, A.-M.; Tousoulis, D.; Pallantza, Z.; Paterakis, G.; Papageorgiou, N.; Oikonomou, E.; Miliou, A.; Vlachopoulou, A.; Stefanadis, C. Comparable Effects of Pioglitazone and Perindopril on Circulating Endothelial Progenitor Cells, Inflammatory Process and Oxidative Stress in Patients with Diabetes Mellitus. *Int. J. Cardiol.* **2012**, *157*, 413–415. [CrossRef]
126. Fadini, G.P.; Boscaro, E.; Albiero, M.; Menegazzo, L.; Frison, V.; De Kreutzenberg, S.; Agostini, C.; Tiengo, A.; Avogaro, A. The Oral Dipeptidyl Peptidase-4 Inhibitor Sitagliptin Increases Circulating Endothelial Progenitor Cells in Patients with Type 2 Diabetes: Possible Role of Stromal-Derived Factor-1α. *Diabetes Care* **2010**, *33*, 1607–1609. [CrossRef]
127. Xu, M.; Zhao, X.; Zheng, M.; Deng, D.; Zhang, S.; Wang, Y.; Fang, Z.; Chen, M. Acute Effects of Sitagliptin on Progenitor Cells and Soluble Mediators in Newly Diagnosed Type 2 Diabetes. *Int. J. Clin. Pharmacol. Ther.* **2020**, *58*, 491. [CrossRef]
128. Nakamura, K.; Oe, H.; Kihara, H.; Shimada, K.; Fukuda, S.; Watanabe, K.; Takagi, T.; Yunoki, K.; Miyoshi, T.; Hirata, K.; et al. DPP-4 Inhibitor and Alpha-Glucosidase Inhibitor Equally Improve Endothelial Function in Patients with Type 2 Diabetes: EDGE Study. *Cardiovasc. Diabetol.* **2014**, *13*, 110. [CrossRef]
129. Fadini, G.P.; Bonora, B.M.; Cappellari, R.; Menegazzo, L.; Vedovato, M.; Iori, E.; Marescotti, M.C.; Albiero, M.; Avogaro, A. Acute Effects of Linagliptin on Progenitor Cells, Monocyte Phenotypes, and Soluble Mediators in Type 2 Diabetes. *J. Clin. Endocrinol. Metab.* **2016**, *101*, 748–756. [CrossRef]
130. De Boer, S.A.; Reijrink, M.; Abdulahad, W.H.; Hoekstra, E.S.; Slart, R.H.; Heerspink, H.J.; Westra, J.; Mulder, D.J. Angiogenic T Cells Are Decreased in People with Type 2 Diabetes Mellitus and Recruited by the Dipeptidyl Peptidase-4 Inhibitor Linagliptin: A Subanalysis from a Randomized, Placebo-Controlled Trial (RELEASE Study). *Diabetes Obes. Metab.* **2020**, *22*, 1220–1225. [CrossRef]
131. Awal, H.B.; Nandula, S.R.; Domingues, C.C.; Dore, F.J.; Kundu, N.; Brichacek, B.; Fakhri, M.; Elzarki, A.; Ahmadi, N.; Safai, S.; et al. Linagliptin, When Compared to Placebo, Improves CD34+ ve Endothelial Progenitor Cells in Type 2 Diabetes Subjects with Chronic Kidney Disease Taking Metformin and/or Insulin: A Randomized Controlled Trial. *Cardiovasc. Diabetol.* **2020**, *19*, 72. [CrossRef]
132. Negro, R.; Greco, E.L.; Greco, G. Alogliptin and Gliclazide Similarly Increase Circulating Endothelial Progenitor Cells in Type 2 Diabetes Patients. *Exp. Clin. Endocrinol. Diabetes* **2019**, *127*, 215–219. [CrossRef] [PubMed]
133. Li, F.; Chen, J.; Leng, F.; Lu, Z.; Ling, Y. Effect of Saxagliptin on Circulating Endothelial Progenitor Cells and Endothelial Function in Newly Diagnosed Type 2 Diabetic Patients. *Exp. Clin. Endocrinol. Diabetes* **2017**, *125*, 400–407. [CrossRef] [PubMed]
134. Dore, F.J.; Domingues, C.C.; Ahmadi, N.; Kundu, N.; Kropotova, Y.; Houston, S.; Rouphael, C.; Mammadova, A.; Witkin, L.; Khiyami, A.; et al. The Synergistic Effects of Saxagliptin and Metformin on CD34+ Endothelial Progenitor Cells in Early Type 2 Diabetes Patients: A Randomized Clinical Trial. *Cardiovasc. Diabetol.* **2018**, *17*, 65. [CrossRef] [PubMed]
135. Akashi, N.; Umemoto, T.; Yamada, H.; Fujiwara, T.; Yamamoto, K.; Taniguchi, Y.; Sakakura, K.; Wada, H.; Momomura, S.; Fujita, H. Teneligliptin, a DPP-4 Inhibitor, Improves Vascular Endothelial Function via Divergent Actions Including Changes in Circulating Endothelial Progenitor Cells. *Diabetes Metab. Syndr. Obes.* **2023**, *16*, 1043–1054. [CrossRef]
136. De Ciuceis, C.; Agabiti-Rosei, C.; Rossini, C.; Caletti, S.; Coschignano, M.A.; Ferrari-Toninelli, G.; Ragni, G.; Cappelli, C.; Cerudelli, B.; Airò, P.; et al. Microvascular Density and Circulating Endothelial Progenitor Cells before and after Treatment with Incretin Mimetics in Diabetic Patients. *High Blood Press. Cardiovasc. Prev.* **2018**, *25*, 369–378. [CrossRef]
137. Ahmad, E.; Waller, H.L.; Sargeant, J.A.; Webb, M.A.; Htike, Z.Z.; McCann, G.P.; Gulsin, G.; Khunti, K.; Yates, T.; Henson, J.; et al. Effects of Liraglutide versus Sitagliptin on Circulating Cardiovascular Biomarkers, Including Circulating Progenitor Cells, in Individuals with Type 2 Diabetes and Obesity: Analyses from the LYDIA Trial. *Diabetes Obes. Metab.* **2021**, *23*, 1409–1414. [CrossRef]
138. Xie, D.; Li, Y.; Xu, M.; Zhao, X.; Chen, M. Effects of Dulaglutide on Endothelial Progenitor Cells and Arterial Elasticity in Patients with Type 2 Diabetes Mellitus. *Cardiovasc. Diabetol.* **2022**, *21*, 200. [CrossRef]

139. Bonora, B.M.; Cappellari, R.; Albiero, M.; Avogaro, A.; Fadini, G.P. Effects of SGLT2 Inhibitors on Circulating Stem and Progenitor Cells in Patients with Type 2 Diabetes. *J. Clin. Endocrinol. Metab.* **2018**, *103*, 3773–3782. [CrossRef]
140. Luo, L.; Dong, B.; Zhang, J.; Qiu, Y.; Liu, X.; Zhou, Z.; He, J.; Zhang, X.; Chen, L.; Xia, W. Dapagliflozin Restores Diabetes-Associated Decline in Vasculogenic Capacity of Endothelial Progenitor Cells via Activating AMPK-Mediated Inhibition of Inflammation and Oxidative Stress. *Biochem. Biophys. Res. Commun.* **2023**, *671*, 205–214. [CrossRef]
141. Hess, D.A.; Terenzi, D.C.; Trac, J.Z.; Quan, A.; Mason, T.; Al-Omran, M.; Bhatt, D.L.; Dhingra, N.; Rotstein, O.D.; Leiter, L.A.; et al. SGLT2 Inhibition with Empagliflozin Increases Circulating Provascular Progenitor Cells in People with Type 2 Diabetes Mellitus. *Cell Metab.* **2019**, *30*, 609–613. [CrossRef]
142. Nandula, S.R.; Kundu, N.; Awal, H.B.; Brichacek, B.; Fakhri, M.; Aimalla, N.; Elzarki, A.; Amdur, R.L.; Sen, S. Role of Canagliflozin on Function of CD34+ ve Endothelial Progenitor Cells (EPC) in Patients with Type 2 Diabetes. *Cardiovasc. Diabetol.* **2021**, *20*, 44. [CrossRef]
143. Fadini, G.; De Kreutzenberg, S.; Mariano, V.; Boscaro, E.; Bertolini, F.; Mancuso, P.; Quarna, J.; Marescotti, M.; Agostini, C.; Tiengo, A.; et al. Optimized Glycaemic Control Achieved with Add-on Basal Insulin Therapy Improves Indexes of Endothelial Damage and Regeneration in Type 2 Diabetic Patients with Macroangiopathy: A Randomized Crossover Trial Comparing Detemir versus Glargine. *Diabetes Obes. Metab.* **2011**, *13*, 718–725. [CrossRef] [PubMed]
144. Oikonomou, D.; Kopf, S.; von Bauer, R.; Djuric, Z.; Cebola, R.; Sander, A.; Englert, S.; Vittas, S.; Hidmark, A.; Morcos, M.; et al. Influence of Insulin and Glargine on Outgrowth and Number of Circulating Endothelial Progenitor Cells in Type 2 Diabetes Patients: A Partially Double-Blind, Randomized, Three-Arm Unicenter Study. *Cardiovasc. Diabetol.* **2014**, *13*, 137. [CrossRef] [PubMed]
145. Piatti, P.M.; Marone, E.; Mantero, M.; Setola, E.; Galluccio, E.; Lucotti, P.; Shehaj, E.; Villa, V.; Perticone, F.; Venturini, M.; et al. Effect of Normalization of Fasting Glucose by Intensified Insulin Therapy and Influence of eNOS Polymorphisms on the Incidence of Restenosis after Peripheral Angioplasty in Patients with Type 2 Diabetes: A Randomized, Open-Label Clinical Trial. *Acta Diabetol.* **2013**, *50*, 373–382. [CrossRef] [PubMed]
146. UK Prospective Diabetes Study (UKPDS) Group. Effect of Intensive Blood-Glucose Control with Metformin on Complications in Overweight Patients with Type 2 Diabetes (UKPDS 34). *Lancet* **1998**, *352*, 854–865. [CrossRef]
147. Yu, J.-W.; Deng, Y.-P.; Han, X.; Ren, G.-F.; Cai, J.; Jiang, G.-J. Metformin Improves the Angiogenic Functions of Endothelial Progenitor Cells via Activating AMPK/eNOS Pathway in Diabetic Mice. *Cardiovasc. Diabetol.* **2016**, *15*, 88. [CrossRef]
148. Horsdal, H.T.; Johnsen, S.P.; Søndergaard, F.; Jacobsen, J.; Thomsen, R.W.; Schmitz, O.; Sørensen, H.T.; Rungby, J. Sulfonylureas and Prognosis after Myocardial Infarction in Patients with Diabetes: A Population-Based Follow-up Study. *Diabetes Metab. Res. Rev.* **2009**, *25*, 515–522. [CrossRef]
149. Johnsen, S.P.; Monster, T.; Olsen, M.L.; Thisted, H.; McLaughlin, J.; Sørensen, H.T.; Lervang, H.; Rungby, J. Risk and Short-Term Prognosis of Myocardial Infarction among Users of Antidiabetic Drugs. *Am. J. Ther.* **2006**, *13*, 134–140. [CrossRef]
150. Filipova, E.; Uzunova, K.; Kalinov, K.; Vekov, T. Effects of Pioglitazone Therapy on Blood Parameters, Weight and BMI: A Meta-Analysis. *Diabetol. Metab. Syndr.* **2017**, *9*, 90. [CrossRef]
151. Sarafidis, P.A.; Georgianos, P.I.; Lasaridis, A.N. PPAR-γ Agonism for Cardiovascular and Renal Protection. *Cardiovasc. Ther.* **2011**, *29*, 377–384. [CrossRef]
152. Lehrke, M.; Marx, N. Diabetes Mellitus and Heart Failure. *Am. J. Cardiol.* **2017**, *120*, S37–S47. [CrossRef] [PubMed]
153. Sheikh, I.M.; Hassan, O.A.; Adam, S.M.; Ali, A.I.; Ogedegbe, O.J.; Tabowei, G.; Barbarawi, A.; Yussuf, F.M.; Nor, M.A.; Adam, S.M.; et al. Association of Pioglitazone with Major Adverse Cardiovascular Events, All-Cause Mortality, and Heart Failure Hospitalizations: A Systematic Review. *Cureus* **2023**, *15*, e46911. [CrossRef] [PubMed]
154. Erdmann, E.; Dormandy, J.; Wilcox, R.; Massi-Benedetti, M.; Charbonnel, B. PROactive 07: Pioglitazone in the Treatment of Type 2 Diabetes: Results of the PROactive Study. *Vasc. Health Risk Manag.* **2007**, *3*, 355–370. [PubMed]
155. Wilcox, R.; Kupfer, S.; Erdmann, E.; PROactive Study Investigators. Effects of Pioglitazone on Major Adverse Cardiovascular Events in High-Risk Patients with Type 2 Diabetes: Results from PROspective pioglitAzone Clinical Trial in Macro Vascular Events (PROactive 10). *Am. Heart J.* **2008**, *155*, 712–717. [CrossRef]
156. Sorrentino, S.A.; Bahlmann, F.H.; Besler, C.; Müller, M.; Schulz, S.; Kirchhoff, N.; Doerries, C.; Horváth, T.; Limbourg, A.; Limbourg, F.; et al. Oxidant Stress Impairs in Vivo Reendothelialization Capacity of Endothelial Progenitor Cells from Patients with Type 2 Diabetes Mellitus: Restoration by the Peroxisome Proliferator-Activated Receptor-γ Agonist Rosiglitazone. *Circulation* **2007**, *116*, 163–173. [CrossRef]
157. Green, J.B.; Bethel, M.A.; Armstrong, P.W.; Buse, J.B.; Engel, S.S.; Garg, J.; Josse, R.; Kaufman, K.D.; Koglin, J.; Korn, S.; et al. Effect of Sitagliptin on Cardiovascular Outcomes in Type 2 Diabetes. *N. Engl. J. Med.* **2015**, *373*, 232–242. [CrossRef]
158. Rosenstock, J.; Kahn, S.E.; Johansen, O.E.; Zinman, B.; Espeland, M.A.; Woerle, H.J.; Pfarr, E.; Keller, A.; Mattheus, M.; Baanstra, D.; et al. Effect of Linagliptin vs Glimepiride on Major Adverse Cardiovascular Outcomes in Patients with Type 2 Diabetes: The CAROLINA Randomized Clinical Trial. *JAMA* **2019**, *322*, 1155–1166. [CrossRef]
159. Scirica, B.M.; Bhatt, D.L.; Braunwald, E.; Steg, P.G.; Davidson, J.; Hirshberg, B.; Ohman, P.; Frederich, R.; Wiviott, S.D.; Hoffman, E.B.; et al. Saxagliptin and Cardiovascular Outcomes in Patients with Type 2 Diabetes Mellitus. *N. Engl. J. Med.* **2013**, *369*, 1317–1326. [CrossRef]
160. White, W.B.; Bakris, G.L.; Bergenstal, R.M.; Cannon, C.P.; Cushman, W.C.; Fleck, P.; Heller, S.; Mehta, C.; Nissen, S.E.; Perez, A.; et al. EXamination of cArdiovascular outcoMes with alogliptIN versus Standard of carE in Patients with Type 2 Diabetes Mellitus

and Acute Coronary Syndrome (EXAMINE): A Cardiovascular Safety Study of the Dipeptidyl Peptidase 4 Inhibitor Alogliptin in Patients with Type 2 Diabetes with Acute Coronary Syndrome. *Am. Heart J.* **2011**, *162*, 620–626.

161. Zhong, J.; Rajagopalan, S. Dipeptidyl Peptidase-4 Regulation of SDF-1/CXCR4 Axis: Implications for Cardiovascular Disease. *Front. Immunol.* **2015**, *6*, 477. [CrossRef]
162. Marso, S.P.; Daniels, G.H.; Brown-Frandsen, K.; Kristensen, P.; Mann, J.F.; Nauck, M.A.; Nissen, S.E.; Pocock, S.; Poulter, N.R.; Ravn, L.S.; et al. Liraglutide and Cardiovascular Outcomes in Type 2 Diabetes. *N. Engl. J. Med.* **2016**, *375*, 311–322. [CrossRef] [PubMed]
163. Gerstein, H.C.; Colhoun, H.M.; Dagenais, G.R.; Diaz, R.; Lakshmanan, M.; Pais, P.; Probstfield, J.; Riesmeyer, J.S.; Riddle, M.C.; Rydén, L.; et al. Dulaglutide and Cardiovascular Outcomes in Type 2 Diabetes (REWIND): A Double-Blind, Randomised Placebo-Controlled Trial. *Lancet* **2019**, *394*, 121–130. [CrossRef]
164. Marso, S.P.; Bain, S.C.; Consoli, A.; Eliaschewitz, F.G.; Jódar, E.; Leiter, L.A.; Lingvay, I.; Rosenstock, J.; Seufert, J.; Warren, M.L.; et al. Semaglutide and Cardiovascular Outcomes in Patients with Type 2 Diabetes. *N. Engl. J. Med.* **2016**, *375*, 1834–1844. [CrossRef] [PubMed]
165. Holman, R.R.; Bethel, M.A.; Mentz, R.J.; Thompson, V.P.; Lokhnygina, Y.; Buse, J.B.; Chan, J.C.; Choi, J.; Gustavson, S.M.; Iqbal, N.; et al. Effects of Once-Weekly Exenatide on Cardiovascular Outcomes in Type 2 Diabetes. *N. Engl. J. Med.* **2017**, *377*, 1228–1239. [CrossRef] [PubMed]
166. Zinman, B.; Wanner, C.; Lachin, J.M.; Fitchett, D.; Bluhmki, E.; Hantel, S.; Mattheus, M.; Devins, T.; Johansen, O.E.; Woerle, H.J.; et al. Empagliflozin, Cardiovascular Outcomes, and Mortality in Type 2 Diabetes. *N. Engl. J. Med.* **2015**, *373*, 2117–2128. [CrossRef] [PubMed]
167. Ferdinand, K.C.; Arora, N. SGLT2 Inhibition for Outcomes: Is This the Panacea? *Am. Heart J. Plus Cardiol. Res. Pract.* **2022**, *21*, 100159. [CrossRef]

biomedicines

MDPI

Review

Advances and Perspectives in Relation to the Molecular Basis of Diabetic Retinopathy—A Review

Michał Błaszkiewicz [1], Agata Walulik [1,*], Kamila Florek [1], Ignacy Górecki [1], Olga Sławatyniec [1] and Krzysztof Gomułka [2]

[1] Student Scientific Group of Adult Allergology, Wroclaw Medical University, 50-369 Wroclaw, Poland
[2] Clinical Department of Internal Medicine, Pneumology and Allergology, Wroclaw Medical University, 50-369 Wroclaw, Poland
* Correspondence: agata.walulik@gmail.com; Tel.: +48-667171892

Abstract: Diabetes mellitus (DM) is a growing problem nowadays, and diabetic retinopathy (DR) is its predominant complication. Currently, DR diagnosis primarily relies on fundoscopic examination; however, novel biomarkers may facilitate that process and make it widely available. In this current review, we delve into the intricate roles of various factors and mechanisms in DR development, progression, prediction, and their association with therapeutic approaches linked to the underlying pathogenic pathways. Specifically, we focus on advanced glycation end products, vascular endothelial growth factor (VEGF), asymmetric dimethylarginine, endothelin-1, and the epigenetic regulation mediated by microRNAs (miRNAs) in the context of DR.

Keywords: diabetes; proliferative diabetic retinopathy; retina; vascular endothelial growth factor; asymmetric dimethylarginine; microRNAs; endothelin-1; advanced glycation end products

1. Aim

The study aimed to indicate the vital biomarkers and molecules involved in the pathomechanism of diabetic retinopathy, evaluate their impact, assess their diagnostic value for staging or risk assessment of DR, and specify the potential point of grasp for therapeutic methods.

2. Introduction

Diabetic retinopathy (DR) remains a major ocular complication of diabetes mellitus (DM) and is the leading cause of irreversible yet preventable vision loss among the working-age adult population, particularly in low- and middle-income areas [1]. Among the 537 million adults (20–79 years) with DM, approximately one-third have signs of DR, and one-third of this group may go on to develop severe retinopathy or macular edema [2,3]. Apart from ocular effects, the presence of DR also signifies an evaluated future risk of myocardial infarction, heart failure, and cerebrovascular accidents [4].

As the worldwide prevalence of diabetes mellitus has significantly increased over the past twenty years, the persistently high incidence of diabetic retinopathy among individuals with diabetes makes screening crucial. This screening is necessary for the early detection of individuals displaying signs of visual impairment due to chronic hyperglycemia, who require a comprehensive ophthalmic examination and appropriate treatment [5].

The COVID-19 pandemic had a significant impact on DR screening, monitoring, and treatment process. According to a study performed in 2020, the Cole Eye Institute, USA, the average delay in care for patients who missed their appointments during the pandemic was 5.34 weeks [6]. Another retrospective study of DR patients who attended the DR screening program at Hospital Universitari Sant Joan de Reus revealed that the number of screened patients decreased to 3286 (57.89%) in 2020, compared to an average 5676.40 ± 439.75 of screened patients between 2015 and 2019. In 2021, this number increased again, resulting in

6804 screened patients [7]. Centers for Disease Control and Prevention (CDC) reports that the prevalence of DR in 2019 in the USA was 3.11% of the USA population [8]. Whereas, 2021 screening programs reported by CDC resulted in a decrease of 2.89% of DR patients [8]. However, the COVID-19 pandemic accelerated the development of screening tools like digital ophthalmoscopes (DOs) for DR diagnosis. Those solutions can be used without prior extensive traineeship in that field by general practitioners or patients by themselves. Although the pandemic is over, there is a possibility to take advantage of using those telemedicine devices in areas with limited access to ophthalmologists. Nevertheless, there are no international guidelines concerning DO usage, but the inclusion of those techniques should be considered [9]. There are different DOs, desktop-based DOs, handheld DOs, and smartphone-based retinal imaging DOs, and their sensitivity ranged from 61% to 81% between different studies considered in the most recent systematic review [10]. However, the NO BLIND study showed 100% specificity and 94.3% sensitivity for digital ophthalmoscope usage by ophthalmology specialists as compared to standard fundus oculi examination in mydriasis [11]. The role of telemedicine in the field of DR should be highlighted as it is a cost-effective approach and it is a tool that enables broad screening and faster diagnosis making [9].

This article provides a summary of the current knowledge regarding diabetic retinopathy, especially emphasizing the molecules that could serve as markers of ongoing pathological processes in the retina.

3. Risk Factors

The most relevant risk factors for the development of diabetic retinopathy include the duration of diabetes, greater uncontrolled hyperglycemia as indicated by high HbA1c levels, and the presence of hypertension [12]. Research showed that maintaining proper blood glucose control has a notably stronger effect on DR prevention compared to controlling blood pressure [13,14]. Research suggests that the risk gradually increases over time, making regular eye examinations essential for individuals with diabetes identified for more than a decade.

Other well-known risk factors for DR are nephropathy and high BMI index [12,15]. Although there are no definite associations between traditional lipid markers and DR, several studies over the years have suggested that lipid-lowering therapy might be an effective adjunctive agent for DR and may reduce the risk of its development [16–20]. Both diabetic retinopathy and nephropathy are complications of DM resulting from microvascular damage through, i.e., inflammation and oxidative stress attributed to uncontrolled blood glucose levels. These mechanisms can result in the simultaneous occurrence of nephropathy and DM, consequently, it is important to regularly screen patients with severe nephropathy for eventual DR development [3,21].

Smoking is an additional risk factor for DR. Xiaoling et al., in the study identifying and comparing 73 studies involving type 1 and type 2 diabetes patients, established a clear association between smoking and DR. In type 1 diabetes, the risk of DR significantly increased among smokers compared to non-smokers. Surprisingly, in type 2 diabetes, the risk of DR was found to be lower in smokers than in non-smokers [22]. However, this result should not change the importance of smoking cessation for overall health benefits.

Research findings indicate that for women with diabetes, pregnancy can pose an additional risk factor for developing or worsening already existing DR. The prevalence of DR in women with type 1 diabetes is higher than in type 2 and it tends to worsen in type 1 diabetic women compared to type 2 [21,23]. Consequently, it is crucial for pregnant women with diabetes to closely monitor blood glucose levels and manage the condition effectively.

Diabetic retinopathy is a complex condition that requires diligent management to prevent or slow down its progression. By understanding the risk factors associated with diabetic retinopathy, presented in Figure 1, individuals with diabetes can take proactive measures to protect their vision. Consistently managing blood sugar levels, blood pressure, and cholesterol and making healthy lifestyle choices, such as quitting smoking, are crucial steps in reducing the risk and severity of diabetic retinopathy.

Risk factors for diabetic retinopathy

- Diabetes duration
- Hyperglycaemia
  1% decrease in HbA1c equates to a decreased risk of retinopathy by 40%
- Hypertension
  10 mmHg decreased SBP equated to a decreased risk of retinopathy progression by 35%
- Dyslipidemia
- Nephropathy
- High BMI index
- Smoking
- Pregnancy

Figure 1. Risk factors for diabetic retinopathy development.

4. Pathophysiology

Diabetic retinopathy is primarily associated with microvascular abnormalities and retinal neurodegeneration [24]. The neurovascular unit comprises endothelial cells and pericytes, basement membrane, glial cells (including astrocytes and Müller cells), microglia, and neurons. The degeneration of this unit is considered a primary indicator of diabetic retinopathy [25].

Hyperglycemia induces non-enzymatic advanced glycation end products creation, increases oxidative stress, and promotes the growth in proinflammatory cytokines, leukocyte migration, and adhesion, which may lead to leukostasis (microcapillaries blockade with leukocytes), moreover, it influences epigenetic modifications [26,27]. Hyperglycemia, chronic inflammation, and microthrombi induce hypoxia and via hypoxia-inducible factor (HIF-1α) upregulates growth factors, mainly VEGF (vascular endothelial growth factor) [28]. The VEGF isoforms promote endothelial cell proliferation during early angiogenesis, and some of its isoforms take part in pathological neovascularization. Furthermore, VEGF increases vascular permeability by disrupting the tight-junction between retinal endothelial cells [29,30].

Hypertension and local retinal vasoconstriction also play a role in DR development and are associated with increased VEGF production [31].

The clinical classification divides DR into non-proliferative diabetic retinopathy (NPDR) and proliferative diabetic retinopathy (PDR) [32]. In the pathogenesis of NPDR, there is a loss of pericytes, a decrease in their protective role, damage to endothelial cells, and excessive thickening of the basement membrane. These changes lead to vascular leakage and cellular damage [28,33]. The clinical manifestation of NPDR in the fundoscopic examination typically reveals microaneurysms, which may rupture and cause hemorrhages. Additionally, vascular leakage can result in the appearance of hard exudates. Macular edema can also occur, and due to the occlusion of microcapillaries, ischemia may develop, leading to nerve fiber infarcts that are visible as "cotton-wool spots" [28]. PDR can occur as a progression from NPDR, but it can also manifest without a preceding NPDR stage. This severe clinical presentation is associated with pathological neovascularization and fibrous proliferation, manifesting as epiretinal or vitreous hemorrhages causing temporal vision loss and retinal detachment leading to permanent blindness [28,34]. Macular edema can be a cause of both NPDR and PDR and is considered reversible damage [35].

5. Molecular Biomarkers

In recent years, the exploration of biomarkers has gained significant momentum, offering novel insights into the pathogenesis and progression of diabetic retinopathy. Biomarkers are measurable biological indicators that reflect normal or pathological processes within the body. They can be used to diagnose, stage, characterize, and monitor diseases, individualize therapeutic interventions, and monitor responses to the therapies [36]. They can be detected in various bodily fluids, such as blood, tears, or even ocular tissues, offering a non-invasive and precise means of diagnosis and monitoring. This article delves into the topic of possible biomarkers in diabetic retinopathy, shedding light on the advancements, challenges, and prospects of these innovative diagnostic tools. We will explore the potential role of biomarkers in detecting the disease at its earliest stages, predicting its progression and tailoring personalized treatment strategies.

5.1. Vascular Endothelial Growth Factor

Angiogenesis is a complex biological process that underlies the development of proliferative diabetic retinopathy, which represents the advanced stage of diabetic retinopathy [37]. Among the many pro-angiogenic factors, vascular endothelial growth factor (VEGF) is notably significant. VEGF is a homodimer glycoprotein with a molecular weight of 46 kDa connected by three disulphide bonds (cystine-knot form). The VEGF family consists of the following members: VEGF-A (also called VEGF or vascular permeability factor as the first discovered molecule of the whole family in 1983), VEGF-B, VEGF-C (essential for the formation of lymphatic vessels) [38], VEGF-D (known as c-Fos-induced growth factor, FIGF), VEGF-E (connected with parapoxvirus Orf, which causes pustular dermatitis) [39], and placenta growth factor (PGF) molecules [40,41]. VEGF production is stimulated by ischemia and hypoxia. Low pO_2 induces the production of the crucial mediator of hypoxic responses—DNA-binding protein called hypoxia-induced factor 1 (HIF-1). HIF-1 binds to specific enhancer elements, which stimulates the transcription of the VEGF gene and, in turn, VEGF mRNA production and decreased mRNA degradation. Accumulated intracellular VEGF is transported from endoplasmic reticulum to Golgi bodies by a chaperone protein known as ORP 150 (oxygen-regulated protein 150), whose secretion is augmented in a hypoxic environment [42,43] (Figure 2).

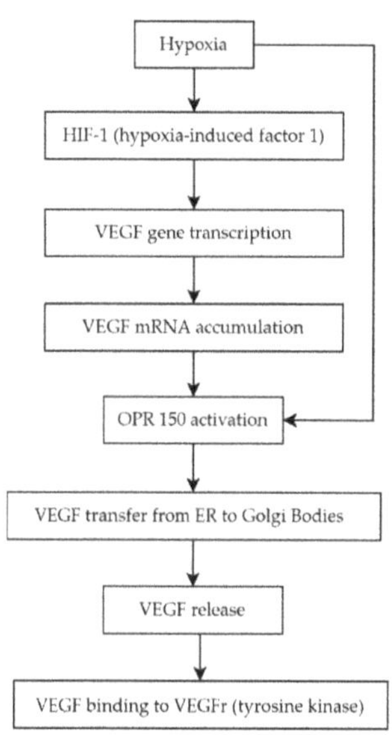

Figure 2. VEGF production and secretion pathway.

VEGF has been shown to play a role in physiological processes such as vasculogenesis—de novo formation of blood vessels during embryogenesis, angiogenesis—vessels formation from already existing vasculature, and pathological processes like tumor growth, tissue remodeling, and metastasis. VEGF mediates its effects by binding to the tyrosine kinase receptors (VEGFRs). The family of VEGFRs consists of the following members: VEGFR1 and VEGFR2 (mainly located on blood vessels endothelial cells) and VEGFR3 (expressed in lymphatic endothelium) (Table 1). The molecular structure of each receptor is similar [44].

Table 1. VEGF receptors and their ligands.

Receptor	VEGFR1	VEGFR2	VEGFR3
VEGF variant	VEGF-A, -B, and PGF	VEGF-A, -C, and -D	VEGF-C and -D

VEGFR1 can be secreted in the soluble form (sFlt1—expressed in the placenta during gestation) to prevent endothelial overproliferation due to VEGF accumulation. There are known VEGF coreceptors as well: the neuropilins, neuropilin-1 and neuropilin-2. Their main role is to enhance the binding of VEGF to the VEGFR2 and the migration of endothelial cells stimulated by VEGF [45]. Heparan sulfate and integrins can also modulate the signal from VEGFR. VEGFR1 is a crucial factor in providing a proper level of VEGF-A, and it plays an important role in the negative regulation of vascular modification. VEGFR1 is also necessary for the process of monocyte migration. PGF bound to VEGFR1 is responsible for initiating inflammatory-related angiogenesis, which is vital in the pathogenesis of various diseases. VEGF-B characteristically binds to VEGFR1 in tissues with high metabolic activity such as myocardial cells. VEGFR2, the most comprehensively studied among the VEGF receptors, binds with VEGF-A, VEGF-C, and VEGF-D. It is known that the activation of VEGFR2 kinase through VEGF-induced VEGFR2 homodimerization is responsible for the majority, if not all, of the known VEGF-related processes such as mitosis stimulation, migration, and survival of endothelial cells, ultimately leading to the formation of new blood vessels [46]. The crucial functions of VEGFR2 in endothelial biology are evident from the various processes involved in its tight regulation such as internalization to early endosomes for the activation of specific pathways and the involvement of phosphatases like vascular endothelial protein tyrosine phosphatase. VEGFR3 has an affinity to VEGF-C and VEGF-D. Although the main function of VEGFR3 was initially identified as the regulation of lymphatic endothelial development and biology, it has also been observed to be present in blood vascular endothelial cells. Angiogenesis-involved endothelial cells exhibit the expression of both VEGFR2 and VEGFR3. VEGFR3 activation is not solely dependent on VEGF-C/VEGF-D binding, as it can also be activated through integrin-mediated mechanisms, it leads to lymphatic vessel expansion and the absorption of interstitial fluid [47]. In addition, VEGF is critical for ensuring the proper morphology and function of vascular structures [46]. Notably, mutations that result in the loss of the VEGF gene allele have been found to be lethal [48]. The development of PDR is linked to relative retinal ischemia, which creates a hypoxic environment, which favors HIF-1 activation and VEGF production. The pathological revascularization in the retina has been attributed to VEGF-A165, a specific splice variant of VEGF-A [49].

As opposed to levels of plasma VEGF, elevated intraocular VEGF has been strongly associated with macular edema and retinal angiogenesis [50]. It has been proven that the aqueous VEGF level is correlated with this in the vitreous [51,52]. What is more, current research revealed that in DR patients, vitreous and aqueous VEGF levels are significantly higher than the plasma levels and they are both associated with DR progression [52]. However, some studies show that the median serum VEGF levels are found to be greater in patients with DM, PDR, and NPDR than in the matched control groups [53,54]. Furthermore, the serum VEGF levels are significantly higher in PDR than in NPDR patients [55]. According to current studies, serum VEGF seems to be an appropriate biomarker for DR onset and severity as well [55,56]. Nonetheless, changes in circulating VEGF-A levels cannot be used as a predictive factor of DR progression [50,53]. Moreover, the increase in serum PGF levels has been observed in NPDR patients treated with aflibercept (anti-VEGF antibody). In PDR patients who underwent the same therapy, PGF remained stable. Increased PGF levels may result from a counter-regulatory mechanism, due to VEGFR2 inhibition. However, in PDR patients, permanent uncontrolled expression of VEGF probably masks the counter-regulated PGF secretion [53]. Current studies reveal that the tear VEGF level is elevated in patients with DR and substantially different between NPDR and PDR patients. What is more, the VEGF level in tears is significantly associated with DR stage and severity [57–59]. There are studies presenting useful methods for tear VEGF level measurements characterized by high sensitivity and specificity [60,61]. Recent studies indicate the importance of anti-VEGF therapy, especially intraocular injections of those drugs [62].

5.2. *Asymmetric Dimethylarginine*

Arginine is an amino acid essential for normal growth and development. Endogenous synthesis is adequate in healthy people but might be deficient in many pathological states [63]. The earliest sign of vascular complications is endothelial dysfunction [64]. Nitric oxide (NO) is an important vasodilator that is crucial in maintaining the health of the vascular endothelium. Studies demonstrate that endothelial dysfunction plays a critical role in the development of diabetes-associated microvascular complications and often precedes advanced diabetic retinopathy (DR) [65–67]. NO is synthesized from the guanidine group of arginine by the enzyme family NO synthases (NOSs), which consist of three isoforms [68,69]. Asymmetric dimethylarginine (ADMA) is an active endogenous methylated amino acid, a structural analogue of L-arginine, which inhibits the activity of all isoforms of NOS, inhibiting the formation of nitric oxide in tissues and blood plasma [70,71]. ADMA is synthesized by the protein arginine N-methyltransferase 1 (PRMT1), mainly metabolized by the dimethylarginine dimethylaminohydrolases (DDAHs) pathway, and eliminated from the body by kidneys [72,73]. ADMA enters cells through cationic amino-acid transporters (CATs) [74]. Plasma levels of ADMA in healthy people vary between 0.3 and 0.5 μmol/L [75], but in pathological states, it may increase even tenfold [76]. ADMA has a negative effect on cells, contributing to oxidative stress, shortening telomeres, inhibiting the release of NO, and increasing the secretion of interleukin-8 and monocyte chemotaxis factor 1 [75]. Under normal conditions, endothelial NOS is inhibited by 10%, but in pathological situations, even by 30–70% [76]. When the plasma ADMA level increases, the NO synthesis in the environment decreases, vascular homeostasis degrades due to vasoconstriction, and endothelial dysfunction begins [69]. Endothelial dysfunction and impaired ocular hemodynamics prime diabetic retinopathy development are associated with decreased NOS activity and NO bioavailability, thus resulting in increased reactive oxygen species (ROS) and vasoconstriction [76,77]. Oxidative stress is closely related to DDAH activity, which further affects ADMA concentrations in patients with diabetes [78,79]. Increased oxidative stress contributes to elevated ADMA, and by the up-regulation of circulating markers of oxidative stress, increased serum ADMA concentration is associated with increased vascular oxidative stress [80–82]. ADMA accumulation was first reported in patients characterized by endothelial dysfunction including hyperglycemia, hypercholesterolemia, and hypertension [83,84]. Impaired liver or renal function could also have an impact on the plasma concentration of ADMA. The significance of ADMA in the inhibition of vascular endothelial growth factor-mediated angiogenesis has been demonstrated in numerous studies. Some evidence suggests that diabetes mellitus with microvascular complications has increased serum levels of ADMA [85–88]. Elevated ADMA was detected in aqueous humor in diabetic patients, especially those with severe retinopathy [89]. The plasma ADMA level is elevated in patients with diabetic microangiopathy such as DR [66,86,90–93]. Lowering ADMA levels may delay the progression of DR by reducing the formation of neovascularization, providing protective advantages for the blood–retinal barrier [92]. Some clinical studies have shown that ADMA levels in diabetic patients with retinopathy were higher than among individuals without retinopathy, and this increase was directly proportional to the severity of diabetes [65,94–96]. High levels of ADMA have been identified not only in advanced DR but also in individuals at the prediabetic and diabetic stages. This observation suggests that ADMA likely plays a crucial role in both the initiation and advancement of DR [81,97]. Further studies that involve larger patient populations to better understand the role of plasma ADMA levels in the development and progression of DR are needed. The serum ADMA level was accepted as a marker of endothelial dysfunction because of its high values in coronary artery disease, end-stage renal failure, stroke, hypertension, and DM [98–101]. In the present moment, there are no drugs targeting ADMA levels in the context of diabetes management [102].

5.3. MicroRNAs

MicroRNAs (miRNAs) are single-strengthened, non-coding RNA, which affect gene expression regulation. Their suppressor interaction with mRNA usually is associated with 3′ untranslated regions (3′ UTRs), although data claim as well its interaction potential according to different sequences such as gene promoters. Moreover, they also have a regulatory role in transcription and translation processes [103]. The creation process of those micromolecules goes from DNA transcription to primary miRNA (pri-mRNA) through precursor miRNA (pre-miRNA) leading to mature miRNA formation [104]. The role of miRNA in signalization pathways is studied nowadays excessively because of those particles' multiplicity. Furthermore, their remarkable stability in circulation makes them attractive potential non-invasive biomarkers and therapeutic grip points [105]. Their role as a biomarker may be a useful tool in the DR diagnostic process because currently assessment is based only on ophthalmological examination and the inclusion of non-invasive objective tests into guidelines could enhance DR detectability.

Molecular bases of miRNA mechanisms of action are distinct for different miRNAs, and it is possible to distinguish which particles affect which pathway leading to DR, such as affecting cell proliferation, angiogenesis, apoptosis, or basement membrane thickening [106]. It has been proven that directly or indirectly particles such as miRNA-9, miRNA-152, miRNA-15b, miRNA-29b-3p, miRNA-199a-3p, miRNA-203a-3p, miRNA-200b-3p, and miRNA-30a-3p downregulate VEGF expression, which lowers the range of active cell-cycle-related proteins and by that protects RMECs (retinal microvascular endothelial cells) from abnormal proliferation [107]. In addition, from previously mentioned biomolecules, the alternative pathway to downregulate VEGF is SIRT1 (nicotinamide adenosine dinucleotide (NAD+)-dependent deacetylase) upregulation, which is possible by miRNA-29b-3p and miRNA-34a inhibition, moreover, causing an increase in proinflammatory cytokines [107]. MiRNA-34a was evaluated to be an interesting therapeutic target, as in rats with induced DR, its silencing was observed as an apoptosis regulation [108]. Relatedly, the miRNA overexpressed in DR upregulating SIRT1 is miRNA-195, which inhibits RMEC and accelerates apoptosis [109]. In addition, miRNA-210 was assessed as a potential biomarker able to distinguish PDR from NPDR; moreover, it refers to DR severity, and progression as well is considered a therapeutic target according to vascular endothelial cells pathological proliferation [110].

MiRNA-20a and miRNA-20b were revealed to downregulate VEGF as well but in different mechanisms—first act by Yse-associated protein (YAP)/hypoxia-inducible factor 1α (HIF1α)/VEGF axis, and second was revealed in the study on rats to be correlated with downregulation of AKT3, lowering VEGF expression [111,112]. Moreover, it was assessed that Resolvin D1 modulates the intracellular VEGF-related miRNAs—miRNA-20a-3p, miRNA-20a-5p, miRNA-106a-5p, and miRNA-20b—expression of retinal photoreceptors challenged with high glucose [113]. Another pathway included in DR pathogenesis and connected to miRNA function is the thickening of basement membrane by increased synthesis of RMEC extracellular matrix—especially the abnormal synthesis of collagen type 4 due to miRNA-29a inhibition by inflammatory factor OPN (osteopontin) also known as secreted phospho-protein 1 (SPP1) [114]. It is needed to mention that there was a confirmed association between OPN and vascular hyperpermeability in human diabetic retinal tissues, and by a blockade of OPN, vascular continuity was preserved, in contrast, by the miRNA-148a-3p action-TGFβ2 expression was lowered and by that basement membrane thickening was decreased [115,116] (Figure 3).

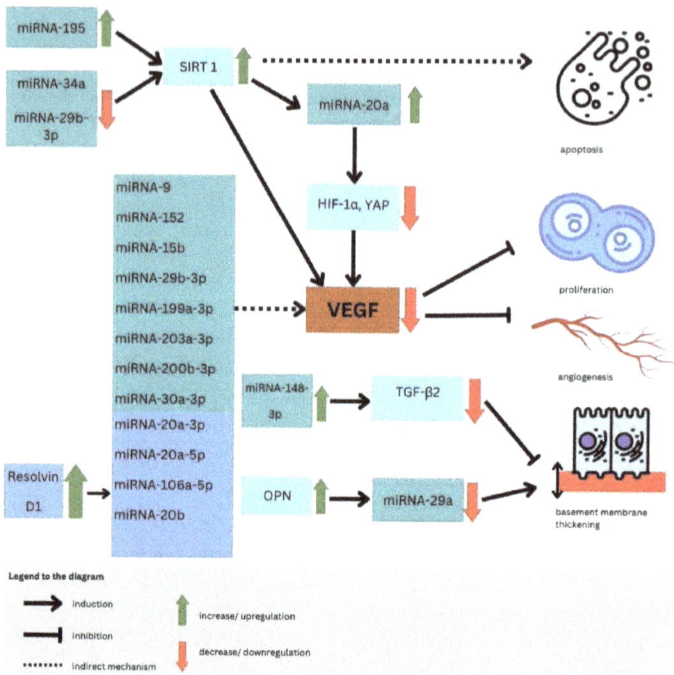

Figure 3. MiRNA impact on apoptosis, angiogenesis, proliferation, and basement membrane thickening in DR.

The role of the miRNA was investigated as a DR biomarker using different sample types and designs compared to various groups according to diabetes type 1 or 2, T1DM or T2DM, patients with DM and healthy individuals, as well studies referring to DR progression. In blood serum samples in T1DM patients with DR and those without retinopathy, the most significant was miRNA-211. Then, miRNA-18b and miRNA-19b were revealed as upregulated; additionally, miRNA-29a, miRNA-148a, miRNA-181a, and miRNA-200a were revealed to have such an impact [117,118]. Furthermore, miRNA-93, miRNA-21, and miRNA-146a are downregulated in T1DM patients [119]. Trials which evaluated biomarkers correlation with DR progression among T1DM revealed as the most important factors certain macromolecules, for PREVENT-1-higher, miRNA-320a concentration, and in PROTECT-1-lower, miRNA-27b expression [120].

According to T2DM, a study was performed and the differences in the following particles were noted: hsa-let-7a-5p, hsa-miRNA-novel-chr5_15976, hsa-miRNA-28-3p, hsa-miRNA-151a-5p, and hsa-miRNA-148a-3p were upregulated compared to DM group with no retinopathy; however, a panel of the first three of them were the closest to help in assessing the diagnosis as its sensitivity and specificity were as follows: 0.92 and 0.94 [121]. Another study showed that in T2DM patients, DR was associated with increased circulating levels of miRNA-25-3p and miRNA-320b and decreased levels of miRNA-495-3p [122]. In addition, it was revealed in the study performed on rats with induced diabetes that miRNA-200b in DR diseases is lower than in the healthy group [123]. According to the vitreous humor, there were studies suggesting changes in several particle concentrations in

PDR groups: miRNA-125, miRNA-21, hsa-miRNA-6734-5p, and hsa-miRNA-1297 [124,125]. MiRNAs, such as hsa-miRNA-3184-3p, hsa-miRNA-24-3p, and hsa-miRNA-197-3p, were assessed to be upregulated in the vitreous humor of PDR patients; furthermore, anti-VEGF-factor administration led to lower expression of those particles [124]. However, vitreous humor parameter measurements are not easy to perform.

Plasma results among T2DM patients gave an insight into lower levels of miRNA-29b in the DR group and miRNA-21 as biomarkers that were significantly associated with PDR. Other parameters that were increased in T2DM patients with DR were miRNA-93 via SIRT1 and miRNA-21, as well as miRNA-152 [126,127]. On the contrary, miRNA-15a, miRNA-20b, miRNA-21, miRNA-24, miRNA-320, miRNA-486, and miRNA-150, miRNA-126, miRNA-191, miRNA-197 are downregulated in that group of patients' plasma samples [128]. Importantly, miRNA-150 is observed in both T1DM and T2DM patients' circulation and in the neutral retina. That factor by Elk1 upregulation stimulates proinflammatory, proangiogenic, and apoptotic influences. Otherwise, a lower range of miRNA-150 in serum impacts Elk1 and Myb overexpression, resulting in the same as the previously mentioned pathway in microvascular complications and neovascularization leading to DR; so, according to that analysis, it is not only a diagnostic biomarker but as well is significantly involved in DR pathogenesis [129]. Importantly, there were two meta-analyses performed according to miRNAs role in DR diagnosis, which revealed its significance and utility. The first study included eight trials with 93 parameters and even though six miRNAs were consistently reported in at least two studies and in the same direction, after stratification by the type of biological samples, miRNA-320a and miRNA-423-5p were consistently reported to be upregulated in two studies using serum samples and two studies using vitreous humor samples, respectively. It was consistently shown that miRNA-27b was downregulated in two experiments using serum samples [130]. However, most recently, analysis assessed miRNA panels' superior diagnostic value to single parameters results [131]. Furthermore, another result is the fact that miRNA-21 in five studies was revealed to be a useful tool in the diagnosis of DR and an early predictor of reactive oxygen species-mediated damage among patients at high risk for diabetes [130,131] (Figure 4).

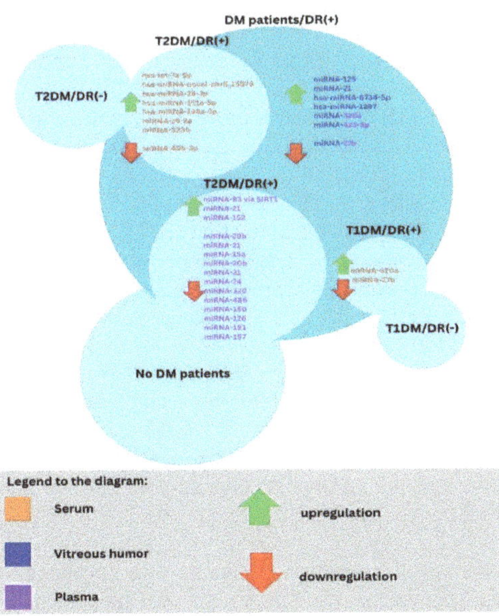

Figure 4. Changes in miRNA regulation depending on DM type and presence of DR in specific sample types. Overlapping circles constitute the study and control groups, while the increase or decrease in regulation of miRNAs was marked only in the study group.

5.4. Endothelin-1

Endothelin-1 (ET-1) in its active form is a 21-amino acid hormone that helps to maintain basal vascular tone and metabolic function in healthy individuals [132]. ET-1 is an endothelium-derived factor with proliferative, profibrotic, and proinflammatory properties [133], and it is the most abundantly expressed member of the endothelin family of proteins (ET-1, ET-2, and ET-3). Immature ET-1 undergoes extensive post-transcriptional processing that concludes with cleavage by endothelin converting enzymes (ECEs) and subsequent release of mature ET-1 primarily toward the interstitial space, and in smaller proportion, into the circulation [132]. ET-1 works on two different ET-1 receptor subtypes, ETA and ETB, to produce its various biological effects [134]. The first subtype, ETA receptors, is predominantly localized on vascular smooth muscle cells (VSMCs) of blood vessels where they mediate contractile and proliferative response to ET-1, whereas ETB receptors have a more composite relation to vascular regulation. ETB receptors can lead to vasodilation via the release of relaxing factors if they are present on endothelial cells or vasoconstriction when they are located on VSMCs in certain vascular beds [133]. Therefore, the overall effect of ET-1 on different tissues is largely dependent on the expression and relative densities of individual receptor subtypes. ET-1 is one of the important markers of endothelial dysfunction, a state characterized by disturbed balance between vasoconstrictors and vasodilators [135]. Due to its vasoconstrictive properties, ET-1 has been widely studied in terms of its role in hypertension and proved clinically significant, e.g., with the use of endothelin receptor antagonists for the treatment of patients with pulmonary arterial hypertension [136]. The vasoconstrictive and in turn hypertensive properties of ET-1 can explain a possible link between elevated plasma ET-1 level and retinopathy under ischemia, a finding relevant to diabetic retinopathy, which is thought to be the consequence of retinal ischemia. Animal models have shown that administration of ET-1 into the posterior vitreous body or the optic nerve leads to physiological and cellular damages of ischemic origin, including obstruction of retinal blood flow, elevated scotopic b-wave in electroretinogram, and apoptosis of cells in ganglion cell layer of the retina [137]. Moreover, in the retina, ET-1 and its ETA receptor have been shown to mediate decreased retinal blood flow during hyperglycemia and in DR. Chen et al. described that hyperglycemia augments ET-1-induced constriction of human retinal venules by activation of ETA receptors [138]. A direct link has been established between hyperglycemia and increased ET-1 secretion from endothelial cells [139]. Various studies demonstrated elevated plasma ET-1 in patients with type 1 or type 2 diabetes [133]. Additionally, patients with advanced DR appear to exhibit elevated ET-1 concentrations in the aqueous of the eye compared to those with early DR and the control group, with exact concentrations varying among individuals, although the severity of DR seems to be a major factor relating to baseline aqueous ET-1 levels [140]. Another study measuring aqueous humor ET-1 found higher concentrations of ET-1 and reduced total retinal blood flow in subjects with early non-proliferative diabetic retinopathy than in age-matched controls [141]. These findings support the claim that ET-1 dysregulation may contribute to the pathogenesis of DR, though aqueous humor ET-1 is still not an exhaustively studied topic. Ottoson-Seeberger et al. demonstrated that exogenous ET-1 causes peripheral insulin resistance in healthy humans [142]. Insulin itself can regulate vascular tone through the increase in ET-1 synthesis and release among other mechanisms [143]. Strong evidence regarding the role of ET-1 in the pathogenesis of diabetic microangiopathy showcases the potential of endothelin receptor antagonists in the treatment of DR. Studies on animal models support this presumption. The use of endothelin receptor A antagonist, atrasentan, in streptozotocin-induced diabetic mice showed attenuation of microvascular changes in the retina [144]. Chou et al. also examined the effects of atrasentan on diabetic mice with similar results, additionally noting significantly reduced retinal pericyte loss [145]. The application of endothelin receptor antagonists via intravitreal administration showed decreased vascular leakage and expression of VEGF and inflammatory factors [146]. Topical administration of bosentan, a dual endothelin receptor antagonist, appeared to prevent neurodegeneration induced by diabetes in mice by blocking and downregulating ETB receptors and shows a viable alternative route to oral administration [147]. There is a clear limitation to extrapolating results of animal studies to human subjects, and more investigation needs to be conducted to fully understand the potential of using ET-1 receptor antagonists as novel therapeutic agents in the treatment of DR.

5.5. Advanced Glycation End Products

One of the mechanisms connecting chronic hyperglycemia with diabetic retinopathy is the formation and accumulation of advanced glycation end products (AGEs). Advanced glycation end products are heterogeneous groups of molecules formed from post-translational non-enzymatic modifications of proteins, lipids, or nucleic acids by saccharides including glucose, fructose, and pentose through the Maillard reaction represented by Figure 5 [148,149]. There are over 20 AGEs identified in human tissues, but some of the most common ones are carboxymethyl-lysine (CML), carboxyethyl-lysine (CEL), pentosidine, pyrraline, and methylglyoxal-derived hydroimidazolone (MG-H1) [150]. The characteristic factor of AGEs that distinguishes them from early glycation products, such as glycohemoglobin A1c (HbA1c), is the lack of spontaneous reversion ability, which once derived results in the accumulation in tissues over time [151]. Even though the discovery of AGEs dates to the early 20th century, not until the 1980s, the role of AGEs in aging and chronic diseases was recognized [152]. The first mention of AGEs and their accumulation in human tissues and their potential role in diabetic complications appeared in 1988 in a scientific article published by Helen Vlassara et al. [153]. Since then, AGEs and their involvement in pathophysiological processes have been the subject of extensive research.

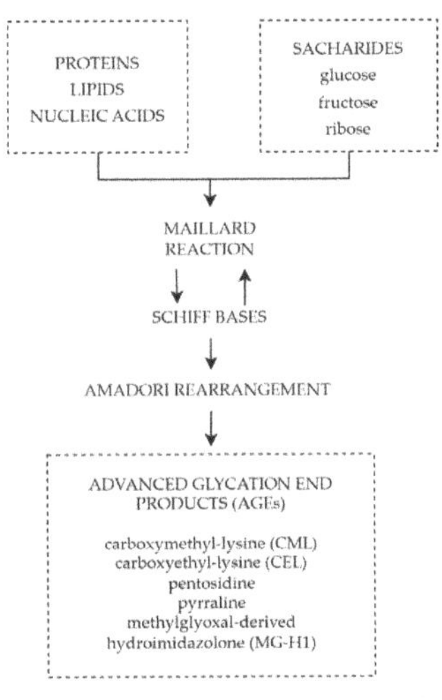

Figure 5. Forming of AGEs through Maillard reaction.

Excessive accumulation of AGEs in tissues has been found in aging processes and various chronic oxidative-based diseases, such as cardiovascular disease, neurodegenerative disorders, chronic renal failure, and most importantly in light of the following considerations, diabetes mellitus [154,155]. While in normal physiological conditions, the production of AGEs is controlled and moderate; however, under persistent hyperglycemia in diabetic patients, AGEs serum levels are much higher compared to the normal non-diabetic population. However, some endogenous factors such as oxidative stress and inflammation can also contribute to AGE formation [156]. AGEs accumulation may be as well through exogenous environmental and dietary sources. Only about 10–30% of AGEs present in food are fully absorbed through gastrointestinal mechanisms [157]. Many foods (e.g., red meat, aged cheeses, highly processed, packaged foods, and food with added sugars) contribute to increased AGEs levels in the body [158,159]. Besides, UV light, ionizing radiation, and air pollution induce high AGE production [160]. Advanced glycation end products play a significant role in the pathophysiology of diabetic retinopathy, one of the most common complications of diabetes mellitus. Even though the precise pathomechanism of its impact on the retina has not been already determined, it is associated with impairment of the neurovascular units (NVUs) through reactive oxygen species, inflammatory reactions, and cell death pathways [161]. AGEs can promote oxidative stress in retinal cells through binding with the receptor for AGEs (RAGE)—ubiquitously expressed in various retinal cells, including endothelial cells, pericytes, and neurons—leading to activation of various pro-oxidant and proinflammatory signaling pathways. A couple of major RAGE signaling pathways have been identified that can start key signaling cellular cascades to various ligands: mitogen-activated protein kinases (MAPKs) including p44/42 (ERK1/2), p38, and c-Jun N-terminal kinases (JNK); Janus kinase (JAK), signal transducer and activator of transcription (STAT); Ras-Rac-Cdc42; and phosphoinositide 3-kinase (P13-K)-Akt/PKB. Activation of the above mechanisms can induce DNA-binding activity among nuclear transcription factors such as STAT1/STAT3/STAT5, nuclear factor κB (NF-κB), and activator protein 1 (AP-1). RAGE under the condition of persistent hyperglycemia is mostly expressed in Müller cells—the ones highly susceptible to damage during DR. AGEs activate Müller cells, subsequently leading to increased production of VEGF, responsible for neovascularization, production of inflammatory cytokines, and monocyte chemoattractant protein-1 (MCP-1) [162–165]. Increased levels of AGEs lead to another pathological pathway: cross-link formation with proteins, resulting in the reduction in energy production, activation of endoplasmic reticulum (ER) stress, and macrophage activation [165]. AGE molecules have also been linked to the loss of pericytes and blood–retinal barrier (BRB) breakdown. The exact understanding of the mechanisms induced by AGEs in the pathophysiology of diabetic retinopathy is crucial for finding an effective treatment for this condition and should be the subject of future research. Analytical methods for the identification of AGEs include both instrumental and immunochemical methods. Spectrofluorometer, high-performance liquid chromatography coupled with mass spectrometry (HPLC/MS), gas chromatography coupled with mass spectrometry (GC–MS), liquid chromatography coupled with tandem mass spectrometry (LC–MS/MS), HPLC with fluorescent detection, and ultra-high-pressure liquid chromatography (UHPLC) are instrumental methods used to detect AGEs. Immunochemical methods contain enzyme-linked immunosorbent assay (ELISA) and Western blotting [166]. The measurement method is based on their chemical structure and ability to emit fluorescence. There are four groups as follows: (1) fluorescent and cross-linked (e.g., pentosidine); (2) fluorescent non-cross-linked; (3) non-fluorescent protein cross-linked; and (4) non-fluorescent and non-cross-linked (CML, CEL, pyrraline). These are especially important in vivo and may be used as biomarkers of pathological conditions such as diabetes and its complications. CML is frequently used as the AGE marker [160,167]. In recent years, research showed that it is more reliable to measure AGEs accumulation in accessible tissue using non-invasive methods than interpret their serum concentration since it does not necessarily reflect tissue AGE levels and depends on the half-time of the molecules [168]. The best choice for an AGE measurement method seems to be skin or lens autofluorescence since the lens crystallins and skin collagen are long-lived proteins reflecting long-term hyperglycemia exposure. Meerwaldt et al. in their research using the Autofluorescent Reader, measured the fluorescence of the skin in patients with type 1 and type 2 diabetes, correlating results with skin biopsies [169]. Autofluorescence clearly correlated with CEL, CML, and pentosidine levels with values higher than in control non-diabetic subjects. For comparison, Gerrits et al. during over 3 years of follow-up research involving 973 type 2 diabetic patients showed that skin autofluorescence was significantly higher in patients with microvascular, neuropathy complications developed but did not have predictive value for those with DR [170]. In the research of Osawa et al. involving patients with type 2 diabetic patients, skin AF was significantly increased with neuropathy, nephropathy, and diabetic retinopathy unlike the patients in the control non-diabetic group [171]. These findings suggest that skin autofluorescence may be a useful tool in identifying patients who are at risk of developing diabetic retinopathy. By measuring skin autofluorescence, it might be possible to identify patients with higher levels of AGEs—biomarkers of diabetes retinopathy and who may be at a higher risk of developing serious optic complications of persistent hyperglycemia. A deep understanding of the mechanisms leading to diabetic retinopathy through AGEs involvement completed via appropriate diagnostics could provide disease diagnosis, prognosis prediction, and therapeutic strategies.

6. Discussion

Diabetic retinopathy is a crucial ocular complication of diabetes mellitus and the major cause of vision deterioration among the working-age adult population, particularly in low- and middle-income areas. Many factors, particularly the duration of diabetes, adversely affect the development and progression of DR. In recent years, interest in identifying factors that contribute to the development of diabetic retinopathy has increased significantly, as well as a better understanding of their role and mechanisms in its further progression. Moreover, the COVID-19 pandemic had a profound impact on the diagnostic and screening protocols for patients with diabetic retinopathy (DR). The restrictions imposed during the pandemic presented considerable challenges for both patients and healthcare professionals. These challenges compelled us to innovate and develop novel telemedicine solutions. Even though the COVID-19 pandemic has subsided, it is crucial that we continue to leverage modern tools and technologies, as they can prove invaluable for patients residing in remote or underserved areas, ensuring better access to quality healthcare. In this cross-sectional survey, we found molecular pathways and biomarkers important in diagnostic and therapeutic processes as well as in the prevention of DR. VEGF is one of the most crucial pro-angiogenic factors, which plays an important role in PDR. Ischemia and hypoxia stimulate VEGF production, and through its many tyrosine kinase receptors, they accelerate the angiogenesis and vascular remodeling in the retina. According to current PDR studies, understanding the complex mechanisms of VEGF signaling pathways is necessary to indicate targets for biological treatment, which can be a milestone in DR therapy. VEGF seems to be an appropriate biomarker, helpful in diagnosing and differentiating the severity of DR. Samples for VEGF level measurements might be taken from blood, vitreous or aqueous fluid, and tears as well. Especially tear VEGF levels might be used as a non-invasive tool to expedite screening programs and assess the severity of DR in patients with diabetes. Using VEGF as a predictive factor of DR development or as a marker of therapeutic management notably in anti-VEGF therapy needs further analysis in dedicated studies. Other factors affecting VEGF levels should be investigated.

ADMA inhibits the activity of NOS, which results in decreased levels of NO and leads to vasoconstriction and endothelial dysfunction. Increased ADMA levels may be considered an early prognostic factor of diabetes complications such as PDR. The use of ADMA as a biomarker may help in early diagnosis, monitoring, and effective therapeutic management of the disease. Reducing ADMA levels in patients with diabetes may be a new therapeutic target to prevent the development of diabetic retinopathy. Endothelin-1 is another factor with an undoubted relationship to diabetic retinopathy. Increased serum and aqueous humor levels are observed in patients with ET-1 elevation dependent on the severity of the progression of the disease. This, juxtaposed with promising results of ET-1 receptor antagonist animal studies, showcases the potential of ET-1 as a possible target for future therapy. It is important to note that miRNAs are not only supposed to be an innovative predictive biomarker and progression indicator in DR but also a potential therapeutic target. Different miRNAs can be found in T1DM and T2DM as well depending on sample type, moreover, some of them differ depending on DR type. The variety of miRNAs and frequently high amounts of particles involved in several pathogenesis pathways can be at the same time the advantage and disadvantage of that prospective novel biomarkers group; hence, miRNAs panels are more adequate than a single biomarker rating. Finally, advanced glycation end products play a significant role in the pathophysiology of diabetic retinopathy causing impairment of the neurovascular units through reactive oxygen species, inflammatory reactions, and cell death pathways. All the above mechanisms play a significant role not only in diabetic retinal disorders, but also other chronic oxidative-based diseases; therefore, a thorough understanding of their properties and mechanisms will allow advances in the diagnosis and treatment of chronic diseases and most importantly diabetic retinopathy. The above factors and signaling pathways can help to create multimodal and highly specified therapies for patients suffering from DR. It is crucial to investigate molecular agents participating in DR pathogenesis. Hopefully, it will provide the ability to inhibit this progressive disease at its early stage.

7. Conclusions

DR as a serious complication of DM needs an advanced diagnostic and therapeutic process. We pointed out the vital biomarkers, which can be helpful in DR investigation.

VEGF is an important pro-angiogenic factor in DR progression. Amid all analyzed techniques, tear VEGF level especially seems to be a promising innovative diagnostic method, mainly because of its non-invasiveness, high sensitivity, and specificity. However, studies suggest that VEGF levels should not be considered as a predictive factor of DR development.

ADMA has significant clinical relevance, and it seems to be reasonable to investigate all possible factors responsible for its level in the organism. Elevated ADMA levels are associated with endothelial dysfunction, oxidative stress, and may contribute to the development and progression of DR. Further research is warranted to explore medications aimed at lowering ADMA, and additional clinical studies are essential to assess whether reducing ADMA levels can effectively decelerate the progression of diabetic microvascular complications and yield improved prognoses.

MiRNAs are promising biomarkers, however, their numerousness may be their disadvantage according to the number of results that would be needed to obtain as well as an advantage. Thanks to this there is a possibility to distinguish various miRNAs panels accurate for specific DM types.

ET-1 is a multifaceted hormone with a crucial role in vascular regulation and endothelial dysfunction, particularly in the context of DR. Elevated ET-1 levels in diabetic patients, especially those with advanced DR, suggest its involvement in the pathogenesis of this condition. While promising findings from animal studies and early human trials indicate the potential therapeutic value of ET-1 receptor antagonists in mitigating DR-related microvascular changes and neurodegeneration, further research is needed to validate their efficacy and safety for clinical use.

Using the biochemical properties of AGEs, which play a significant role in the pathogenesis of DR, as a biomarker is a promising direction in the diagnosis of diabetic retinopathy. A method based on skin autofluorescence testing would provide an easy, accessible, non-invasive, and relatively rapid way to identify patients at risk of developing diabetic retinopathy.

8. Limitations

Our study has several limitations. The results of some of the publications used in the process of writing the above paper present outcomes based on small groups of patients or homogeneous populations, which raises the need for studies on groups both more numerous and diverse in age, gender, and ethnicity. There is a lack of studies focused on a practical clinical approach rather than on the biochemical characteristics of the molecules presented. Further systematic review and meta-analysis should be conducted to confirm the diagnostic value of the above biomarkers.

Author Contributions: Conceptualization, M.B., A.W., K.F., I.G., O.S. and K.G.; writing—original draft preparation, M.B., A.W., K.F., I.G. and O.S.; writing—review and editing, K.G.; visualization—M.B., A.W., K.F., I.G. and O.S.; supervision, K.G.; funding acquisition, K.G. All authors have read and agreed to the published version of the manuscript.

Funding: This research received no external funding.

Institutional Review Board Statement: Not applicable.

Informed Consent Statement: Not applicable.

Data Availability Statement: Data sharing is not applicable as no datasets were generated or analyzed during the current study.

Acknowledgments: Figures were created with BioRender.com (accessed on 4 April 2023).

Conflicts of Interest: The authors declare no conflict of interest.

References

1. Tan, T.E.; Wong, T.Y. Diabetic retinopathy: Looking forward to 2030. *Front. Endocrinol.* **2023**, *13*, 1077669. [CrossRef] [PubMed]
2. International Diabetes Federation. International Diabetes Federation—Facts & Figures. Idf.org. Published 12 September 2021. Available online: https://www.idf.org/aboutdiabetes/what-is-diabetes/facts-figures.html (accessed on 15 May 2023).
3. Cheung, N.; Mitchell, P.; Wong, T.Y. Diabetic retinopathy. *Lancet* **2010**, *376*, 124–136. [CrossRef] [PubMed]
4. Modjtahedi, B.S.; Wu, J.; Luong, T.Q.; Gandhi, N.K.; Fong, D.S.; Chen, W. Severity of Diabetic Retinopathy and the Risk of Future Cerebrovascular Disease, Cardiovascular Disease, and All-Cause Mortality. *Ophthalmology* **2021**, *128*, 1169–1179. [CrossRef] [PubMed]
5. Teo, Z.L.; Tham, Y.C.; Yu, M.; Chee, M.L.; Rim, T.H.; Cheung, N.; Bikbov, M.M.; Wang, Y.X.; Tang, Y.; Lu, Y.; et al. Global Prevalence of Diabetic Retinopathy and Projection of Burden through 2045: Systematic Review and Meta-analysis. *Ophthalmology* **2021**, *128*, 1580–1591. [CrossRef] [PubMed]
6. Ahmed, I.; Liu, T.Y.A. The Impact of COVID-19 on Diabetic Retinopathy Monitoring and Treatment. *Curr. Diabetes Rep.* **2021**, *21*, 40. [CrossRef]
7. Romero-Aroca, P.; Baget-Bernaldiz, M.; Sagarra, R.; Hervás, E.; Blasco, R.; Molina, J.; Moreno, E.F.; Garcia-Curto, E. Impact of the COVID-19 Pandemic on the Metabolic Control of Diabetic Patients in Diabetic Retinopathy and Its Screening. *J. Clin. Med.* **2022**, *11*, 7121. [CrossRef] [PubMed]
8. Centers for Disease Control and Prevention. Vision & Eye Health Surveillance System (VEHSS), Vision Health Initiative. Available online: https://www.cdc.gov/visionhealth/vehss/project/index.html (accessed on 26 October 2023).
9. Galiero, R.; Pafundi, P.C.; Nevola, R.; Rinalida, L. The Importance of Telemedicine during COVID-19 Pandemic: A Focus on Diabetic Retinopathy. *J. Diabetes Res.* **2020**, *2020*, 9036847. [CrossRef]
10. Robles, R.; Patel, N.; Neag, E.; Mittal, A.; Markatia, Z.; Ameli, K.; Lin, B. A Systematic Review of Digital Ophthalmoscopes in Medicine. *Clin. Ophthalmol.* **2023**, *17*, 2957–2965. [CrossRef] [PubMed]
11. Sasso, F.C.; Pafundi, P.C.; Gelso, A.; Bono, C. Telemedicine for screening diabetic retinopathy: The NO BLIND Italian multicenter study. *Diabetes Metab. Res. Rev.* **2019**, *35*, e3113. [CrossRef]
12. Lin, K.Y.; Hsih, W.H.; Lin, Y.B.; Wen, C.Y.; Chang, T.J. Update in the epidemiology, risk factors, screening, and treatment of diabetic retinopathy. *J. Diabetes Investig.* **2021**, *12*, 1322–1325. [CrossRef]
13. Chew, E.Y.; Davis, M.D.; Danis, R.P.; Locato, J.F. The effects of medical management on the progression of diabetic retinopathy in persons with type 2 diabetes: The Action to Control Cardiovascular Risk in Diabetes (ACCORD) Eye Study. *Ophthalmology.* **2014**, *121*, 2443–2451. [CrossRef]
14. Action to Control Cardiovascular Risk in Diabetes Follow-On (ACCORDION) Eye Study Group; The Action to Control Cardiovascular Risk in Diabetes Follow-On (ACCORDION) Study Group. Persistent effects of intensive glycemic control on retinopathy in type 2 diabetes in the Action to Control Cardiovascular Risk in Diabetes (ACCORD) follow-on study. *Diabetes Care* **2016**, *39*, 1089–1100. [CrossRef] [PubMed]
15. Kaštelan, S.; Tomić, M.; Gverović Antunica, A.; Ljubić, S.; Salopek Rabatić, J.; Karabatić, M. Body mass index: A risk factor for retinopathy in type 2 diabetic patients. *Mediat. Inflamm.* **2013**, *2013*, 436329. [CrossRef] [PubMed]
16. Chang, Y.C.; Wu, W.C. Dyslipidemia and diabetic retinopathy. *Rev. Diabet. Stud.* **2013**, *10*, 121–132. [CrossRef]
17. Kohner, E.M.; Aldington, S.J.; Stratton, I.M.; Manley, S.E.; Holman, R.R.; Matthews, D.R.; Turner, R.C. United Kingdom Prospective Diabetes Study 30. Diabetic retinopathy at diagnosis of non-insulin-dependent diabetes mellitus and associated risk factors. *Arch. Ophthalmol.* **1998**, *116*, 297–303. [CrossRef] [PubMed]
18. Klein, R.; Sharrett, A.R.; Klein, B.E.; Moss, S.E.; Folsom, A.R.; Wong, T.Y.; Brancati, F.L.; Hubbard, L.D.; Couper, D.; ARIC Group. The association of atherosclerosis, vascular risk factors, and retinopathy in adults with diabetes: The Atherosclerosis Risk in Communities study. *Ophthalmology* **2002**, *109*, 1225–1234. [CrossRef] [PubMed]

19. Klein, R.; Marino, E.K.; Kuller, L.H.; Polak, J.F.; Tracy, R.P.; Gottdiener, J.S.; Burke, G.L.; Hubbard, L.D.; Boineau, R. The relation of atherosclerotic cardiovascular disease to retinopathy in people with diabetes in the Cardiovascular Health Study. *Br. J. Ophthalmol.* **2002**, *86*, 84–90. [CrossRef] [PubMed]
20. van Leiden, H.A.; Dekker, J.M.; Moll, A.C.; Nijpels, G.; Heine, R.J.; Bouter, L.M.; Stehouwer, C.D.; Polak, B.C. Blood pressure, lipids, and obesity are associated with retinopathy: The Hoorn study. *Diabetes Care* **2002**, *25*, 1320–1325. [CrossRef]
21. Vujosevic, S.; Aldington, S.J.; Silva, P.; Peto, P. Screening for diabetic retinopathy: New perspectives and challenges. *Lancet Diabetes Endocrinol.* **2020**, *8*, 337–347. [CrossRef]
22. Cai, X.; Chen, Y.; Yang, W.; Gao, X.; Han, X.; Ji, L. The association of smoking and risk of diabetic retinopathy in patients with type 1 and type 2 diabetes: A meta-analysis. *Endocrine* **2018**, *62*, 299–306. [CrossRef]
23. Rasmussen, K.L.; Laugesen, C.S.; Ringholm, L.; Vestgaard, M.; Damm, P.; Mathiesen, E.R. Progression of diabetic retinopathy during pregnancy in women with type 2 diabetes. *Diabetologia* **2010**, *53*, 1076–1083. [CrossRef] [PubMed]
24. Rubsam, A.; Parikh, S.; Fort, P.E. Role of Inflammation in Diabetic Retinopathy. *Int. J. Mol. Sci.* **2018**, *19*, 942. [CrossRef] [PubMed]
25. Simo, R.; Stitt, A.W.; Gardner, T.W. Neurodegeneration in diabetic retinopathy: Does it really matter? *Diabetologia* **2018**, *61*, 1902–1912. [CrossRef]
26. Ansari, P.; Tabasumma, N.; Snigdha, N.N.; Siam, N.H.; Panduru, R.V.N.R.S.; Azam, S.; Hannan, J.M.A.; Abdel-Wahab, Y.H.A. Diabetic Retinopathy: An Overview on Mechanisms, Pathophysiology and Pharmacotherapy. *Diabetology* **2022**, *3*, 159–175. [CrossRef]
27. Kowluru, R.A.; Santos, J.M.; Mishra, M. Epigenetic modifications and diabetic retinopathy. *Biomed. Res. Int.* **2013**, *2013*, 635284. [CrossRef] [PubMed]
28. Kollias, A.N.; Ulbig, M.W. Diabetic retinopathy: Early diagnosis and effective treatment. *Dtsch. Arztebl. Int.* **2010**, *107*, 75–83. [CrossRef]
29. Carmeliet, P. Mechanisms of angiogenesis and arteriogenesis. *Nat. Med.* **2000**, *6*, 389–395. [CrossRef] [PubMed]
30. Ishida, S.; Usui, T.; Yamashiro, K.; Kaji, Y.; Ahmed, E.; Carrasquillo, K.G.; Amano, S.; Hida, T.; Oguchi, Y.; Adamis, A.P. VEGF164 is proinflammatory in the diabetic retina. *Investig. Ophthalmol. Vis. Sci.* **2003**, *44*, 2155–2162. [CrossRef]
31. Williams, B.; Baker, A.Q.; Gallacher, B.; Lodwick, D. Angiotensin II increases vascular permeability factor gene expression by human vascular smooth muscle cells. *Hypertension* **1995**, *25*, 913–917. [CrossRef]
32. Viswanath, K.; McGavin, D.D. Diabetic retinopathy: Clinical findings and management. *Community Eye Health* **2003**, *16*, 21–24.
33. Roy, S.; Kim, D. Retinal capillary basement membrane thickening: Role in the pathogenesis of diabetic retinopathy. *Prog. Retin. Eye Res.* **2021**, *82*, 100903. [CrossRef]
34. Kern, T.S.; Huang, S.S. Vascular damage in diabetic retinopathy. *Ocul. Dis. Mech. Manag.* **2010**, *2010*, 506–513.
35. Bakri, S.J.; Kaiser, P.K. Chapter 21—Diabetic Retinopathy. In *Retinal Imaging*; Huang, D., Kaiser, P.K., Lowder, C.Y., Elias, I., Traboulsi, E.I., Eds.; Mosby: Maryland Heights, MO, USA, 2006; pp. 233–240.
36. Aronson, J.K.; Ferner, R.E. Biomarkers—A General Review. *Curr. Protoc. Pharmacol.* **2017**, *76*, 9.23.1–9.23.17. [CrossRef] [PubMed]
37. Nawaz, I.M.; Rezzola, S.; Cancarini, A.; Russo, A.; Costagliola, C.; Semeraro, F.; Presta, M. Human vitreous in proliferative diabetic retinopathy: Characterization and translational implications. *Prog. Retin. Eye Res.* **2019**, *72*, 100756. [CrossRef]
38. Homsi, J.; Daud, A.I. Spectrum of activity and mechanism of action of VEGF/PDGF inhibitors. *Cancer Control* **2007**, *14*, 285–294. [CrossRef] [PubMed]
39. Shibuya, M. Vascular endothelial growth factor receptor-2: Its unique signaling and specific ligand, VEGF-E. *Cancer Sci.* **2005**, *94*, 751–756. [CrossRef]
40. Arrigo, A.; Aragona, E.; Bandello, F. VEGF-targeting drugs for the treatment of retinal neovascularization in diabetic retinopathy. *Ann. Med.* **2022**, *54*, 1089–1111. [CrossRef]
41. Holmes, D.I.; Zachary, I. The vascular endothelial growth factor (VEGF) family: Angiogenic factors in health and disease. *Genome Biol.* **2005**, *6*, 209. [CrossRef]
42. Gupta, N.; Mansoor, S.; Sharma, A.; Sapkal, A.; Sheth, J.; Falatoonzadeh, P.; Kuppermann, B.; Kenney, M. Diabetic retinopathy and VEGF. *Open Ophthalmol. J.* **2013**, *7*, 4–10. [CrossRef] [PubMed]
43. Ferrara, N. Vascular Endothelial Growth Factor: Basic Science and Clinical Progress. *Endocr. Rev.* **2004**, *25*, 581–611. [CrossRef] [PubMed]
44. Stuttfeld, E.; Ballmer-Hofer, K. Structure and function of VEGF receptors. *IUBMB Life* **2009**, *61*, 915–922. [CrossRef] [PubMed]
45. Clauss, M. Molecular Biology of the VEGF and the VEGF Receptor Family. *Semin. Thromb. Hemost.* **2000**, *26*, 561–570. [CrossRef]
46. Wang, X.; Bove, A.M.; Simone, G.; Ma, B. Molecular Bases of VEGFR-2-Mediated Physiological Function and Pathological Role. *Front. Cell Dev. Biol.* **2020**, *8*, 599281. [CrossRef] [PubMed]
47. Claesson-Welsh, L. VEGF receptor signal transduction—A brief update. *Vasc. Pharmacol.* **2016**, *86*, 14–17. [CrossRef]
48. Carmeliet, P.; Ferreira, V.; Breier, G.; Harpal, K. Abnormal blood vessel development and lethality in embryos lacking a single VEGF allele. *Nature* **1996**, *380*, 435–439. [CrossRef] [PubMed]
49. Bucolo, C.; Barbieri, A.; Vigano, I.; Band, F. Short-and Long-Term Expression of Vegf: A Temporal Regulation of a Key Factor in Diabetic Retinopathy. *Front. Pharmacol.* **2021**, *12*, 707909. [CrossRef]
50. Hirano, T.; Toriyama, Y.; Iesato, Y.; Imai, A.; Murata, T. Changes in plasma vascular endothelial growth factor level after intravitreal injection of Bevacizumab, Aflibercept, or Ranibizumab for diabetic macular edema. *Retina* **2018**, *38*, 1801–1808. [CrossRef]

51. Wu, F.; Phone, A.; Lamy, R.; Chen, Y. Correlation of Aqueous, Vitreous, and Plasma Cytokine Levels in Patients with Proliferative Diabetic Retinopathy. *Investig. Ophthalmol. Vis. Sci.* **2020**, *61*, 26. [CrossRef]
52. Midena, E.; Frizziero, L.; Midena, G.; Pilotto, T. Intraocular fluid biomarkers (liquid biopsy) in human diabetic retinopathy. *Graefes Arch. Clin. Exp. Ophthalmol.* **2021**, *259*, 3549–3560. [CrossRef]
53. Bonfiglio, V.; Platania, C.B.M.; Lazzara, F.; Conti, F.; Pizzo, C.; Reibaldi, M.; Russo, A.; Fallico, M.; Ortisi, E.; Pignatelli, F.; et al. TGF-β Serum Levels in Diabetic Retinopathy Patients and the Role of Anti-VEGF Therapy. *Int. J. Mol. Sci.* **2020**, *21*, 9558. [CrossRef]
54. Nalini, M.; Raghavulu, B.V.; Annapurna, A.; Chandl, V. Correlation of various serum biomarkers with the severity of diabetic retinopathy. *Diabetes Metab. Syndr. Clin. Res. Rev.* **2017**, *11*, S451–S454. [CrossRef]
55. Nakhleh, E.; Abu, Y.; Nafez, M.; Abu, T.; Ala MAbojaradeh, A.S.; Al-Akily, E.M.; Abdo, L.; Emoush, O. Relationship between Serum Vascular Endothelial Growth Factor Levels and Stages of Diabetic Retinopathy and Other Biomarkers. *J. Ophthalmol.* **2020**, *2020*, 8480193. [CrossRef]
56. Ahuja, S.; Saxena, S.; Akduman, L.; Khanna, V. Serum vascular endothelial growth factor is a biomolecular biomarker of severity of diabetic retinopathy. *Int. J. Retin. Vitr.* **2019**, *5*, 29. [CrossRef] [PubMed]
57. Ang, W.J.; Zunaina, E.; Norfadzillah, A.J.; Lewin, A.S. Evaluation of vascular endothelial growth factor levels in tears and serum among diabetic patients. *PLoS ONE* **2019**, *14*, e0221481. [CrossRef] [PubMed]
58. Kaštelan, S.; Orešković, I.; Bišćan, F.; Kaštelan, H.; Gverović Antunica, A. Inflammatory and angiogenic biomarkers in diabetic retinopathy. *Biochem. Medica* **2020**, *30*, 385–399. [CrossRef] [PubMed]
59. Majidreza, S.; Alizadeh, M.; Saeid, A. The tear VEGF and IGFBP3 in healthy and diabetic retinopathy. *Int. J. Diabetes Dev. Ctries.* **2019**, *40*, 93–98. [CrossRef]
60. Mei, C.; Pan, L.; Xu, W.; Li, Z. An ultrasensitive reusable aptasensor for noninvasive diabetic retinopathy diagnosis target on tear biomarker. *Sens. Actuators B Chem.* **2021**, *345*, 130398. [CrossRef]
61. Wang, J.Y.; Kwon, J.S.; Hsu, S.M.; Chuang, H.S. Sensitive tear screening of diabetic retinopathy with dual biomarkers enabled using a rapid electrokinetic patterning platform. *Lab A Chip* **2020**, *20*, 356–362. [CrossRef]
62. Hashimoto, Y.; Okada, A.; Matsui, H.; Obata, R. Recent trends in anti-vascular endothelial growth factor intravitreal injections: A large claims database study in Japan. *Jpn. J. Ophthalmol.* **2023**, *67*, 109–118. [CrossRef]
63. Grillo, M.A.; Colombatto, S. Arginine revisited: Minireview article. *Amino Acids* **2004**, *26*, 345–351. [CrossRef]
64. Endemann, D.H.; Schiffrin, E.L. Endothelial dysfunction. *J. Am. Soc. Nephrol.* **2004**, *15*, 1983–1992. [CrossRef] [PubMed]
65. Yonem, A.; Duran, C.; Unal, M.; Ipcioglu, O.M.; Ozcan, O. Plasma apelin and asymmetric dimethylarginine levels in type 2 diabetic patients with diabetic retinopathy. *Diabetes Res. Clin. Pract.* **2009**, *84*, 219–223. [CrossRef]
66. Narayanan, P.S.; Rojas, M.; Suwanpradid, J.; Toque, H.A.; Caldwell, W.R.; Caldwell, R.B. Arginase in retinopathy. *Prog. Retin. Eye Res.* **2013**, *36*, 260–280. [CrossRef] [PubMed]
67. Sena, C.M.; Pereira, A.M.; Seica, R. Endothelial dysfunction—A major mediator of diabetic vascular disease. *Biochim. Biophys. Acta* **2013**, *1832*, 2216–2231. [CrossRef]
68. Forstermann, U.; Closs, E.I.; Pollock, J.S.; Nakane, M.; Schwarz, P.; Gath, I.; Kleinert, H. Nitric oxide synthase isozymes. Characterization, purification, molecular cloning, and functions. *Hypertension* **1994**, *23*, 1121–1131. [CrossRef]
69. Toutouzas, K.; Riga, M.; Stefanadi, E.; Stefanadis, C. Asymmetric dimethylarginine (ADMA) and other endogenous nitric oxide synthase (NOS) inhibitors as an important cause of vascular insulin resistance. *Horm. Metab. Res.* **2008**, *40*, 655–659. [CrossRef] [PubMed]
70. Bode-Boger, S.M.; Scalera, F.; Martens-Lobenhoffer, J. Asymmetric dimethylarginine (ADMA) accelerates cell senescence. *Vasc. Med.* **2005**, *10*, 65–71. [CrossRef]
71. Sirman, Y.V.; Savytskyi, I.V. Study of endothelial dysfunction and asymmetric dimethylarginine levels. *J. Educ. Health Sport* **2019**, *9*, 395–412. [CrossRef]
72. Leiper, J.M.; Vallance, P. The synthesis and metabolism of asymmetric dimethylarginine (ADMA). *Eur. J. Clin. Pharmacol.* **2006**, *62*, 33–38. [CrossRef]
73. Morris, S.M. Arginine metabolism revisited. *J. Nutr.* **2016**, *146*, 2579–2586. [CrossRef]
74. Trocha, M.; Merwid-Lad, A.; Szuba, A.; Sozanski, T.; Magdalan, J.; Szelag, A. Asymmetric dimethylarginine synthesis and degradation under physiological and pathological conditions. *Adv. Clin. Exp. Med.* **2010**, *19*, 233–243.
75. Vallance, P.; Leone, A.; Calver, A.; Collier, J.; Moncada, S. Accumulation of an endogenous inhibitor of nitric oxide synthesis in chronic renal failure. *Lancet* **1992**, *339*, 572–575. [CrossRef] [PubMed]
76. Sydow, K.; Munzel, T. ADMA and oxidative stress. *Atheroscler. Suppl.* **2003**, *4*, 41–51. [CrossRef]
77. Cardounel, A.J.; Cui, H.; Samouilov, A.; Johnson, W.; Kearns, P.; Tsai, A.-L.; Berka, V.; Zweier, J.L. Evidence for the pathophysiological role of endogenous methylarginines in regulation of endothelial NO production and vascular function. *J. Biol. Chem.* **2007**, *282*, 879–887. [CrossRef]
78. Jian, Q.; Wu, Y.; Zhang, F. Metabolomics in diabetic retinopathy: From potential biomarkers to molecular basis of oxidative stress. *Cells* **2022**, *11*, 3005. [CrossRef] [PubMed]
79. Peters, K.S.; Rivera, E.; Warden, C.; Harlow, P.A.; Mitchell, S.L.; Calcutt, M.W.; Samuels, D.C.; Brantley, M.A. Plasma arginine and citrulline are elevated in diabetic retinopathy. *Am. J. Ophthalmol.* **2022**, *235*, 154–162. [CrossRef]

80. Sumarriva, K.; Uppal, K.; Ma, C.; Herren, D.J.; Wang, Y.; Chocron, I.M.; Warden, C.; Mitchell, S.L.; Burgess, G.L.; Goodale, M.P.; et al. Arginine and carnitine metabolites are altered in diabetic retinopathy. *Investig. Ophthalmol. Vis. Sci.* **2019**, *60*, 3119–3126. [CrossRef]
81. Dag, U.; Caglayan, M.; Alakus, M.F.; Oncul, H. The relationship between reduced choroidal thickness due to high plasma asymmetrical dimethylarginine level and increased severity of diabetic retinopathy. *Arq. Bras. Oftalmol.* **2023**, *86*, 27–32. [CrossRef]
82. Lamprou, S.; Koletsos, N.; Mintziori, G.; Anyfanti, P.; Trakatelli, C.; Kotsis, V.; Gkaliagkousi, E.; Triantafyllou, A. Microvascular and endothelial dysfunction in prediabetes. *Life* **2023**, *13*, 644. [CrossRef] [PubMed]
83. Krasnicki, P.; Proniewska-Skretek, E.; Dmuchowska, D.A.; Dobrzycki, S.; Mariak, Z. Asymmetric dimethylarginine (ADMA) as a marker of blood flow disturbances in ocular circulation in patients with type 2 diabetes and coronary artery disease. *Mag. Lek. Okulisty* **2009**, *3*, 325–331.
84. Tousoulis, D.; Kampoli, A.-M.; Stefanadis, C. Diabetes mellitus and vascular endothelial dysfunction: Current perspectives. *Curr. Vasc. Pharmacol.* **2012**, *10*, 19–32. [CrossRef]
85. Stepien, E.; Szuscik, I.; Tokarz, A.; Enguita, F.J.; Solnica, B.; Zurakowski, A.; Malecki, M. The role of microparticles in pathomechanisms of diabetic retinopathy—Analysis of intercellular communication mechanisms in endothelial aging. Case control study in patients with metabolic syndrome, diabetes type 1 and type 2. *J. Med. Sci.* **2014**, *83*, 322–327. [CrossRef]
86. Huang, C.-Y.; Zhou, T.; Li, G.; Li, M.-Y.; Xiong, X.-M.; Wu, M.-T.; Jiang, J.-L. Asymmetric dimethylarginine aggravates blood-retinal barrier breakdown of diabetic retinopathy via inhibition of intercellular communication in retinal pericytes. *Amino Acids* **2019**, *51*, 1515–1526. [CrossRef] [PubMed]
87. Liu, J.; Li, C.; Chen, W.; He, K.; Ma, H.; Ma, B.; Zhao, P.; Tian, L. Relationship between serum asymmetric dimethylarginine level and microvascular. *Bio. Med. Res. Int.* **2019**, *2019*, 2941861. [CrossRef]
88. Alpay, A.; Ozcan, O.; Ugurbas, S.C.; Ugurbas, S.H. Investigated of vitreous and serum asymmetric dimethylarginine levels in diabetic. *Res. Sq.* **2019**, *2019*. [CrossRef]
89. Sugai, M.; Ohta, A.; Ogata, Y.; Nakanishi, M.; Ueno, S.; Kawata, T.; Saito, N.; Tanaka, Y. Asymmetric dimethylarginine (ADMA) in the aqueous humor of diabetic patients. *Endocr. J.* **2007**, *54*, 303–309. [CrossRef]
90. Abhary, S.; Kasmeridis, N.; Burdon, K.P.; Kuot, A.; Whiting, M.J.; Yew, W.P.; Petrovsky, N.; Craig, J.E. Diabetic retinopathy is associated with elevated serum asymmetric and symmetric dimethylarginines. *Diabetes Care* **2009**, *32*, 2084–2086. [CrossRef]
91. Eliana, F.; Suwondo, P.; Makmun, L.H.; Harbuwono, D.S. ADMA as a marker of endothelial dysfunction in prediabetic women. *Acta Medica Indones.* **2011**, *43*, 92–98.
92. Du, M.-R.; Yan, L.; Li, N.-S.; Wang, Y.-J.; Zhou, T.; Jiang, J.-L. Asymmetric dimethylarginine contributes to retinal neovascularization of diabetic retinopathy through EphrinB2 pathway. *Vasc. Pharmacol.* **2018**, *108*, 46–56. [CrossRef]
93. Yun, J.H.; Kim, J.-M.; Jeon, H.J.; Oh, T.; Choi, H.J.; Kim, B.-J. Metabolomics profiles associated with diabetic retinopathy in type 2 diabetes patients. *PLoS ONE* **2020**, *15*, e241365. [CrossRef]
94. Malecki, M.T.; Undas, A.; Cyganek, K.; Mirkiewicz-Sieradzka, B.; Wolkow, P.; Osmenda, G.; Walus-Miarka, M.; Guzik, T.J.; Sieradzki, J. Plasma asymmetric dimethylarginine (ADMA) is associated with retinopathy in type 2 diabetes. *Diabetes Care* **2007**, *30*, 2899–2901. [CrossRef] [PubMed]
95. Hernandes, C.; Porta, M.; Bandello, F.; Grauslund, J.; Harding, S.P.; Aldington, S.J.; Egan, C.; Frydkjaer-Olsen, U.; Garcia-Arumi, J.; Gibson, J.; et al. The usefulness of serum biomarkers in the early stages of diabetic retinopathy: Results of the EUROCONDOR clinical trial. *J. Clin. Med.* **2020**, *9*, 1233. [CrossRef] [PubMed]
96. Aydogan, S.; Dilli, D.; Kabatas, E.U.; Akduman, H.; Sah Ipek, M.; Oguz, B.; Atlas, N.; Zenciroglu, A. The serum levels of asymmetric dimethylarginine, vascular endothelial growth factor, and insulin-like growth factor-1 in preterms with retinopathy of prematurity. *Fetal Pediatr. Pathol.* **2022**, *41*, 634–639. [CrossRef] [PubMed]
97. Wieczor, R.; Wieczor, A.M.; Kulwas, A.; Rosc, D. ADMA (asymmetric dimethylarginine) and angiogenic potential in patients with type 2 diabetes and prediabetes. *Exp. Biol. Med.* **2021**, *246*, 153–162. [CrossRef] [PubMed]
98. Sibal, L.; Agarwal, S.C.; Home, P.D.; Boger, R.H. The role of asymmetric dimethylarginine (ADMA) in endothelial dysfunction and cardiovascular disease. *Curr. Cardiol. Rev.* **2010**, *6*, 82–90. [CrossRef]
99. Jaroszynski, A.J.; Jaroszynska, A.; Wysokinski, A. Asymmetric dimethylarginine—The link between hart and kidney diseases. *Chor. Serca I Naczyń* **2012**, *9*, 225–229.
100. Celik, M.; Cerrah, S.; Arabul, M.; Akalin, A. Relation of asymmetric dimethylarginine levels to macrovascular disease and inflammation markers in type 2 diabetic patients. *J. Diabetes Res.* **2014**, *2014*, 139215. [CrossRef]
101. Kawata, T.; Daimon, M.; Hasegawa, R.; Teramoto, K.; Toyoda, T.; Sekine, T.; Yamamoto, K.; Uchida, D.; Himi, T.; Yoshida, K.; et al. Effect of angiotensin-converting enzyme inhibitor on serum asymmetric dimethylarginine and coronary circulation in patients with type 2 diabetes mellitus. *Int. J. Cardiol.* **2009**, *132*, 286–288. [CrossRef]
102. Guo, X.; Xing, Y.; Jin, W. Role of ADMA in the pathogenesis of microvascular complications in type 2 diabetes mellitus. *Front. Endocrinol.* **2023**, *14*, 1183586. [CrossRef]
103. O'Brien, J.; Hayder, H.; Zayed, Y.; Peng, C. Overview of MicroRNA Biogenesis, Mechanisms of Actions, and Circulation. *Front. Endocrinol.* **2018**, *9*, 402. [CrossRef]
104. Ha, M.; Kim, V. Regulation of microRNA biogenesis. *Nat. Rev. Mol. Cell Biol.* **2014**, *15*, 509–524. [CrossRef] [PubMed]

105. Glinge, C.; Clauss, S.; Boddum, K.; Jabbari, R.; Jabbari, J.; Risgaard, B.; Tomsits, P.; Hildebrand, B.; Kaab, S.; Wakili, R.; et al. Stability of Circulating Blood-Based MicroRNAs—Pre-Analytic Methodological Considerations. *PLoS ONE* **2017**, *12*, e0167969. [CrossRef] [PubMed]
106. Karbasforooshan, H.; Karimi, G. The role of SIRT1 in diabetic retinopathy. *Biomed. Pharmacother.* **2018**, *97*, 190–194. [CrossRef] [PubMed]
107. Chang, X.; Zhu, G.; Cai, Z.; Wang, Y.; Lian, R.; Tang, X.; Ma, C.; Fu, S. miRNA, lncRNA and circRNA: Targeted Molecules Full of Therapeutic Prospects in the Development of Diabetic Retinopathy. *Front. Endocrinol.* **2021**, *12*, 771552. [CrossRef] [PubMed]
108. Ji, Q.; Han, J.; Wang, L.; Liu, J.; Dong, Y.; Zhu, K.; Shi, L. MicroRNA-34a promotes apoptosis of retinal vascular endothelial cells by targeting SIRT1 in rats with diabetic retinopathy. *Cell Cycle* **2020**, *19*, 2886–2896. [CrossRef] [PubMed]
109. Shan, L.; Zhang, H.; Han, Y.; Kuang, R. Expression and mechanism of microRNA 195 in diabetic retinopathy. *Endocr. J.* **2022**, *69*, 529–537. [CrossRef]
110. Yin, C.; Lin, X.; Sun, Y.; Ji, X. Dysregulation of miR210 is involved in the development of diabetic retinopathy and serves a regulatory role in retinal vascular endothelial cell proliferation. *Eur. J. Med. Res.* **2020**, *25*, 20. [CrossRef]
111. Pan, Q.; Gao, Z.; Zhu, C.; Peng, Z.; Song, M.; Li, L. Overexpression of histone deacetylase SIRT1 exerts an antiangiogenic role in diabetic retinopathy via miR-20a elevation and YAP/HIF1α/VEGFA depletion. *Am. J. Physiol. Endocrinol. Metab.* **2020**, *319*, 932–943. [CrossRef]
112. Qin, B.; Liu, J.; Liu, S.; Li, B.; Ren, J. MiR-20b targets AKT3 and modulates vascular endothelial growth factor-mediated changes in diabetic retinopathy. *Acta Biochim. Biophys. Sin.* **2016**, *48*, 732–740. [CrossRef]
113. Maisto, R.; Trotta, M.C.; Petrillo, F.; Izzo, S.; Cuomo, G.; Alfano, R.; Hermenean, A.; Barcia, J.M.; Galdiero, M.; Platania, C.B.M.; et al. Resolvin D1 Modulates the Intracellular VEGF-Related miRNAs of Retinal Photoreceptors Challenged With High Glucose. *Front. Pharmacol.* **2020**, *11*, 235. [CrossRef]
114. Duan, P.; Chen, S.; Zeng, Y.; Xu, H.; Liu, Y. Osteopontin Upregulates Col IV Expression by Repressing miR-29a in Human Retinal Capillary Endothelial Cells. *Mol. Ther. Nucleic Acids* **2020**, *20*, 242–251. [CrossRef]
115. Someya, H.; Ito, M.; Nishio, Y.; Sato, T.; Harimoto, K.; Takeuchi, M. Osteopontin-induced vascular hyperpermeability through tight junction disruption in diabetic retina. *Exp. Eye Res.* **2022**, *220*, 1090–1094. [CrossRef] [PubMed]
116. Wang, J.; Yao, Y.; Wang, K.; Chu, T. MicroRNA-148a-3p alleviates high glucose-induced diabetic retinopathy by targeting TGFB2 and FGF2. *Acta Diabetol.* **2020**, *57*, 1435–1443. [CrossRef] [PubMed]
117. Liu, H.N.; Cao, N.J.; Li, X.; Qian, W.; Chen, X.L. Serum microRNA-211 as a biomarker for diabetic retinopathy via modulating Sirtuin 1. *Biochem. Biophys. Res. Commun.* **2018**, *505*, 1236–1243. [CrossRef]
118. Miao, C.; Chang, J.; Zhang, G.; Fang, Y. MicroRNAs in type 1 diabetes: New research progress and potential directions. *Biochem. Cell Biol.* **2018**, *96*, 498–506. [CrossRef] [PubMed]
119. Margaritis, K.; Margioula-Siarkou, G.; Giza, S.; Kotanidou, E.P.; Tsinopoulou, V.R.; Christoforidis, A.; Galli-Tsinopoulou, A. Micro-RNA Implications in Type-1 Diabetes Mellitus: A Review of Literature. *Int. J. Mol. Sci.* **2021**, *22*, 2165. [CrossRef]
120. Li, E.H.; Huang, Q.Z.; Li, G.C.; Xiang, Z.Y.; Zhang, X. Effects of miRNA-200b on the development of diabetic retinopathy by targeting VEGFA gene. *Biosci. Rep.* **2017**, *37*, 2016572. [CrossRef]
121. Liang, Z.; Gao, K.P.; Wang, Y.X.; Liu, Z.C.; Tian, L.; Yang, X.Z.; Ding, J.Y.; Wu, W.T.; Yang, W.H.; Li, Y.L.; et al. RNA sequencing identified specific circulating miRNA biomarkers for early detection of diabetes retinopathy. *Am. J. Physiol. Endocrinol. Metab.* **2018**, *315*, 374–385. [CrossRef]
122. Santovito, D.; Toto, L.; De Nardis, V.; Ces, D. Plasma microRNA signature associated with retinopathy in patients with type 2 diabetes. *Sci Rep.* **2021**, *11*, 4136. [CrossRef]
123. McArthur, K.; Feng, B.; Wu, Y.; Chen, S.; Chakrabarti, S. MicroRNA-200b regulates vascular endothelial growth factor-mediated alterations in diabetic retinopathy. *Diabetes* **2011**, *60*, 1314–1323. [CrossRef]
124. Yang, Y.; Yue, W.; Wang, N.; Wang, Z.; Li, B.; Zeng, J.; Yoshida, S.; Ding, C.; Zhou, Y. Altered Expressions of Transfer RNA-Derived Small RNAs and microRNAs in the Vitreous Humor of Proliferative Diabetic Retinopathy. *Front. Endocrinol.* **2022**, *13*, 913370. [CrossRef] [PubMed]
125. Kot, A.; Kaczmarek, R. Exosomal miRNA Profiling in Vitreous Humor in Proliferative Diabetic Retinopathy. *Cells* **2022**, *12*, 123. [CrossRef]
126. Guo, J.; Zhou, P.; Liu, Z.; Dai, F.; Pan, M.; An, G.; Han, J.; Du, L.; Jin, X. The Aflibercept-Induced MicroRNA Profile in the Vitreous of Proliferative Diabetic Retinopathy Patients Detected by Next-Generation Sequencing. *Front. Pharmacol.* **2021**, *12*, 781276. [CrossRef] [PubMed]
127. Saleh, A.A.; El-Hefnawy, S.M.; Kasemy, Z.A.; Alhagaa, A.A.; Nooh, M.Z.; Arafat, E.S. Mi-RNA-93 and Mi-RNA-152 in the Diagnosis of Type 2 Diabetes and Diabetic Retinopathy. *Br. J. Biomed. Sci.* **2022**, *79*, 10192. [CrossRef] [PubMed]
128. Zampetaki, A.; Kiechl, S.; Drozdov, I.; Willeit, P.; Mayr, U.; Prokopi, M.; Mayr, A.; Weger, S.; Oberhollenzer, F.; Bonora, E.; et al. Plasma microRNA profiling reveals loss of endothelial miR-126 and other microRNAs in type 2 diabetes. *Circ. Res.* **2010**, *107*, 810–817. [CrossRef]
129. Ko, G.Y.; Yu, F.; Bayless, K.J.; Ko, M.L. MicroRNA-150 (miR-150) and Diabetic Retinopathy: Is miR-150 Only a Biomarker or Does It Contribute to Disease Progression? *Int. J. Mol. Sci.* **2022**, *23*, 99. [CrossRef]
130. Zhou, H.; Peng, C.; Huang, D.S.; Liu, L.; Guan, P. microRNA Expression Profiling Based on Microarray Approach in Human Diabetic Retinopathy: A Systematic Review and Meta-Analysis. *DNA Cell Biol.* **2020**, *39*, 441–450. [CrossRef]

131. Ma, L.; Wen, Y.; Li, Z.; Wu, N.; Wang, Q. Circulating MicroRNAs as Potential Diagnostic Biomarkers for Diabetic Retinopathy: A Meta-Analysis. *Front. Endocrinol.* **2022**, *13*, 929924. [CrossRef]
132. Jenkins, H.N.; Rivera-Gonzalez, O.; Gibert, Y.; Speed, J.S. Endothelin-1 in the pathophysiology of obesity and insulin resistance. *Obes. Rev.* **2020**, *21*, e13086. [CrossRef]
133. Ergul, A. Endothelin-1 and diabetic complications: Focus on the vasculature. *Pharmacol. Res.* **2011**, *63*, 477–482. [CrossRef]
134. Stow, L.R.; Jacobs, M.E.; Wingo, C.S.; Cain, B.D. Endothelin-1 gene regulation. *FASEB J.* **2010**, *25*, 16–28. [CrossRef] [PubMed]
135. Kostov, K. The causal relationship between endothelin-1 and hypertension: Focusing on endothelial dysfunction, arterial stiffness, vascular remodeling, and Blood Pressure Regulation. *Life* **2021**, *11*, 986. [CrossRef] [PubMed]
136. Abman, S.H. Role of endothelin receptor antagonists in the treatment of pulmonary arterial hypertension. *Annu. Rev. Med.* **2009**, *60*, 13–23. [CrossRef] [PubMed]
137. Cheung, S.S.; Leung, J.W.; Lam, A.K.; Acy, L. Selective over-expression of endothelin-1 in endothelial cells exacerbates inner retinal edema and neuronal death in ischemic retina. *PLoS ONE* **2011**, *6*, e26184. [CrossRef] [PubMed]
138. Chen, Y.-L.; Rosa, R.H.; Kuo, L.; Hein, T.W. Hyperglycemia augments endothelin-1–induced constriction of human retinal venules. *Transl. Vis. Sci. Technol.* **2020**, *9*, 1. [CrossRef] [PubMed]
139. Chang, W.; Lajko, M.; Fawzi, A.A. Endothelin-1 is associated with fibrosis in proliferative diabetic retinopathy membranes. *PLoS ONE* **2018**, *13*, e0191285. [CrossRef]
140. Kang, H.M.; Hasanuzzaman, M.; Kim, S.W.; Koh, H.J.; Lee, S.C. Elevated aqueous endothelin-1 concentrations in advanced diabetic retinopathy. *PLoS ONE* **2022**, *17*, e0268353. [CrossRef]
141. Khuu, L.-A.; Tayyari, F.; Sivak, J.M.; Singer, S. Aqueous humor endothelin-1 and total retinal blood flow in patients with non-proliferative diabetic retinopathy. *Eye* **2017**, *31*, 1443–1450. [CrossRef]
142. Ottosson-Seeberger, A.; Lundberg, J.M.; Alvestrand, A.; Ahlborg, G. Exogenous endothelin-1 causes peripheral insulin resistance in healthy humans. *Acta Physiol. Scand.* **1997**, *161*, 211–220. [CrossRef]
143. Anfossi, G.; Russo, I.; Doronzo, G.; Trovati, M. Relevance of the vascular effects of insulin in the rationale of its therapeutical use. *Cardiovasc. Hematol. Disord. Drug Targets* **2007**, *7*, 228–249. [CrossRef]
144. Wang, Z.; Yadav, A.S.; Leskova, W.; Harris, N.R. Attenuation of streptozotocin-induced microvascular changes in the mouse retina with the endothelin receptor A antagonist atrasentan. *Exp. Eye Res.* **2010**, *91*, 670–675. [CrossRef] [PubMed]
145. Chou, J.C.; Rollins, S.D.; Ye, M.; Batlle, D.; Fawzi, A.A. Endothelin receptor-a antagonist attenuates retinal vascular and neuroretinal pathology in diabetic mice. *Investig. Opthalmology Vis. Sci.* **2014**, *55*, 2516–2525. [CrossRef] [PubMed]
146. Alrashdi, S.F.; Deliyanti, D.; Wilkinson-Berka, J.L. Intravitreal administration of endothelin type A receptor or endothelin type B receptor antagonists attenuates hypertensive and diabetic retinopathy in rats. *Exp. Eye Res.* **2018**, *176*, 1–9. [CrossRef]
147. Bogdanov, P.; Simo-Servat, O.; Sampedro, J.; Garcia, M. Topical administration of Bosentan prevents retinal neurodegeneration in experimental diabetes. *Int. J. Mol. Sci.* **2018**, *19*, 3578. [CrossRef] [PubMed]
148. Shen, C.Y.; Lu, C.H.; Wu, C.H.; Li, K.J. The Development of Maillard Reaction, and Advanced Glycation End Product (AGE)-Receptor for AGE (RAGE) Signaling Inhibitors as Novel Therapeutic Strategies for Patients with AGE-Related Diseases. *Molecules* **2020**, *25*, 5591. [CrossRef]
149. Ruiz, H.H.; Ramasamy, R.; Schmidt, A.M. Advanced Glycation End Products: Building on the Concept of the "Common Soil" in Metabolic Disease. *Endocrinology* **2020**, *161*, bqz006. [CrossRef]
150. Reddy, V.P.; Aryal, P.; Darkwah, E.K. Advanced Glycation End Products in Health and Disease. *Microorganisms* **2022**, *10*, 1848. [CrossRef]
151. Khalid, M.; Petroianu, G.; Adem, A. Advanced Glycation End Products and Diabetes Mellitus: Mechanisms and Perspectives. *Biomolecules* **2022**, *12*, 542. [CrossRef]
152. Mao, L.; Yin, R.; Yang, L.; Zhao, D. Role of advanced glycation end products on vascular smooth muscle cells under diabetic atherosclerosis. *Front. Endocrinol.* **2022**, *13*, 983723. [CrossRef]
153. Vlassara, H.; Bucala, R.; Striker, L. Pathogenic effects of advanced glycosylation: Biochemical, biologic, and clinical implications for diabetes and aging. *Lab. Investig.* **1988**, *58*, 317–326.
154. Zhang, Q.; Wang, Y.; Fu, L. Dietary advanced glycation end-products: Perspectives linking food processing with health implications. *Compr. Rev. Food Sci. Food Saf.* **2020**, *19*, 2559–2587. [CrossRef] [PubMed]
155. Vistoli, G.; De Maddis, D.; Cipak, A.; Zarkovic, N.; Carini, M.; Aldini, G. Advanced glycoxidation and lipoxidation end products (AGEs and ALEs): An overview of their mechanisms of formation. *Free Radic. Res.* **2013**, *47*, 3–27. [CrossRef] [PubMed]
156. Uribarri, J.; Woodruff, S.; Goodman, S.; Cai, W. Advanced glycation end products in foods and a practical guide to their reduction in the diet. *J. Am. Diet. Assoc.* **2010**, *110*, 911–916. [CrossRef] [PubMed]
157. Garay-Sevilla, M.E.; Rojas, A.; Portero-Otin, M.; Uribarri, J. Dietary AGEs as Exogenous Boosters of Inflammation. *Nutrients* **2021**, *13*, 2802. [CrossRef] [PubMed]
158. Gill, V.; Kumar, V.; Singh, K.; Kumar, A.; Kim, J.J. Advanced Glycation End Products (AGEs) May Be a Striking Link Between Modern Diet and Health. *Biomolecules* **2019**, *9*, 888. [CrossRef] [PubMed]
159. Zawada, A.; Machowiak, A.; Rychter, A.M.; Rata, A.E. Accumulation of Advanced Glycation End-Products in the Body and Dietary Habits. *Nutrients* **2022**, *14*, 3982. [CrossRef]
160. Perrone, A.; Giovino, A.; Benny, J.; Martinelli, F. Advanced Glycation End Products (AGEs): Biochemistry, Signaling, Analytical Methods, and Epigenetic Effects. *Oxid. Med. Cell. Longev.* **2020**, *2020*, 3818196. [CrossRef]

161. Oshitari, T. Advanced Glycation End-Products and Diabetic Neuropathy of the Retina. *Int. J. Mol. Sci.* **2023**, *24*, 2927. [CrossRef]
162. Stitt, A.W. AGEs and diabetic retinopathy. *Investig. Ophthalmol. Vis. Sci.* **2010**, *51*, 4867–4874. [CrossRef]
163. Mokini, Z.; Marcovecchio, M.L.; Chiarelli, F. Molecular pathology of oxidative stress in diabetic angiopathy: Role of mitochondrial and cellular pathways. *Diabetes Res. Clin. Pract.* **2010**, *87*, 313–321. [CrossRef]
164. Safi, S.Z.; Qvist, R.; Kumar, S.; Batumalaie, K.; Ismail, I.S. Molecular mechanisms of diabetic retinopathy, general preventive strategies, and novel therapeutic targets. *Biomed. Res. Int.* **2014**, *2014*, 801269. [CrossRef] [PubMed]
165. Chung, Y.R.; Choi, J.A.; Koh, J.Y.; Yoon, Y.H. Ursodeoxycholic Acid Attenuates Endoplasmic Reticulum Stress-Related Retinal Pericyte Loss in Streptozotocin-Induced Diabetic Mice. *J. Diabetes. Res.* **2017**, *2017*, 1763292. [CrossRef] [PubMed]
166. Stirban, A.; Heinemann, L. Skin Autofluorescence—A Non-invasive Measurement for Assessing Cardiovascular Risk and Risk of Diabetes. *Eur. Endocrinol.* **2014**, *10*, 106–110. [CrossRef] [PubMed]
167. Vlassara, H.; Uribarri, J. Advanced glycation end products (AGE) and diabetes: Cause, effect, or both? *Curr. Diab. Rep.* **2014**, *14*, 453. [CrossRef]
168. Meerwaldt, R.; Links, T.; Zeebregts, C.; Tio, R.; Smit, O. The clinical relevance of assessing advanced glycation endproducts accumulation in diabetes. *Cardiovasc. Diabetol.* **2008**, *7*, 29. [CrossRef] [PubMed]
169. Meerwaldt, R.; Graaff, R.; Oomen, P.H.N.; Jagger, J.J. Simple non-invasive assessment of advanced glycation endproduct accumulation. *Diabetologia* **2004**, *47*, 1324–1330. [CrossRef] [PubMed]
170. Gerrits, E.G.; Lutgers, H.L.; Kleefstra, N.; Gano, N.O. Skin autofluorescence: A tool to identify type 2 diabetic patients at risk for developing microvascular complications. *Diabetes Care* **2008**, *31*, 517–521. [CrossRef]
171. Osawa, S.; Katakami, N.; Sato, I.; Sakamoto, F. Skin autofluorescence is associated with vascular complications in patients with type 2 diabetes. *J. Diabetes Complicat.* **2018**, *32*, 839–844. [CrossRef]

biomedicines

Review

Suppressing Inflammation for the Treatment of Diabetic Retinopathy and Age-Related Macular Degeneration: Dazdotuftide as a Potential New Multitarget Therapeutic Candidate

Brice Nguedia Vofo and Itay Chowers *

Department of Ophthalmology, Hadassah—Hebrew University Medical Center, Jerusalem 91120, Israel; vofo@hadassah.org.il
* Correspondence: chowers@hadassah.org.il; Tel.: +972-2-6776365

Abstract: Diabetic retinopathy (DR) and age-related macular degeneration (AMD) are major causes of blindness globally. The primary treatment option for DME and neovascular AMD (nAMD) is anti-vascular endothelial growth factor (VEGF) compounds, but this treatment modality often yields insufficient results, and monthly injections can place a burden on the health system and patients. Although various inflammatory pathways and mediators have been recognized as key players in the development of DR and AMD, there are limited treatment options targeting these pathways. Molecular pathways that are interlinked, or triggers of multiple inflammatory pathways, could be promising targets for drug development. This review focuses on the role of inflammation in the pathogenesis of DME and AMD and presents current anti-inflammatory compounds, as well as a potential multitarget anti-inflammatory compound (dazdotuftide) that could be a candidate treatment option for the management of DME and AMD.

Keywords: diabetic retinopathy; diabetic macula edema; age related macular degeneration; anti-inflammatory compounds; anti-vascular endothelial growth factor; dazdotuftide

1. Introduction

Diabetic retinopathy (DR), and age-related macular degeneration (AMD) are the major causes of blindness in the developed world [1]. The international diabetes federation estimates that the global population with diabetes mellitus will approximately double between 2019 and 2045 [2]. The global prevalence of DR and clinically significant diabetic macular edema (DME) amongst diabetic patients is estimated to be 22.27% and 4.07%, respectively [3]. In DME, macular thickening and exudation of lipids alter the macular structure and are associated with vision loss. AMD is the leading cause of central vision loss in people age over 50 years in developed countries [4]. Since age is a major risk factor for AMD, with a rapidly aging population and increasing lifespan, the prevalence of AMD is also expected to rise [5]. In 2020, it was estimated that 196 million people live with AMD, and these numbers were projected to rise to 288 million by 2040. AMD accounts for 8.7% of all blindness worldwide [5,6]. It is classified into non-neovascular/atrophic or "dry" AMD (aAMD) and neovascular AMD (nAMD). In aAMD, atrophy is defined as complete retinal pigment epithelium and outer retina atrophy, which is referred to as geographic atrophy once it becomes confluent. In nAMD, macular neovascularization develops, leading to exudation and subsequent scaring and atrophy.

Anti-vascular endothelial growth factor (VEGF) compounds are the main treatment modality used for DME and nAMD, while suppressing complement activation is the only available treatment modality for aAMD. While anti-VEGF therapy proved to be efficient for DME and nAMD, insufficient response is common in these conditions [7,8]. In aAMD, available complement inhibitors achieve only modest inhibition of atrophy growth. Thus, an important need for additional more effective therapies exists for these conditions. Inflammation is a major pathway involved in the pathogenesis of DME and both forms of AMD. Here, we describe the rational for anti-inflammatory treatment in these conditions as well as available and future potential treatments.

2. Inflammation in the Pathogenesis of DME

Hyperglycemia in diabetic patient triggers several biochemical processes leading to inflammation, ischemia, and a pro-angiogenic state in the retina, with subsequent complications of vascular leakage, edema, neovascularization, and neurodegeneration [9,10]. Several pathways have been involved in the process.

2.1. Toll-Like Receptor Activation

Hyperglycemia enhances the expression and activation of Toll-like receptor 4 (TLR4) in human endothelial cells that may play an important role in DR. TLR4 is a pattern recognition receptor normally found in different types of cells in the retina, such as RPE, photoreceptors, microglial cells, astrocytes, Müller cells, and retinal vascular endothelial cells [11,12]. Hyperglycemia also upregulates endogenous TLR4 ligands, including the high-mobility group box 1 (HMGB1) [13–15]. TLR4 activation contributes to increased leukostasis through myeloid differentiation factor 88 (MyD88)-dependent pathways in leukocytes, with subsequent adhesion to retinal vessel walls [16]. Such adhesion triggers further inflammation, leading to endothelial cell death, pericyte loss, and vascular occlusion; all of which will lead to ischemia, hypoxia, and neovascularization [16,17]. The HMGB1-TLR4 signaling cascade also leads to translocation of nuclear factor kappa-light-chain enhancer of activated B cells (NF-κB) into the nucleus, resulting in the release of pro-inflammatory and pro-angiogenic cytokines, such as VEGF, basic fibroblast growth factor (bFGF), tumor necrosis factor (TNF)-α, interleukin (IL)-1, IL-6, and IL-8 [18]. Upregulation of these cytokines has multiple pro-inflammatory consequences including macrophage and endothelial cell activation. Upregulation of TLR4 has also been associated with increased levels of biomarkers of oxidative stress such as malondialdehyde, over-production of reactive oxygen species (ROS), and diminished antioxidant activities of super-oxide dismutase, catalase, and glutathione peroxidase [19–21]. TLR4 is also involved in glia (astrocyte and Müller cells) activation, contributing to neovascularization in hypoxic retina [22–24]. These glial cells have been shown to secrete VEGF [25]. Interestingly, TLR4 and its ligand HMGB1, are in a positive feedback loop, possibly perpetuating a chronic inflammatory and angiogenic state in the retina [26].

2.2. Polyol Pathway and Advanced Glycation End Products

Excess glucose is metabolized by the polyol pathway through aldose reductase which produces sorbitol. Sorbitol is impermeable to the cellular membrane, it accumulates in cells and induces osmotic damage [27,28]. Sorbitol can be metabolized into fructose-3-phosphate and deoxyglucosone via the sorbitol dehydrogenase-mediated pathway. These bi-products are glycolyzing agents that will lead to the deposition of advanced glycation end products (AGEs) [29–31]. The biochemical process involved in the sorbitol dehydrogenase-mediated pathway, and the upregulation of the polyol pathway, result in increased ROS and oxidative stress. Accumulated AGEs might crosslink proteins, altering their function, and affecting blood vessel wall components, the basement membrane, and cellular receptors [30]. AGEs could further induce damage by activating the cognate receptors to induce pro-inflammatory and pro-oxidant events that will drive oxidative stress and leukocyte adhesion in DR [30], leading to pericyte and capillary loss, and microaneurysm formation [32,33].

2.3. Protein Kinase C Pathway

The increased flux of glucose via the glycolytic pathway leads to elevated diacylglycerol levels that activate the protein kinase C (PKC). Apart from the plethora of biochemical processes triggered by this pathway that drives overexpression of nicotinamide adenine dinucleotide phosphate oxidase and NFkB in a number of vascular cells, exacerbating oxidative stress and inflammatory processes [34], the PKC-β isoform also drives VEGF expression [34].

2.4. RAAS System

The expression of the angiotensin-converting enzyme (ACE) in the retina has been reported to adversely affect capillary perfusion and vascular structure, and mediate VEGF upregulation. The accumulation of glucose and its metabolite, succinate, has been shown to activate the renin–angiotensin–aldosterone system in DR eyes [35]. Treatment with fosinopril (an ACE inhibitor) was found to improve the pathological and biochemical markers of DR in streptozotocin-induced diabetes in rats. Moreover, the upregulation of ACE in their serum and TGF-β1 in their pathological outer and inner nuclear layers of the retina were reduced. Hence, ACE-mediated TGF-β1 activation seem to play a role in the destruction of the blood-retina barrier during DR [36]. Moreover, high ACE concentrations were recently found in the blood serum of both DME and PDR patients by Neroev et al. [37].

2.5. Macrophage Polarization

Macrophages can progressively aggravate an inflammatory state under hyperglycemic conditions. Sofia et al. found that under long-term hyperglycemic treatment, macrophages secreted excessive inflammatory mediators while their phagocytosis and bactericidal functions were damaged at the same time [38]. Castro et al. also showed that macrophages exhibited a pro-inflammatory M1 phenotype after being exposed to high glucose both in vitro and in patients with hyperglycemia [39]. Glucose transporter 1-mediated glucose uptake in macrophages promotes glycolysis and ROS production, further inducing a pro-inflammatory phenotype of macrophages [40]. In mouse peritoneal macrophages, exposure to a high concentration of glucose (25 mM d-glucose) resulted in the increased levels of mRNA transcription of IL-1b, TNF-α, IL-6, IL-12, and iNOS through JUN N-terminal kinase/NF-κB [41].

2.6. Oxidative Stress

Oxidative stress mediated by the production of superoxide has been proposed as the unifying mechanism that links all the hyperglycemia-induced biochemical and molecular pathways discussed above [42,43]. Parallel to its ability to induce VEGF expression, there is evidence that oxidative stress can increase NF-κB, resulting in upregulation of genes involved in the immune and inflammatory processes as well as cellular proliferation and apoptosis; upregulate adhesion molecules (ICAM-1, VCAM-1, Integrins, and selectins); activate microglial cells to secrete inflammatory mediators (IL-1, IL-2, IL-6, IL-8, TNF-α); and increase expression of Monocyte Chemoattractant Protein 1 and Macrophage Inflammatory Protein 1 α gene [44].

Inflammation and leukostasis, resulting from the above mentioned mechanisms, induce capillary occlusion and hypoxia, which further stimulate VEGF expression and the accompanying vascular abnormalities that characterize DR [45]. Indeed, the use of various anti-inflammatory drugs, such as Nepafenac and triamcinolone, have all been shown to reduce VEGF expression, diminish leukostasis, reduce vascular permeability, inhibit retinal cell death, and improve VA [46–48]. Although VEGF expression and breakdown of the blood–retinal barrier has been well documented as a cause of DR and DME, there are other pathways through which retinal inflammatory mediators can affect vascular hyperpermeability and leakage, such as TLR4, interleukin-1β, and TNFα [11,49,50].

3. Inflammation in the Pathogenesis of AMD

3.1. Complement Activation

Inflammation is a major pathway in the pathogenesis of aAMD and nAMD. Several lines of evidence implicate the complement cascade and mononuclear cells in AMD. Components of the complement system were identified in AMD eyes, particularly in the retinal pigment epithelium (RPE) and drusen, the hallmark lesions of the disease. Systemic activation of the complement cascade was also detected, and genetic variants in complement genes which lead to accelerated complement activation are associated with increased risk for developing AMD [51–53]. The excessive activation of complement can lead to RPE and photoreceptor cell death, as well as chronic inflammation, oxidative stress, and angiogenesis, which ultimately contribute to vision loss [54,55]. Thus, targeting the complement cascade has emerged as a promising therapeutic approach for AMD, with several drug and gene therapy strategies currently in development that aim to reduce complement activation in AMD. Recently, the first compound based on complement inhibition (pegcetacoplan) was approved by the FDA for the treatment of aAMD. Monthly or bi-monthly intravitreal injections of this compound are associated with approximately 20% reduction of the progression of atrophy [56,57].

3.2. Mononuclear Cells

Mononuclear cells, such as macrophages and microglia, were also implicated in AMD. Macrophages accumulate in the vicinity of AMD lesions, where they can phagocytose debris and secrete pro-inflammatory and proangiogenic cytokines and chemokines. These cells can also interact with the complement system and modulate its activity, further exacerbating the immune response and tissue damage [58,59]. M1 macrophages are known to promote inflammation and angiogenesis, while M2 macrophages are associated with the resolution of inflammation and tissue repair [60]. Studies have suggested that a shift from M1 to M2 macrophages is anti-inflammatory. In vitro M2 macrophages have been shown to reduce the production of pro-inflammatory cytokines, such as IL-1β and TNF-α, and promote the production of anti-inflammatory cytokines, such as IL-10 and TGF-β, in response to RPE cells and choroidal endothelial cells [61,62]. In addition, M2 macrophages can inhibit the proliferation, migration, and tube formation of choroidal endothelial cells, which are critical for the development of CNV, the hallmark of nAMD [63]. In vivo, a shift from M1 to M2 macrophages also demonstrated anti-inflammatory properties, for example, the intravitreal injection of IL-4, a cytokine that promotes the activation of M2 macrophages, resulted in reduced CNV lesion size and vascular leakage in a mouse model of nAMD [64]. Similarly, the depletion of M1 macrophages or the polarization of macrophages towards an M2-like phenotype resulted in a reduction in CNV lesion size and vascular leakage in mouse models of nAMD [63,65]. Polarized macrophages can excrete cytotoxicity and/or increase abnormal neovascularization (CNV) and may thus be targeted to treat AMD [66–71].

3.3. TLR4

TLR was reported to be expressed in many cells, including RPE, photoreceptors, astrocytes, microglia, and retinal vascular endothelial cells [72]. RPE cells are activated to secrete pro-inflammatory and pro-angiogenic cytokines [73,74]. TLR activation in the retina induces cell death, and degenerating retina cells further stimulate TLR cells [75–78]. This leads to a vicious cycle of TLR activation, pro-inflammatory and angiogenic signaling, cell death, and further activation. In a systematic review by Klettner et al., the potential role of TLR activation of RPE in the development of AMD was summarized into the following: complement activation, pro-inflammation and pro-angiogenesis, neuronal degeneration, reduced RPE cell functions (barrier function, phagocytosis, function in visual cycle), and RPE cell degeneration leading to more TLR4 activation [79]. Amyloid-β, a component of drusen, can upregulate TLR4 and NF-κB expression and lead to progression of AMD [80,81]. TLR4 inhibition could attenuate expression of inflammatory and angiogenic factors, particularly IL-6, IL-8, IL-33, bFGF, and VEGF [82]. Moreover, a VEGF and CNV suppressive effect of calcium supplementation has been reported and associated to its ability to decrease the expression of TLR4, NF-κB, and Hif-1α in RPE cells [83].

3.4. Additional Factors

Other factors exacerbating inflammation in AMD are oxidative injury and smoking [84–86]. The components of drusen, A2E, oxidative stress, and VEGF-A expression, have been shown to activate NLRP3, leading to the activation of caspase-1 cascade [80,87–89]. Caspase-1 activates IL-18 and IL-1β [90]. IL-1β is a potent activator and mediator of inflammation, it is also a strong pro-angiogenic factor that drives VEGF production [91]. Il-18 has also been implicated in several inflammatory conditions [92]. Oxidative stress, and ROS, NLRP3, complement cascade, Ang2, macrophage recruitment and polarization, hypoxia of the RPE are all factors that promote the production of VEGF, angiogenesis, and the progression in nAMD. VEGF-A strongly induces vascular proliferation and migration of the endothelial cells essential for both physiological and pathological angiogenesis [93]. Currently the mainstay of treatment for nAMD is anti-VEGF therapy. However, more efforts in the development of therapies targeting the upstream triggers of VEGF and additional pro-angiogenic factors could complement and supplement current therapies for nAMD.

4. Anti-Inflammatory Compounds for the Treatment of DME and AMD

4.1. Anti-Inflammatory Effect of Anti-VEGF Compounds

Intravitreal injection of anti-VEGF compounds is the standard of care treatment of DME. Pivotal studies have demonstrated the efficacy and safety of several biologic anti VEGF compounds among them aflibercept [7], ranibizumab [94], and faricimab [95], as well as more recently biosimilar compounds such as Formycon and Bioeq's FYB201, MYL-1701, Razumab, ranibizumab-nuna, and ranibizumab-eqrn [96–98]. Interestingly, many studies have demonstrated that anti-VEGF compounds were not only anti-angiogenic, but also possess anti-inflammatory properties which may contribute in part in their success in the management of retinal pathologies [99–101]. By inhibiting VEGF, anti-VEGF compounds can reduce the recruitment of immune cells and the production of pro-inflammatory cytokines, thereby exerting their anti-inflammatory effects [102]. Additionally, VEGF has been shown to enhance the permeability of blood vessels, which can contribute to the accumulation of inflammatory cells and fluid in tissues. By inhibiting VEGF, anti-VEGF compounds can reduce vascular permeability and thereby limit the accumulation of inflammatory cells and fluid in tissues [103].

4.2. Corticosteroids

Corticosteroids have long been recognized as a potential treatment option for DME. Dexamethasone, triamcinolone, and fluocinolone have been used in many forms, including particulate suspension, viscoelastic mixtures, and solid slow-release devices [46,104–106]. The enthusiasm was initially high using different dosages and treatment intervals [107]. However, while protocol B trial of the DRCR network proved that focal laser led to higher VA gains at three years compared to intravitreal triamcinolone injections, protocol I compared the effectiveness of intravitreal ranibizumab, intravitreal triamcinolone acetonide, and focal/grid laser photocoagulation for the treatment of diabetic macular edema, and it concluded that intravitreal ranibizumab and intravitreal triamcinolone acetonide were both superior to focal/grid laser photocoagulation for improving visual acuity in patients with DME. However, the study also found that the use of intravitreal triamcinolone acetonide was associated with a higher risk of complications, including increased intraocular pressure and cataract progression [47,108,109]. The protocol U of the DRCR network demonstrated that combining a dexamethasone implant with anti-VEGF therapy (ranibizumab) resulted in moderate gains in VA compared to continuous anti-VEGF treatment alone, in the short term [110]. A literature review of articles comparing dexamethasone implants to anti-VEGF therapy in DME also reported similar VA outcome in observational studies, and superior VA gains in the dexamethasone implant group, in real life studies, although the authors argue that these differences could be due to differences in the baseline VA and the number of anti-VEGF injections in different studies [111]. However, according to the findings reported in a recent meta-analysis, intravitreal steroid treatment for DME was associated with no significant difference in BCVA compared to anti-VEGF treated eyes, although with a significantly lower retinal thickness [112]. Corticosteroid therapy has also been shown to be potentially useful in DME eyes that respond poorly to anti-VEGF [113–115].

Intravitreal injections of triamcinolone (as off-label use) were demonstrated to yield a two-step reversal in the DR severity score compared to focal/grid laser at three years [116]. The DR-Pro-DEX study and others also indicated that dexamethasone and fluocinolone implants significantly delayed the progression and reduced the severity of DR [117,118]. The anti-inflammatory effect of steroids is thought to be due to their ability to reduce the levels of several pro-inflammatory cytokines, including IL-1β, IL-6, IL-8, tumor TNF-α, and VEGF in the vitreous of patients with DR [104,119]. In addition to reducing cytokine levels, steroids have also been shown to modulate several other molecular pathways involved in the pathogenesis of DR, including the regulation of extracellular matrix proteins, the suppression of ROS production, and the modulation of cellular apoptosis and survival pathways [120,121].

The side effects of corticosteroids remain the main limitation to their use for the management of these ocular pathologies. Cataract in phakic eyes and intraocular pressure elevation regardless of lens status has been reported in varying degrees in all studies [122–127]. Studies indicate that up to 32% of eyes treated with corticosteroids may develop high ($\geq$25 mmHg) intraocular pressure [127–129]. In addition, steroid treatments induce lens opacification. The Score study [5] estimated the 12 month incidence of new onset lens opacities or progression of lens opacities to be up to 33%, and by 24 months, over 33% of patients required cataract surgery [130]. In addition, there are other less frequent complications of steroid use, such as non-infectious endophthalmitis, and pseudo-endophthalmitis, activation of ocular and peri-ocular infections, and steroid-induced central serous chorioretinopathy [131].

4.3. *Rho-Associated Protein Kinase Inhibition*

Ripasudil is a Rho-associated kinase inhibitor developed originally for the treatment of glaucoma and ocular hypertension. Rho-associated protein kinase (ROCK) 1 and 2 determine macrophage polarization into M1 and M2 subtypes. Aging is known to increase ROCK2 signaling, thereby leading to the over-expression of proangiogenic macrophages associated with increased IL-4 production and angiogenesis. A recent study showed that NLRP3, apoptosis-associated speck-like proteins containing a CARD (ASC), caspase1, IL-1β, and IL-18 were inhibited by ripasudil [132].

4.4. *None-Steroidal Anti-Inflammatory Drugs*

NSAIDS are potent inhibitors of cyclooxygenase enzymes and therefore suppress the synthesis of pro-inflammatory prostaglandins. Studies have also described the role of pro-inflammatory prostaglandins in the pathogenesis of DR and AMD, with recent studies searching for the therapeutic role of NSAIDs for these disorders [133]. Moreover, NSAIDS have been detected and measured in the vitreous cavity after topical application, making them more attractive as a convenient route of intravitreal drug administration [134].

In AMD, the use of NSAIDS has been mentioned in the management of nAMD, but only in combination with anti-VEGF. For example, in 2015, a pilot study described higher efficacy in terms of visual acuity improvement when a topical NSAID (bromfenac) was associated to aflibercept injection (EYLEA®, 2 mg, Regeneron Pharmaceuticals, Inc., New York, NY, USA) compared with a single anti-VEGF therapy (EYLEA®, 2 mg), although the anatomical outcome was the same. Cox-2 has been detected in human CNV membranes and there is scientific evidence that it is a promoter of CNV [135,136]. Hence, the pharmacological inhibition of COX appears to reduce VEGF expression in mice models [137].

In DR, scientific evidence indicates that retina cells consistently upregulate COX and prostaglandins [138,139], hence the potential place of NSAIDS in their management. The therapeutic potential of NSAIDS was first suspected a century ago, when rheumatoid arthritis patients on salicylates had reduced incidence of DR [140], since then, several studies have examined the clinical benefit of NSAIDS given both systemically [141], topically [142], and even intravitreally [143]. However, most of these studies are small, retrospective, uncontrolled studies [144]. Despite the considerable scientific rational, Protocol R of the DRCR network examined the effect of topical NSAIDS for non-central DME in a multi-center double-masked randomized trial, and concluded that, at one year, there was no meaningful effect on OCT measured retinal thickness [145]. Due consideration must also be given to the potential side effects associated with the long term use of NSAIDS, especially amongst patients whose corneas are compromised by diabetes, ocular surgery, or auto-immune disease. For example, although rare, corneal melting secondary to NSAIDS use is a potential complication in this patient population and could be sight threatening [146].

5. Dazdotuftide

Dazdotuftide is a novel, small synthetic molecule. It is a peptide conjugate comprised of tuftsin and phosphorylcholine that are covalently attached. The phosphorylcholine (PPC) moiety is based on a sequence from helminths' secretory molecules which has been shown to be responsible for their immunoregulatory functions [147]. Tuftsin is a naturally occurring endogenous immunomodulatory tetra-peptide (Thr-Lys-Pro-Arg) produced in the spleen by enzymatic cleavage of the Fc-domain of the heavy chain of IgG. The peptide is coupled to diazotized 4-aminophenyphosphorylchloride to form an azo bond between the tuftsin and PC [148]. Extensive research has been done on Tuftsin and PPC separately, and the activities of each of them towards immune regulation. Dazdotuftide has been suggested to provide a strong synergistic effect, far surpassing the efficacy of the compounds given separately [149].

5.1. *Dazdotuftide In Vivo and In Vitro Studies*

Dazdotuftide and its components demonstrated in various autoimmune animal models and in vitro test systems its inhibitory effect on TLR-4 (inhibition of NfKb cascade), NRP-1 (inhibition of VEGF 165), and ACE2. In vivo studies have demonstrated Dazdotuftide to be effective in the treatment of inflammation in autoimmune animal models: rheumatoid arthritis [150], lupus nephritis [148], and colitis [151]. Dazdotuftide' ability to prevent and treat the disease in these models was accompanied by reduction of pro-inflammatory cytokine levels and an increase of anti-inflammatory cytokine expression, as well as expansion of T and B regulatory cells. It is proposed that the dual functionality of dazdotuftide is due to its binding to different receptors via its two moieties: the PPC targeting TLR4 [152], and leading to NF-κB inhibition and suppression of inflammatory cytokine synthesis, and the tuftsin end of Dazdotuftide targeting neuropilin-1 [153], leading to inhibition of VEGF 165 activity [154] and macrophage shift towards M2 anti-inflammatory macrophages that secrete IL-10 and induce Treg activation [155].

In vitro, dazdotuftide was tested on specimens of peripheral blood mononuclear cells (PBMCs) and temporal artery biopsies (TABs) obtained from patients with giant cell arthritis and age-matched controls. The PBMCs were activated by CD3/CD28 beads and tests were conducted to depict inflammatory cytokine secession and IL-10 anti-inflammatory cytokines. Upon treatment with dazdotuftide, there was a decrease in the production of IL-1β, IL-2, IL-5, IL-6, IL-9, IL-12(p70), IL-13, IL-17A, IL-18, IL-21, IL-22, IL-23, IFNγ, TNFα, and GM-CSF by activated PBMCs, with negligible effect on cell viability. Likewise, in inflamed TABs, treatment with dazdotuftide reduced the production of IL-1β, IL-6, IL-13, IL-17A, and CD68 gene expression. The effects of Dazdotuftide were considered superior to dexamethasone as a standard of care due to its greater reduction of IL-2, IL-18, and IFNγ in CD3/CD28-activated PBMCs, and CD68 gene in inflamed TABs [156]. Moreover, recent analysis by molecular docking has demonstrated the strong binding and inhibitory ability of tuftsin on ACE2 and NRP1 [157].

5.2. Dazdotuftide Inhibition of TLR and NRP-1

TLR (inhibition of NfKb), NRP-1 (increase reactivity of VEGF 165), and ACE activation have been demonstrated to play key roles in the cascade of events that leads to inflammation and contributes to the progression of DR and nAMD. In a diabetic retina, hyperglycemia enhances the expression and activation of TLR4 in human endothelial cells that may play an important role in DR [11] Cells exposed to high glucose had an increased expression of downstream factors of TLR4 including myeloid differentiation factor 88, an inflammatory cytokine inducer, and NF-κB [158,159], which may lead to the secretion of more inflammatory cytokines like IL-1β [160]. TLR4 polymorphisms were associated with a higher prevalence of retinopathy, further supporting the role of this gene in DR [161,162]. In an oxygen-induced retinopathy model, the absence of TLR4 was seen to be associated with low glial activation and low expression of HMGB-1, the endogenous ligand for TLR4. The expression of HMGB-1 in ischemic retina was shown to promote the production of pro-inflammatory factors and also initiate TLR4-dependent responses that contribute to neovascularization [23]. In fact, TLR4 signaling was implicated in inflammation, leukostasis, angiogenesis, blood–retinal barrier breakdown, hypoxia, cellular apoptosis, neurodegeneration, and oxidative stress in a diabetic retina. This is, therefore, a potential therapeutic target for DR, that has stimulated research around several compounds hypothesized to inhibit this receptor [10]. ACE activation has been implicated in the pathogenesis of DR and DME, potentially causing a disruption of the blood–retinal barrier in diabetic eyes [35–37]. Tuftsin, a component of dazdotuftide, has a strong binding affinity to ACE2 [157]. This is therefore another pathological pathway to DR and DME that could be inhibited by dazdotuftide (see Figure 1).

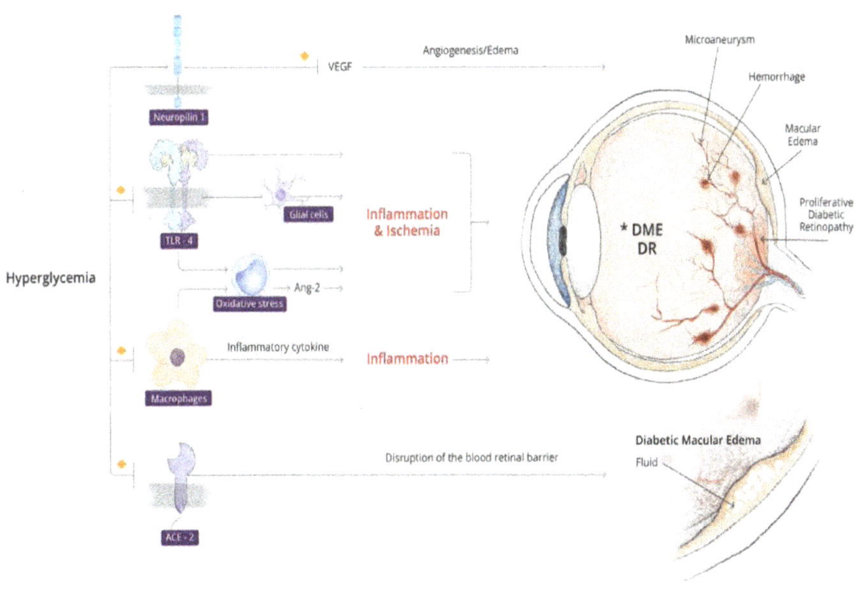

Figure 1. Illustration of potential sites for dazdotuftide inhibition along the pathogenic pathway of diabetic macula oedema and diabetic retinopathy (DR). * Diabetic macula oedema.

In the context of nAMD, TLR inhibition could prevent complement activation, inhibiting RPE cell loss in aAMD and downplaying the RPE cell-driven BRB breakdown, leukocyte recruitment, VEGF production, angiogenesis, and exudation in nAMD [79]. TLR inhibition could also break the vicious cycle of retina cell death and degeneration that leads to pro-inflammatory and angiogenic signaling and further TLR activation. In both DR and nAMD, neovascularization is driven by VEGF, and this cytokine may be suppressed via Dazdotuftide activity [75–78].

NRP1 functions as a co-receptor for VEGF and its inhibition would diminish VEGF bioactivity [154]. For example, NRP1 has been found to be present, alongside VEGFR-2, in the endothelial and RPE cells in nAMD eyes demonstrating subfoveal CNV [163], and variations in the NRP1 gene were associated with treatment response to anti-VEGF therapy in nAMD [164].

6. Conclusions

While anti-VEGF compounds are effective and useful for the treatment of DR/DME and nAMD, many eyes experience an insufficient effect, and these compounds are ineffective for aAMD. Inflammation is a major pathway in the pathogenesis of DR/DME, aAMD, and nAMD. Corticosteroids are the only anti-inflammatory compounds approved for the treatment of DR/DME, and anti-complement biologics are the only approved therapy for aAMD. While these therapies are effective, both are associated with significant side effects and have limited efficacy. Dazdotuftide combines several functions including anti-VEGF, anti-TLR, and M1 to M2 macrophage polarization which could be an added advantage in the management of DME, DR, and nAMD. Dazdotuftide's ability to inhibit NRP1, TLR, and activate anti-inflammatory macrophages makes this multi-target new drug a potential new therapeutic option for DR/DME and AMD. Targeting TLR, an upstream molecule implicated in the pathogenesis of these posterior ocular pathologies, may also yield better durability of the therapeutic effect, with a lower intra-vitreal injection frequency required than the current anti-VEGF therapies. Additionally, dazdotuftide may be formulated as a slow-release implant, thereby further reducing treatment burden and increasing patient compliance, which is a crucial factor for successful treatment in chronic conditions such as DR/DME and nAMD. Clinical trials should now test the hypothesis that this compound may be useful for these indications.

Author Contributions: Conceptualization, B.N.V. and I.C.; literature search, B.N.V. and I.C.; writing—original draft preparation, B.N.V. and I.C.; writing—review and editing, B.N.V. and I.C. All authors have read and agreed to the published version of the manuscript.

Funding: This research received no external funding.

Institutional Review Board Statement: Not applicable.

Informed Consent Statement: Not applicable.

Data Availability Statement: No new data were created or analyzed in this study. Data sharing is not applicable to this article.

Conflicts of Interest: B.N.V. and I.C. are both consultants of Tarsier™ Pharma, (Massachusetts, United States) a pharmaceutical company developing a drug with dazdotuftide.

References

1. Common Eye Disorders and Diseases | CDC. Available online: https://www.cdc.gov/visionhealth/basics/ced/index.html (accessed on 26 February 2023).
2. Saeedi, P.; Petersohn, I.; Salpea, P.; Malanda, B.; Karuranga, S.; Unwin, N.; Colagiuri, S.; Guariguata, L.; Motala, A.A.; Ogurtsova, K.; et al. Global and regional diabetes prevalence estimates for 2019 and projections for 2030 and 2045: Results from the International Diabetes Federation Diabetes Atlas, 9th edition. *Diabetes Res. Clin. Pract.* **2019**, *157*, 107843. [CrossRef] [PubMed]
3. Teo, Z.L.; Tham, Y.-C.; Yu, M.; Chee, M.L.; Rim, T.H.; Cheung, N.; Bikbov, M.M.; Wang, Y.X.; Tang, Y.; Lu, Y.; et al. Global Prevalence of Diabetic Retinopathy and Projection of Burden through 2045: Systematic Review and Meta-analysis. *Ophthalmology* **2021**, *128*, 1580–1591. [CrossRef] [PubMed]

4. Ferris, F.L.; Wilkinson, C.P.; Bird, A.; Chakravarthy, U.; Chew, E.; Csaky, K.; Sadda, S.R. Beckman Initiative for Macular Research Classification Committee Clinical classification of age-related macular degeneration. *Ophthalmology* **2013**, *120*, 844–851. [CrossRef]
5. Wong, W.L.; Su, X.; Li, X.; Cheung, C.M.G.; Klein, R.; Cheng, C.-Y.; Wong, T.Y. Global prevalence of age-related macular degeneration and disease burden projection for 2020 and 2040: A systematic review and meta-analysis. *Lancet Glob. Health* **2014**, *2*, e106–e116. [CrossRef] [PubMed]
6. Chapman, N.A.; Jacobs, R.J.; Braakhuis, A.J. Role of diet and food intake in age-related macular degeneration: A systematic review. *Clin. Experiment. Ophthalmol.* **2019**, *47*, 106–127. [CrossRef]
7. Brown, D.M.; Schmidt-Erfurth, U.; Do, D.V.; Holz, F.G.; Boyer, D.S.; Midena, E.; Heier, J.S.; Terasaki, H.; Kaiser, P.K.; Marcus, D.M.; et al. Intravitreal Aflibercept for Diabetic Macular Edema: 100-Week Results from the VISTA and VIVID Studies. *Ophthalmology* **2015**, *122*, 2044–2052. [CrossRef]
8. Heier, J.S.; Brown, D.M.; Chong, V.; Korobelnik, J.-F.; Kaiser, P.K.; Nguyen, Q.D.; Kirchhof, B.; Ho, A.; Ogura, Y.; Yancopoulos, G.D.; et al. Intravitreal aflibercept (VEGF trap-eye) in wet age-related macular degeneration. *Ophthalmology* **2012**, *119*, 2537–2548. [CrossRef]
9. Whitehead, M.; Wickremasinghe, S.; Osborne, A.; Van Wijngaarden, P.; Martin, K.R. Diabetic retinopathy: A complex pathophysiology requiring novel therapeutic strategies. *Expert Opin. Biol. Ther.* **2018**, *18*, 1257–1270. [CrossRef]
10. Bayan, N.; Yazdanpanah, N.; Rezaei, N. Role of toll-like receptor 4 in diabetic retinopathy. *Pharmacol. Res.* **2022**, *175*, 105960. [CrossRef]
11. Wang, L.; Wang, J.; Fang, J.; Zhou, H.; Liu, X.; Su, S.B. High glucose induces and activates Toll-like receptor 4 in endothelial cells of diabetic retinopathy. *Diabetol. Metab. Syndr.* **2015**, *7*, 89. [CrossRef]
12. Du, M.; Martin, A.; Hays, F.; Johnson, J.; Farjo, R.A.; Farjo, K.M. Serum retinol-binding protein-induced endothelial inflammation is mediated through the activation of toll-like receptor 4. *Mol. Vis.* **2017**, *23*, 185. Available online: https://pubmed.ncbi.nlm.nih.gov/28400700/ (accessed on 21 June 2022). [PubMed]
13. Zhang, T.-H.; Huang, C.-M.; Gao, X.; Wang, J.-W.; Hao, L.-L.; Ji, Q. Gastrodin inhibits high glucose-induced human retinal endothelial cell apoptosis by regulating the SIRT1/TLR4/NF-κBp65 signaling pathway. *Mol. Med. Rep.* **2018**, *17*, 7774–7780. [CrossRef]
14. Jiang, S.; Chen, X. HMGB1 siRNA can reduce damage to retinal cells induced by high glucose in vitro and in vivo. *Drug Des. Devel. Ther.* **2017**, *11*, 783–795. [CrossRef] [PubMed]
15. Mohammad, G.; Siddiquei, M.M.; Othman, A.; Al-Shabrawey, M.; Abu El-Asrar, A.M. High-mobility group box-1 protein activates inflammatory signaling pathway components and disrupts retinal vascular-barrier in the diabetic retina. *Exp. Eye Res.* **2013**, *107*, 101–109. [CrossRef]
16. Tang, J.; Allen Lee, C.; Du, Y.; Sun, Y.; Pearlman, E.; Sheibani, N.; Kern, T.S. MyD88-dependent pathways in leukocytes affect the retina in diabetes. *PLoS ONE* **2013**, *8*, e68871. [CrossRef] [PubMed]
17. Bandello, F.; Lattanzio, R.; Zucchiatti, I.; Del Turco, C. Pathophysiology and treatment of diabetic retinopathy. *Acta Diabetol.* **2013**, *50*, 1–20. [CrossRef]
18. Liu, T.; Zhang, L.; Joo, D.; Sun, S.-C. NF-κB signaling in inflammation. *Signal Transduct. Target. Ther.* **2017**, *2*, 17023. [CrossRef] [PubMed]
19. Hui, Y.; Yin, Y. MicroRNA-145 attenuates high glucose-induced oxidative stress and inflammation in retinal endothelial cells through regulating TLR4/NF-κB signaling. *Life Sci.* **2018**, *207*, 212–218. [CrossRef]
20. Li, W.; Jin, L.; Cui, Y.; Nie, A.; Xie, N.; Liang, G. Bone marrow mesenchymal stem cells-induced exosomal microRNA-486-3p protects against diabetic retinopathy through TLR4/NF-κB axis repression. *J. Endocrinol. Investig.* **2021**, *44*, 1193–1207. [CrossRef]
21. Wang, Y.; Tao, J.; Jiang, M.; Yao, Y. Apocynin ameliorates diabetic retinopathy in rats: Involvement of TLR4/NF-κB signaling pathway. *Int. Immunopharmacol.* **2019**, *73*, 49–56. [CrossRef]
22. van Beijnum, J.R.; Buurman, W.A.; Griffioen, A.W. Convergence and amplification of toll-like receptor (TLR) and receptor for advanced glycation end products (RAGE) signaling pathways via high mobility group B1 (HMGB1). *Angiogenesis* **2008**, *11*, 91–99. [CrossRef]
23. He, C.; Sun, Y.; Ren, X.; Lin, Q.; Hu, X.; Huang, X.; Su, S.-B.; Liu, Y.; Liu, X. Angiogenesis mediated by toll-like receptor 4 in ischemic neural tissue. *Arterioscler. Thromb. Vasc. Biol.* **2013**, *33*, 330–338. [CrossRef]
24. Fu, H.; Liu, H. Deletion of toll-like receptor 4 ameliorates diabetic retinopathy in mice. *Arch. Physiol. Biochem.* **2020**, *129*, 519–525. [CrossRef] [PubMed]
25. Ishida, S.; Shinoda, K.; Kawashima, S.; Oguchi, Y.; Okada, Y.; Ikeda, E. Coexpression of VEGF receptors VEGF-R2 and neuropilin-1 in proliferative diabetic retinopathy. *Investig. Ophthalmol. Vis. Sci.* **2000**, *41*, 1649–1656.
26. Hirschfeld, M.; Weis, J.J.; Toshchakov, V.; Salkowski, C.A.; Cody, M.J.; Ward, D.C.; Qureshi, N.; Michalek, S.M.; Vogel, S.N. Signaling by toll-like receptor 2 and 4 agonists results in differential gene expression in murine macrophages. *Infect. Immun.* **2001**, *69*, 1477–1482. [CrossRef]
27. Gabbay, K.H. Hyperglycemia, polyol metabolism, and complications of diabetes mellitus. *Annu. Rev. Med.* **1975**, *26*, 521–536. [CrossRef]
28. Gabbay, K.H. The sorbitol pathway and the complications of diabetes. *N. Engl. J. Med.* **1973**, *288*, 831–836. [CrossRef]
29. Szwergold, B.S.; Kappler, F.; Brown, T.R. Identification of fructose 3-phosphate in the lens of diabetic rats. *Science* **1990**, *247*, 451–454. [CrossRef] [PubMed]

30. Hammes, H.P.; Martin, S.; Federlin, K.; Geisen, K.; Brownlee, M. Aminoguanidine treatment inhibits the development of experimental diabetic retinopathy. *Proc. Natl. Acad. Sci. USA* **1991**, *88*, 11555–11558. [CrossRef] [PubMed]
31. Peppa, M.; Vlassara, H. Advanced glycation end products and diabetic complications: A general overview. *Horm. Athens Greece* **2005**, *4*, 28–37. [CrossRef]
32. Stitt, A.; Gardiner, T.A.; Alderson, N.L.; Canning, P.; Frizzell, N.; Duffy, N.; Boyle, C.; Januszewski, A.S.; Chachich, M.; Baynes, J.W.; et al. The AGE inhibitor pyridoxamine inhibits development of retinopathy in experimental diabetes. *Diabetes* **2002**, *51*, 2826–2832. [CrossRef]
33. Zong, H.; Ward, M.; Stitt, A.W. AGEs, RAGE, and diabetic retinopathy. *Curr. Diab. Rep.* **2011**, *11*, 244–252. [CrossRef]
34. Koya, D.; King, G.L. Protein kinase C activation and the development of diabetic complications. *Diabetes* **1998**, *47*, 859–866. [CrossRef]
35. Peti-Peterdi, J.; Kang, J.J.; Toma, I. Activation of the renal renin-angiotensin system in diabetes—New concepts. *Nephrol. Dial. Transplant. Off. Publ. Eur. Dial. Transpl. Assoc.-Eur. Ren. Assoc.* **2008**, *23*, 3047–3049. [CrossRef] [PubMed]
36. Sun, P.; Xu, N.; Li, Y.; Han, Y. Destruction of the blood-retina barrier in diabetic retinopathy depends on angiotensin-converting enzyme-mediated TGF-β1/Smad signaling pathway activation. *Int. Immunopharmacol.* **2020**, *85*, 106686. [CrossRef] [PubMed]
37. Neroev, V.V.; Chesnokova, N.B.; Kost, O.A.; Okhotsimskaya, T.D.; Pavlenko, T.A.; Beznos, O.V.; Binevsky, P.V.; Lisovskaya, O.A. Bradykinin and angiotensin-converting enzyme in serum of patients with diabetic retinopathy and the prognosis of diabetic macular edema development (pilot study). *Probl. Endocrinol.* **2021**, *67*, 13–19. [CrossRef]
38. Pavlou, S.; Lindsay, J.; Ingram, R.; Xu, H.; Chen, M. Sustained high glucose exposure sensitizes macrophage responses to cytokine stimuli but reduces their phagocytic activity. *BMC Immunol.* **2018**, *19*, 24. [CrossRef]
39. Torres-Castro, I.; Arroyo-Camarena, Ú.D.; Martínez-Reyes, C.P.; Gómez-Arauz, A.Y.; Dueñas-Andrade, Y.; Hernández-Ruiz, J.; Béjar, Y.L.; Zaga-Clavellina, V.; Morales-Montor, J.; Terrazas, L.I.; et al. Human monocytes and macrophages undergo M1-type inflammatory polarization in response to high levels of glucose. *Immunol. Lett.* **2016**, *176*, 81–89. [CrossRef] [PubMed]
40. Freemerman, A.J.; Johnson, A.R.; Sacks, G.N.; Milner, J.J.; Kirk, E.L.; Troester, M.A.; Macintyre, A.N.; Goraksha-Hicks, P.; Rathmell, J.C.; Makowski, L. Metabolic reprogramming of macrophages: Glucose transporter 1 (GLUT1)-mediated glucose metabolism drives a proinflammatory phenotype. *J. Biol. Chem.* **2014**, *289*, 7884–7896. [CrossRef] [PubMed]
41. Pan, Y.; Wang, Y.; Cai, L.; Cai, Y.; Hu, J.; Yu, C.; Li, J.; Feng, Z.; Yang, S.; Li, X.; et al. Inhibition of high glucose-induced inflammatory response and macrophage infiltration by a novel curcumin derivative prevents renal injury in diabetic rats. *Br. J. Pharmacol.* **2012**, *166*, 1169–1182. [CrossRef]
42. Du, X.L.; Edelstein, D.; Rossetti, L.; Fantus, I.G.; Goldberg, H.; Ziyadeh, F.; Wu, J.; Brownlee, M. Hyperglycemia-induced mitochondrial superoxide overproduction activates the hexosamine pathway and induces plasminogen activator inhibitor-1 expression by increasing Sp1 glycosylation. *Proc. Natl. Acad. Sci. USA* **2000**, *97*, 12222–12226. [CrossRef] [PubMed]
43. Nishikawa, T.; Edelstein, D.; Du, X.L.; Yamagishi, S.; Matsumura, T.; Kaneda, Y.; Yorek, M.A.; Beebe, D.; Oates, P.J.; Hammes, H.P.; et al. Normalizing mitochondrial superoxide production blocks three pathways of hyperglycaemic damage. *Nature* **2000**, *404*, 787–790. [CrossRef] [PubMed]
44. Sheemar, A.; Soni, D.; Takkar, B.; Basu, S.; Venkatesh, P. Inflammatory mediators in diabetic retinopathy: Deriving clinicopathological correlations for potential targeted therapy. *Indian J. Ophthalmol.* **2021**, *69*, 3035–3049. [CrossRef]
45. Kaul, K.; Hodgkinson, A.; Tarr, J.M.; Kohner, E.M.; Chibber, R. Is inflammation a common retinal-renal-nerve pathogenic link in diabetes? *Curr. Diabetes Rev.* **2010**, *6*, 294–303. [CrossRef] [PubMed]
46. Kuppermann, B.D.; Blumenkranz, M.S.; Haller, J.A.; Williams, G.A.; Weinberg, D.V.; Chou, C.; Whitcup, S.M.; Dexamethasone DDS Phase II Study Group. Randomized controlled study of an intravitreous dexamethasone drug delivery system in patients with persistent macular edema. *Arch. Ophthalmol.* **2007**, *125*, 309–317. [CrossRef] [PubMed]
47. Gillies, M.C.; Sutter, F.K.; Simpson, J.M.; Larsson, J.; Ali, H.; Zhu, M. Intravitreal triamcinolone for refractory diabetic macular edema: Two-year results of a double-masked, placebo-controlled, randomized clinical trial. *Ophthalmology* **2006**, *113*, 1533–1538. [CrossRef]
48. Kern, T.S.; Miller, C.M.; Du, Y.; Zheng, L.; Mohr, S.; Ball, S.L.; Kim, M.; Jamison, J.A.; Bingaman, D.P. Topical administration of nepafenac inhibits diabetes-induced retinal microvascular disease and underlying abnormalities of retinal metabolism and physiology. *Diabetes* **2007**, *56*, 373–379. [CrossRef]
49. Simo, R.; Hernandez, C. Novel approaches for treating diabetic retinopathy based on recent pathogenic evidence. *Prog. Retin. Eye Res.* **2015**, *48*, 160–180. [CrossRef]
50. Liu, X.; Ye, F.; Xiong, H.; Hu, D.-N.; Limb, G.A.; Xie, T.; Peng, L.; Zhang, P.; Wei, Y.; Zhang, W.; et al. IL-1β induces IL-6 production in retinal Müller cells predominantly through the activation of p38 MAPK/NF-κB signaling pathway. *Exp. Cell Res.* **2015**, *331*, 223–231. [CrossRef]
51. Fritsche, L.G.; Igl, W.; Bailey, J.N.C.; Grassmann, F.; Sengupta, S.; Bragg-Gresham, J.L.; Burdon, K.P.; Hebbring, S.J.; Wen, C.; Gorski, M.; et al. A large genome-wide association study of age-related macular degeneration highlights contributions of rare and common variants. *Nat. Genet.* **2016**, *48*, 134–143. [CrossRef]
52. Yehoshua, Z.; de Amorim Garcia Filho, C.A.; Nunes, R.P.; Gregori, G.; Penha, F.M.; Moshfeghi, A.A.; Zhang, K.; Sadda, S.; Feuer, W.; Rosenfeld, P.J. Systemic complement inhibition with eculizumab for geographic atrophy in age-related macular degeneration: The COMPLETE study. *Ophthalmology* **2014**, *121*, 693–701. [CrossRef]

53. de Garcia Filho, C.A.A.; Yehoshua, Z.; Gregori, G.; Nunes, R.P.; Penha, F.M.; Moshfeghi, A.A.; Zhang, K.; Feuer, W.; Rosenfeld, P.J. Change in drusen volume as a novel clinical trial endpoint for the study of complement inhibition in age-related macular degeneration. *Ophthalmic Surg. Lasers Imaging Retin.* **2014**, *45*, 18–31. [CrossRef]
54. Anderson, D.H.; Radeke, M.J.; Gallo, N.B.; Chapin, E.A.; Johnson, P.T.; Curletti, C.R.; Hancox, L.S.; Hu, J.; Ebright, J.N.; Malek, G.; et al. The pivotal role of the complement system in aging and age-related macular degeneration: Hypothesis re-visited. *Prog. Retin. Eye Res.* **2010**, *29*, 95–112. [CrossRef] [PubMed]
55. Hageman, G.S.; Anderson, D.H.; Johnson, L.V.; Hancox, L.S.; Taiber, A.J.; Hardisty, L.I.; Hageman, J.L.; Stockman, H.A.; Borchardt, J.D.; Gehrs, K.M.; et al. A common haplotype in the complement regulatory gene factor H (HF1/CFH) predisposes individuals to age-related macular degeneration. *Proc. Natl. Acad. Sci. USA* **2005**, *102*, 7227–7232. [CrossRef] [PubMed]
56. Liao, D.S.; Grossi, F.V.; El Mehdi, D.; Gerber, M.R.; Brown, D.M.; Heier, J.S.; Wykoff, C.C.; Singerman, L.J.; Abraham, P.; Grassmann, F.; et al. Complement C3 Inhibitor Pegcetacoplan for Geographic Atrophy Secondary to Age-Related Macular Degeneration: A Randomized Phase 2 Trial. *Ophthalmology* **2020**, *127*, 186–195. [CrossRef] [PubMed]
57. Jaffe, G.J.; Westby, K.; Csaky, K.G.; Monés, J.; Pearlman, J.A.; Patel, S.S.; Joondeph, B.C.; Randolph, J.; Masonson, H.; Rezaei, K.A. C5 Inhibitor Avacincaptad Pegol for Geographic Atrophy Due to Age-Related Macular Degeneration: A Randomized Pivotal Phase 2/3 Trial. *Ophthalmology* **2021**, *128*, 576–586. [CrossRef] [PubMed]
58. Nebel, C.; Aslanidis, A.; Rashid, K.; Langmann, T. Activated microglia trigger inflammasome activation and lysosomal destabilization in human RPE cells. *Biochem. Biophys. Res. Commun.* **2017**, *484*, 681–686. [CrossRef]
59. Ambati, J.; Anand, A.; Fernandez, S.; Sakurai, E.; Lynn, B.C.; Kuziel, W.A.; Rollins, B.J.; Ambati, B.K. An animal model of age-related macular degeneration in senescent Ccl-2- or Ccr-2-deficient mice. *Nat. Med.* **2003**, *9*, 1390–1397. [CrossRef]
60. Ambati, J.; Atkinson, J.P.; Gelfand, B.D. Immunology of age-related macular degeneration. *Nat. Rev. Immunol.* **2013**, *13*, 438–451. [CrossRef]
61. Yang, Y.; Guo, Z.; Chen, W.; Wang, X.; Cao, M.; Han, X.; Zhang, K.; Teng, B.; Cao, J.; Wu, W.; et al. M2 Macrophage-Derived Exosomes Promote Angiogenesis and Growth of Pancreatic Ductal Adenocarcinoma by Targeting E2F2. *Mol. Ther.* **2021**, *29*, 1226–1238. [CrossRef]
62. Ma, W.; Zhao, L.; Fontainhas, A.M.; Fariss, R.N.; Wong, W.T. Microglia in the Mouse Retina Alter the Structure and Function of Retinal Pigmented Epithelial Cells: A Potential Cellular Interaction Relevant to AMD. *PLoS ONE* **2009**, *4*, e7945. [CrossRef] [PubMed]
63. Yang, Y.; Liu, F.; Tang, M.; Yuan, M.; Hu, A.; Zhan, Z.; Li, Z.; Li, J.; Ding, X.; Lu, L. Macrophage polarization in experimental and clinical choroidal neovascularization. *Sci. Rep.* **2016**, *6*, 30933. [CrossRef] [PubMed]
64. Sakurai, E.; Anand, A.; Ambati, B.K.; van Rooijen, N.; Ambati, J. Macrophage depletion inhibits experimental choroidal neovascularization. *Investig. Ophthalmol. Vis. Sci.* **2003**, *44*, 3578–3585. [CrossRef] [PubMed]
65. Cao, X.; Shen, D.; Patel, M.M.; Tuo, J.; Johnson, T.M.; Olsen, T.W.; Chan, C.-C. Macrophage polarization in the maculae of age-related macular degeneration: A pilot study. *Pathol. Int.* **2011**, *61*, 528–535. [CrossRef] [PubMed]
66. Grunin, M.; Hagbi-Levi, S.; Chowers, I. The role of monocytes and macrophages in age-related macular degeneration. *Adv. Exp. Med. Biol.* **2014**, *801*, 199–205. [CrossRef] [PubMed]
67. Hagbi-Levi, S.; Grunin, M.; Jaouni, T.; Tiosano, L.; Rinsky, B.; Elbaz-Hayoun, S.; Peled, A.; Chowers, I. Proangiogenic characteristics of ac-tivated macrophages from patients with age-related macular degeneration. *Neurobiol. Aging.* **2017**, *51*, 71–82. [CrossRef]
68. Hagbi-Levi, S.; Abraham, M.; Tiosano, L.; Rinsky, B.; Grunin, M.; Eizenberg, O.; Peled, A.; Chowers, I. Promiscuous Chemokine Antago-nist (BKT130) Suppresses Laser-Induced Choroidal Neovascularization by Inhibition of Monocyte Recruitment. *J. Immunol. Res.* **2019**, *2019*, 8535273. [CrossRef]
69. Rinsky, B.; Hagbi-Levi, S.; Elbaz-Hayoun, S.; Grunin, M.; Chowers, I. Characterizing the effect of supplements on the phenotype of cultured macrophages from patients with age-related macular degeneration. *Mol. Vis.* **2017**, *23*, 889–899.
70. Elbaz-Hayoun, S.; Rinsky, B.; Hagbi-Levi, S.; Grunin, M.; Tammy HayaYedid Chowers, I. Evaluation of antioxidant treatments for the modulation of macrophage function in the context of retinal degeneration. *Mol. Vis.* **2019**, *25*, 479–488.
71. Hagbi-Levi, S.; Tiosano, L.; Rinsky, B.; Levinger, N.; Elbaz-Hayoun, S.; Carmi, S.; Grunin, M.; Chowers, I. Anti-tumor necrosis factor alpha reduces the proangiogenic effects of activated macrophages derived from patients with age-related macular degeneration. *Mol. Vis.* **2021**, *27*, 622–631.
72. Ko, M.K.; Saraswathy, S.; Parikh, J.G.; Rao, N.A. The role of TLR4 activation in photoreceptor mitochondrial oxidative stress. *Investig. Ophthalmol. Vis. Sci.* **2011**, *52*, 5824–5835. [CrossRef] [PubMed]
73. Jonas, J.B.; Tao, Y.; Neumaier, M.; Findeisen, P. Cytokine concentration in aqueous humour of eyes with exudative age-related macular degeneration. *Acta Ophthalmol.* **2012**, *90*, e381–e388. [CrossRef]
74. Miao, H.; Tao, Y.; Li, X.X. Inflammatory cytokines in aqueous humor of patients with choroidal neovascularization. *Mol. Vis.* **2012**, *18*, 574. Available online: https://pubmed.ncbi.nlm.nih.gov/22419849/ (accessed on 27 June 2022).
75. Bernard, J.J.; Cowing-Zitron, C.; Nakatsuji, T.; Muehleisen, B.; Muto, J.; Borkowski, A.W.; Martinez, L.; Greidinger, E.L.; Yu, B.D.; Gallo, R.L. Ultraviolet radiation damages self noncoding RNA and is detected by TLR3. *Nat. Med.* **2012**, *18*, 1286–1290. [CrossRef]
76. Fujimoto, T.; Sonoda, K.H.; Hijioka, K.; Sato, K.; Takeda, A.; Hasegawa, E.; Oshima, Y.; Ishibashi, T. Choroidal neovascularization enhanced by Chlamydia pneumoniae via Toll-like receptor 2 in the retinal pigment epithelium. *Investig. Ophthalmol. Vis. Sci.* **2010**, *51*, 4694–4702. [CrossRef]

77. Klettner, A.; Koinzer, S.; Meyer, T.; Roider, J. Toll-like receptor 3 activation in retinal pigment epithelium cells—Mitogen-activated protein kinase pathways of cell death and vascular endothelial growth factor secretion. *Acta Ophthalmol.* **2013**, *91*, e211–e218. [CrossRef] [PubMed]
78. Kleinman, M.E.; Kaneko, H.; Cho, W.G.; Dridi, S.; Fowler, B.J.; Blandford, A.D.; Albuquerque, R.J.C.; Hirano, Y.; Terasaki, H.; Kondo, M.; et al. Short-interfering RNAs induce retinal degeneration via TLR3 and IRF3. *Mol. Ther. J. Am. Soc. Gene Ther.* **2012**, *20*, 101–108. [CrossRef] [PubMed]
79. Klettner, A.; Roider, J. Retinal Pigment Epithelium Expressed Toll-like Receptors and Their Potential Role in Age-Related Macular Degeneration. *Int. J. Mol. Sci.* **2021**, *22*, 8387. [CrossRef] [PubMed]
80. Liu, R.T.; Gao, J.; Cao, S.; Sandhu, N.; Cui, J.Z.; Chou, C.L.; Fang, E.; Matsubara, J.A. Inflammatory mediators induced by amyloid-beta in the retina and RPE in vivo: Implications for inflammasome activation in age-related macular degeneration. *Investig. Ophthalmol. Vis. Sci.* **2013**, *54*, 2225–2237. [CrossRef]
81. Zhou, X.; Yuan, L.; Zhao, X.; Hou, C.; Ma, W.; Yu, H.; Xiao, R. Genistein antagonizes inflammatory damage induced by β-amyloid peptide in microglia through TLR4 and NF-κB. *Nutrition* **2014**, *30*, 90–95. [CrossRef]
82. Chen, L.; Bai, Y.; Zhao, M.; Jiang, Y. TLR4 inhibitor attenuates amyloid-β-induced angiogenic and inflammatory factors in ARPE-19 cells: Implications for age-related macular degeneration. *Mol. Med. Rep.* **2016**, *13*, 3249–3256. [CrossRef]
83. Sung, I.S.; Park, S.Y.; Jeong, K.-Y.; Kim, H.M. Investigation of the preventive effect of calcium on inflammation-mediated choroidal neovascularization. *Life Sci.* **2019**, *233*, 116727. [CrossRef] [PubMed]
84. Marie, M.; Bigot, K.; Angebault, C.; Barrau, C.; Gondouin, P.; Pagan, D.; Fouquet, S.; Villette, T.; Sahel, J.-A.; Lenaers, G.; et al. Light action spectrum on oxidative stress and mitochondrial damage in A2E-loaded retinal pigment epithelium cells. *Cell Death Dis.* **2018**, *9*, 287. [CrossRef] [PubMed]
85. Klein, R.; Knudtson, M.D.; Cruickshanks, K.J.; Klein, B.E.K. Further Observations on the Association Between Smoking and the Long-term Incidence and Progression of Age-related Macular Degeneration: The Beaver Dam Eye Study. *Arch. Ophthalmol.* **2008**, *126*, 115–121. [CrossRef] [PubMed]
86. Davies, K.J. Oxidative stress, antioxidant defenses, and damage removal, repair, and replacement systems. *IUBMB Life* **2000**, *50*, 279–289. [CrossRef]
87. Anderson, O.A.; Finkelstein, A.; Shima, D.T. A2E induces IL-1ß production in retinal pigment epithelial cells via the NLRP3 inflammasome. *PLoS ONE* **2013**, *8*, e67263. [CrossRef]
88. Marneros, A.G. NLRP3 inflammasome blockade inhibits VEGF-A-induced age-related macular degeneration. *Cell Rep.* **2013**, *4*, 945–958. [CrossRef]
89. Shimada, K.; Crother, T.R.; Karlin, J.; Dagvadorj, J.; Chiba, N.; Chen, S.; Ramanujan, V.K.; Wolf, A.J.; Vergnes, L.; Ojcius, D.M.; et al. Oxidized mitochondrial DNA activates the NLRP3 inflammasome during apoptosis. *Immunity* **2012**, *36*, 401–414. [CrossRef]
90. Voronov, E.; Carmi, Y.; Apte, R.N. The role IL-1 in tumor-mediated angiogenesis. *Front. Physiol.* **2014**, *5*, 114. [CrossRef]
91. Krishnan, S.M.; Sobey, C.G.; Latz, E.; Mansell, A.; Drummond, G.R. IL-1β and IL-18: Inflammatory markers or mediators of hypertension? *Br. J. Pharmacol.* **2014**, *171*, 5589–5602. [CrossRef]
92. Kim, E.J.; Cho, D.; Kim, T.S. Efficient induction of T helper type 1-mediated immune responses in antigen-primed mice by anti-CD3 single-chain Fv/interleukin-18 fusion DNA. *Immunology* **2004**, *111*, 27–34. [CrossRef] [PubMed]
93. Oommen, S.; Gupta, S.K.; Vlahakis, N.E. Vascular endothelial growth factor A (VEGF-A) induces endothelial and cancer cell migration through direct binding to integrin α9β1: Identification of a specific α9β1 binding site. *J. Biol. Chem.* **2011**, *286*, 1083–1092. [CrossRef]
94. Wykoff, C.C.; Elman, M.J.; Regillo, C.D.; Ding, B.; Lu, N.; Stoilov, I. Predictors of Diabetic Macular Edema Treatment Frequency with Ranibizumab During the Open-Label Extension of the RIDE and RISE Trials. *Ophthalmology* **2016**, *123*, 1716–1721. [CrossRef] [PubMed]
95. Wells, J.A.; Wykoff, C.C.; Willis, J.R.; Haskova, Z.; Lin, H.; Silverman, D.; Adamis, A.P.; Ives, J.; Abreu, F.; Basu, K.; et al. Efficacy, durability, and safety of faricimab in diabetic macular edema (DME): One-year results from the phase 3 YOSEMITE and RHINE trials. *Investig. Ophthalmol. Vis. Sci.* **2021**, *62*, 1037.
96. Kaiser, P.K.; Schmitz-Valckenberg, M.S.; Holz, F.G. Anti–Vascular Endothelial Growth Factor Biosimilars in Ophthalmology. *Retina* **2022**, *42*, 2243–2250. [CrossRef]
97. Kumar, A.; Agarwal, D.; Kumar, A. Commentary: Use of biosimilars for retinal diseases in India: Challenges and concerns. *Indian J. Ophthalmol.* **2021**, *69*, 357–358. [CrossRef]
98. Sharma, A.; Kumar, N.; Parachuri, N.; Bandello, F.; Kuppermann, B.D.; Loewenstein, A. Biosimilars for Retinal Diseases: An Update. *Am. J. Ophthalmol.* **2021**, *224*, 36–42. [CrossRef]
99. Mérida, S.; Sancho-Tello, M.; Almansa, I.; Desco, C.; Peris, C.; Moreno, M.-L.; Villar, V.M.; Navea, A.; Bosch-Morell, F. Bevacizumab Diminishes Inflammation in an Acute Endotoxin-Induced Uveitis Model. *Front. Pharmacol.* **2018**, *9*, 649. Available online: https://www.frontiersin.org/articles/10.3389/fphar.2018.00649 (accessed on 26 March 2023). [CrossRef]
100. Qin, H.-F.; Shi, F.-J.; Zhang, C.-Y.; Luo, D.-W.; Qin, S.-Y.; Wu, J.; Xie, H.; Zhang, J.-T.; Qiu, Q.-H.; Liu, K.; et al. Anti-VEGF reduces inflammatory features in macular edema secondary to retinal vein occlusion. *Int. J. Ophthalmol.* **2022**, *15*, 1296–1304. [CrossRef]
101. Nakao, S.; Arima, M.; Ishikawa, K.; Kohno, R.; Kawahara, S.; Miyazaki, M.; Yoshida, S.; Enaida, H.; Hafezi-Moghadam, A.; Kono, T.; et al. Intravitreal Anti-VEGF Therapy Blocks Inflammatory Cell Infiltration and Re-Entry into the Circulation in Retinal Angiogenesis. *Investig. Ophthalmol. Vis. Sci.* **2012**, *53*, 4323–4328. [CrossRef]

102. Wheeler, K.C.; Jena, M.K.; Pradhan, B.S.; Nayak, N.; Das, S.; Hsu, C.-D.; Wheeler, D.S.; Chen, K.; Nayak, N.R. VEGF may contribute to macrophage recruitment and M2 polarization in the decidua. *PLoS ONE* **2018**, *13*, e0191040. [CrossRef]
103. Ferrara, N. Role of vascular endothelial growth factor in physiologic and pathologic angiogenesis: Therapeutic implications. *Semin. Oncol.* **2002**, *29*, 10–14. [CrossRef] [PubMed]
104. Jonas, J.B.; Söfker, A. Intraocular injection of crystalline cortisone as adjunctive treatment of diabetic macular edema. *Am. J. Ophthalmol.* **2001**, *132*, 425–427. [CrossRef] [PubMed]
105. Campochiaro, P.A.; Brown, D.M.; Pearson, A.; Ciulla, T.; Boyer, D.; Holz, F.G.; Tolentino, M.; Gupta, A.; Duarte, L.; Madreperla, S.; et al. Long-term benefit of sustained-delivery fluocinolone acetonide vitreous inserts for diabetic macular edema. *Ophthalmology* **2011**, *118*, 626–635. [CrossRef] [PubMed]
106. Jonas, J.B.; Kreissig, I.; Söfker, A.; Degenring, R.F. Intravitreal injection of triamcinolone for diffuse diabetic macular edema. *Arch. Ophthalmol.* **2003**, *121*, 57–61. [CrossRef]
107. Michaelides, M.; Kaines, A.; Hamilton, R.D.; Fraser-Bell, S.; Rajendram, R.; Quhill, F.; Boos, C.J.; Xing, W.; Egan, C.; Peto, T.; et al. A prospective randomized trial of intravitreal bevacizumab or laser therapy in the management of diabetic macular edema (BOLT study) 12-month data: Report 2. *Ophthalmology* **2010**, *117*, 1078–1086.e2. [CrossRef]
108. Diabetic Retinopathy Clinical Research Network. A randomized trial comparing intravitreal triamcinolone acetonide and focal/grid photocoagulation for diabetic macular edema. *Ophthalmology* **2008**, *115*, 1447–1449.e10. [CrossRef]
109. Diabetic Retinopathy Clinical Research Network; Elman, M.J.; Aiello, L.P.; Beck, R.W.; Bressler, N.M.; Bressler, S.B.; Edwards, A.R.; Ferris, F.L.; Friedman, S.M.; Glassman, A.R.; et al. Randomized trial evaluating ranibizumab plus prompt or deferred laser or triamcinolone plus prompt laser for diabetic macular edema. *Ophthalmology* **2010**, *117*, 1064–1077.e35. [CrossRef]
110. Maturi, R.K.; Glassman, A.R.; Liu, D.; Beck, R.W.; Bhavsar, A.R.; Bressler, N.M.; Jampol, L.M.; Melia, M.; Punjabi, O.S.; Salehi-Had, H.; et al. Effect of Adding Dexamethasone to Continued Ranibizumab Treatment in Patients with Persistent Diabetic Macular Edema: A DRCR Network Phase 2 Randomized Clinical Trial. *JAMA Ophthalmol.* **2018**, *136*, 29–38. [CrossRef]
111. Kodjikian, L.; Bellocq, D.; Mathis, T. Pharmacological Management of Diabetic Macular Edema in Real-Life Observational Studies. *BioMed Res. Int.* **2018**, *2018*, 8289253. [CrossRef]
112. Patil, N.S.; Mihalache, A.; Hatamnejad, A.; Popovic, M.M.; Kertes, P.J.; Muni, R.H. Intravitreal Steroids Compared with Anti-VEGF Treatment for Diabetic Macular Edema: A Meta-Analysis. *Ophthalmol. Retin.* **2023**, *7*, 289–299. [CrossRef] [PubMed]
113. Cicinelli, M.V.; Cavalleri, M.; Querques, L.; Rabiolo, A.; Bandello, F.; Querques, G. Early response to ranibizumab predictive of functional outcome after dexamethasone for unresponsive diabetic macular oedema. *Br. J. Ophthalmol.* **2017**, *101*, 1689–1693. [CrossRef]
114. Kim, J.H.; Lee, T.G.; Lew, Y.J. Short-term efficacy of intravitreal triamcinolone acetonide for bevacizumab-resistant diabetic macular oedema. *Acta Ophthalmol.* **2015**, *93*, e178–e179. [CrossRef] [PubMed]
115. Hatz, K.; Ebneter, A.; Tuerksever, C.; Pruente, C.; Zinkernagel, M. Repeated Dexamethasone Intravitreal Implant for the Treatment of Diabetic Macular Oedema Unresponsive to Anti-VEGF Therapy: Outcome and Predictive SD-OCT Features. *Ophthalmologica* **2018**, *239*, 205–214. [CrossRef] [PubMed]
116. Bressler, N.M.; Edwards, A.R.; Beck, R.W.; Flaxel, C.J.; Glassman, A.R.; Ip, M.S.; Kollman, C.; Kuppermann, B.D.; Stone, T.W. Diabetic Retinopathy Clinical Research Network Exploratory analysis of diabetic retinopathy progression through 3 years in a randomized clinical trial that compares intravitreal triamcinolone acetonide with focal/grid photocoagulation. *Arch. Ophthalmol.* **2009**, *127*, 1566–1571. [CrossRef]
117. Iglicki, M.; Zur, D.; Busch, C.; Okada, M.; Loewenstein, A. Progression of diabetic retinopathy severity after treatment with dexamethasone implant: A 24-month cohort study the "DR-Pro-DEX Study". *Acta Diabetol.* **2018**, *55*, 541–547. [CrossRef]
118. Wykoff, C.C.; Chakravarthy, U.; Campochiaro, P.A.; Bailey, C.; Green, K.; Cunha-Vaz, J. Long-term Effects of Intravitreal 0.19 mg Fluocinolone Acetonide Implant on Progression and Regression of Diabetic Retinopathy. *Ophthalmology* **2017**, *124*, 440–449. [CrossRef]
119. Arimura, N.; Otsuka, H.; Yamakiri, K.; Sonoda, Y.; Nakao, S.; Noda, Y.; Hashiguchi, T.; Maruyama, I.; Sakamoto, T. Vitreous mediators after intravitreal bevacizumab or triamcinolone acetonide in eyes with proliferative diabetic retinopathy. *Ophthalmology* **2009**, *116*, 921–926. [CrossRef]
120. Semeraro, F.; Morescalchi, F.; Cancarini, A.; Russo, A.; Rezzola, S.; Costagliola, C. Diabetic retinopathy, a vascular and inflammatory disease: Therapeutic implications. *Diabetes Metab.* **2019**, *45*, 517–527. [CrossRef]
121. Rodríguez, M.L.; Millán, I.; Ortega, Á.L. Cellular targets in diabetic retinopathy therapy. *World J. Diabetes* **2021**, *12*, 1442–1462. [CrossRef]
122. Gillies, M.C.; Simpson, J.M.; Billson, F.A.; Luo, W.; Penfold, P.; Chua, W.; Mitchell, P.; Zhu, M.; Hunyor, A.B.L. Safety of an intravitreal injection of triamcinolone: Results from a randomized clinical trial. *Arch. Ophthalmol.* **2004**, *122*, 336–340. [CrossRef] [PubMed]
123. Storey, P.P.; Obeid, A.; Pancholy, M.; Goodman, J.; Borkar, D.; Su, D.; Regillo, C. Ocular Hypertension after Intravitreal Injection of 2-mg Triamcinolone. *Retina* **2020**, *40*, 75–79. [CrossRef] [PubMed]
124. Bakri, S.J.; Beer, P.M. Intravitreal triamcinolone injection for diabetic macular edema: A clinical and fluorescein angiographic case series. *Can. J. Ophthalmol.* **2004**, *39*, 755–760. [CrossRef]

125. Haller, J.A.; Bandello, F.; Belfort, R., Jr.; Blumenkranz, M.S.; Gillies, M.; Heier, J.; Loewenstein, A.; Yoon, Y.H.; Jiao, J.; Li, X.Y.; et al. Dexamethasone intravitreal implant in patients with macular edema related to branch or central retinal vein occlusion twelve-month study results. *Ophthalmology* **2011**, *118*, 2453–2460. [CrossRef] [PubMed]
126. Boyer, D.S.; Yoon, Y.H.; Belfort, R.; Bandello, F.; Maturi, R.K.; Augustin, A.J.; Li, X.-Y.; Cui, H.; Hashad, Y.; Whitcup, S.M.; et al. Three-year, randomized, sham-controlled trial of dexamethasone intravitreal implant in patients with diabetic macular edema. *Ophthalmology* **2014**, *121*, 1904–1914. [CrossRef]
127. Smithen, L.M.; Ober, M.D.; Maranan, L.; Spaide, R.F. Intravitreal triamcinolone acetonide and intraocular pressure. *Am. J. Ophthalmol.* **2004**, *138*, 740–743. [CrossRef] [PubMed]
128. Vasconcelos-Santos, D.V.; Nehemy, P.G.; Schachat, A.P.; Nehemy, M.B. Secondary ocular hypertension after intravitreal injection of 4 mg of triamcinolone acetonide: Incidence and risk factors. *Retina* **2008**, *28*, 573–580. [CrossRef]
129. Roth, D.B.; Verma, V.; Realini, T.; Prenner, J.L.; Feuer, W.J.; Fechtner, R.D. Long-term incidence and timing of intraocular hypertension after intravitreal triamcinolone acetonide injection. *Ophthalmology* **2009**, *116*, 455–460. [CrossRef]
130. Ip, M.S.; Scott, I.U.; VanVeldhuisen, P.C.; Oden, N.L.; Blodi, B.A.; Fisher, M.; Singerman, L.J.; Tolentino, M.; Chan, C.K.; Gonzalez, V.H.; et al. A randomized trial comparing the efficacy and safety of intravitreal triamcinolone with observation to treat vision loss associated with macular edema secondary to central retinal vein occlusion: The Standard Care vs. Corticosteroid for Retinal Vein Occlusion (SCORE) study report 5. *Arch. Ophthalmol.* **2009**, *127*, 1101–1114. [CrossRef]
131. Fung, A.T.; Tran, T.; Lim, L.L.; Samarawickrama, C.; Arnold, J.; Gillies, M.; Catt, C.; Mitchell, L.; Symons, A.; Buttery, R.; et al. Local delivery of corticosteroids in clinical ophthalmology: A review. *Clin. Experiment. Ophthalmol.* **2020**, *48*, 366–401. [CrossRef]
132. Ripasudil Alleviated the Inflammation of RPE Cells by Targeting the miR-136-5p/ROCK/NLRP3 Pathway—PubMed. Available online: https://pubmed.ncbi.nlm.nih.gov/32252692/ (accessed on 27 June 2022).
133. Kim, S.J.; Flach, A.J.; Jampol, L.M. Nonsteroidal anti-inflammatory drugs in ophthalmology. *Surv. Ophthalmol.* **2010**, *55*, 108–133. [CrossRef]
134. Heier, J.S.; Awh, C.C.; Busbee, B.G.; Waterbury, L.D.; Daniel, P.; Stoller, G.L.; Cleary, T.S. Vitreous nonsteroidal antiinflammatory drug concentrations and prostaglandin E2 levels in vitrectomy patients treated with ketorolac 0.4%, bromfenac 0.09%, and nepafenac 0.1%. *Retina* **2009**, *29*, 1310–1313. [CrossRef]
135. Monnier, Y.; Zaric, J.; Rüegg, C. Inhibition of angiogenesis by non-steroidal anti-inflammatory drugs: From the bench to the bedside and back. *Curr. Drug Targets Inflamm. Allergy* **2005**, *4*, 31–38. [CrossRef]
136. Gately, S.; Kerbel, R. Therapeutic potential of selective cyclooxygenase-2 inhibitors in the management of tumor angiogenesis. *Prog. Exp. Tumor Res.* **2003**, *37*, 179–192. [CrossRef]
137. Takahashi, K.; Saishin, Y.; Saishin, Y.; Mori, K.; Ando, A.; Yamamoto, S.; Oshima, Y.; Nambu, H.; Melia, M.B.; Bingaman, D.P.; et al. Topical nepafenac inhibits ocular neovascularization. *Investig. Ophthalmol. Vis. Sci.* **2003**, *44*, 409–415. [CrossRef] [PubMed]
138. Johnson, E.I.; Dunlop, M.E.; Larkins, R.G. Increased vasodilatory prostaglandin production in the diabetic rat retinal vasculature. *Curr. Eye Res.* **1999**, *18*, 79–82. [CrossRef]
139. Amrite, A.C.; Ayalasomayajula, S.P.; Cheruvu, N.P.S.; Kompella, U.B. Single periocular injection of celecoxib-PLGA microparticles inhibits diabetes-induced elevations in retinal PGE2, VEGF, and vascular leakage. *Investig. Ophthalmol. Vis. Sci.* **2006**, *47*, 1149–1160. [CrossRef]
140. Powell, E.D.; Field, R.A. Diabetic Retinopathy and Rheumatoid Arthritis. *Lancet Lond. Engl.* **1964**, *2*, 17–18. [CrossRef] [PubMed]
141. The DAMAD Study Group. Effect of aspirin alone and aspirin plus dipyridamole in early diabetic retinopathy. A multicenter randomized controlled clinical trial. *Diabetes* **1989**, *38*, 491–498. [CrossRef]
142. Hariprasad, S.M.; Callanan, D.; Gainey, S.; He, Y.-G.; Warren, K. Cystoid and diabetic macular edema treated with nepafenac 0.1%. *J. Ocul. Pharmacol. Ther. Off. J. Assoc. Ocul. Pharmacol. Ther.* **2007**, *23*, 585–590. [CrossRef]
143. Soheilian, M.; Karimi, S.; Ramezani, A.; Peyman, G.A. Pilot study of intravitreal injection of diclofenac for treatment of macular edema of various etiologies. *Retina* **2010**, *30*, 509–515. [CrossRef]
144. Schoenberger, S.D.; Kim, S.J. Nonsteroidal Anti-Inflammatory Drugs for Retinal Disease. *Int. J. Inflamm.* **2013**, *2013*, 281981. [CrossRef]
145. Friedman, S.M.; Almukhtar, T.H.; Baker, C.W.; Glassman, A.R.; Elman, M.J.; Bressler, N.M.; Maker, M.P.; Jampol, L.M.; Melia, M. Topical Nepafenec in Eyes with Non-Central Diabetic Macular Edema. *Retina* **2015**, *35*, 944–956. [CrossRef] [PubMed]
146. Rigas, B.; Huang, W.; Honkanen, R. NSAID-induced corneal melt: Clinical importance, pathogenesis, and risk mitigation. *Surv. Ophthalmol.* **2020**, *65*, 1–11. [CrossRef] [PubMed]
147. Harnett, M.M.; Kean, D.E.; Boitelle, A.; McGuiness, S.; Thalhamer, T.; Steiger, C.N.; Egan, C.; Al-Riyami, L.; Alcocer, M.J.; Houston, K.M.; et al. The phosphorycholine moiety of the filarial nematode immunomodulator ES-62 is responsible for its anti-inflammatory action in arthritis. *Ann. Rheum. Dis.* **2008**, *67*, 518–523. [CrossRef]
148. Bashi, T.; Blank, M.; Ben-Ami Shor, D.; Fridkin, M.; Versini, M.; Gendelman, O.; Volkov, A.; Barshak, I.; Shoenfeld, Y. Successful modulation of murine lupus nephritis with tuftsin-phosphorylcholine. *J. Autoimmun.* **2015**, *59*, 1–7. [CrossRef] [PubMed]
149. Shemer, A.; Kivity, S.; Shovman, O.; Bashi, T.; Perry, O.; Watad, A.; Ben-Ami Shor, D.; Volkov, A.; Barshack, I.; Bragazzi, N.L.; et al. Tuftsin–phosphorylcholine (TPC) equally effective to methylprednisolone in ameliorating lupus nephritis in a mice model. *Clin. Exp. Immunol.* **2018**, *193*, 160–166. [CrossRef]
150. Bashi, T.; Shovman, O.; Fridkin, M.; Volkov, A.; Barshack, I.; Blank, M.; Shoenfeld, Y. Novel therapeutic compound tuftsin-phosphorylcholine attenuates collagen-induced arthritis. *Clin. Exp. Immunol.* **2016**, *184*, 19–28. [CrossRef]

151. Ben-Ami Shor, D.; Bashi, T.; Lachnish, J.; Fridkin, M.; Bizzaro, G.; Barshak, I.; Blank, M.; Shoenfeld, Y. Phosphorylcholine-tuftsin compound prevents development of dextransulfate-sodium-salt induced murine colitis: Implications for the treatment of human inflammatory bowel disease. *J. Autoimmun.* **2015**, *56*, 111–117. [CrossRef] [PubMed]
152. Blank, M.; Shoenfeld, Y. Helminth-Related Tuftsin-Phosphorylcholine Compound and its Interplay with Autoimmune Diseases. *Isr. Med. Assoc. J. IMAJ* **2019**, *21*, 158–162.
153. Nissen, J.C.; Selwood, D.L.; Tsirka, S.E. Tuftsin signals through its receptor neuropilin-1 via the transforming growth factor beta pathway. *J. Neurochem.* **2013**, *127*, 394–402. [CrossRef] [PubMed]
154. von Wronski, M.A.; Raju, N.; Pillai, R.; Bogdan, N.J.; Marinelli, E.R.; Nanjappan, P.; Ramalingam, K.; Arunachalam, T.; Eaton, S.; Linder, K.E.; et al. Tuftsin binds neuropilin-1 through a sequence similar to that encoded by exon 8 of vascular endothelial growth factor. *J. Biol. Chem.* **2006**, *281*, 5702–5710. [CrossRef]
155. Blank, M.; Bashi, T.; Lachnish, J.; Ben-Ami-Shor, D.; Shovman, O.; Fridkin, M.; Eisenstein, M.; Volkov, A.; Barshack, I.; Shoenfeld, Y. Helminths-based bi-functional molecule, tuftsin-phosphorylcholine (TPC), ameliorates an established murine arthritis. *PLoS ONE* **2018**, *13*, e0200615. [CrossRef]
156. Croci, S.; Bonacini, M.; Muratore, F.; Caruso, A.; Fontana, A.; Boiardi, L.; Soriano, A.; Cavazza, A.; Cimino, L.; Belloni, L.; et al. The therapeutic potential of tuftsin-phosphorylcholine in giant cell arteritis. *J. Autoimmun.* **2019**, *98*, 113–121. [CrossRef] [PubMed]
157. Huang, J.; Wang, J.; Li, Y.; Wang, Z.; Chu, M.; Wang, Y. Tuftsin: A Natural Molecule Against SARS-CoV-2 Infection. *Front. Mol. Biosci.* **2022**, *9*, 859162. [CrossRef]
158. Dasu, M.R.; Devaraj, S.; Zhao, L.; Hwang, D.H.; Jialal, I. High glucose induces toll-like receptor expression in human monocytes: Mechanism of activation. *Diabetes* **2008**, *57*, 3090–3098. [CrossRef] [PubMed]
159. Quagliaro, L.; Piconi, L.; Assaloni, R.; Martinelli, L.; Motz, E.; Ceriello, A. Intermittent high glucose enhances apoptosis related to oxidative stress in human umbilical vein endothelial cells: The role of protein kinase C and NAD(P)H-oxidase activation. *Diabetes* **2003**, *52*, 2795–2804. [CrossRef]
160. Dasu, M.R.; Jialal, I. Free fatty acids in the presence of high glucose amplify monocyte inflammation via Toll-like receptors. *Am. J. Physiol. Endocrinol. Metab.* **2011**, *300*, E145–E154. [CrossRef]
161. Yang, W.-J.; Hu, J.; Uemura, A.; Tetzlaff, F.; Augustin, H.G.; Fischer, A. Semaphorin-3C signals through Neuropilin-1 and PlexinD1 receptors to inhibit pathological angiogenesis. *EMBO Mol. Med.* **2015**, *7*, 1267–1284. [CrossRef]
162. Buraczynska, M.; Baranowicz-Gaszczyk, I.; Tarach, J.; Ksiazek, A. Toll-like receptor 4 gene polymorphism and early onset of diabetic retinopathy in patients with type 2 diabetes. *Hum. Immunol.* **2009**, *70*, 121–124. [CrossRef]
163. Lim, J.I.; Spee, C.; Hangai, M.; Rocha, J.; Ying, H.S.; Ryan, S.J.; Hinton, D.R. Neuropilin-1 expression by endothelial cells and retinal pigment epithelial cells in choroidal neovascular membranes. *Am. J. Ophthalmol.* **2005**, *140*, 1044–1050. [CrossRef] [PubMed]
164. Lorés-Motta, L.; van Asten, F.; Muether, P.S.; Smailhodzic, D.; Groenewoud, J.M.; Omar, A.; Chen, J.; Koenekoop, R.K.; Fauser, S.; Hoyng, C.B.; et al. A genetic variant in NRP1 is associated with worse response to ranibizumab treatment in neovascular age-related macular degeneration. *Pharmacogenet. Genom.* **2016**, *26*, 20–27. [CrossRef] [PubMed]

MDPI AG
Grosspeteranlage 5
4052 Basel
Switzerland
Tel.: +41 61 683 77 34

Biomedicines Editorial Office
E-mail: biomedicines@mdpi.com
www.mdpi.com/journal/biomedicines

www.ingramcontent.com/pod-product-compliance
Lightning Source LLC
Chambersburg PA
CBHW040312270926
51850CB00007BC/1104
9783725874309